MANAGEMENT OF HEART DISEASES WITH CONVENTIONAL, COMPLIMENTARY AND ALTERNATIVE GROUP OF THERAPIES

(An Integrative Approach)

A Useful Guide For Ayurvedic Physicians, Cardiologists And Medical Students

Volume - 2

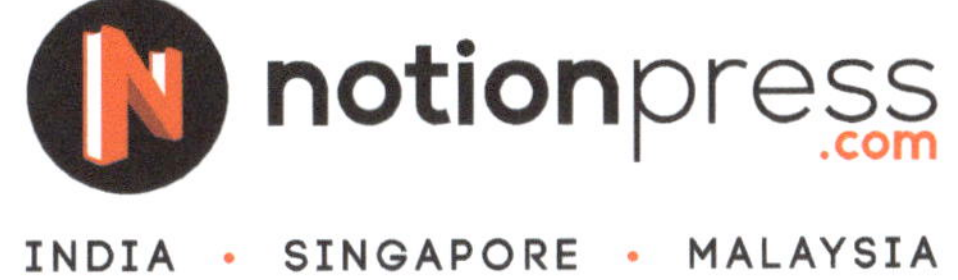

ISBN
Paperback 979-8-89415-326-1
Hardcase 979-8-89446-823-5

MANAGEMENT OF HEART DISEASES WITH CONVENTIONAL, COMPLIMENTARY AND ALTERNATIVE GROUP OF THERAPIES

(An Integrative Approach)

A Useful Guide For Ayurvedic Physicians, Cardiologists And Medical Students

Prof. (Dr) K.C.Verma
MBBS, DCH, MD, DM (Cardiology)
FICP(USA), FRSTM&H (Lond), FCSI (India)
Senior Consulting Heart Specialist
Formerly Prof. in Cardiovascular and
Thoracic Unit, Govt. Medical College,
Jammu (J & K)

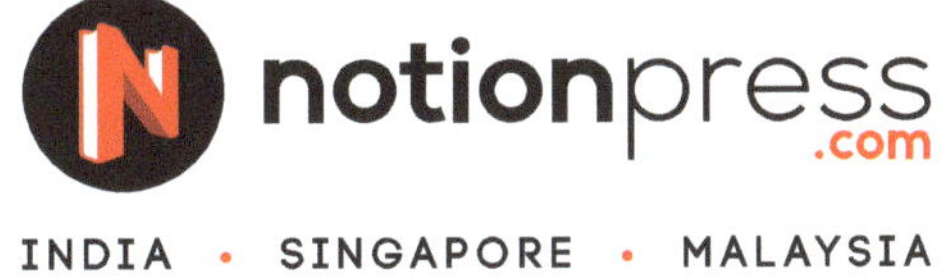

INDIA • SINGAPORE • MALAYSIA

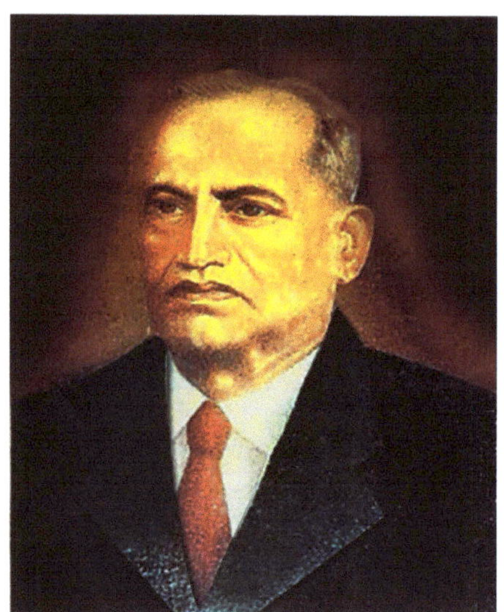

Portrait of Col. Sir Ram Nath Chopra (1882-1973) popularly known as Father of Indian Pharmacology and Doyen of Science and Medicine.

In Memory of Sir Ram Nath Chopra

Col. Sir Ram Nath Chopra S/O Dewan Raghu Nath Chopra, was born in August 17, 1882 at Gujranwala, Punjab. Schooling at Jammu and Srinagar; College studies at Government College, Lahore; In England Chopra joined in Downing College, Cambridge in 1903. He worked with famous Dr. Walter E. Dixon, a famous pharmacologist and first professor of pharmacology in that college. R.N.Chopra's thesis title was "Action of drugs on ciliary movement in the respiratory tract". In 1905 he was admitted in B.A. after qualifying for Natural Sciences Tripos. While studying at Cambridge he joined in Barthelomew's Hospital, London and competed for the Indian Medical Service (1908) and got third place in merit. He also obtained Cambridge M.B. and M.D. and the London M.R.C.P. He was awarded the Sc.D. degree of Cambridge University for his contributions to the science of medicine. The Royal College of Physicians of London elected him as a Fellow. For about 12 years he worked as young IMS officer first in East Africa and then in Afghan war. In 1921, he joined as First Professor of Pharmacology in Calcutta School of Tropical Medicine to teach PG students, became director of the institution in 1934. Along with this position he also chaired the Pharmacology at Calcutta Medical College to teach UG students. His hand in developing the Pharmacology laboratory at School made it a well equipped best laboratory equal to those in UK. He served the school till 1941 (i.e., for 20 years). After retirement in the same year the Government of J & K appointed him as Director of Medical Services and then appointed as Director of Drug Research Laboratory where he served the lab till 1960. His ambition was observed as bringing modern pharmacology from the traditional materia medica. He is well known for his Experimental Pharmacology. He is the First person in establishing a research centre for pharmacological work. He enormously worked in the area of General Pharmacology and Chemotherapy. Most particularly his work areas covered studies on Indigenous drugs covering their chemical composition, invitro & invivo tests for the active principles, biochemical & biophysical changes in mammalian organism; surveys on drug addiction, Drug analysis etc.

The department of Pharmacology at Calcutta School of Tropical Medicines stood as land mark for other researches also covering clinical evaluation of drugs, tropical medicine, therapeutics, experimental pharmacology, toxicology, drug standardization and biological assays, diagnostic services etc. His work on indigenous drugs inspired many other institutions to join their hands in the research of that area. With his continuous research various indigenous drugs like ispaghula, kurchi, rauwolfia, psoralea, cobra venom, etc. were proved to have pharmacologically active principles and got place in Indian Pharmacopoeial List 1946 and Pharmacopoeia of India 1955.

He also contributed a lot for Indian systems of medicine. One of his great contributions was utilize under the chairmanship of Drug Enquiry Committee in 1930-31 during which period he roamed throughout India and given provoking recommendations to the Govt. of India due to which a seed of pharmacy profession has taken birth. With his recommendations Prof. Mahadev Lal Schroff got inspired and started Pharmacy course first time in India in 1932 at Banarus Hindu University. And also Drugs Act 1940 was framed which was later changed as Drugs and Cosmetics Act in 1962. Later Ayurvedic (including Siddha) and Unani drugs were also under its coverage in 1964. Government of J & K appointed him as Director of Medical Services and then appointed as Director of Drug Research Laboratory (his personal Laboratory which he donated to the Government of India, Previously called Drug Research laboratory then Regional Research Laboratory and now it is known as Indian Institute of Integrative Medicines) where he served the lab till 1960. He died in Srinagar, in june 13,1973.

(K C VERMA)

Foreword

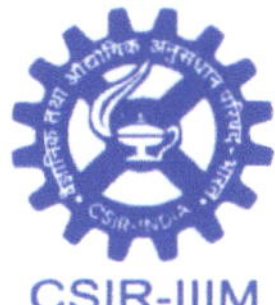

CSIR-IIIM

डॉ. राम विश्वकर्मा
निदेशक
Dr. Ram Vishwakarma
Director

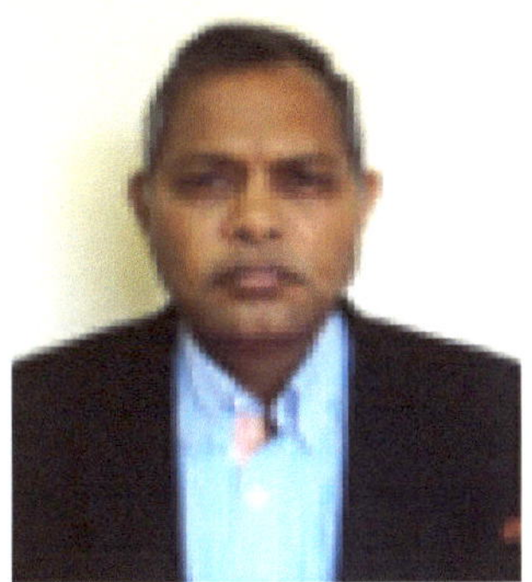

Tel. : +91-191-2584999, 2585222 (O), 2586333 (F)
Resi. : +91-191-2581444
EPABX : +91-191-2585006 - 2585013
E-mail : director@iiim.res.in; ram@iiim.res.in
Website : www.iiim.res.in

सीएसआईआर–भारतीय समवेत औषध संस्थान
(वैज्ञानिक तथा औद्योगिक अनुसंधान परिषद)
केनाल रोड, जम्मू – 180 001 (भारत)
CSIR-Indian Institute of Integrative Medicine
(Council of Scientific & Industrial Research)
Canal Road, Jammu - 180 001 (INDIA)

Prof (Dr) K.C Verma MBBS, DCH, MD, DM has a brilliant record of academic achievements and vast teaching experience in the discipline of medicine and cardiology and has held different positions in medical education at Govt. Medical College, Jammu. Dr Verma is practicing medicine for more than 30 years in the city of temples at Jammu Heart Clinic, Jammu (J&K). Besides his clinical practice, he is also very much interested in clinical research and non-invasive techniques in cardiology. He has published more than forty research papers in the medical Journals of repute which has brought him due appreciations from medical fraternity from all over the world. In recognition to his contributions in medical field, he was awarded prestigious Fellow of International College of Physicians, USA and Fellow of Royal Society of Tropical Medicine and Hygiene, London. In the year 2008, he was conferred the prestigious 'Glory of India Award' by India International Friendship Society on the day of Parvasi, Bhartiya Divas during international conference at New Delhi and award of Gold medal & Fellowship of Cardiological Society of India (FCSI). In addition, he is also recipient of Best Citizen of India award by international publishing House, New Delhi. Dr Verma has written 10 books on different aspects of cardiovascular medicine which are published by reputed Indian Publishing houses. His current book is on "Management of Heart Diseases with Conventional, Complimentary and Alternative Group of Therapies" (An Integrative Approach). It has been written with basic concept of integrating systems of traditional medicine and modern medicine so that patient with particular disease is treated confidently with the application of either stand alone or combined therapeutic techniques with least cost and minimal side effects. Opening chapters of present volume details the introduction of alternative, complimentary and modern medicine, where the author explains the classification, pathogenesis, diagnosis and treatment according to the ancient disciplines of Chinese, Buddha and Indian Ayurveda. The author also enlightens the readers regarding three doshas i.e. kapha, pitta and vatta and five natural elements i.e. fire, water, air, akash and earth which become the key factors for not only the causation of different bodily ailments but also guides us in their management

Dr Verma not only discusses the diagnosis and management of various cardiovascular diseases by modern medicine but he also integrated these with oldest discipline of Ayurveda and AYUSH. He has proved his point by citing research where patients with angina, heart attack and rhythm irregularities can be effectively managed through therapies under AYUSH systems of medicine. Similarly he has also touched upon the diseases like obesity, diabetes mellitus, venous insufficiencies, menopause, hematological disorders, vitamin/mineral deficiencies and mental stress which can be very well treated with AYUSH therapies.

I am sure this book would be of immense interest to both undergraduate and postgraduate students, physicians and general practitioners of AYUSH. It will also prove to be a handy guide to the students and physicians of modern medicine who would like to integrate AYUSH systems with allopathy in the management of their patients with least complications and minimal cost.

(Ram Vishwakarma)

ANNOTATION

Biotechnology and its Role in Complimentary and Alternative Medicine (CAM)

Most of the healthcare modalities accompanying CAM practices have been poorly accepted by the medical group owing to poor understanding or lack of scientific evidences regarding their productiveness as potential therapeutic interventions. The use of CAM in public healthcare domain has, thus, remained a controversial issue generating a huge debate. There is a reasonable requirement of another, evidence-based research approach for evaluation of productiveness and effectiveness of the CAM therapies and their development which would further influence people's individual choices regarding exertion of certain CAM therapies in accordance to their clinical condition. Researchers across the globe have been conducting scruplous research on a large-scale on several natural products and alternative therapeutics for the betterment of current CAM industry. There are number of examples can be cited which could possibly indicate the essentiality of Biotechnology in understanding the putative efficacy and effectiveness of CAM in certain diseases. Some of these are as follow:

1 . Various studies are being carried out by the Johns Hopkins Center for Cancer Complementary Medicine for assessing the antioxidant, anti-inflammatory, pain relieving of certain herbals and prayer in African women with breast cancer.

2. The clinical productiveness, mechanism of action and safety of hyperbaric oxygen therapy is being assessed by the University Of Pennsylvania Specialized Center Of Research in Hyperbaric Oxygen Therapy for the treatment of various types of cancer of head and neck and its putative negative effect on the disease progression.

3. Andrographolide, a bioactive chemical found in Andrographis paniculata and its derivatives have been found to have important therapeutic activities such as anti-inflammatory, antibacterial, antidiabetic, antitumor, anti-viral, anti-feedent. It is also known to have important activities that fights against cardiovascular disease, platelet activatrion, infertility and NF-ƙB activation (Jayakumar, Hsieh et al. 2013).

4.. S-adenosyl-L-methionine (SAMe), a major methyl component found in the brain and involved in many metabolic pathways, is found to have anti-depressant properties and helps in treating dementia (Mischoulon and Fava 2002).

5. Mind-body interventions like yoga and meditation has found to have an important role in fighting depression sleep disorders etc., and increasing youthfulness and longevity. Detailed research has indicated that they have significant effect on the levels of certain mind-body hormones such as dopamine, serotonin, cortisol, DHEA, GABA, endorphins, melatonin, growth hormones etc.

6. A recent study by the Universities of Coventry and Radbound have shown that mind-body interventions like meditation, yoga and Tai Chi influence molecular changes in DNA and can help reverse the molecular changes related to various ailments (Buric, Farias *et al.* 2017). Activity (Epel, Puterman *et al.* 2016; Conklin, King *et al.* 2018).

I have been associated with DR. K C VERMA DM, cardiologist of repute for more than 20 years and from time to time saught his guidance in selected projects on human genetic particularily human genome. Currently I am associated with him on a newer project highlighting the role of telomere length in chronic cardiovascular disorders such as hypertension, stroke, myocardial infarction and diabetes mellitus. Dr verma has also written a chapter in this book "management of heart diseases with conventional,complimentary and alternative group of therapies." on telomere shortening in chronic cardiovascular ailments and its recovery by administration of various herbal medicines. I have gone through the various topics of this integrative cardiology and found it very informative in managing the heart ailments with combined approach of modern medicine and traditional medicine under the main discipline of AYUSH. This book is a power house of knowledge in integrative medicine and would be of immense help to the researchers of biotechnology, undergraduate and postgraduate students of both modern medicine and AYUSH disciplines

Vijaeshwar Verma Ph.D., M.N.A.Sc., FAMI.
Professor & Dean, Faculty of Engineering, Head,
Department of Biotechnology. Co-ordinator Bioinformatics Centre,
Shri Mata Vaishno Devi University (SMVDU), Kakryal, Katra-182320 (J&K)

Preface

Indian ancient methods of treatment ie AYUSH (Ayurveda, Unani, Siddha and Homopathy), almost disappeared from India in a phased manner or restictricted to only a few clergy people, sadhus and Hakeems and that too for the benefit of influential personalities like Raja, maharajas and top rich individuals of this country. English rule which lasted more than 100 years brought lots of changes not only in administration but also in workings of common man's, life. During this peried, among many other alterations and modifications, they also shifted the discipline of Allopathy, also called modern medicine for the treatment of various illnesses prevailing in this country. Discipline of modern medicine became more popular than AYUSH due to its well planned research on animals and human volunteers, teaching in medical colleges and training of doctors and specialists. Medicines for different diseases were manufactured and classified after 5-10 years of research. Treatment prescribed to patients was later monitored for their curative effects and various side effects. Currently, physcians of modern medicine, practicing more than 30 years, did find that modern medicines and its techniques alone are not free from life threatening complications. With renewed thinking over the past one decade or so, AYUSH has become a well planned discipline and almost introduced in each state of united India. This discipline too like allopathy hac been supported with research, teachings in colleges and inventing newer medicines and techniques and therefore, is being accepted as an alternative system to allopathy with greater confidence.

This book has been written with basic concept of integrating both disciplines of AYUSH and modern medicine so that patient of particular disease is treated confidently with the application of either alone or combined therapeutic techniques with least cost and minimal side effects. Starting chapters details the introduction of alternative and complimentary medicine when compared to modern medicine and classification, pathogenesis, clinical features and categorization of different medicines of AYUSH according to three Doshas i.e. Kapha, Pitta and Vatta and five natural elements i.e. Fire, water, air, akash and earth. Research has shown that patients with angnia, heart attach and rhythm irregularities can be effectively managed with AYUSH technology including acupuncture. Similarily diseases like obesity, diabetes mellitus, venous insufficiencies, menopause, hematological disorders, vitamins minerals deficiencies and mental stress can be very well treated with AYUSH group of therapies. Heart failure which is the end result of many diseases like congenital, acquired heart diseases and hemodynamic disturbances is usually managed with modern and AYUSH medicines, but can also be treated with specially designed devices as alternative to conventional therapies. As an alternative to surgical intervention in the management of valvular heart diseases, non-surgical percutaneous transcatheter fitting of artificial valves has been the procedure of choice. Enhanced External Counter Pulsation (EECP) therapy which is a simple, non-invasive and alternative solution to the complex problem of angina pectoris has been briefly discussed. To keep our body fit and healthy, an account of balanced diet, calories and exercise have been cited with illustrations Role of homeopathy, aromatherapy, Transcendental Meditation, Electromagnetic Waves, Reiki and Acupuncture in maintaining human health has been briefly outlined. Kundalini Awakening and Yoga as alternative methods are being frequently combined with conventional treatment with better results in heart patients with open heart surgery. Application of TAI CHI AND QIGONG discipline, music and Herbal therapies for the prevention and management of cardiovascular disorders has been thoroughly discussed.

AI, or Artificial Intelligence, refers to the simulation of human intelligence in machines that are programmed to think like humans and mimic their actions. The term may also be applied to any machine that exhibits traits associated with a human mind such as learning and problem-solving.Since it is a newer technology its wider application in medical science is well established ,I there,added a few chapters such as Ocular images-based Artificial Intelligence In Diagnosis of Systemic Diseases Including Cardiovascular Ailments ,Artificial Intelligence-Based Smart Comrade Robot for Elders Healthcare,Applications of ChatGPT In Medical Practice, Education and Research and Health Implications of human body earthing to the Earth's surface electrons .

(K C VERMA)

Foreword by :- Director Dr Ram Vishavkarma
Dedication:- Sir ,Ram Nath Chopra
Preface

Volume - 1

CONTENTS

Chapter No..	Name of Chapter	Page No.

Volume - 2

Chapter No. | Name of the Chapter

Electromagnetic Therapy is an Alternative Natural Treatment for Human Ailments

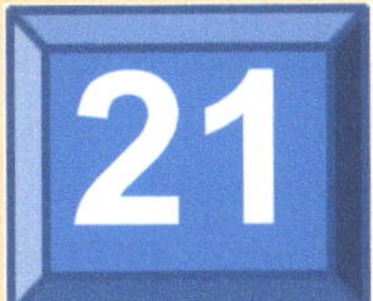

Electromagnetic waves are produced by the motion of electrically charged particles. These waves are also called electromagnetic radiation because they radiate from the electrically charged particles. They travel through empty space as well as through air and other substances.

Electromagnetic waves at low frequencies are referred to as electromagnetic fields and those at very high frequencies are called electromagnetic radiations .Energy therapies use magnets and therapeutic touch to manipulate the body's energy fields and improve health. Here's a round-up of some common energy therapies:

Effects of Electromagnetic waves on Human Health

While the positive aspect of technologic innovation makes the life easier, it may also involve components that impair the quality of life via its certain negative effects. A discussion about the adverse effects of electromagnetic waves on the biological life has been ongoing since the discovery of electricity in the 19th century Electromagnetic waves generated by many natural and human-made sources can travel for long distances and play a very important role in daily life. In particular, the electromagnetic fields in the Radiofrequency (RF) zone are used in communications,

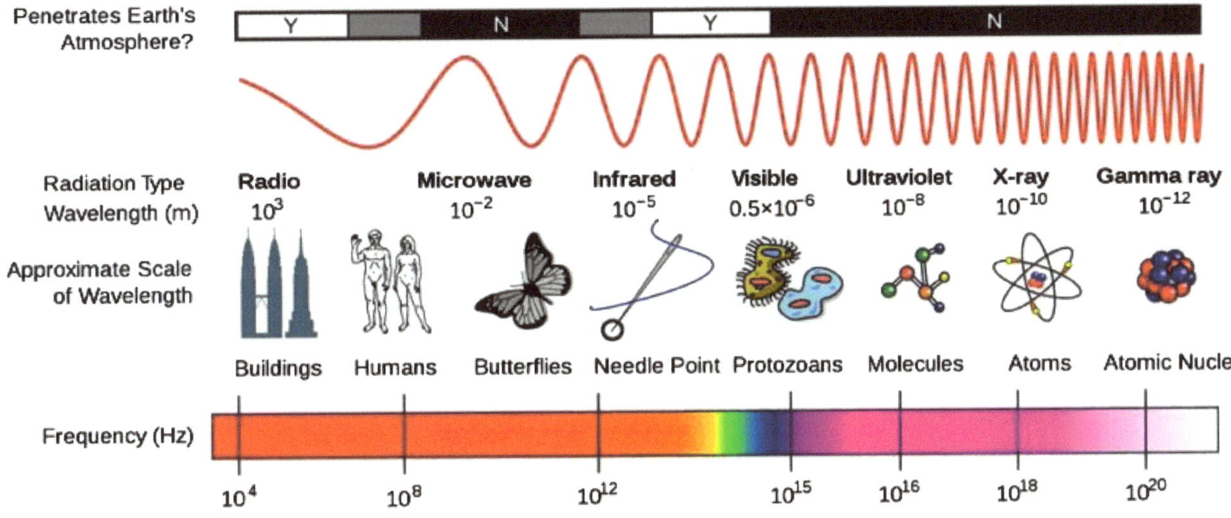

Fig. 21.1: *Electromagnetic spectrum and been introduced to a few of the waves from within it. The complete spectrum contains many key areas ranging from radio to gamma. Remember that the speed of light is constant so as frequency gets larger, wavelength must get shorter and vice versa.*

radio and television broadcasting, cellular networks and indoor wireless systems. Resulting from the technological innovations, the use of electromagnetic fields gradually increases and thus people are exposed to electromagnetic waves at levels much higher than those present in the nature. Along with the widespread use of technological products in daily life, the biological effects of electromagnetic waves started to be discussed. Particularly, the dramatically increasing number of mobile phones users rise significant concerns due to its potential damage on people exposed by radiofrequency waves. Since mobile phones are used in positions very close to the human body and require a large number of base station antennas, the public and the scientists have question marks in their mind about the impact of mobile phone networks on health

What is Magnetic Therapy ?

Magnetic therapy is widely used in Rheumatic disorders, nonarticular rheumatism, leucoderma, menstrual disorders, hypertension and asthma. Even cancer is becoming amenable to magneto therapy, use of magnetism in Agriculture is a pioneer work of Russians. Magnets increase and improve the shelf life of fruits, vegetables. Human body is transparent to magnetic field which acts at once on the body as a whole. The sugar, oil, protein content of seeds and fruits increases with south pole magnetized water. Cooked foods remains us-spoiled for longer periods if kept on North pole. While south pole increase fermentation.

South pole helps fermentation of liquors and increases Growth of moulds and bacteria. It promotes dense vegetable growth and gives bigger size flowers and fruits.

North pole retards growth of bacteria and plants and causes sparse vegetative growth, decreases fermentation rate of alcohol. It increases shelf-life of cooked foods.

1. North pole arrests growth of bacteria, so putrefaction of cells is decreased while South Pole increase putrefaction. So North Pole is applied over infected wounds. Human life span can be extended up to 400 yrs with suitable power of magnetic fields. So magnet is the best answer to ageing process.
2. Cancer cannot exist in a magnetic field. North pole applied to tumour causes shrinkage of the tumour, cancer cells have excessive frequency of cell vibration, which is normalized by magnet.
3. Cows yield more milk with magnet therapy using North Pole.
4. In Japan, effects of magnet in high blood pressure, Bursitis, constipation and fatigue were studied in detail and this led to the commercial production of cosmetic articles like wrist bands for hypertension, Belts for constipation, neck-laces to keep ladies young and belts for lumbago.
5. Magnet is good for Rheumatism, myalgia, kidney stones. In such cases use magnetized water.
6. Magnet is used to separate RBC from blood.

How Magnet Works: (Figs. 21.2 and 21.3)

There is a continuous influence of celestial magnetism on lower and higher forms of life. Human body is also affected by natural magnetism. If also acts as a magnet unit. Every cell works as a magnet unit. Every cell works as a micromagnet. So different organs have different powers of magnetic field depending on their biological activity.

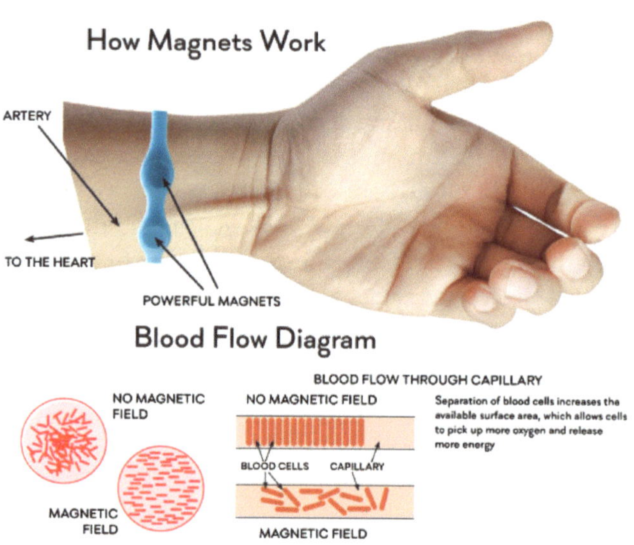

Fig.21.2: *Illustration explains that when magnet is applied to the obstructed artery ,its magnetic field separates blood cells with increase of surface area which in turns allows cells to pick up more oxygen and release more energy.*

1. Magnetic dowsing or Radiesthesia is study of disease, where distant diagnosis is important. It is becoming popular all over world. It is based on the principle that magnetic emanations form our body concentrate on the little pendulum used in magnetic dowsing. The pendulum thus utilizes the subtle variations in the altered magnetic emanation of different organs and tells you about any morbidity in any organ. For health, there should be harmony between the different groups of cells in the body. Geomagnetic activity has definite control over this harmony.
2. Heart attacks occur when there is fluctuation in terrestrial magnetism. Increased solar activity as shown by sunspots or sun storms or solar flares increase solar magnetic field producing increased

violent behaviour in man and animals. Sudden Geomagnetic disturbances cause increased effect on the biomagnetic potentials of all living beings. This leads to increased Cardiovascular diseases in man and increased Neuropsychic disorders. There is increased incidence of various types of epileptic attacks also during such solar storms. This is an example of its toxic pathogenic effects on all organisms. Heart attacks occur when he Earth's magnetic field increase by 3-4 times, and the pulsating fields, react with human heart of brain and trigger heart-attacks and mental symptoms.

The permanent magnets now made, have stabilizing effect on human organism. They bring about harmony and equilibrium in the biomagnetic potential in the various organs of the body. This explains the soothing effect of magnet in mental diseases.

All human tissues, brain heart, kidney, skin, lungs, gastro-intestinal and genito-urinary tracts have a 24 hour biorhythm, during which thousands of biochemical reactions occur in a predetermined manner and provide proper energy for that organism. In disease, the biorhythm of various organs is disturbed. This is particularly so in cancer.

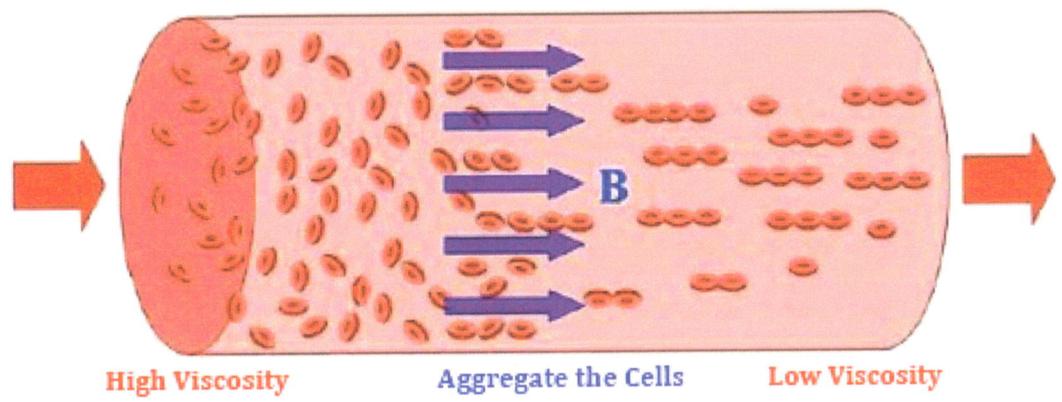

Fig. 21.3: *It is found that the magnetic field (B) polarises the red blood cells causing them to link together in short chains, streamlining the movement of the blood*

3. Magneto-therapy is to restore this to normal biomagnetic rhythm and potential. Blood is the most important medium of magnetic therapy. Magnet influences the conductivity and other properties of blood, including separation of RBCs, which are greatly influenced because of iron in haemoglobin. The increased circulation in various organs produces enhanced metabolic activity and quick disposal of waste. Improved circulation leads to quick all-round healing. Magneto therapy increase wound healing, promotes health and sense of well-being, improves circulation and increases resistance power to disease, decreases fatigue and improves vigour. ESR is markedly affected by magneto therapy, north pole magneto helps arrest infection. South pole on Right hand slows heart rate, while south pole on left palm, increases heart rate. Regular use of magnetized water help to dissolve our atherosclerotic plaque.
4. Magnet helps speedy and effective disposal of waste (Pus and inflammatory exudates) giving relief in arthritis, septicaemia and urinary infection. There is also increased Na excretion in urine. Considerable improvement occurs in respiration with magneto therapy. The increased oxygen of blood helps in Asthma, bronchitis and lung congestion South Pole opens up the spastic bronchii and bronchioles and increases the ease of breathing in asthma.
5. Different types of aches and pains from tooth ache to dysuria and dysmenorrhoea quickly respond to magneto-therapy, it gives sure positive effects in alleviating pain. The magnet is also known as Instant Pain Killer - sciatica, Osteo-arthritis, and Rheumatiod arthritis responds best to Magneto therapy.
6. Positive effects of Magneto-therapy can also be observed in various cases of endocrinopathies. Magnets help improve memory, intelligence, concentration and understanding. It also helps in Psychosomatic disorders, tension and stress states. It has soothing effect in insomnia. Skin and hair get their form corrected by Magnet. Magneto-therapy is effective in Leucoderma, Seborrhoea, Psoriasis, greying of hair, hair-falling etc.

7. Magneto-therapy is effective in obesity. It helps in harmonizing the functions of various organs heart, lungs, kidney, brain etc. It improves the immunological system and self-regulating faculty of human body.
8. For common disorders like dyspepsia, flatulence, diarrhoea good results are obtained by the use of magnet. Magnetised water is effective in many digestive and urinary complaints, painful urination, kidney stones etc.
9. Systematic use of magnet in cancers is very effective to arrest growth and spread. Cancers cannot exist in a strong magnet field. North pole has powerful effect in hard and cystic and malignant tumours.

   Herring's laws of cure state that disease is a subtle force which deranges the vital force of an organism. Natural flow of this in disease is from outer to inner, so for cure redirect this force from within to without. Disease travels downwards from above and so for cure, from below up. Don't attempt to interrupt nature's efforts at cure or reverse the natural direction of disease. So treat in consonance with natural laws, match subtle natural force to tackle subtle disease force. Here lies the importance of magnet. Magneto therapy works on the natural laws of magnet. It affects the whole body by effecting magnetic equilibrium between various organs and their functions.
10. Jesus Christ on whom the 7 wise men of the East bestowed the knowledge of healing the sick, used the faculty of human magnetism to cure human ailments. It was not mere magical cure.

What is magnetic field therapy?

Magnetic field therapy uses magnets to maintain health and treat illness. The human body and the earth naturally produce electric and magnetic fields. Electromagnetic fields also can be technologically produced, such as radio and television waves. Practitioners of magnetic field therapy believe that interactions between the body, the earth, and other electromagnetic fields cause physical and emotional changes in humans. They also believe that the body's electromagnetic field must be in balance to maintain good health. Practitioners apply magnetic field therapy to the outside of the body. The magnets may be:

- Electrically charged, to deliver an electrical pulse to the treated area.
- Used with acupuncture needles, to treat energy pathways in the body.
- Static (not electrically charged) and stationary on the treated area for periods of time, to deliver continuous treatment.

Clinical Applications of Magnet Therapy

People use magnet therapy for a wide range of health problems, including:

- Joint problems, such as arthritis.
- Migraine headaches.
- Pain, including mild to moderate pain after surgery as well as long-term (chronic) pain.
- Depression.
- Cancer.
- Overstretched muscles or injuries to muscles, ligaments, andtendons (strains and sprains).
- Magnetic treatment for high blood pressure
- Magnets could prevent heart attacks by thinning the blood as effectively as aspirin
- Magnetically Targeted Stem Cell Delivery for Regenerative Medicine
- Non invasive tecknique of MRI

If a person's blood becomes too thick it can damage blood vessels and increase the risk of heart attacks. But a Temple University physicist has discovered that he can thin the human blood by subjecting it to a magnetic field. Rongjia Tao, professor and chair of physics at Temple University, has pioneered the use of electric or magnetic fields to decrease the viscosity of oil in engines and pipelines. Now, he is using the same magnetic fields to thin human blood in the circulation system.

Because red blood cells contain iron, Tao has been able to reduce a person's blood viscosity by 20-30 percent by subjecting it to a magnetic field of 1.3 Telsa (about the same as an MRI) for about one minute.

Tao and his collaborator tested numerous blood samples in a Temple lab and found that the magnetic field polarizes the red blood cells causing them to link together in short chains, streamlining the movement of the blood. Because these chains are larger than the single blood cells, they flow down the center, reducing the friction against the walls of the blood vessels. The combined effects reduce the viscosity of the blood, helping it to flow more freely. When the magnetic field was taken away, the blood's original viscosity state slowly returned, but over a period of several hours.

"By selecting a suitable magnetic field strength and pulse duration, we will be able to control the size of the aggregated red-cell chains, hence to control the blood's viscosity," said Tao. "This method of magneto-rheology provides an effective way to control the blood viscosity within a selected range."

Currently, the only method for thinning blood is through drugs such as aspirin; however, these drugs often produce unwanted side effects. Tao said that the magnetic field method is not only safer, it is repeatable. The magnetic fields may be reapplied and the viscosity reduced again. He also added that the viscosity reduction does not affect the red blood cells' normal function.

Tao said that further studies are needed and that he hopes to ultimately develop this technology into an acceptable therapy to prevent heart disease.

Electromagnetic Fields and the Heart : Basic Science and Clinical Use

Heart disease is the number one cause of mortality in the United States and Canada. The heart is a very electrically dynamic organ. Heart disease includes many causes. These range from vascular disease, electrical conduction defects, muscle problems, valvular effects, congenital defects, infectious problems, trauma and pericardial problems, all as the direct or primary cause of the cardiac disease. Other non-direct problems can also affect the heart secondary to other systemic issues, including, but not limited to, hypertension, kidney disease, lung disease, autoimmune diseases, toxicities of various kinds, etc. Finding nonpharmacologic and noninvasive ways of managing heart disease in a safe, effective, nontoxic way is always a goal.

Magnetocardiography

Magnetocardiography (MCG) is a technique to measure the magnetic fields produced b y e lectrical a ctivity in the heart using extremely sensitive devices such as the superconducting quantum interference device (SQUID). If the magnetic field is m easured u sing a multichannel device, a map of the magnetic field is obtained over the chest; from such a map, using mathematicalalgorithms that take into account the conductivity structure of the torso, it is possible to locate the source of the activity. For example, sources of abnormal rhythms or arrhythmia may be located using MCG.

History

The first MCG m easurements w ere m ade b y Baule and McFee using two large coils placed over the chest, connected in opposition to cancel out the relatively large magnetic background. Heart signals were indeed seen, but were very noisy. The next development was by David Cohen, who used a magnetically shielded room to reduce the background, and a smaller coil with better electronics; the heart signals were now less noisy, allowing a magnetic map to be made, verifying the magnetic properties and source of the signal. However, the use of an inherently noisy coil detector discouraged widespread interest in the MCG. The turning point came with the development of the sensitive detector called the SQUID (superconducting quantum interference device) by James Zimmerman. The combination of this detector and Cohen's new shielded room at MIT allowed the MCG signal to be seen as clearly as the conventional electrocardiogram, and the publication of this resultmarked the real beginning of magnetocardiography (as well as biomagnetism generally).

Magnetocardiography is used in various laboratories and clinics around the world, both for research on the normal human heart, and for clinical diagnosis.

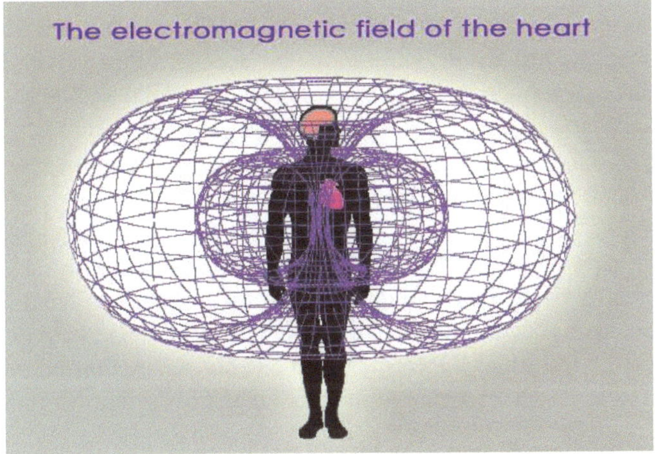

Fig.21.4: *The heart's electromagnetic field*

Magnetic fields have been found to significantly affect cardiac function, in addition to effects on a myriad of other body systems and problems. Not all magnetic fields are the same. Different types of magnetic fields may have different effects on the heart. Treatment of secondary causes can be just as important as the primary management of the heart itself.

It is just to summarize that EMF therapy acts beneficially on the functional state of the cardiovascular, nervous and endocrine systems as well as on tissue metabolism. The heart has been found through numerous studies to be very electromagnetically sensitive. This sensitivity extends to all external fields, whether therapeutic or otherwise, including their interactions with each other and with the body. Some of the benefits to the cardiovascular system are indirect, acting through stress reduction effects, emotional responses, endocrine system, the immune system and especially the autonomic nervous system. Autonomic neural regulation makes the tone of the vascular system normal. Even cardiac muscle blood vessels are dilated. Decreased vascular resistance decreases the workload of the heart, reducing strain, which if applied over long periods of time could lead to decreased cardiac wear and tear. EMFs have a moderating effect on cardiac function as well as the microcirculatory system. Pulsed magnetic fields, versus sinusoidal fields, appear to be less aggressive towards the heart. Much of their actions depend on cellular Ca++ ion changes.

There are multiple other actions of EMFs on the cardiovascular system. One is an anti-atherogenic effect and a reduction of platelet adhesion factors, which could reduce the possibility of cardiac vascular occlusions and cardiac damage. Because of actions on stress proteins, cardio-protection is now a feasible use, not only for treating or reducing cardiac ischemia but also for the trauma created by cardiac surgery. EMFs are even useful post-operatively in facilitating and accelerating recovery through wound healing effects, for superficial and even deep tissues.

There are significant differences between clinical ELF PEMF systems and high frequency (microwave or cell phone levels) sources. Indeed, there are many clinical therapy systems that use high frequencies, but they are usually used for tissue destruction, for tumors and colon, bladder, skin and heart arrhythmia lesions, etc. General or public use of EMFs for personal use should be limited to low strength ELFs or high frequency EMFs that do not create heating.

The evidence reviewed here gives reasonable support for wider medical application of magnetic field (MF) therapy as a method of non-drug therapy in cardiovascular disease, alone or in a complementary fashion with medical or other modalities.

Magnetically targeted stem cell delivery for regenerative medicine (Fig. 21.5).

Stem cells play a special role in the body as agents of self-renewal and auto-reparation for tissues and organs. Stem cell therapies represent a promising alternative strategy to regenerate damaged tissue when natural repairing and conventional pharmacological intervention fail to do so. A fundamental impediment for the evolution of stem cell therapies has been the difficulty of effectively targeting administered stem cells to the disease foci. Biocompatible magnetically responsive nanoparticles are being utilized for the targeted delivery of stem cells in order to enhance their retention in the desired treatment site. This noninvasive treatment-localization strategy has shown promising results and has the potential to mitigate the problem of poor long-term stem cell engraftment in a number of organ systems post-delivery. In addition, these same nanoparticles can be used to track and monitor the cells in vivo, using magnetic resonance imaging. In the present review we underline the principles of magnetic targeting for stem cell delivery, with a look at the logic behind magnetic nanoparticle systems, their manufacturing and design variants, and their applications in various pathological models.

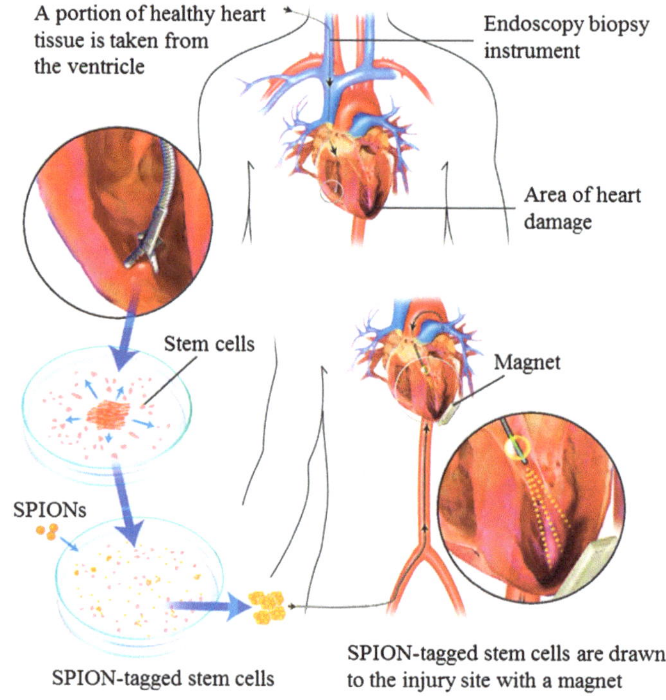

Fig.21.5: *Illustration showing magnetically targeted stem cell delivery for regenerative medicine*

Magnets could prevent heart attacks by thinning the blood as effectively as aspirin

People at risk of heart attacks are often prescribed aspirin to thin the blood, but now scientists believe that Magnets could one day be used instead. Scientists at Temple University in Michigan found that a device that uses a magnetic field to thin fuel, can have the same effect on human blood. Professor Rongjia Tao pioneered the use of electric or magnetic fields to decrease the viscosity of oil in engines in 2008. He realised that this could work on our own circulation system in a similar way. (Fig. 21.6)

Because red blood cells contain iron, Tao has been able to reduce a person's blood viscosity (resistance to flow) by 20-30 per cent by subjecting it to a magnetic field for about one minute. The field measured 1.3 Telsa which is about the same as an MRI machine.

Abbreviations:

EMF = Electro-magnetic field

ELF = Extremely low frequency

PEMF = Pulsed electromagnetic field

ERI = Elective replacement indication

EOL = End of life
LRL = Lower rate limit
ERN = Elective replacement near
ERT = Elective replacement time

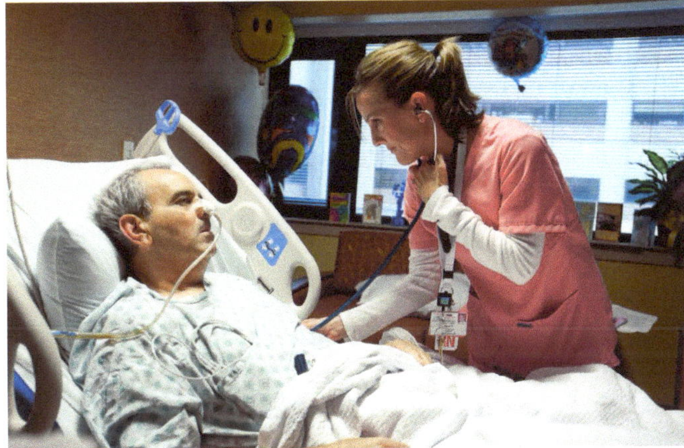

Fig. 21.6: *Heart attacks occur when blood is stopped from reaching the organ. A magnetic device could help increase blood low*

After testing numerous blood samples in a laboratory, Tao found that the magnetic field polarises the red blood cells causing them to link together in short chains, streamlining the movement of the blood. As these chains are larger than the single blood cells, they flow down the centre, reducing the friction against the walls of the blood vessels. The combined effects reduce the viscosity of the blood, helping it to flow more freely. When the magnetic field was taken away, the blood's original viscosity state slowly returned over a period of several hours. (Fig. 24.6) 'By selecting a suitable magnetic field strength and pulse duration, we will be able to control the size of the aggregated red-cell chains, hence to control the blood's viscosity,' said Tao. Currently, the only method for thinning blood is through drugs such as aspirin; however, these drugs often produce unwanted side effects. Tao said that the magnetic field method is not only safer, it is repeatable. The magnetic fields may be reapplied and the viscosity reduced again. He also added that the viscosity reduction does not affect the red blood cells' normal function. Tao said that further studies are needed and that he hopes to ultimately develop this technology into an acceptable therapy to prevent heart disease.

Clinical Applications of Magnets on Cardiac Rhythm Management Devices

All pacemakers respond to a magnet by switching to an asynchronous pacing mode at a programmed atrioventricular (AV) delay and a fixed magnet rate depending on the manufacturer, device model, and the status of the battery. The programmed mode DDD switches to DOO, VVI switches to VOO, and AAI switches to AOO. The rate response feature is switched to 'OFF' on magnet application in pacemakers. In biventricular pacemakers, both the right and left ventricles continue to be paced in the above modes with magnet application so long as the device is at or above ERI. However, from below ERI voltage, this response is unpredictable.

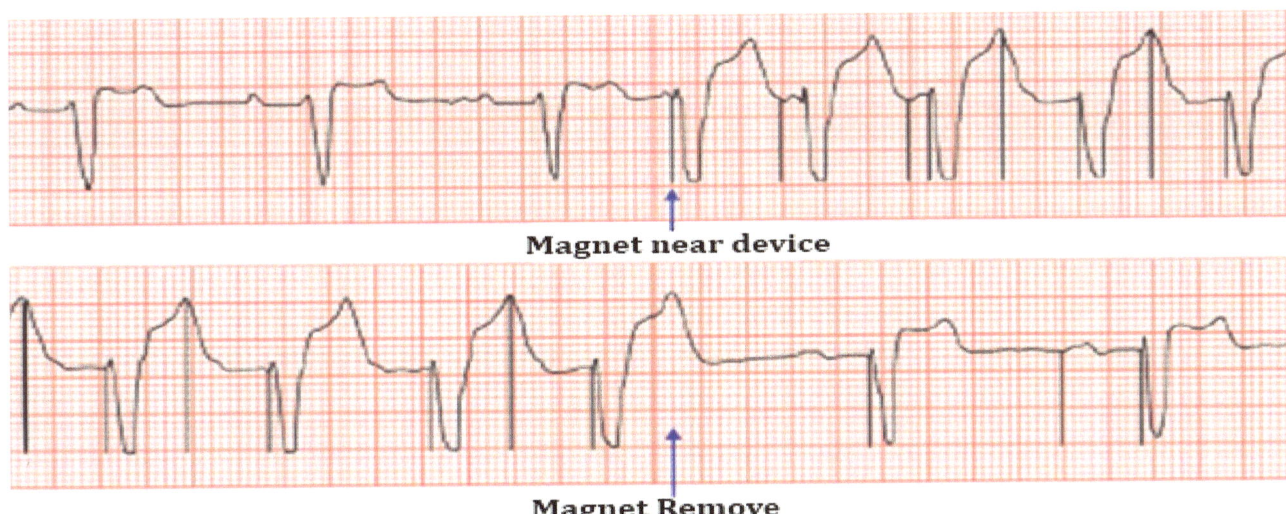

Fig.21.7: *Example of asynchronous pacing induced when a portable headphone was placed on a patient's chest overlying the pacemaker (top : arrow "Magnet Near Device"). Removal of the headphone (bottom:arrow "Magnet Removed") resulted in an immediate return of normal pacemaker function.*

If magnet application on a pacemaker site does not produce any response on the surface ECG pacing rate or mode, the magnet may be repositioned. If no change is still observed, the following reasons may apply :

(i) a depleted pacemaker battery;
(ii) the pacemaker is programmed to ignore the magnet (St. Jude, Boston Scientific, and Biotronik synchronous mode);
(iii) the magnetic field does not reach the device, as in the case of those with deeper (abdominal or submuscular) implants or in very obese patients;
(iv) EOL or lower battery life. Additionally, with Biotronik pacemakers in a synchronous mode, if the patient's intrinsic heart rate is higher than the lower rate limit (LRL) programmed, there will be no ECG response.

In almost all pacemakers, removal of the magnet causes the device to revert to pacing at the normal preprogrammed rate with the exception of Sorin pacemakers as described below.

Boston Scientific

Boston Scientific pacemakers are designed to switch to an asynchronous pacing mode on magnet application if the device is not programmed to a magnet 'OFF' mode. It also has a battery test mode and an electrogram (EGM) mode to initiate ECG storage without any effect on pacing.

In the magnet response mode, Boston Scientific pacemakers are paced at a magnet rate of 100 bpm at EOL with an AV delay of 100 ms. The third pulse during the magnet test is issued at 50% of the programmed pulse width to allow the clinician to evaluate the safety margin. The magnet rate is 100, 95, and 85 beats per minute (bpm) at EOL, elective replacement near (ERN), and ERT, respectively, in Boston Scientific pacemakers.

Medtronic

Medtronic pacemakers do not have a magnet 'OFF' mode and asynchronous pacing can always be expected on magnet application. With the exception of EnRhythm® (Medtronic, Minneapolis, MN, USA), asynchronous pacing is preceded by three paced pulses at 100 bpm, with the pulse width of the last pacing reduced by 20%. This is known as the TMT and is used to ascertain adequate pacing capture safety margin. In Medtronic devices, the magnet rates are 85 and 65 bpm at EOL and ERI, respectively. A rate of 65 bpm is specifically reserved for providing information about battery life (ERI) with magnet application. Thus, Medtronic pacemakers cannot be programmed to pace at a rate of 65 bpm.

St. Jude Medical

St. Jude Medical pacemakers may be programmed to ignore the magnet ('OFF' mode) or have one of the following three manufacturer-programmed modes :

(i) Battery test mode, in which there is a switch to asynchronous pacing immediately on magnet application;
(ii) Battery test + EGM mode, in which an ECG is stored if the magnet is held over the device for less than 5 s and a switch is made to asynchronous pacing if held for >5 s; and
(iii) EGM mode, in which an ECG is stored without any effect on pacing.

An additional VARIO mode is present in some older models (Microny® and Regency®, St. Jude Medical Inc., St. Paul, MN, USA). This feature was available in some Pacesetter devices, which are currently under St. Jude Medical but are being phased out. This mode is to check battery life and adequate pacing capture safety margin. It involves a repetitive cycle of 32 asynchronous events on magnet application with the first 16 paced events at 100 bpm (85 bpm at ERI) followed by 15 events at 119 bpm with successive reduction in pacing voltage and the last paced event at no output.

Biotronik

Biotronik devices respond differently to magnets depending on manufacturer-programmed modes that could be

(i) asynchronous,
(ii) synchronous (which demands pacing in programmed mode at LRL), or
(iii) auto (i.e. 10 asynchronous events followed by reversion to synchronous mode). A synchronous mode is also used for a patient-triggered recording. The magnet rates for different modes vary according to the available battery life.

Sorin

Sorin pacemakers also switch to asynchronous pacing in response to magnet application with a pulse width of 0.5 ms and rest AV delay (original programmed sensed AV delay). When the magnet is removed, the 'capture test' is initiated comprising six asynchronous pulses at magnet rate, programmed amplitude, and pulse width with an AV delay of 94 ms. This is used to verify adequate capture with programmed pulse width and amplitude. This is followed by the 'rate test' comprising two asynchronous pulses at programmed rate and AV delay to demonstrate sufficient capture at these values. Capture and rate tests are followed by pacing at the original programmed rate.

Magnetic Treatment for High Blood Pressure

Although there is no known cure for the majority of people suffering with high blood pressure, it is possible to treat it very successfully. Mainstream treatments include water tablets (diuretics) and high blood pressure tablets (anti hypertensives : beta blockers, ace inhibitors and calcium channel blockers).

Magnetic therapy can also be used to treat high blood pressure by eliminating excess fluid in the body. When a person is first diagnosed with high blood pressure the first course of treatment a doctor will try is diuretics, the aim of water tablets is to eliminate fluid from the body this is a side effect of high blood pressure (particularly the extremities : hands, feet and ankles). The excess fluid puts pressure in the heart and this in turn increases blood pressure.

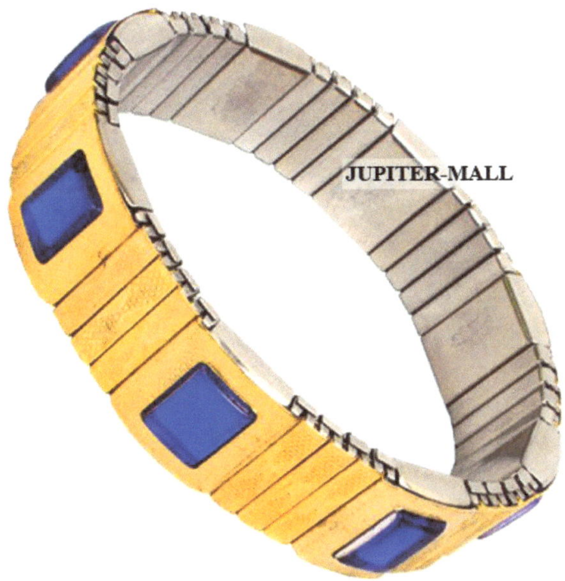

Fig. 21.8: *Wrist bracelet which can be applied in the treatment of systemic hypertension*

The primary aim of diuretics is to get rid of the extra fluid so that blood pressure is reduced, as the workload of the heart reduces. Magnetised water has a natural detoxification effect on the body, drinking at least 4 glasses a day will eliminate excess fluid (plus toxins stored in the fluid) from the body. This has the same effect a that of diuretics in that as the fluid is "off loaded" the workload of the heart is decreased and blood pressure is reduced. In addition to drinking magnetised water, blood pressure can also be reduced by wearing a magnetic bracelet or magnetic strap around the wrist. The radial artery is situated in the wrist and is one of the bodies main arteries. When a magnetic field is applied over the radial artery, the magnetism is rapidly absorbed and distributed around the whole body. Blood flow is improved around the whole body and the heart ,the whole circulatory system receives increased oxygen which in turn increases oxygenation of the organs and tissues, as a result of the improved oxygenation the heart does not have to pump so many times a minute to ensure enough oxygen is supplied to the body and this reduces the workload which will automatically reduce blood pressure. Although these 2 magnetic treatments for high blood pressure are extremely effective and will give results very quickly, it is important to remember that high blood pressure medication should not be stopped suddenly. If you use magnets to treat your high blood pressure ensure that your blood pressure is checked regularly by the GP or practice nurse. When your blood pressure has reduced your doctor will reduce your medication accordingly.

Is magnetic field therapy safe?

Young children and pregnant women should not use magnetic field therapy, because the safety of this therapy is not proved. People who have medical devices or implants with a magnetic field, such as a pacemaker, should not use magnet therapy, because it could interfere with the function of the implant.

Magnet therapy is not thought to have negative side effects or complications when it is combined with conventional medical treatment. Always tell your doctor if you are using an alternative therapy or if you are thinking about combining an alternative therapy with your conventional medical treatment. It may not be safe to forgo your conventional medical treatment and rely only on an alternative therapy.

The MRI uses powerful magnets to create its images. For your safety, anyone undergoing a scan should be free of any metallic or magnetic items. Inform the MRI staff if you have any metallic implants or any metal under the skin. Most metallic implants, such as sternal wires and clips used for heart surgery, pose no problem.

Some conditions may make an MRI inadvisable. Tell your doctor if you have any of the following conditions:

- Implanted pacemaker or defibrillator
- Older model Starr-Edwards (metallic ball/cage type) heart valve implant
- Cerebral aneurysm clip (metal clip in a blood vessel in the brain)
- Pregnancy
- Implanted insulin pump, narcotic pump, or implanted nerve stimulators (TENS) for back pain

- Metal in the eye or eye socket
- Cochlear (ear) implant for hearing impairment

Getting too close to magnets can have fatal consequences for heart patients

According to Swiss researchers some magnets which are used in many new commercial products can interfere with implanted heart devices such as pacemakers and the consequences can be fatal.

It appears that magnets made from neodymium-iron-boron are increasingly being used in computer hard drives and "in-ear" headphones, and this is of concern because being close to such magnets can disrupt the normal functioning of cardiac devices.

Ordinary iron or ferrite magnets, which are a dull grey colour with a low magnetic strength, such as those used to stick badges on fridges are apparently not a problem; it is the powerful magnets made from neodymium-iron-boron, which are shiny and silver in colour that are the worry.

What is magnetic resonance imaging (MRI) of the heart?

Magnetic resonance imaging (MRI) is a diagnostic exam that uses a combination of a large magnet, radio waves, and a computer to produce detailed images of organs and structures within the body.

How does MRI work?

The MRI machine is a large, cylindrical (tube-shaped) machine that creates a strong magnetic field around the patient. This magnetic field, along with radio waves, alters the hydrogen atoms' natural alignment in the body. Computers are then used to form 2-dimensional (2D) images of the heart's structure based on the activity of the hydrogen atoms. Cross-sectional views can be obtained to reveal further details. MRI does not use ionizing radiation.

A magnetic field is created and pulses of radio waves are sent from a scanner. The radio waves knock the nuclei of the atoms in your body out of their normal position. As the nuclei realign into proper position, they send out radio signals. These signals are received by a computer that analyzes and converts them into an image of the part of the body being examined. This image appears on a viewing monitor. Some MRI machines look like narrow tunnels, while others are more spacious or wider.

Other related procedures that may be used to assess the heart include resting or exerciseelectrocardiogram (ECG), Holter monitor, signal-averaged ECG, cardiac catheterization,chest X-ray, computed tomography (CT scan), electrophysiological studies, myocardial perfusion **scans, radionuclide angiography, and ultrafast CT scan.**

Clinical Utility of MRI of the Heart

MRI of the heart may be performed for further evaluation of signs or symptoms that may suggest:

- Atherosclerosis: A gradual clogging of the arteries over many years by fatty materials and other substances in the blood stream
- Cardiomyopathy: An enlargement of the heart due to thickening or weakening of the heart muscle
- Congenital heart disease: Defects in one or more heart structures that occur during formation of the fetus, such as a ventricular septal defect (hole in the wall between the two lower chambers of the heart)
- Congestive heart failure: A condition in which the heart muscle has become weakened to an extent that blood cannot be pumped efficiently, causing buildup (congestion) in the blood vessels, lungs, feet, ankles, and other parts of the body
- Aneurysm: A dilation of a part of the heart muscle or the aorta (the large artery that carries oxygenated blood out of the heart to the rest of the body), which may cause weakness of the tissue at the site of the aneurysm
- Valvular heart disease: Malfunction of one or more of the heart valves that may cause an obstruction of the blood flow within the heart
- Cardiac tumor: A tumor of the heart that may occur on the outside surface of the heart, within one or more chambers of the heart (intracavitary), or within the muscle tissue of the heart
- There may be other reasons for your doctor to recommend an MRI of the heart.

What are the risks of an MRI?

Because radiation is not used, there is no risk of exposure to ionizing radiation during an MRI procedure. Each patient must be screened before exposure to the MRI magnetic field.

Due to the use of the strong magnet, special precautions must be taken to perform an MRI on patients with certain implanted devices such as pacemakers or cochlear implants. The MRI technologist will need some information regarding the implanted decide, such as the make and model number, to determine if it is safe for you to have an MRI. Patients who have internal metal objects, such as surgical clips, plates, screws or wire mesh, might not be eligible for an MRI exam.

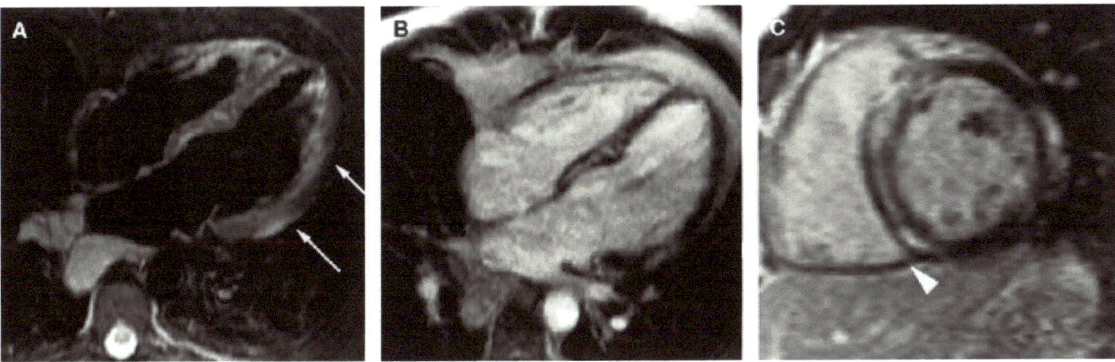

Fig. 21.9: *Serial late gadolinium-enhanced cardiac MRI scans of the patient with tubercular myocarditis. (A) Horizontal long axis view using black blood T2-weighted imaging, demonstrating patchy areas of high-intensity signal, most notably in the basal lateral wall of the left ventricle (arrows). (B) Horizontal long axis and (C) short axis view showing corresponding areas of fibrosis in the lateral wall of the basal left ventricle. Myocardial fibrosis is seen in the basal septal wall (arrowhead).*

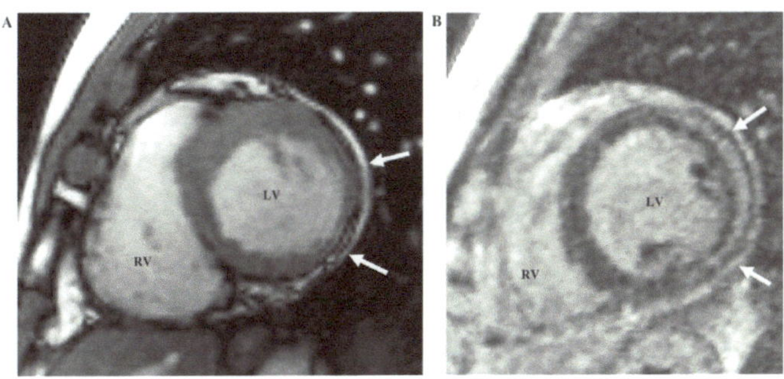

Fig. 21.10: *Cardiac MRI in myocarditis in patient with SLE. (A) Hypocontractility is demonstrated in the lateral wall of the left ventricle in cine TrueFISP sequence as an evidence of ongoing inflammation (arrows). (B) Late enhancement image shows intramural high signal intensity areas (arrows) due to focal inflammatory necrosis. LV, left ventricle; RV, right ventricle.*

- If there is a possibility that you are claustrophobic then you should ask your physician to provide you with anti-anxiety medication that you can take prior to your MRI examination. You should plan to have someone drive you home afterwards.
- If you are pregnant or suspect that you may be pregnant, you should notify your health care provider. To date there is no information indicating that MRI is harmful to an unborn child, however MRI testing during the first trimester is discouraged.
- A doctor may order a contrast dye to be used during some MRI exams in order for the radiologist to better view internal tissues and blood vessels on the completed images.
- If contrast is used, there is a risk for allergic reaction to the contrast. Patients who are allergic or sensitive to contrast dye or iodine should notify the radiologist or technologist.
- If you have severe kidney disease or are on kidney dialysis, there is a risk of a condition called "nephrogenic systemic fibrosis" from the contrast dye. You should discuss this risk with your doctor prior to the test.
- Nephrogenic Systemic Fibrosis (NSF) is a very rare but serious complication of MRI contrast use in patients with kidney disease or kidney failure. If you have a history of kidney disease, kidney failure, kidney transplant, liver disease or are on dialysis, you must inform the MRI technologist or radiologist prior to receiving contrast.
- MRI contrast may have an effect on other conditions, such as allergies, asthma, anemia, hypotension (low blood pressure), kidney disease, and sickle cell disease.

There may be other risks depending on your specific medical condition. Be sure to discuss any concerns with your doctor prior to the procedure.

Conclusions

Although electronic devices and the development in communications makes the life easier, it may also involve negative effects. These negative effects are particularly important in the electromagnetic fields in the Radiofrequency (RF) zone which are used in communications, radio and television broadcasting, cellular networks and indoor wireless systems. Along with the widespread use of technological products in daily life, the biological effects of electromagnetic waves has began to be more widely discussed.

The general opinion is that there is no direct evidence of hazardous effects on human health incurred by low-frequency radiofrequency waves. Studies at the cellular level, which uses relatively higher frequencies, demonstrate undesirable effects. In recent years there are a lot of studies about effects of EMF on cellular level; DNA, RNA molecules, some proteins, and hormones, intracellular free radicals, and ions are shown.

Particularly, the dramatically increasing number of mobile phones users rise significant concerns due to its potential damage on people exposed by radiofrequency waves. There are increasing number of in vivo, in vitro, and epidemiologic studies on the effects of mobile phones, base stations and other EMF sources in last decade.

Epidemiologic evidence compiled in the past ten years starts to indicate an increased risk, in particular for brain tumor, from mobile phone use. Because of mobile phones used close the brain tissue, electromagnetic waves affects it the most.The magnitude of the brain tumor risk is moderate.

A literature search on 'mobile phone use and cancer 'in Pubmed lists 350 studies. More than half of all of these studies is related to brain tumors. At present, evidence for a causal relationship between mobile phone use and brain tumors relies predominantly on epidemiology, in particular on the large studies on this subject. However, the etiopathogenesis of this causal relationship is not clear. The absence of this clear etiology even raise doubts about the cause itself. Weak evidence in favor of a causal relationship is provided by some animal and in vitro studies, but overall, genotoxicity assays, both in vivo and in vitro, are inconclusive to date.

Bibliography and Acknowledgement

- AJ Kastin, W. Pan, 2003 Peptide transport across the blood-brain barrier. In: Prokai L, Prokai-Tatrai K (Eds.) Peptide transport and delivery into the central nervous system. Birkhauser, Basel
- Antonella, V. Branca, 2010 Heavy metals exposure and electromagnetic hypersensitivity. Science of the Total Enviroment 408 2010 4919 4920
- Baldi, G. Coureau, A. Jaffre, A. Gruber, S. Ducamp, D. Provost, P. Leabilly, A. Vital, H. Loiseau, R. Salamon, 2010 Occupational and Residential Exposure to Electromagnetic Fields and Risk of Brain Tumours in adults: a case-control study in Gronde, France. *International journal of cancer.*
- Balmori, 2009 Electromagnetic pollution from phone masts. Effects on wildlife. *Pathophysiology*. **16**(2-3):191-9.
- D. Brusick, R. Albertini, D. Mc Ree, D. Peterson, *et al.* 1998 Genotoxicity of radiofrequency radiation. DNA/Genetox Espert Panel. *Environ Mol Mutagen*. **32** 1 1 16
- DA. Savitz, 1993 Overview of epidemiologic research on electric and magnetic fields and cancer. *Am Ind Hyg Assoc J.* **54** 4 197 204 .
- DJ Panagopoulos, LH. Margaritis, 2010 The effect of exposure duration on the biological activity of mobile telephone radiation. Mutation Research/genetic Toxicology and Environmental Mutagenesis. 17 22
- Draper, T. Vincent, ME. Kroll, J. Swanson, 2005 Childhood cancer in relation to distance from high voltage power lines in England and Wales: a case-control study. *BMJ.*; 330(7503):1290.
- Exposure to high frequency electromagnetic fields, biological effects and health consequences 2009100 kHz-300 GHz). Review of the scientific evidence on dosimetry, biological effects, epidemiological observations, and health consequences concerning exposure to high frequency electromagnetic fields. Editors: Vecchia P, Matthes R, Ziegelberger G, Lin J, Saunders R, Swerdlow A. International Commission on Non-Ionizing Radiation Protection. ICNIRP 16/2009
- F. Tian, T. Nakahara, M. Yoshida, N. Honda, H. Hirose, J. Miyakoshi, 2002 Exposure to power frequency magnetic fields suppresses X-ray-induced apoptosis transiently in Ku80 -deficient xrs5cells. *Biocemical and Biophysical Research Communications* **292** (2), 355-361.
- Foletti, A. Lisi, M. Ledda, *et al.* 2009 Cellular ELF signals as a possible tool in informative medicine. Electromagnetic *Biology and Medicine*. **28** (1), 71 EOF 79 EOF -79
- Ghezel-Ahmadi, A. Engel, J. Weidermann, L. T. Budnik, X. Baur, U. Frick, S. Hauser, N. Dahmen, 2010 Heavy metal exposure in patients suffering from electromagnetic hypersensitivity. **408** 4 774 8 .
- Guidelines On Limits Of Exposure To Static Magnetic Fields. In: International Commission On Non-Ionizing Radiation Protection ICNIRP Guidelines *Health Physics* 2009 96 4
- Hocking, I. R. Gordon, H. L. Grain, G. E. Hatfield, 1996 Cancer incidence and mortality and proximity to TV towers. *Med J Aust*; **165** (11 12).
- HS Burr, F.S.C. Northrop, 1935 The electro-dynamic theory of life. *The quarterly Review of Biology* **10**(3), 322-325
- J. Begley, M. W. Brightman, 2003 Structural and functional aspects of the blood-brain barrier. In: Prokai L., Prokai-Tatrai K (Eds.)., Peptide transport an delivery into the central nervous system. Birkhauser, Basel.
- J. C. Lin, M.F. Lin, 1982 Microwave hyperthermia-induced blood-brain barrier alterations. *Radiat. Res.* **89** 77 87
- J. Martinez-Samano, V. P. Torres-Duran, M. A. Juarez-Oropeza, D. Elias-Vinas, L. Verdugo-Diaz, 2010 Effects of acute electromagnetic field exposure and movement restraint on antioxidant system in liver, hearth, kidney and plasma of Wistar rats: A preliminary report. *Int. J. Radiat. Biol.,* 86 12 1088 1094

- J. Schüz, Ahlbom, 2008 Exposure to electromagnetic fields and the risk of childhood leukaemia: a review. *Radiat Prot Dosimetry*. **132** 2 202 11. Epub
- J. Schüz, P. Elliott, A. Auvinen, *et al.* 2010 An International prospective cohort study of mobile phone users and health (Cosmos): Design considerations and enrolement. *Cancer Epidemiology. 101016*
- Johansen, J. Boice, J. Jr Mc Laughlin, J. Olsen, 2001 Cellular telephones and cancer a nationwide cohort study in Denmark. *J Natl Cancer Inst*; **93** (3): 203 EOF 7 EOF .
- K. Paksy, G. Thuroczy, Z. Forgacs, P. Lazar, I. Gaati, 2000 Influence of sinusoidal 50 -Hz magnetic field on cultured human ovarian granulosa cells. *Electromagnet Biology and Medicine* 19(1), 95-99.
- K. Takahashi, I. Kaneko, M. Date, E. Fukada, 1986 Effect of pulsing electromagnetic fields on DNA syntesis in mammalian cells in culture. *Cellular and Molecular Life Sciences* **42** (2), 185-186
- Kula, A. Sobczak, R. Kuska, 2000 Effects of static and ELF magnetic fields on free-radical processes in rat liver and kidney. *Electromagnetic Biology and Medicine* **19** (1), 99-105.
- L. Kheifets, A. Ahlbom, C. M. Crespi, *et al.* 2010 Pooled analysis of recent studies on magnetic fields and childhood leukemia. *British Journal of Cancer*. 03 1128 1135
- M. Cifra, J. Z. Fields, A. Farhadi, 2010 Electromagnetic cellular interactions. *Progress In Biophysics and Molecular Biology*. 1 24
- M. Röösli, Patrizia. Frei, E. Mohler, K. Hug, 2010 Systematic review on the health effects of exposure to radiofrequency electromagnetic fields from mobile phone base stations. Bull World health Organ: 88 887 896 .
- Marino, R. Becker, 1977 /9 Biological effects of extremely low frequency electric and magnetic fields: a review. *Physiological Chemistry and Physics (*2), 131.
- Murray MT . Osteoarthritis. In JE Pizzorno, MT Murray, eds., Textbook of Natural Medicine, 4th ed., pp. 1651-1661.2013
- N. Wertheimer, E. Leeper, 1979 Electrical wiring configurations and childhood cancer. *Am J Epidemiol*. 109 3 273 84 .
- P. Elliott, M. B. Toledano, J. Bennett, L. Beale, K. de Hoogh, N. Best, D. J. Brigggs, 2010 Mobile phone base stations and early childhood cancers: case-control study. *BMJ*. 22;340.
- P. Michelozzi, A. Capon, U. Kirchmayer, *et al.* 2002 Adult and Parkash. Sharma Ved, R. Kumar Neelima, 2010 Changes in honeybee behaviour and Biology under the influence of cellphone radiations. *Current Science*, 98 10
- R. Cooke, S. Laing, A. J. Swerdlow, 2010 A case- control study of risk of leukaemia in relation to mobile phone use. *Br. J. Cancer*. ;103 11 1729 35 .
- R. Goodman, A. Henderson, 1988 Exposure of salivary gland cells to low-frequency electromagnetic fields alters polypeptide synhtesis. Proceedings of the National Academy of Sciences of the United States of America **85** (11), 3928.
- R. Goodman, C. Basett, A. Henderson, 1983 Pulsing electromagnetic fields induce cellular transcription. *Science 220*(4603), 1283 EOF 1285 EOF .
- R. R. Shivers, J. A. Wijsman, 1998 Blood-brain barrier permeability during hyperthermia. *Prog. Brain Res.* **115** 413 424 .
- R. W. Morgan, MA Kelsh, K. Zhao, K. A. Exuzides, S. Heringer, W. Negrete, 2000 Radiofrequency exposure and mortality from cancer of the brain and lymphatic/hematopoietic systems. *Epidemiology;* **11** (2): 118 EOF 127.
- S. Coskun, B. Balabanli, A. Canseven, N. Seyhan, 2009 Effects of continous and intermittent magnetic fields on oxidative parameters. ?n vivo. *Neurochemical Research* **34.** 238 243
- S. M. Mortazavi, E. Daiee, A. Yazdi, *et al.* 2008 Mercury release from dental amalgam restorations after magnetic resonance imaging and following mobile phone use. *Pak. J Biol Sci.* **11** 8 1142 6 .
- T. Hawkins, R. D. Egleton, 2008 Pathophysiology of the blood-brain barrier: animal models and methods. *Curr Top. Dev. Biol.* **80** 277 309 .
- T. Hawkins, T. P. Davis, 2005 The blood-brain barrier / neurovasculer unit in health and disease. *Pharmacol. Rev*. **57** 173 185 .
- V. G. Khurana, C. Teo, M. Kundi, L. Hardell, M. Carlberg, 2009 Sep Cell phones and brain tumors. *Surg Neurol.,* **72** 3 205 14.
- Weintraub M, *et al.* (2008). Complementary and Alternative Medicine for Pain Management. New York: Springer.
- Zrimec, I. Jerman, G. Lahajnar, 2002 Alternating electric fields stimulate ATP synthesis in Esherichia Coli. *Cellular and Molecular Biology Letters* **7**(1), 172-175.

Reiki and Pranic Healing In Health and Disease

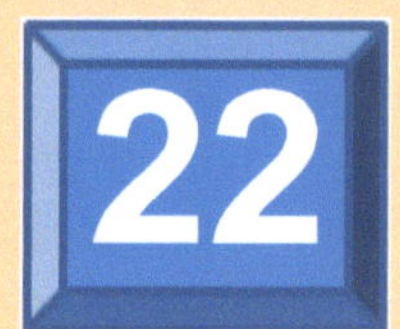

Reiki is a spiritual healing art with its roots in Japanese origin. The word Reiki comes from the Japanese word (Rei) which means "Universal Life" and (Ki) which means "Energy".

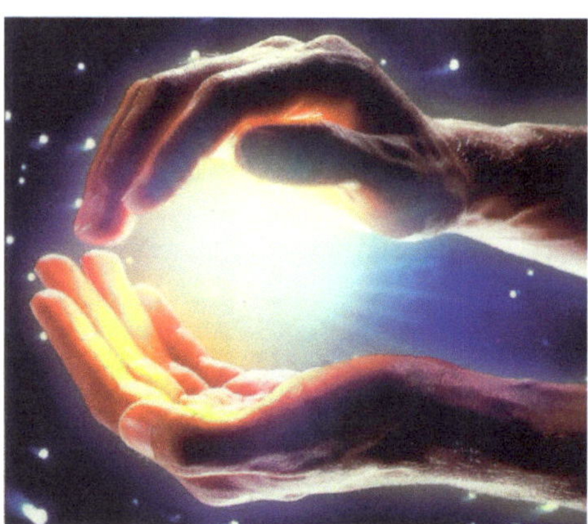

Fig.22.1: *Subtle vibrational field is set to the surroundings which penetrate the body during Reiki practice*

What is Reiki: "Universal Life Force Energy" – is a means of providing access to the unlimited light filled energy inside of us and in our Universe. Reiki is a Japanese technique for stress reduction and relaxation that also promotes healing. It is administered by "laying on of hands" on a fully clothed body and is based on the idea that an unseen "life force energy" flows through us and is what causes u s to be alive. If one's "life force energy" is low, then we are more likely to get sick or feel stress, and if it is high, we are more capable of being happy and healthy. I believe it is important to live and act in a way that promotes harmony with others (Fig.22.1)

A Reiki treatment feels like a wonderful glowing radiance that flows through and around you. Reiki treats the whole person including body, emotions, mind and spirit creating many beneficial effects that include relaxation and feelings of peace, security and well-being. The" Universal Life Force Energy" flows through the practitioner's hands and into the body of the recipient, fostering healing on the physical, mental, emotional and spiritual levels. There is no massage manipulation, unless you choose to combine with a massage

Additional advantages of Reiki:

- Works on all levels including the physical, mental, emotional and spiritual
- Promotes specific healing
- Relieves and reduces pain
- Reduces stress and increases relaxation
- Increases energy and vitality
- Creates inner harmony and awareness
- Works on mental and emotional disorders
- Promotes calmness and serenity, feelings of well-being
- Loosens blocked energy
- Pets, plants, and children love it
- Does not require a belief or faith
- Works on relationships
- Brings joy and centering to user as well as recipient

Reiki is a simple, natural and safe method of spiritual healing and self-improvement that everyone can use. It has been effective in helping virtually every known illness and malady and always creates a beneficial effect. It also works in conjunction with all other medical or therapeutic techniques to relieve side effects and promote recovery. While Reiki is spiritual in nature, it is not a religion. In fact, Reiki is not dependent on belief at all and will work whether you believe in it or not. Because Reiki comes from God, many people find that using Reiki puts them more in touch with the experience of their religion rather than having only an intellectual concept of it. The purpose is to help people realize that healing the spirit by consciously deciding to improve oneself is a necessary part of the Reiki healing experience. In order for the Reiki healing energies to have lasting results, the client must accept responsibility for her or his healing and take an active part in it. Guidelines for living a gracious life and virtues worthy of practice for their inherent value

The evidence: There is something to be said for the healing touch when it comes to bringing about a state of calm. One study checked the effect of Reiki on people hospitalized with heart disease. It showed that Reiki was effective in bringing about an increase in:

- Happiness
- Relaxation
- Feeling of calm

Reiki is a spiritual, vibrational healing practice used to promote balance throughout the human system. Reiki does not involve physical manipulation or the ingestion or application of any substances, but works with the subtle vibrational field thought to surround and penetrate the body. (Reiki is commonly translated from the Japanese as universal life energy.)

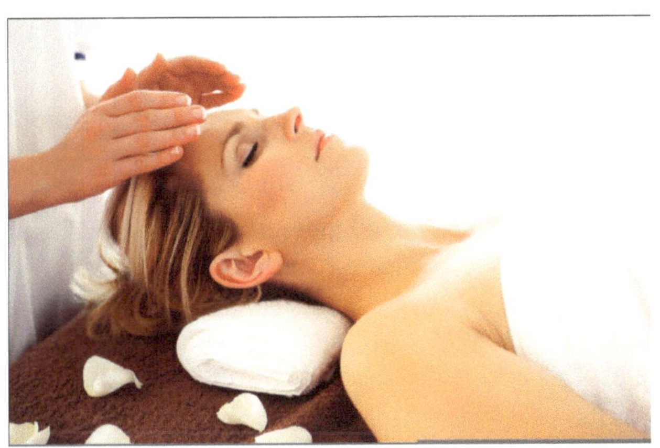

Fig. 22.2: *A young lady is feeling sense of calmness after healing touch of Reiki*

Reiki treatment is usually facilitated by light, non-manipulative touch to a clothed recipient. You can get Reiki treatments from a either a professional or a friend who has been trained, or you can learn to give yourself Reiki-treatment as a daily wellness practice.

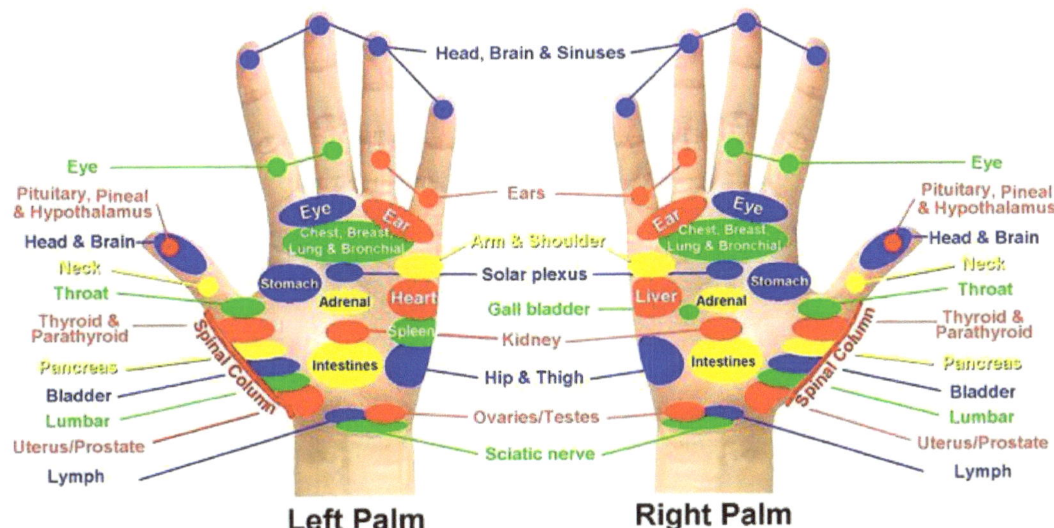

Fig. 22.3: *Illistrations of palms of both hands depicting anatomical Location of various organs of the body which transmit energy to the receipient during Reiki session*

People receiving Reiki often express a sense of connection to their own innatespirituality, or inner source of meaning. There is, however, no religious belief system attached to Reiki. Reiki was originally developed as a practice for self-care, and students were encouraged to give treatment to and receive treatment from others. The practice can be easily learned by anyone who is interested, regardless of age (children through seniors) or condition of health.

Some people practice or receive Reiki to strengthen their wellness; others use it to help cope with symptoms, such as pain or fatigue, or to support their medical care, even in the case of chronic illness or at the end-of-life. According to a national survey published in 2007, 1.2 million adults and 161,000 children received one or more sessions of an energy therapy such as Reiki in the previous year.

Historical Aspects of Reiki

Reiki, as it is practiced in the U.S. today, dates back to the teachings of Mikao Usui in Japan in the early 1920's. Usui was a lifelong spiritual aspirant, a lay monk with a wife and two children. In Usui's time, various lineages of Buddhist, Taoist, and Shinto practices coexisted as the dominant themes in Japanese spirituality and culture.

Usui's intense spiritual practices culminated in a profound revelation that led to the practice now commonly called Reiki. This realization most likely occurred in 1922.

Usui traveled widely in Japan during the last four years of his life, offering his spiritual teachings to more than 2,000 beginning students, but training only 16 as Reiki masters. One of his master students, Chujiro Hayashi, was a retired naval officer. Hayashi worked with Usui to excerpt the healing practices from Usui's larger body of teachings so that they could be more widely disseminated. With Usui's blessings, Hayashi opened a Reiki clinic in Tokyo where 16 practitioners gave treatment in pairs. Hawayo Takata, a first generation Japanese-American, came to Hayashi's clinic for relief from a number of medical conditions, including asthma. Months of treatment restored Takata's health, and she became a devoted student. With Hayashi's active guidance and support, Takata brought Reiki to Hawaii in 1937 and eventually to the US mainland. Takata practiced and taught Reiki for 40 years before she began training Reiki masters (practitioners empowered to teach others). Since Takata's death in December 1980, her 22 Reiki masters have spread her teachings. Reiki has become very popular and is now practiced around the world, although not usually in the traditional form Takata taught.

Learnings in Using Reiki Hand Positions (Fig.22.3)

Before you switch to intuitive work, the hand positions comes in handy. As well as the knowledge of the treatment tricks and tips :). As you approach the Reiki treatment, you should keep in mind the following:

- Remember that when you send Reiki, you're a channel. Clear your mind, relax, and if you wish, focus on your Hara – that is, your abdomen. As a channel, Reiki flows through you. When you place your hands on the body, whether it's your body or the body of another person, it's not like you're sending anything – the body itself feels Reiki and draws it through your hands in such quantity that is required by this particular area of the body.
- Usually,for Reiki beginners to spend from 3 upto 5 minutes "giving" Reiki to the given hand position, and then switch the position to another one. Of course, physical touch is not mandatory. If you wish or if the other person wishes, you may simple "hover" your hands an inch or so above the body. Reiki will flow nevertheless.
- When you channel Reiki, your hands can be placed in two separate parts of the body, yet your fingers should stick together). When you wish to switch the hand position, just do so, move your hands to another part of the body.
- Reiki will flow whenever your focused or distracted. It is possible to talk during Reiki treatment and get distracted. Actually, it's pretty useful. For example, when something distract you, it won't really affect the flow of Reiki. Or when the person you're sending Reiki to wishes to chat, you can socialize with this person). But, on the other hand, Reiki flows better through a clear and calm mind. You shouldn't force yourself to focus on Reiki, but at the same time you shouldn't get distracted too much. Practice Reiki Gassho meditation and focus on the Hara region – this will help you achieve a calm and relaxed mind during Reiki treatments.Don't get tense. Make sure both your mind and muscles are relaxed. And make sure your body position is comfortable

Reiki Healing Massage (Fig. 22.4)

Reiki massage therapy promotes mental calm, interior, peace and general wellbeing by transferring "the universal energy" to your own "vital force."

What is Reiki massage therapy

Reiki healing is an alternative medicine practice that transfers universal energy through the palms of aReiki practitioner and to your body to promote healing and balance.

During your Reiki treatment you will lie on a massage table, and our Reiki practitioner will place his or her hands on you in various positions. The practitioner will focus on a position for several minutes before moving on to another position. These hand positions will focus on the head, the torso, the knees and feet. Overall, the Reiki massage therapy experience is designed help your body heal itself, focusing on not only on the physical but also mental, emotional and energy healing as well. It's not uncommon to feel warmth or a tingling in your body during a treatment. After a treatment session you can expect to be in a deep state of relaxation and have a general feeling of wellbeing and contentedness.

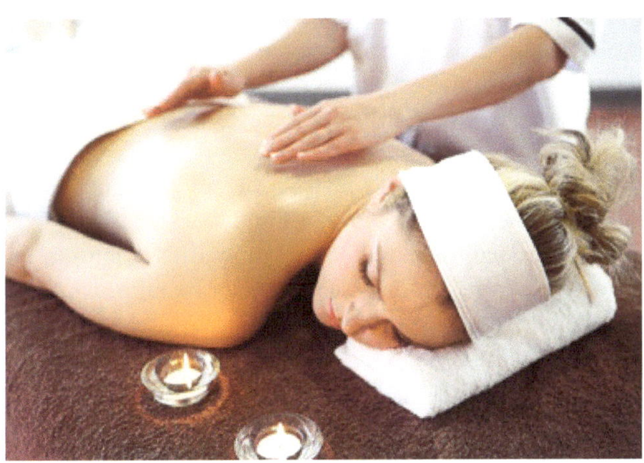

Fig. 22.4: *Lady is undergoing Reiki massage for getting feeling of wellbeing.*

Reiki as a complementary and alternative medical practice

Reiki as a complementary and alternative medicine practice that uses putative (yet to be measured) energy fields, or biofields, to affect health. Energy biofield therapies "generally reflect the concept that human beings are infused with subtle forms of energy," which are believed to surround and interpenetrate human form. Energy therapies, such as therapeutic touch and healing touch, are believed to balance these subtle energy fields.

Some Reiki practitioners find that Reiki is different from other energy therapies and is actually closer to meditation. For example, while most energy therapies use techniques to assess the recipient's biofield and make specific corrections, Reiki practitioners do not diagnose and do not deliberately reorganize the biofield.

Reiki practice is extremely passive. The Reiki practitioner's hands are still for most of the treatment, moving only to change hand placements. The Reiki practitioner is neutral, making no attempt to fix the recipient or to change the biofield. Additionally, the practitioner does not in any way control Reiki energy; she/he merely rests her hands lightly on the body (or just above the body if needed, for example, in the presence of an open wound or burn).

Reiki energy in the practitioner's hands arises spontaneously in response to the individual recipient's need for balance at that particular time. In this way, each Reiki treatment is automatically customized to the immediate need of that particular recipient, even though the practitioner may use the same sequence of hand placements for each treatment. Reiki is optimally given in a full treatment format but can also be administered in abbreviated treatments to a specific area or areas of the body. In urgent situations, even moments of Reiki touch can be soothing.

The Health Benefits of Reiki Healing

One of the greatest Reiki healing health benefits is stress reduction and relaxation, which triggers the bodies natural healing abilities, and improves and maintains health. Reiki healing is a natural therapy that gently balances life energies and brings health and well being to the recipient.

Reiki healing practice would like to support the individual under the following circumstances such as :-

- When you have a medical condition and want to feel better while supporting your health care
- When you are healthy but not sleeping well, may be adding unwanted pounds
- When You would like to feel more engaged, more in control of your life and your health
- When you feel sometimes isolated, hopeless to address the challenges of your life
- When you want to develop your inner spiritual connection, on your own terms

How Does Reiki practice help.

Because Reiki practice is balancing at every level, it can help anyone who receives a treatment or learns self practice. If you are tired, you'll feel refreshed. If you are anxious, you'll feel serene. If you are distressed, you'll feel comforted. Instead of feeling overwhelmed, you'll discover a renewed clarity and purpose. And these subjective changes come with physical changes associated with deep relaxation, such as a slower heart rate and easier breathing.

The first session usually brings improvement, and the benefits grow with repeated sessions. In emergencies or during intensive care, patients often show benefit within a few minutes.

Reiki supports your health care.

Reiki practice is safe, and cannot interfere with any medical care you are receiving. during surgery, and to people in the infusion suite as they receive chemotherapy.

Many of patients who adopt Reiki treatment are happy and healthy, and smart. Others want to develop themselves spiritually and discover greater meaning in life. And of course many have sought Reiki treatment or training realizing that balancing their systems can help them to cope better with a wide range of health conditions, including:

- Cancer
- Heart disease
- Anxiety
- Depression
- Chronic pain

- Infertility
- Neurodegenerative disorders
- ADD/ADHD
- Autism/developmental delays
- HIV/AIDS
- Crohn's Disease
- Irritable Bowel Syndrome
- Traumatic brain injury
- Emotional illness, including mild psychosis
- Fatigue syndromes
- End-of-life care and bereavement

The following are commonly reported benefits of Reiki practice. Although at this time, the evidence for most of these benefits is anecdotal, there are research data showing Reiki treatment can be effective for:

- Relaxation
- Pain management
- Reduced anxiety
- Reduced depression
- Improved sleep
- Improved digestion
- Enhanced well-being
- Stronger self-esteem
- Support for substance abuse recovery
- Accelerated surgical recovery
- Reduced side effects from radiation, chemotherapy and Other medications
- Greater self awareness
- Greater ease and satisfaction in relationship
- Heightened intuition

When you receive Reiki healing, you'll lie fully clothed on a treatment table while the Reiki practitioner places hands lightly on or just above your head and torso.

Pranic Healing

"A time will come when science will make tremendous advances, not because of better instruments for discovering things, but because a few people will have at their command great spiritual powers, which at the present are seldom used. Within a few centuries, the art of spiritual healing will be increasingly developed and universally used."

Astronomer, Man, Mind, and the Universe. -Gustaf Stromberg, Mt. Wilson

'Prana' is the Sanskrit word for life force. It is called 'chi' in China and 'ki' in Japan.

Pranic Healing is a revolutionary and comprehensive system of natural healing techniques that uses prana to treat illness. It is a synthesis of ancient, esoteric healing methods that have been rediscovered, researched and tested over decades with proven success by the founder of Modern Pranic Healing, Grand Master Choa Kok Sui. Pranic Healing has been described as a simple and yet very powerful technology that can be employed with immediate benefits to the patient.

Historical Background

Grand Master Choa Kok Sui, modern founder of Pranic Healing®, developed Pranic Healing over a 20 year period using experimentation and evidence-based research. He formulated an easy-to-learn system which has shown to have immediate positive results contributing to better health, quality-of-life and wellbeing. There are currently over 100 Pranic Healing centers across the globe. Pranic Healing combined with medical treatments continues to help millions globally. It is not intended to replace conventional medicine, but rather to complement it.

Pranic Healing was developed by Master Choa Kok Sui and was based on his observation that vital energy does in fact exists which constantly affects the health and well-being of our body. People with less vital energy and contaminated aura tend to be weak and sick, while people with more energy and brighter aura tend to be healthier.

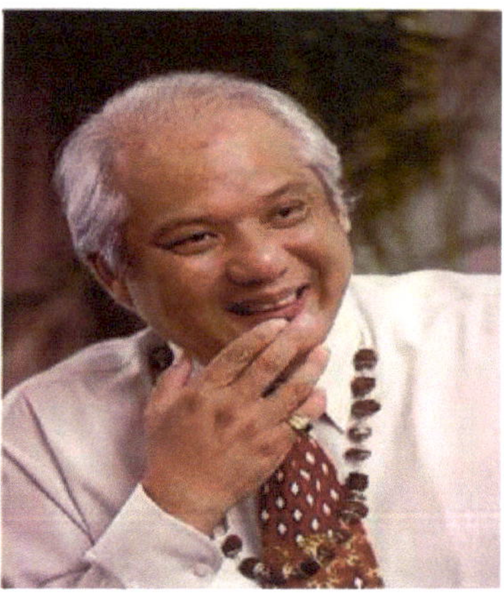

Fig. 22.5: *Photograph of Master Choa Kok Sui who is an excellent teacher of Pranic healing and Arhatic Yoga*

His clairvoyant observations and case studies on patients also showed that people with certain energetic patterns tend to have similar ailments. For example, all patients with hypertension were observed to have over-activated Meng Mein chakra as well as congested and over-activated Solar Plexus chakra.

His vast body of knowledge and study on various healing modalities, spiritual technologies and traditional sciences including Yoga, Chinese Chi Kung, Theosophy and Psychic Phenomenon helped him understand the matter deeply and design experiments to further validate his findings.

The experiments were conducted on real patients with various health issues and ailments. The results of healing techniques were investigated through clairvoyant observations and interviews.

Master Choa Kok Sui spent more than 20 years of research to conceptualize Pranic Healing as a science with principles, techniques and steps with the aim that whoever follows the procedures, comes up with the expected results.

Finally in 1987, Pranic Healing was introduced to the public through the publication of a book called "The Ancient Science and Art of Pranic Healing;" its name was later changed to "Miracles through Pranic Healing."

By Pranic Healing becoming more and more popular in various countries, more people started applying it on patients and recording their testimonials; and Master Choa Kok Sui was encouraging such experiments and observations to further validate the effectiveness of his system. Some of the testimonials were included at the last chapter of the Miracles through Pranic Healing book for the public to view.

It's simplicity, sophistication, non-sectarianism and intellectual approach in describing the ailments and providing solutions to scan and improve them, made Pranic Healing a popular method, even among medical doctors.

Pranic Healing workshops were soon conducted in universities, hospitals, churches and corporations. California Neurosurgery hospital was among the first hospitals where Pranic Healing workshops were conducted to complement medical treatments.

Departments of Pranic Healing were later put up in a number of hospitals including Apollo Speciality Hospitals in Chennai, Bangalore and Delhi, Sir Charles Gairdner Hospital Nedlands Western Australia, and Cancer Center of Ventura County Oxnard California to help the patients recover faster.

Master Choa Kok Sui introduced Pranic Healing as a complementary therapy to medical treatment, not a replacement, as it deals with energy body and the energy centers rather than physical organs. Based on the Principle of Correspondence, he observed that what affects the energy body, affects the physical body and vice versa, which is one of the reasons why it works.

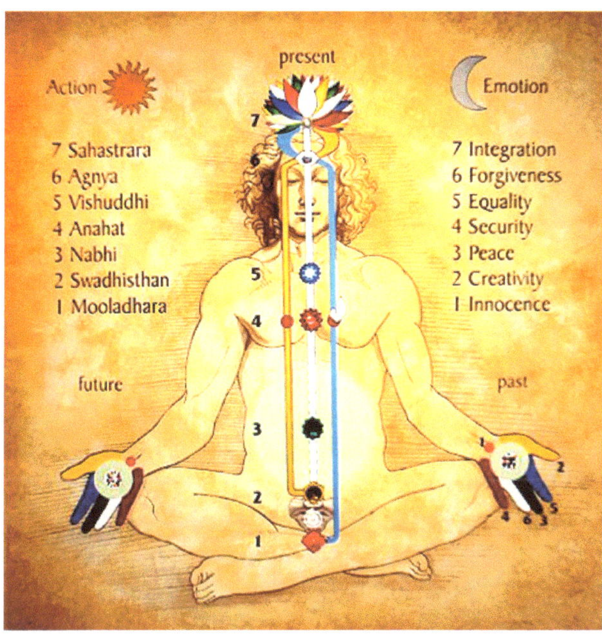

Fig. 22.6: *Illustration showing 7 majors human energy chakaras and subltebodies*

Pranic Healing is an energy "no-touch"force

Pranic Healing is an energy "no-touch" healing system based on the fundamental principle that the body has the innate ability to heal itself. Pranic Healing utilizes "life force," "energy," or prana to accelerate the body's inborn ability to heal itself. It is practiced by hundreds of thousands across the world.

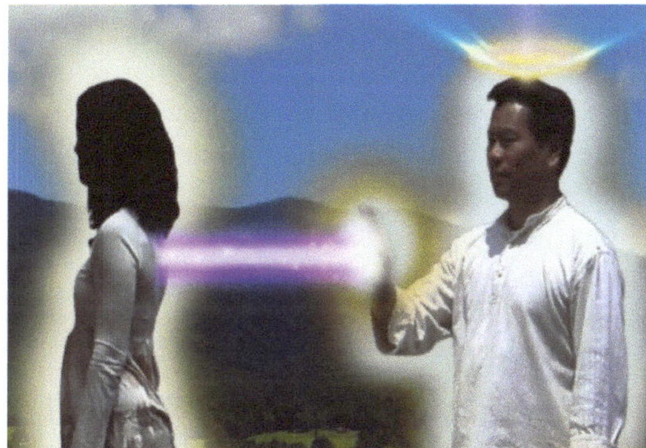

Fig. 22.7: *Demonstrates automatic transmission of pranic healing force from pranic healer specialist to his patient*

Energy can be transformed:- Science explains to us that energy can neither be created nor destroyed but can be transformed from one form to another. Think about what this could mean to you? If you can understand how to work with energy, it can help transform all the negative results in your life into positive results – sickness into well-being, lack into abundance, stress into peace of mind and failing relationships into healthy, strong bonds. So since Pranic Healing uses energy, there is a lot more to it than just the healing part. It not only makes you aware of the aura around the human body – the 'chakras' (energy centers) and their effects on our health, but also teaches us how to feel or scan the aura and determine which parts of the chakras may be affected. By learning about energy, we become more conscious about its ubiquitous presence, be it in people, buildings or even objects.

The Essence of Prana

What is the fundamental difference between a living and dead person? Both people have a body, a set of organs and billions of cells. What differentiates them is an 'unseen' force that gives one person the awareness and consciousness to experience living while causing the other person ro experience a permanent black-out. Call it Breath of Life or Vitality of the Soul, Prana is the life sustaining force found within the body of every living thing. Without Prana, we cease to exist as "living beings". Grand Master Choa Kok Sui explains : "Life Energy or Prana is all around us. It is pervasive; we are actually in an ocean of Life Energy"

Principles Behind Pranic Science:- The fundamental principles of Pranic Healing are:

Principle of Self- Recovery: The innate ability of every living being to heal itself

Principle of Life Force: Healing process can be accelerated by increasing the pranic life force of the individual

How does it work?

- Pranic Healing corrects imbalances in the body's energy field and transfers life force to the patient. This life force can also be characterized as universal energy; it is not the healer's energy. Trained Pranic Healers access and transmit universal energy to the patient using specific frequencies and techniques for specific diseases and conditions
- Pranic Healing is done without touching.
- Pranic Healing is a three step process that substantially accelerates the body's innate ability to heal at all levels: physical, emotional, mental and spiritual.

1. Checking - Scanning for energy abnormalities
2. Cleansing - Removing energy abnormalities: used to remove dirty or diseased energy in the body and to eradicate blockages in the energy channels
3. Replenishing and revitalizing with life force- Energizing: the transference of fresh 'prana' or life energy to the body and is applied once the cleansing process is completed.

To give an example, when we cut our fingers or bruise our legs, our body automatically takes the necessary steps to prevent blood loss and repair the damaged tissues. Our bodies are constantly exposed to a variety of toxins, chemicals and pollutants from the environments we live in but our 'in-built' defense system fights of all these germs and protects us. When we are healthy and happy, we feel all charged up and are full of energy. When we are sick or upset, we feel down or drained out. In other words, a healthy body has an abundance of prana while a sick or diseased body is low on prana.

The healing process of an individual is accelerated by increasing the prana life force in them which is readily available from the sun, air and earth.

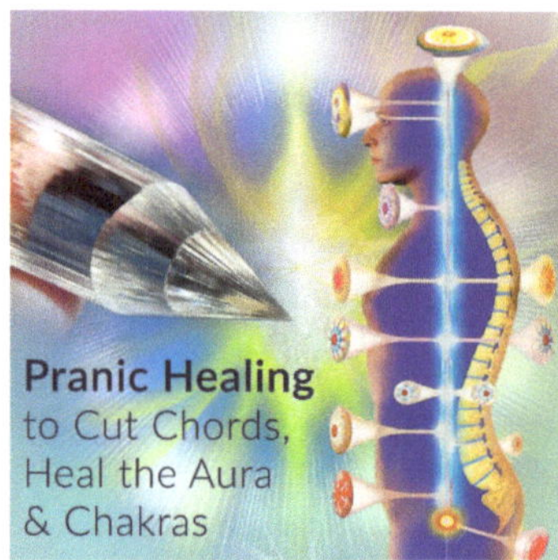

Fig. 22.8: *Cut Chords, Heal Aura-Seal Holes and Cracks, Cleanse & Energize Chakras for Well being*

Some Benefits of Pranic Healing

- In cases of fever, parents can bring down the temperature of their children in just a few hours
- Coughs and colds can usually be alleviated in a day
- Major illnesses such as eye, liver, kidney, and heart problems can be partially or substantially relieved in a few sessions
- Improved health and increased stamina
- Inner peace and happiness
- Better memory and concentration
- Rapid spiritual growth
- Reduced stress
- Better interpersonal skills
- Greater self-esteem
- Attain the ability to attract good luck and become more prosperous

What is Difference between Reiki and Pranic Healing?

Reiki and Pranic Healing are the ways of holistically treating a person or living being. The principle behind both these treatments is similar, but there is a huge difference between both these healing therapies. Undoubtedly, the main principle is same, but the way of doing the treatment is different for practitioners.

This is a quick and easy to comprehend article to understand the difference between pranic healing and Reiki. The intent of healing a person and use of hands is common in these treatment procedures, but there are still a lot of things different in both modes of healing.

Energy Flow Procedure: In Reiki treatment, the flow of energy is undirected and there is free flow of energy. There is full dedication made on the body parts where it is required the most and the main focus is on clearing the blockages in energy field. Pranic healing involves acute awareness of chakras (energy centers) in the body and there is proper focus made on the specific chakras to cleanse and stabilize them. There are specific procedures for handling different diseases or ailments and treatment is made by balancing specific chakra sets.

Side Effects: Reiki has no side effects on healer or the person taking it. Pranic healing also has no side effects, but there are very specific guidelines to be followed for the use of energy transformation and chakra healing. If healer is unsure about treating any particular chakra, they should avoid taking any chance on the client for the same to avoid any sort of serious affects on the body.

Healing Methodology: Reiki healing can be done by reaching through various levels of attunements learnt by masters or practitioners. This way, they can heal by bringing energy levels at a frequency and turning negative impact into positive energy. Pranic healing makes use of free-floating energy (prana) from different resources (air, sun and earth) and activates body chakras to carry forward the healing process. The negative or discarded energy is cleaned off by neutralizing it in mineral salt.

There are many people who know both these procedures and implement one of them on different conditions. Reiki can be used spontaneously and you will not require anything perquisites for your treatment through this mode of healing. On the other hand, pranic healing requires proper time, equipments (like salt) and methodologies to undergo a correct procedure.

Which is preferable: Pranic healing or Reiki?

It is absolutely a personal choice of practitioner and your trust on a particular healing therapy, which decides your preference. Reiki is gentle, warm and doesn't require any intensification. Pranic healing needs skills and practice; and if you require results, you have to be particular about following a right process in a correct way. In simple words, Pranic healing is a package of surgical equipments and Reiki is a multi-purpose healing tool.

Bibliography and Acknowledgement

- Abdi S, Zhou Y. Management of pain after burn injury. *Curr Opin Anaesthesiol* 2002 Oct; **15**(5):563-7.
- Astin JA, Harkness E, Ernst E. The efficacy of "distant healing": a systematic review of randomized trials. *Ann Intern Med* 6-6-2000;**132**(11):903-910.
- Brewitt B, Vittetoe T, Hartwell B. The efficacy of Reiki hands-on healing: improvements in spleen and nervous system function as quantified by electrodermal screening [abstract]. *Alternative Therapies in Health and Medicine* 1997;**3**:89.
- Crawford SE, Leaver VW, Mahoney SD. Using Reiki to decrease memory and behavior problems in mild cognitive impairment and mild Alzheimer's disease. *J Altern Complement Med* 2006 Nov;**12**(9):911-3.
- Global Pranic Healing. (n.d.). Retrieved from http://globalpranichealing.com/about/the-founder/
- Kennedy P. Working with survivors of torture in Sarajevo with Reiki. Complement Ther *Nurs. Midwifery* 2001;**7**(1):4-7.
- Krucoff MW, Crater SW, Gallup D, *et al.* Music, imagery, touch, and prayer as adjuncts to interventional cardiac care: the Monitoring and Actualisation of Noetic Trainings (MANTRA) II randomised study. *Lancet* 7-16-2005; **366**(9481):211-217.
- Mackay N, Hansen S, McFarlane O. Autonomic nervous system changes during Reiki treatment: a preliminary study. *J Altern Complement Med* 2004; **10**(6):1077-1081.
- Mansour AA, Beuche M, Laing G, *et al.* A study to test the effectiveness of placebo Reiki standardization procedures developed for a planned Reiki efficacy study. *J Altern Complement Med.* 1999; **5**(2):153-164.
- Master Choa Kok Sui. The Origin of Modern Pranic Healing and Arhatic Yoga. The Institute for Inner Studies Publishing Foundation.
- Murray, McKinney, Gorrie, Foundations of Maternal-Newborn Nursing, W.B. Saunders Company, Philadelphia
- Murray, McKinney, Gorrie, (Footnote by Wright & Higgins, 1999: Sompson, 1999), Foundations of Maternal-Newborn Nursing, W.B. Saunders Company, Philadelphia 5. Jonas, W.B., Crawford, C.C., Healing Intention and Energy Medicine, Churchill Livingstone
- Olson K, Hanson J. Using Reiki to manage pain: a preliminary report. *Cancer Prev Control* 1997; **1**(2):108-113.
- Olson K, Hanson J, Michaud M. A phase II trial of Reiki for the management of pain in advanced cancer patients. *J Pain Symptom Manage* 2003; **26**(5):990-997.
- Sui, M. C. (2004). Miracles Through Pranic Healing: Practical Manual on Energy Healing. Institute for Inner Studies Publishing Foundation.
- Sui, Choa Kok, Miracles Through Pranic Healing, 1999 2nd edition, Institute For Inner Studies Publishing, Makati City, Philippines
- Sui, Choa Kok, Practical Psychic Self Defense for Home and Office, Institute For Inner Studies Publishing, Makati City, Philippines
- U.S. Pranic Healing Center. (n.d.). Retrieved from http://pranichealing.com/master-choa-kok-sui

Management of Heart Disease with EECP as an Alternative Therapy to Coronary Bypass Surgery

Coronary artery disease is usually treated with modern techniques and is essential in reducing the risk of heart attack or stroke. The following are the different methods employed in its management

1. CAD is treated by reducing the risk factors -High blood pressure, high cholesterol, high blood sugar, smoking, etc.
2. It is treated by taking medications as directed.
3. Percutaneous coronary intervention (PCI) – Angioplasty is the widening of the blocked artery using a small balloon with the deployment of a flexible wire mesh tube (stent) which remains in place holding the artery open.
4. Coronary artery bypass surgery (CABG) open heart surgery.

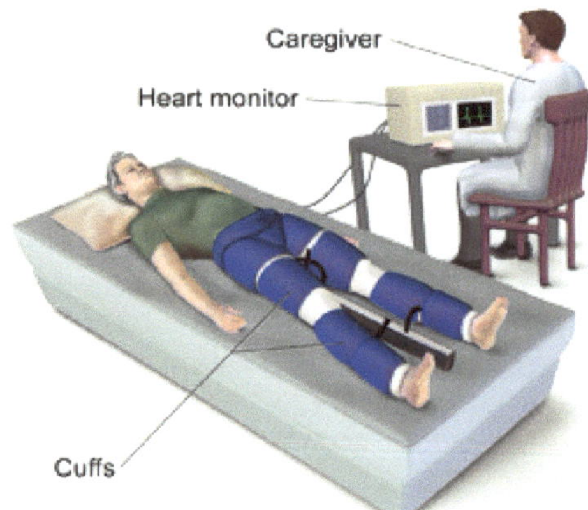

Fig 23.1 *Illustration showing cardiac external counterpulsation.*

When all other treatments have failed to relieve persistent angina (chest pain) symptoms, enhanced external counterpulsation (EECP) may be an option. EECP can help stimulate blood vessels to develop small branches, creating a natural bypass around narrowed or blockedarteries that cause the chest pain.

The EECP treatment uses a series of blood pressure cuffs on both legs to gently but firmly compress the blood vessels in the lower limbs to increase blood flow to the heart. Each wave of pressure is electronically timed to the heartbeat, so that the increased blood flow is delivered to your heart at the precise moment it is relaxing.

What is ECP?

People suffering from angina or heart failure may not do day to day work easily Such as walking, Going in market, climbing steps.For all these heart patients there is a non-invasive treatment called EECP therapy available that clinical experience has shown to be safe and to have benefit for the treatment of angina and heart failure. Around 80% of patients who completed this treatment experienced significant symptom relief that may last longer than bypass surgery or stent. The Science And Art Of Living (SAAOL) was established in 1995 and is the most comprehensive cardiac rehabilitation and reversal program in India. Today Saaol has 42 Hospital branches spread in the Asian sub continent. Aim of Saaol is to change the complete lifestyle and reduce the risk of heart disease.

How EECP Works (Fig 23.1 and 23.2)

EECP works by pumping blood from the legs upward to the heart while the heart is at rest. The mechanism improves circulation throughout the body, promotes angiogenesis, and has long-term, positive effects

- You lie on a comfortable EECP bed.
- You are hooked to a heart monitor.
- Three large blood pressure like cuffs wrap around the calves, thighs, buttocks.
- A continuous electrocardiogram (ECG) is used to set

the timing.

- The cuffs inflate while the heart is at rest, when it normally gets its supply of blood and oxygen.
- The cuffs deflate at the end of that rest period just before the next heart beat.
- The special sensor applied to your finger checks the oxygen level in your blood and monitors the pressure waves created by the cuff inflations and deflations.

What is the equipment of EECP consisting of?

The EECP equipment consists of:

- Air compressor
- A computer console
- A treatment table
- A set of 3 pneumatic cuffs applied to each lower extremity.

How much pressure is applied during inflation?

The pressure applied to the pneumatic cuffs during sequential inflation -from calves to thighs to buttocks is 4 – 6 pounds per square inch (psi) which is the equivalent to 206 to 360 mmHg.

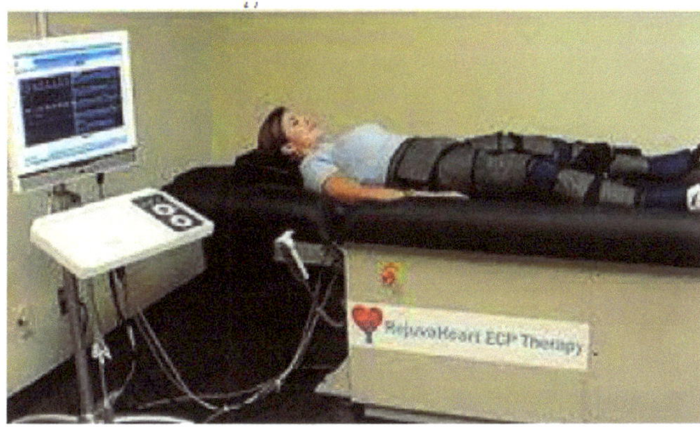

Fig 23. 2:*Patient with chronic angina pectoris has been connected with EECP equipment ready to perform the application. Patient receives treatment of one hour daily for 35 days course.*

Mechanism of EECP

Treats patients in 7 different stages. Once a 35 hours Treatment starts:

- Coronory artery starts filling increases in first 3 to 4 hours.
- Coronary Resistance starts decreases in first 6 to 7 hours treatment
- Coronary Flow Velocity increases and patient start feeling it in first 10 to 12 hours.
- Myocardial perfusion increases in first 15 to 18 hours
- Dormant Collateral opens in first 22 to 25 hours and Patient can feels changes in heart.
- NeoVascularisation of Angio-Genesis happen in first 25 to 28 hours treatment.
- Mayocardial Efficienct expands at the end of 35 hours.
- When the heart pumps again, pressure is released instantaneously. This lowers resistance in the blood vessels in the legs so that blood may be pumped more easily from your heart.
- EECP may encourage some small blood vessels in the heart to open. These collateral blood vessels may eventually become "natural bypass" vessels to provide blood flow to heart muscle. This contributes to the relief of chest pain. (Fig. 23.6)

What Happens During EECP Treatment?

EECP is a non-invasive, outpatient therapy.

During treatment:

- Patients lie down on a padded table in a treatment room.
- Three electrodes are applied to the skin of the chest and connected to an electrocardiograph (ECG). The ECG will display the heart›s rhythm during treatment. Blood pressure is also monitored.
- A set of cuffs is wrapped around the calves, thighs, and buttocks. These cuffs attach to air hoses that connect to valves that inflate and deflate the cuffs. Patients experience a sensation of a strong "hug" moving upward from calves to thighs to buttocks during inflation followed by the rapid release of pressure on deflation. Inflation and deflation are electronically synchronized with the heartbeat and blood pressure

How often are EECP Treatments?

Patients who are accepted for EECP treatment must undergo 35 hours of therapy. Treatment is administered 1-2 hours a day, five days a week, for 7 weeks.

Who is a candidate for EECP?

You may be a candidate for EECP if you:

- Have chronic stable angina
- Are not receiving adequate relief by taking nitrates, calcium channel blockers, and beta-blockers
- Do not qualify as a candidate for invasive procedures (bypass surgery, angioplasty, or stenting)

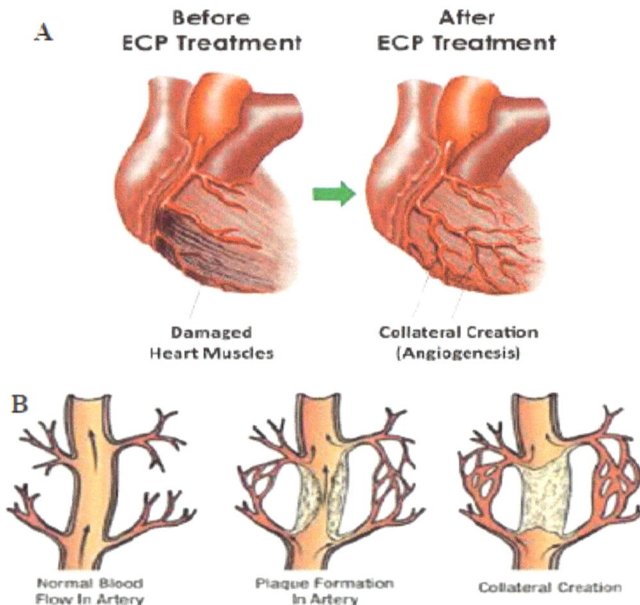

Fig. 23.3: *(A)Showing damaged heart muscle due to heart attack (left)and multiple natural bypass after EECP(Right) (B) Showing normal blood supply of the heart (left) ,plaque formation (middle)and development of natural collateral circulation after EECP (right)*

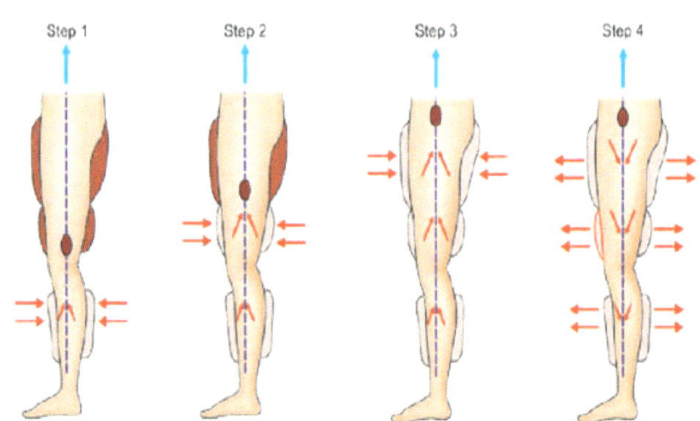

Fig 23.4: *Technique of EECP Three pairs of pneumatic cuffs are applied to the calves, lower thighs, and upper thighs. The cuffs are inflated sequentially during diastole, distal to proximal. The compression of the lower-extremity vascular bed increases diastolic pressure and flow and increases venous return. The pressure is then released at the onset of systole. Inflation and deflation are timed according to the R-wave on the patient's cardiac monitor. The pressures applied and the inflation–deflation timing can be altered by using the pressure waveforms and electrocardiogram on the enhanced external counterpulsation (EECP) therapy monitor.*

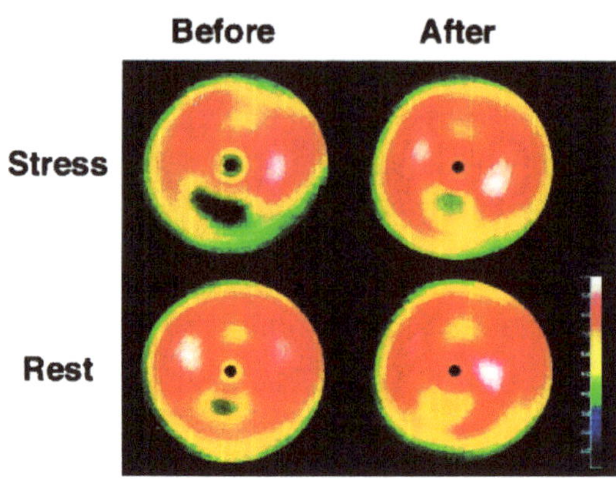

Fig.23.5: *Representative left ventricular polar maps of thallium-201 uptake from a female patient before and after enhanced external counterpulsation treatment. Note that the exercise-induced perfusion defect in an inferior lesion before enhanced external counterpulsation was not apparent after treatment, indicating improved myocardial perfusion.*

Published studies conducted at numerous medical centers have demonstrated benefits for most patients undergoing EECP, including:

- Less need for anti-anginal medication
- Decrease in symptoms of angina
- Increased ability to do activities without onset of symptoms
- Ability to return to enjoyable activities

it is often referred to as the natural Bypass. Unlike bypass surgery, balloon angioplasty, and stenting procedures, EECP is non-invasive, carries no risk, is comfortable, and is administered in outpatient sessions. Patients often watch television during the treatment. Others bring compact disks or cassette players to listen to music. The entire process from the patient's arrival to departure takes between one and one-half to two hours.

Clinical studies and data from the International ECP:

ECP has been around since the 1960's. It was invented at Harvard University and perfected over the years. The Food & Drug Administration (FDA-USA) in the 1970s, also by NHS (England), CE (Europe), Australia, China, has approved EEP for treatment for cardiovascular disease: In 1970, ECP was first approved for Cardiogenic shock (the heart cannot pump blood to the body) and acute myocardial infarction (heart attack). In 1995, ECP was given approval for coronary artery disease (blockages of the arteries), and angina pectoris (chest pain). In June 2002, ECPwas approved for treatment of congestive heart failure (the heart fails to pump enough blood to the organs).

Research

Patient Registry (IEPR) coordinated by the Epidemiology Data Centre at the University of Pittsburgh continues to demonstrate that 84% of patients realise therapeutic benefit immediately upon completion of a course of ECP therapy. At patient follow-up, therapeutic benefit is enhanced at six months and sustained at 24 months. Over the years ECP has undergone rigorous clinical trials at leading Universities around the world. It has been the subject of dozens of scientific studies published in leading medical journals

Expert Opinions

- ECP treatment is a safe, cost-effective, non-invasive method of restoring myocardial perfusion and reducing symptoms of angina. ECP treatment is the perfect disease management tool for chronic coronary artery disease. (Dr.John E. Strobeck, Interventional Cardiologist, Co-founder of the Heart Failure Society of America Medical Director the Heart & Lung Center Hawthorne, NJ)
- ECP treatment helps patients with Ischemic Heart Disease by recruitment of collaterals and increase of blood flow to ischemic regions. It also improves endothelial functions and reduces arterial stiffness. All the above mechanism of action seems to benefit patients of Chronic Stable angina and heart failure (Dr Ashok H Punjabi. Director, Krishna Cardiac Care Centre, Mumbai and honorary cardiologist at the Lilavati Hospital)

EECP has numerous distinct advantages over surgery

1. Outpatient
2. Lowr Risk
3. No additional Medication required
4. No recuperation time required
5. No side effectn

What does EECP stand for?

The acronym EECP stands for Enhanced External Counterpulsation.

What is EECP Therapy?

EECP is a non-invasive, outpatient treatment for heart disease that is used to relieve or eliminate angina. During the treatment, blood pressure cuffs are wrapped around your legs, and squeeze and release in sync with your heartbeat, promoting blood flow throughout your body and particularly to your heart. In the process, EECP develops new pathways around blocked arteries in the heart by expanding networks of tiny blood vessels ("collaterals") that help increase and normalize blood flow to the heart muscle. For this reason, it is often called the natural bypass.

What are the advantages of EECP?

Unlike bypass surgery, balloon angioplasty, and stenting procedures, EECP is non-invasive, carries no risk, is comfortable and is administered in outpatient sessions.

Are there any risks or side effects of EECP?

EECP is safe. Occasionally, some patients experience mild skin irritation under the areas of the blood pressure cuffs. Experienced EECP therapists address this irritation by using extra padding where needed to make the patient comfortable. Some patients experience a bit more fatigue at the beginning of their course of treatment, but it usually subsides after the first few sessions. In fact, patients typically feel energized by EECP.

How long does EECP take?

The standard course of treatment is one hour per day, five days per week, for seven weeks (a total of 35 one-hour sessions). Some patients have two treatments in one day in order to complete the program more quickly. Some patients extend the program beyond 35 treatments, depending on their particular medical situation and goals.

When can I expect to start feeling better from EECP?

Most patients begin to experience beneficial results from EECP between their 15th and 25th day of treatment. These benefits include increased stamina, improved sleeping patterns, decreased angina, and less reliance on nitroglycerin and other medications. There is variation, certainly, and some patients start to feel better as soon as in their first week of treatment

What happens if I miss a treatment?

You are encouraged to come for your EECP treatment every day. However, missing a day will not have a negative effect on your overall results. When you come back, you will simply pick up where you left off, and the missed treatment will be added to the end of your program until you have a total of 35 sessions. Just like exercise, the more consistent you are with your EECP schedule, the better your results will be.

Do the benefits of EECP last?:

Yes. In patients followed for three to five years after treatment, the benefits of EECP, including less angina, less nitroglycerin usage, and improved blood flow patterns documented on stress tests, had lasted.

What does EECP feel like?

EECP feels like a deep muscle massage to your legs. During the treatment, you do not feel anything in the chest or heart. You only feel the cuffs that are wrapped around your legs squeezing in time to your own heartbeat. Our patients have affectionately described this sensation as "gentle hugs." Most of our patients relax, listen to music, or read during their treatments. Some even sleep!

How does EECP compare to angioplasty or bypass surgery?

The five-year outcomes for EECP patients are virtually the same as for angioplasty and bypass surgery patients.

Is EECP FDA-approved? What kind of research has been done on it?

EECP was approved by the FDA in 1995 as a treatment for coronary artery disease and angina, cardiogenic shock and for use during a heart attack. In 2002, the FDA approved EECP as a treatment for congestive heart failure. It has undergone rigorous clinical trials at leading universities and EECP has been the subject of more than 100 scientific studies published in leading medical journals throughout the world.

I have a pacemaker, is that a problem with EECP?

No. Pacemakers and internal defibrillators do not interfere in any way with EECP.

I am on Blood Thinning medicines. Is that a problem with EECP?

No. Patients on Coumadin / Warfarin / Acitrom are able to undergo EECP treatments safely.

I have congestive heart failure (CHF). Is that a problem with EECP?

No. In fact, in July 2002 the FDA approved EECP as a treatment for congestive heart failure (CHF). After completing a course of EECP treatment, patients with CHF typically have less swelling in their legs, less shortness of breath, less fatigue and often require less diuretic medication.

Have already had bypass surgery / angioplasty / stents. Can I still have EECP?

Yes! Most of our patients have already had one (or more) of these procedures. They come for EECP treatment because they still have angina.

Is there an age limit for EECP?

No. We have successfully treated patients as young as 36 and as old as 97 without any difficulties. Many of our patients are in their 70's and 80's and complete the entire EECP program with excellent results.

Are there any patients who are not able to have EECP?

There are very few patients who are unable to have EECP. Those who should not be treated include pregnant women, individuals with a severe leakage in their aortic valve requiring surgical repair and patients with an active blood clot in their leg.

Can EECP dislodge plaque and cause a stroke or heart attack?

No. Our bodies obey the laws of physics, and one principle law is that fluid will follow the path of least resistance. Atherosclerotic plaques are calcified and hard and they create an obstruction that diverts the blood through alternate routes. During EECP, when your blood is flowing to your heart, it will naturally bypass arteries with plaque and enter healthy, non-diseased blood vessels to go around the blockages. Going around the blockages is a longer trip, but it is a much easier one. In time, these new pathways are reinforced and become lasting routes for blood to reach your heart beyond the blockages. Every EECP patient has had multiple, serious blockages. No one has ever had a heart attack or a stroke as a result of the treatment.

I had blood clot in my leg three years ago. Can I have EECP?

Yes. Having a history of a blood clot (deep venous thrombosis or DVT) in your leg does not preclude you from having EECP. It is recommended that you have a Doppler ultrasound of your leg to confirm the blood clot has resolved before beginning the EECP program.

Does EECP aggravate high blood pressure (hypertension)

No. If you have hypertension that is properly managed, you may undergo EECP without difficulty. Oftentimes, patients with hypertension find that their blood pressure improves as they proceed with EECP. If your hypertension is uncontrolled, you must seek medical care to get your blood pressure under control with proper medications before proceeding with EECP.

I have varicose veins. May I still have EECP?

Yes. Varicose veins are typically a cosmetic issue, not a medical one. As such, they do not preclude individuals from receiving EECP. We often use extra padding in patients with varicose veins to ensure maximum comfort.

I have atrial fibrillation and an irregular heartbeat. May I still have EECP?

Yes. An irregular heartbeat, including one caused by atrial fibrillation, will not interfere with EECP if the heart rate is controlled and no faster than 100 beats per minute.

I have bad circulation in my legs (peripheral vascular disease or PVD). May I still have EECP?

Yes, and you should! EECP improves blood flow throughout the entire body, including your legs. If you have poor leg circulation, you might need more than 35 treatments. My patients typically require at least 50 treatments to get the full benefit of the program. In addition to improved stamina, less angina, and less nitroglycerin use, patients with PVD have a marked improvement in their leg circulation in response to EECP

What happens if my angina returns months or years after I finish my EECP treatment course? Can I come back for more?

Yes. EECP is not a once-in-a-lifetime treatment. Heart disease is a chronic illness and symptoms may return at some point in the future. The door is always open for you to return for additional courses of EECP as needed.

What are the advantages of EECP Therapy?

EECP Therapy is not invasive, does not require a hospital stay, has no recovery period, and allows you to return to your routine each day after receiving treatment.

Is EECP Therapy a Safe Option for My Patients?

Yes, it's completely non-invasive, thereby reducing the risk of complications associated with surgery. Complications as a result of treatment are typically minor and rare when compared to other treatments. Most people tolerate EECP Therapy with no major discomfort, side effects or complications. Typical side effects include fatigue or muscle aches. A small number of people develop pressure sores, skin irritation or bruising from the cuff inflation.

What are the benefits of EECP Therapy?

Most patients experience positive results, such as the following:

Having no angina or angina that is less frequent and less intense. Having more energy Being able to take part in more activities of daily living with little or no angina or heart failure symptoms Enjoying a better quality of life Having a more positive outlook

Is EECP® Therapy comfortable?

There is a feeling of pressure from the cuffs around your legs and buttocks. Once you become accustomed to this pressure, the sessions usually pass comfortably.

How will I feel after the treatment?

EECP therapy is often described as being like "passive exercise," so you may feel tired after the first few days of treatment. This is normal, especially if you haven't been exercising. Usually, once this short "training period" is over, you will begin to notice that you have more energy.

How long do the benefits of EECP Therapy last after a course of treatment?

The International EECP Patient Registry (IEPR) collects data on the safety, effectiveness, and long-term benefits of EECP therapy. The IEPR data have shown that benefits of EECP therapy can last up to three years after completing a full course (35 hours) of treatment. Other smaller studies have shown the benefits last up to five years in some patients.

When can I expect to feel improvement?

Each patient responds differently. Most patients report beginning to feel better about halfway through the seven weeks.

Can I have therapy more than once?

Yes. If your symptoms return, your doctor will decide if you need to repeat your EECP treatments.

What if I miss an appointment?

Having your EECP therapy each day of the seven-week treatment course is an important part of receiving the greatest benefit. Missed treatments are usually made up so you receive all 35 hours.

Can I exercise during the weeks I'm receiving EECP Therapy? Your doctor will discuss an exercise program, how and when you should begin, and how much you should do. Exercising can help you keep the benefits of your EECP treatments.

When can I resume sexual activity?

Like exercise, this is an important issue to discuss with your doctor.

Can everyone have EECP Therapy?

Your doctor knows your medical history and condition and will determine if you can have EECP therapy.

What are the risks of EECP Therapy?

Occasionally, patients develop mild skin irritation in the areas under the treatment cuffs or experience muscle or joint discomfort. Some patients feel tired after the first few treatments but this usually ends after the first week. Rarely, patients develop shortness of breath requiring hospitalization and treatment. Your EECP therapist is trained to make your treatments safe and to minimize risk.

Does insurance cover EECP Therapy?

Yes. Medicare covers EECP treatments for the patients who meet the Medicare criteria. Most private insurance companies have coverage policies similar to Medicare.

How can I find out if I'm a candidate for EECP Therapy?

You can start by completing our quick and easy Are You a Candidate? questionnaire. Have your physician review the completed questionnaire to help determine if EECP therapy is the right choice for you.

I have already had bypass surgery/angioplasty/stents. Can I still have EECP ?

Yes. The majority of our patients on EECP therapy have already had coronary angioplasty with stents (PCI) and/or CABG surgery. They received EECP therapy because of recurrent angina pectoris or similar symptoms despite medical therapy and/or revascularization.

How long can last the clinical effects of EECP?

The clinical benefits of EECP extend beyond the time period of any acute hemodynamic beneficial effects. For example, the patients treated with EECP in the Multicenter Study of Enhanced External Counterpulsation reported a reduction in angina episodes and decrease in nitrate use beyond the duration of therapy. It is not fully understood why after the EECP therapy is completed, the patient remains improved and the clinical benefit can last several years.

What is the mechanism of action of EECP ?

Improve endothelial function through increase vasodilatation and decrease of intimal hyperplasia.

- EECP leads to improved coronary blood flow derived from increased shear stress, which leads to increased endothelial nitric oxide release and resultant vasodilatation.
- Enhance collateral capillary development by increasing blood flow to the ischemic region of the myocardium and increase capillary density. Shear stress is a known stimulus for coronary collateral development and recruitment. Vascular endothelial growth factors (VEGF) and platelet-derived growth factors (PDGF) that are crucial in angiogenesis are up regulated by vascular shear stress.

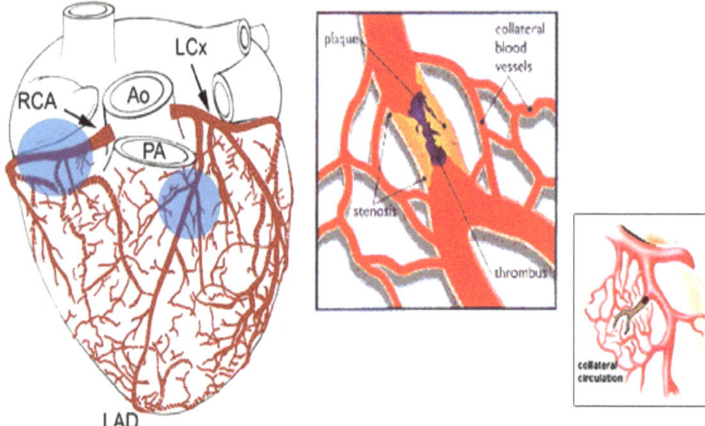

Fig. 23.6: *shows development of collateral circulation after application of EECP in patient with obstructive coronary artery disease*

- Improve neurohormonal factors by increasing nitric oxide and decreasing B-type natriuretic peptide (BNP), atrial natriuretic peptide (ANP), and angiotensin II.
- Reduce arterial stiffness which leads to a decrease in vascular resistance and blood pressure; and an increase in cardiac efficiency.

- EECP may promote improvement in exercise duration with no change in peak double product by reduction in peripheral vascular resistance.

Is there a difference between EECP and ECP?

Yes. EECP is a registered trademark of Vasomedical, Inc., the leading manufacturer of EECP equipment in the U.S. Vasomedical has a patent on the timing mechanism of the machine (when the cuffs squeeze and release in time to the patient's EKG, the most critical part of the treatment). This timing mechanism distinguishes them from those who make other external counterpulsation (ECP) equipment, and makes the EECP machine by far the most clinically effective device on the market. Every published U.S. study and most studies originating in countries around the world and published in the leading English-language medical journals have used the Vasomedical EECP equipment exclusively

Can a patient with atrial fibrillation have EECP therapy?

Uncontrolled atrial fibrillation, atrial flutter, and frequent PVCs may interfere with triggering of the EECPsystem. The average beats should be of 50-100/min. However, if the heart rate is controlled and no faster than 100 bpm, atrial fibrillation will not interfere with EECP .

Frequent and irregular heartbeats with high heart rate (HR) >100 or low HR <50 should delay EECP until rate control has been achieved.

Can a patient with varicose veins have EECP ?

Yes. Varicose veins do not preclude individuals from receiving EECP . We often use extra padding in patients with varicose veins to ensure maximum comfort. However, if the diagnosis of deep vein thrombosis is entertained, a venous US Doppler study of the lower extremities should be performed before EECP .

Can a patient with peripheral artery disease have EECP ?

Yes. EECP improves blood flow throughout the entire body, including the lower extremities. In our experience, patients with this condition –if not severe- may require more than 35 EECP sessions to obtain the full benefit of the therapy. We have documented with arterial Doppler studies the circulation of the lower extremities, before and after EECP in some patients with diabetes -with marked improvement in response to EECP .

What happens if angina returns months or years after a patient finish EECP treatment course? Can he / she come back for more?

Yes. EECP is not an once-in-a-lifetime treatment. Heart disease is a chronic inflammatory illness and symptoms may return at some point in the future. In this case, a myocardial perfusion study is performed to document reversible ischemia, and EECP therapy can be repeated sequentially with three months intervals in between according to Medicare guidelines.

Does EECP aggravate high blood pressure (hypertension)?

No. If you have hypertension that is properly managed, you may undergo EECP without difficulty. Oftentimes, patients with hypertension find that their blood pressure improves as they proceed with EECP . If your hypertension is uncontrolled, you must seek medical care to get your blood pressure under control with proper medications before proceeding with EECP .

As a matter of fact, EECP has a therapeutic role in the management of arterial hypertension and hypertensive heart disease.

Is there an age limit for EECP ?

No. We have successfully treated patients as young as 35 and as old as 86 without any difficulties. Many of our patients are in their 80s and complete the entire EECP program with excellent results.

Can EECP dislodge plaque and cause a stroke or heart attack?

No. Atherosclerotic plaques are calcified and h ard, and they create an obstruction that detours the blood through alternate routes of least resistance. During EECP , when blood is flowing to y our h eart, i t w ill n aturally bypass arteries with significant plaque a nd e nter healthy, non-diseased blood vessels to go around the blockages. In time, these new pathways are reinforced and become lasting routes for blood to reach your heart beyond the blockages. This is why; EECP is often called the "natural bypass."

What happens if a patient misses an EECP session?

Missing a day of EECP therapy will not have a negative effect on the overall treatment. Just like any other therapy, you are encouraged to have EECP every day, except for weekends. The more consistent you are with the EECP schedule, the better the results will be. The missed session will be added to the end of your program until you have a total of 35 sessions.

Besides angina, does EECP have been useful for other non-cardiac conditions?

In our experience, EECP has been useful for other non-cardiac conditions such as erectile dysfunction, renal failure with fluid retention refractory to diuretics, and obesity associated with fluid retention as well. At the present, it has been described that EECP has a therapeutic role in the treatment of restless leg syndrome, hepatorenal syndrome, erectile dysfunction, syndrome X, and retinal artery occlusion.

Why is EECP an underutilized therapy in patients with refractory AP?

Most practicing cardiologists today don't have hands-on experience with this modality. Many of the university medical centers who train cardiology fellows don't have an EECP program. There are some logistic problems involved as well. For example, if you live in Anaheim and there is an EECP program at Cedars Sinai Medical Center in Los Angeles, you will spend about 2-4 hours in going back and forth to this Medical Center for one hour of therapy every day for 35 days.

Lack of exposure to EECP , and the interrupted follow-up of these patients with refractory angina pectoris miss the opportunity to see how much difference EECP can make in the symptoms and quality of life of these patients. In addition, there is not a genuine interest by the academia and/or industry to support new randomized clinical trials. Finally, to make things worse, there are cardiologists who would like to see "a more solid clinical data" to continue practicing "evidence-based medicine." The fact remains that you can't argue with patients getting better and improving the quality of their lives with EECP therapy -as shown in the testimonials.

What is the current status and the expected future of EECP?

Leading technology for treating cardiovascular disease is slowly moving from very invasive methods to less invasive. Medical history is witnesses that in the seventies bypass surgery was the big news in the treatment of coronary artery disease. In the eighties it was balloon angioplasty and in the nineties it was the stent now we can move still a step further to a totally noninvasive treatment with EECP.

The Future belongs to those who succeed and EECP in now provided world wide by leading hospitals. The success of EECP can be judged by the fact that in the US Medicare reimbursement rate for EECP has increased by 7% whereas that for other procedures like angioplasty and bypass surgery decreased by 6%

Bibliography and Acknowledgement

- Arora RR, Chou TM, Jain D, Fleishman B, Crawford L, McKiernan T, and Nesto RW. The Multicenter study of enhanced external counterpulsation (MUST-EECP): effect of EECP on exercise-induced myocardial ischemia and anginal episodes. J Am Coll Cardiol 33: 1833–1840, 1999.
- Barsness G, Feldman AM, Holmes DR, Holubkov R, Kelsey SF, Kennard ED, and the IEPR Investigators. The International EECP Patient Registry (IEPR): design, methods, baseline characteristics, and acute results. Clin Cardiol 24: 435–442, 2001.
- Bonetti PO, Barsness GW, Keelan PC, Schnell TI, Pumper GM, Kuvin JT, Schnall RP, Holmes DR Jr, Higano ST, and Lerman A.Enhanced external counterpulsation improves endothelial function in patients with symptomatic coronary artery disease. J Am Coll Cardiol 41: 1761–1768, 2003.
- Bonetti PO, Holmes DR, Lerman A, and Barsness GW. Enhanced external counterpulsation for ischemic heart disease: what's behind the Curtin? J Am Coll Cardiol 41: 1918–1925, 2003.
- Lawson WE, Hui JCK, and Cohn PF. Long-term prognosis of patients with angina treated with enhanced external counterpulsation: five-year follow-up study. Clin Cardiol 23: 254–258, 2000.
- Lawson W, Hui JCK, Guo T, Burger L, Jiang Lillis L, O, Soroff HS, and Cohn PF. Prior revascularization increases the effectiveness of enhanced external counterpulsation. Clin Cardiol 21: 841–844, 1998.
- Lawson WE, Hui JCK, Soroff HS, Zheng ZS, Kayden DS, Sasvary D, Atkins H, and Cohn PF. Efficacy of enhanced external counterpulsation in the treatment of angina pectoris. Am J Cardiol 70: 859–862, 1992.
- Lawson WE, Hui JCK, Zheng ZS, Burger L, Jiang L, Lillis O, Oster Z, Soroff H, and Cohn PF.Improved exercise tolerance following enhanced external counterpulsation: cardiac or peripheral effect.Cardiology 87: 271–275, 1996.
- Lawson WE, Hui JCK, Zheng ZS, Oster Z, Katz JP, Diggs P, Burger L, Cohn CD, Soroff HS, and Cohn PF. Three-year sustained benefit from enhanced external counterpulsation in chronic angina pectoris.Am J Cardiol 75: 840–841, 1995.
- Lawson WE, Kennard ED, Holubkov R, Kelsey SF, Strobeck JE, Soran O, and Feldman AM. Benefit and safety of enhanced external counterpulsation in treating coronary artery patients with a history of congestive heart failure. Cardiology 96: 78–84, 2001.

Kundalini Awakening with Activation of Seven Chakras In Treatment of Chronic Disorders of Human body

The Rapid Healing Technique along with the chakra meditation

It is a new way to process and heal negative emotions, remove blockages in the meridian system and clear and balance the human energetic system. This process can lead a person into a state of wholeness. Wholeness is achieved through a process of self-remembrance, re-collection and re-union. A person comes back into direct experience with himself or herself as a complete human being, referred by some as the "Higher Self," "Soul," "Superconscious", In this state the conscious and unconscious are one and the person is able to radiate energy fully from all his or her centers of power and consciousness, which includes the 7 chakras. By clearing (removing/transforming) energy blockages and releasing energy trapped in the subtle energy system, an individual feels, recovers and consciously re-experiences old parts of self again that were lost in the original separation from God. In our journey through life many have stored up fear, pain, fear of pain, resentment, hurt and anger. The Rapid Healing Technique transforms negative emotions into love.

What is Kundalini?

In Sanskrit, "kundalini" roughly translates to "coiled life energy." It is believed to be the feminine form of the divine energy or consciousness. The Vedas, the ancient scriptures of Hinduism, describe kundalini as residing in the sacral chakra at the base of the spine. Awakening the kundalini through either mindful meditation or a spontaneous event like a near-death experience is believed to contribute to a spiritual enlightenment that promotes the healing of physical, mental, emotional and spiritual ailments. Yogi and spiritual guru Paramhans Swami Maheshwarananda writes in "The Hidden Power in Humans" that awakening kundalini energy results in a range of physical symptoms. Feelings of extreme hot or cold, tingling sensations in the extremities, increased sensitivity and changes in sexual desire or sensitivity are also associated with release of kundalini energy.

What is Kundalini Yoga ?

Kundalini yoga is a form of gentle exercise that combines traditional yoga poses with mantras and controlled breathing. In kundalini yoga, slow, controlled body movements and poses are coordinated with deep abdominal breathing. While the purpose of other types of yoga like Hatha or Bikram may be strength conditioning or weight loss, kundalini yoga is more concerned with holistic wellness, relaxation and the development of consciousness. Intensive forms of kundalini yoga are typically practiced in groups under the guidance of a yogi or kundalini guru trained in guided meditation, though at-home practices that use a DVD or text guide are also available.

Kundalini Yoga is an ancient science of directing life force, often called Prana or Chi (qi), which is usually depicted as a coiled serpent at the base of the spine. When this life force is directed up the chakras, or spinal centers, and through to the crown chakra and beyond, it is said to *awaken* a state of Nirvana or Bliss. Although this is the term often used, a more correct way of describing the energy would be that it goes from a*tamasic* to a *rajastic* state or from a *static* to an *active* state. A true kundalini awakening is described in Eastern terms as the joining of Shiva and Shakti, or the masculine and feminine states of consciousness. These are yet again, metaphors to describe a phenomenon which happens in the nervous system, when subtle energy flows unimpeded to the Pineal gland, where DMT, a naturally occurring hormone in our brains is set alight, and we bathe in very pleasurable sensations (akin to bliss) that the ancients often spoke of. In more modern terminology,

Kundalini Yoga allows this transition of stagnant energy into active energy which then lights the fire of consciousness through bio-molecular electricity and hormone activation. Jogi Bhajan first brought the ancient teachings of Kundalini Yoga to the United States in the late 1960s, but it was taught for centuries prior and has been alluded to in many great documents from varying cultures throughout the world.

The Yoga Sutras, for example, allude to the efficiency of this type of practice, stating that what is normally achieved in 12 years of Hatha Yoga as well as 6 years of Raja Yoga, plus 3 years of Mantra Yoga practice, can be obtained singularly through just one year of Kundalini practice.

There are references to Kundalini Yoga in ancient texts from Sumeria, Egypt, Africa, and Babylon even, but we find mention of it directly and most prevalently in ancient texts from India.The Hatha Yoga Pradipika refers to breathing techniques that awaken the kundalini (*Bhastrika* and *Shitali*, respectively), while the *Rig Veda* refers to awakening the kundalini as "releasing the waters." One can easily see why this metaphor is used since anytime Kundalini Shakti is given rise, energy flows more easily through the *nadis* of the body. There is even an ashvini mudra, named after Vedic dieties who were well versed in awakening kundalini.

There have been archeological excavations in the Indus Valley which show a man seated in a meditative posture with serpents rising up his legs – the serpent being the commonly accepted symbol of rising kundalini. The teachings of this ancient culture were shrouded in mystery as well as misunderstanding for many centuries, since awakening kundalini prematurely, that is, without cleansing the physical body first, can lead to unfortunate side effects, definitely *not* akin to bliss. Kundalini Yoga practiced with a clean diet, a moral and ethical code (as outlined in the Yamas and Niyamas) and the direction of a qualified Kundalini Yoga Teacher can be safe and effective, however, and one can experience elevated states of consciousness as well as greater clarity of mind and a more perfected physical vessel.

What is the Sannyasin;s Kundalini Path?

The sannyasin balances within himself both the male and female energies. Complete unto himself, he is whole and independent. Having attained an equilibrium of ida and pingala, he becomes a knower of the known. Aum.

Bhashya

These arise within the sannyasin a pure energy, neither masculine nor feminine. This is the sushumna current coming into power through which he gains control of the kundalini force and eventually, after years of careful guidance, attains nirvikalpa samadhi. Eventually, in one life or another, all will turn to the renunciate path. However, it would be equally improper for a renunciate-minded soul to enter family life as for a householder to seek to be a sannyasin. A word of warning. Be cautious of those who promise great kundalini awakenings and spiritual rewards from severe practices without preparation, initiation and renunciation. Those entering the serious life of sannyasa must be prepared to follow the traditional path of unrewarded sadhana through the years, apart from dear family and friends. Such is the way to reach the truth of yoga. It takes many, many years for the soul to thus ripen and mature. The Tirumantiram affirms, "Many are the births and deaths forgotten by souls shrouded in ignorance, enveloped in mala's darkness. At the moment Great Siva's grace is gained, the renunciate attains the splendorous light." Aum Namah Sivaya.

Within every human being there is a subtle body of three energy channels (nadis) and seven energy centres (chakras). At the root of this system lies a creative, protective and nurturing power which is a dormant, maternal energy (Kundalini). When this power is awakened within us, it rises spontaneously through the spinal column, passes through each of the chakras and emits from the fontanelle bone area on top of the head. This process is referred to as Enlightenment (Self-realization). This energy can actually be felt on top of the head and on the palms of the hands. Any imbalances in the subtle system can be felt on various parts of each hand. Through this meditatio none can learn, not only how to diagnose and decode the state of one's own inner subtle system, but one can also learn very simple clearing techniques to rebalance oneself.

There are 7 major chakras within our subtle body

Mooladhara, Swadisthana, Nabhi (Manipura), Hearth (Anahata), Vishuddhi, Agnya, Sahasrara

Each chakra has different qualities and by healing or balancing these chakras, we awaken and enhance their qualities within us, making us more balanced and integrated. Our enlightened chakras give us joy and peace.

Each of these subtle chakras is a storehouse of energy for the gross plexuses supplying the physical, mental and emotional demands of the sympathetic nervous system. For instance, if the Swadisthan chakra looks after the abdominal organs, it also supplies energy to creative action and thought and depth to the aesthetic sensibility. Before Kundalini awakening, the energy in the chakras is limited and exhaustible, as in a battery. After realization, they are connected by Kundalini passing through Sushumna (the middle channel) to the infinite current of the universal superconscious, to the all-pervading power of divine love.

Within every human being there is a subtle body of three energy channels (nadis) and seven energy centres (chakras). At the root of this system lies a creative, protective and nurturing power which is a dormant, maternal energy (Kundalini). When this power is awakened within us, it rises spontaneously through the spinal column, passes through each of the chakras and emits from the fontanelle bone area on top of the head. This process is referred to as Enlightenment (Self-realization). This energy can actually be felt on top of the head and on the palms of the hands. Any imbalances in the subtle system can be felt on various parts of each hand. Through this meditation one can learn, not only how to diagnose and decode the state of one's own inner subtle system, but one can also learn very simple clearing techniques to rebalance oneself.

1. Each chakra has different qualities and by healing or balancing these chakras, we awaken and enhance their qualities within us, making us more balanced and integrated. Our enlightened chakras give us joy and peace.
2. Each of these subtle chakras is a storehouse of energy for the gross plexuses supplying the physical, mental and emotional demands of the sympathetic nervous system. For instance, if the Swadisthan chakra looks after the abdominal organs, it also supplies energy to creative action and thought and depth to the aesthetic sensibility. Before Kundalini awakening, the energy in the chakras is limited and exhaustible, as in a battery. After realization, they are connected by Kundalini passing through Sushumna (the middle channel) to the infinite current of the universal superconscious, to the all-pervading power of divine love.

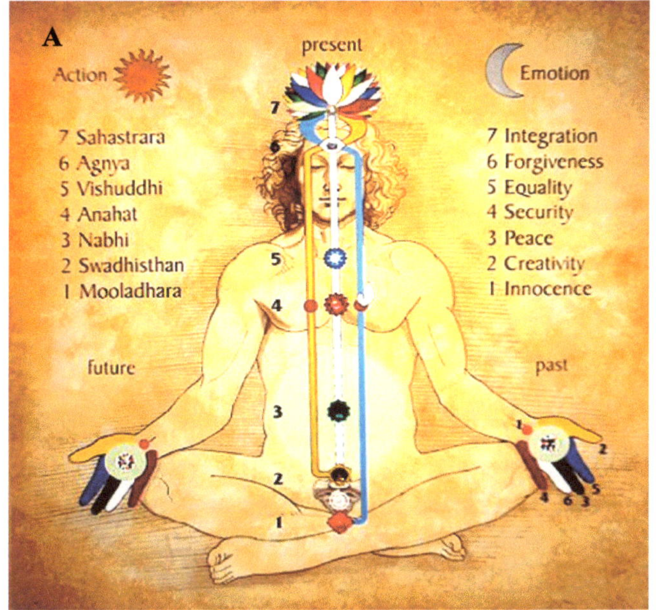

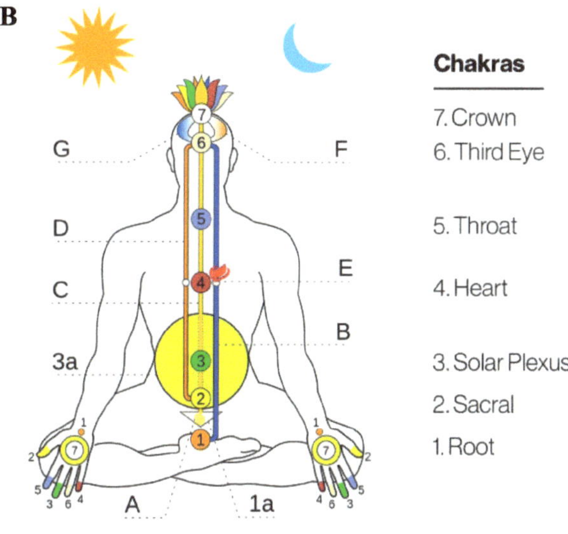

Fig. 24.1: (A &B) Illustrations showing 7 major chakras within our subtle body

1.Mooladhara Chakra

The Root Chakra: It is located at the tail of the spine between anus and sex organs. This chakra rules the organs of elimination. Working on this chakra helps in feelings of insecurity, fear, and sexual perversions. Focusing on it makes you grounded, centered and stable. Yoga Asanas that help in strengthening this chakra are Bakasana, Yoga Mudras, Yoga Asanas, Bhekasana, Utkatasana, and moola bandha asana.

Physical manifestation: Pelvic plexus

Number of petals/sub-plexuses: 4

Element: Earth

Controls: Excretion and reproductive organs

Qualities: Innocence, wisdom, fearlessness

Place on hand: Heel of palm

Situated below the sacrum bone, the awakened Mooladhara chakra gives us innocence and wisdom. Innocence gives us joy without the limitation of conditionings and prejudice, a quality that can be found on small children. This quality diminishes as we grow up and develop a sense of ego and selfish desires. Fortunately this innate innocence is never destroyed and can return to us by practicing Sahaja Meditation. It is like the sun which is obscured by clouds but which shines again after the clouds pass. In India the elephant-headed deity, Shri Ganesha, is worshipped as the essence of innocence and wisdom. He has the body of a child, symbolizing innocence and the head of an elephant, symbolizing humility and wisdom.

2. Swadisthana Chakra

The Sacral Chakra: It is located at reproductive glands, covers kidneys and bladder. Focusing on this chakra helps in maintaining healthy relationships, creativity, and patience. It also helps in overcoming guilt and rigid emotions. Yoga Asanas that help in strengthening of this chakra are Bhujanga asana, Yoga Mudras, Yoga Asanas, Title asana, Marjari asana, Gaumukh asana and Setubandha asana.

Physical manifestation : Aortic plexus

Number of petals/sub-plexuses : 6

Element : Fire

Controls : Kidneys, liver, spleen, pancreas, uterus, intestines

Qualities : Creativity, pure attention. pure desire, pure knowledge

Place on hand : Thumb

The Swadishthana chakra moves like a satellite around the Nabhi chakra and the Void and provides us with our sense of aesthetics, art, music, our appreciation and connection with nature. It looks after our digestive organs and provides us with the dynamic energy to do physical, mental and creative work.

The quality of Swadisthan is pure knowledge (Nirmala Vidya), knowledge of things as they are in the absolute sense. This knowledge needs to be experienced by ourselves directly not through an external agency.

The key to true creativity is in achieving the state of thoughtless awareness (nirvichar samadhi). Like a lake, silent and still, all the beauty of the creation around You, is reflected within. You become the flute, an egoless channel for the divine music of vibrations. You are, in the words of the Poet, 'a heart that watches and receives'.

3. Nabhi (Manipura) Chakra

The Solar Plexus: This chakra is located at the naval and covers digestive organs. Balancing this chakra helps will power and self- esteem. It provides strength for inner balance. Focusing on it helps in controlling feelings of anger, greed and indigestion. Yoga Asanas that help in strengthening this chakra are stretching, Dhanuarasana, Mayurasana, Yoga Mudras, Yoga Asanas, Matsayasana and all exercises involving abdominal muscles.

Physical manifestation : Navel/Solar plexus

Number of petals/sub-plexuses : 10

Element : Water

Controls : Stomach, intestines, liver, spleen

Qualities : Seeking, peace, generosity, satisfaction, pure attention, looking after others

Place on hand : Middle finger

When enlightened by the Kundalini, the Nabhi chakra gives us unconditional generosity, complete contentment and profound inner peace. On the right side, it looks after the upper part of our liver which is the organ of our attention. We seek food, shelter and comfort and ultimately, we seek to evolve into a new state of spiritual awareness and to receive our Self-realization.

"Satisfaction" is actually a key word for Nabhi. Because of liver problems and the consequent irritability people often develop the habit of expressing discontent at the slightest provocation. For them, life without worry is an impossibility.

When the Spirit manifests, you see things in their true perspective, through purified attention, and give up worrying. In the peace of thoughtlessness, you can only be content. Then you know the Spirit is not bothered with passing fads and trends, a button missing here or there. The mantra for Nabhi is : "In my Spirit I am satisfied."

4. Heart Chakra

The Heart Chakra: It is located at the heart, covers lungs and thymus gland. Balancing this chakra helps in maintaining qualities such as love, compassion, forgiveness, kindness, and understanding these qualities in others. Focusing on this chakra helps you awaken to spiritual awareness. Focusing on in is very useful when going through feelings of grief, possessiveness, hurt and rejection. Yoga Asanas that help to balance this chakra are Yoga Mudras, Yoga Asanas, Balasana, all exercises which involve twisting of the upper body and all Pranayamas.

Physical manifestation : Cardiac plexus

Number of petals/sub-plexuses : 12

Element : Air

Controls : Heart, lungs, sternum bone

Qualities : Joy, compassion, sense of security, love, responsibility

Place on hand : Little finger

Within the Heart chakra resides the Self: the spirit or atma. The spirit manifests when our heart is open, at which point we feel the pure joy of existence and the meaning and purpose of our place in creation. The quality of the Heart chakra is pure, unconditional love. Before our realization we rarely love unconditionally-we expect something in return. We mistake feelings of love for physical attraction, infatuation and selfishness. We love our children because they are 'ours' but do not love other children in the same way. Often we expect something back from them later in life as a repayment for our love. Love that expects is emotional attachment. Pure love has no motive. It emanates from the spirit and not from the body or mind. If you see how a small puppy runs to every person it sees in a park just to give them its love and share with them its joy, that is the essence of love. The Heart chakra also manifests in the head at the fontanelle bone so it's important to keep our Heart chakra clean, as this is the entry point to the super consciousness, where the Kundalini escapes from the subtle system and unites us with the Paramachaitanya-the all-pervading power of divine love.

5. Vishuddhi Chakra

The Throat Chakra: It is located at the throat and covers trachea region and thyroid gland. Concentrating on this chakra helps in improving communication and sharing of knowledge. It helps in eliminating laziness, insecurity and weakness in expressive abilities. Focusing on it also helps eliminate the fear of other people's opinion in judgment. Highly beneficial thyroid related problems. Yoga Asanas that help to balance this chakra are Sarvangasana, Bhujangasana, Halasana, Yoga Mudras, Yoga Asanas, Ustrasana, Marjari Asana, Gaumukhasana, Bhrama mudra and all chantings.

Physical manifestation : Cervical plexus

Number of petals/sub-plexuses : 16

Element : Sky/Space/Ether

Controls : Neck, arms, face, tongue, mouth, nose, teeth, thyroid

Qualities : Sweetness of communication, diplomacy, collectivity, detachment, self-respect and respect for others, brother/sister relationship

Place on hand : First finger

The Vishuddhi embodies the qualities which governs our communication with others. As it awakens we discover greater self-respect (left Vishuddhi) and greater respect for others (right Vishuddhi). Our ego is not bloated by praise and we are not upset by aggression or criticism. The Vishuddhi is also the chakra that manifests the power of witnessing. By daily practice of Sahaja Meditation, we become identified with our spirit. In this state of union with our spirit, we become witness of our body, our mind, our thoughts, our emotions, and ultimately the detached witness of the drama of our lives.

6. Agnya, Chakra

The Third Eye: It lies at the center in between eyebrows. It covers brain and pituitary gland. Balancing this helps improve visualization, fantasizing, concentration, and determination. Focusing on it is of great help in feelings of depression, confusion and rejection of spirituality. Yoga Asanas that help in balancing this chakra are Guru Pranama, Yoga Mudras, Yoga Asanas, chanting and Yoga mudra.

Physical manifestation : Optic chiasma

Number of petals/sub-plexuses : 2

Element : Light

Controls : Pineal body/pituitary gland, eyesight, memory, mind

Qualities : Forgiveness

Place on hand : Ring finger

The Agnya is the narrow gate which, when open, allows our kundalini to ascend to the limbic area of the brain. It is the chakra of forgiveness, humility and compassion. Forgiveness is the power to let go of anger, hatred and resentment and to discover, in humility, the nobility and generosity of the spirit. Once we start to see that by not forgiving others we are actually doing no harm to anyone other than ourselves, we start to realize that it is not only wise and generous to forgive but also very practical and pragmatic. By forgiving, we start to feel a tremendous sense of peace and relief. Forgiveness melts away all our ego and conditionings, our false ideas of racism and nationalism and our misidentifications.

7. Sahasrara Chakra

The Crown Chakra: It is located at the crown of the head and covers brain and pituitary gland. Focusing on it helps achieve enlightenment, gives a sense of unity and takes you to the greatest heights of your mind and body by eliminating grief and fear of death. Yoga Asanas that help in balancing this chakra are Sat kriya and Dhyana.

Physical manifestation : Limbic area of brain

Number of petals/sub-plexuses : 1000

Qualities : Joy, thoughtless awareness, union with the Divine, collective consciousness

Place on hand : Centre of palm

Our complete subtle instrument is integrated in the Sahasrara chakra. Each chakra has its seat. As our attention and our kundalini rise to Sahasrara chakra we enter a new dimension of consciousness. We go beyond the relative to the absolute. We rise above the three channels of the subtle system-beyond the past, present and future and into a timeless state and experience the inner joy and bliss of the divine. This is a heavenly place far beyond our imagination.

When the Kundalini reaches the Sahasrara, the thousand petals of this chakra begin to open and enlightenment begins to manifest. We may experience a pulsation at the fontanelle bone, followed by a subtle flow of cool vibrations. The Kundalini unites our individual consciousness to the universal consciousness. Our individual atma, our soul, is connected to the paramatma, the supreme spirit. We are suddenly tuned into the universal wavelength of vibrations, to the subtle joy that is present in nature. These vibrations pervade the universe but before Realization we are unaware of them.

The opening of this chakra is known as second birth. Our human birth can be likened to the hatching of an egg and Self-realization to the breaking of the egg and the emergence of the bird. This is why an egg is given at Easter, to symbolize the second birth.

How you may feel or act when Chakras are Overactive or Underactive

Root Chakra

Overactive:- Fearful, nervous, insecure, or ungrounded; materialistic or greedy; resistant to change

Underactive:- Lacking a sense of being at home or secure anywhere, codependent, unable to get into one's body, fearful of abandonment

Sacral Chakra

Overactive:- Overemotional, very quick to attach and invest in others, attracted to drama, moody, lacking personal boundaries

Underactive:- Stiff, unemotional, closed off to others, lacking self-esteem or self-worth, possibly in an abusive relationship

Navel (Solar Plexus) Chakra

Overactive:- Domineering, aggressive, angry, perfectionistic or overly critical of oneself or others

Underactive:- Passive, indecisive, timid, lacking self-control

Heart Chakra

Overactive:- Loving in a clingy, suffocating way; lacking a sense of self in a relationship; willing to say yes to everything; lacking boundaries, letting everyone in

Underactive:- Cold, distant, lonely, unable or unwilling to open up to others, grudgeful

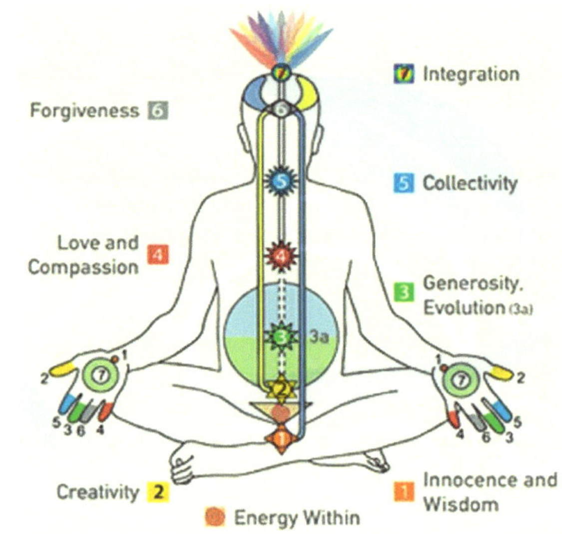

Fig. 24. 2: *illustration showing practice of Sahaja Yoga, a dynamic technique for meditation*

Throat Chakra

Overactive:- Overly talkative, unable to listen, highly critical, verbally abusive, condescending

Underactive:- Introverted, shy, having difficulty speaking the truth, unable to express needs

Third Eye Chakra

Overactive:- Out of touch with reality, lacking good judgment, unable to focus, prone to hallucinations

Underactive:- Rigid in thinking, closed off to new ideas, too reliant on authority, disconnected or distrustful of inner voice, anxious, clinging to the past and fearful of the future

Crown Chakra

Overactive:- Addicted to spirituality, heedless of bodily needs, having difficulty controlling emotions

Underactive:- Not very open to spirituality, unable to set or maintain goals, lacking direction

The Chakras and Associated Glands, Organs and Symptoms

Root Chakra

Adrenal glands, spine, blood, and reproductive organs

Physical Symptoms of Unbalance:- Inability to sit still, restlessness, unhealthy weight (either obesity or eating disorder), constipation, cramps, fatigue or sluggishness

Sacral Chakra

Kidneys and reproductive organs:- ovaries, testes, and uterus

Physical Symptoms of Unbalance:- Lower-back pain or stiffness, urinary issues, kidney pain or infection, infertility, impotence

Navel (Solar Plexus) Chakra

Central nervous system, digestive system (stomach and intestines), liver, pancreas, metabolic system

Physical Symptoms of Unbalance:- Ulcers, gas, nausea, or other digestive problems; eating disorders; asthma or other respiratory ailments; nerve pain or fibromyalgia; infection in the liver or kidneys; other organ problems

Heart Chakra

Thymus gland and immune system, heart, lungs, breasts, arms, hands

Physical Symptoms of Unbalance:- Heart and circulatory problems (high blood pressure, heart palpitations, heart attack), poor circulation or numbness, asthma or other respiratory ailments, breast cancer, stiff joints or joint problems in the hands

Throat Chakra

Thyroid, neck, throat, shoulders, ears, and mouth

Physical Symptoms of Unbalance:- Stiffness or soreness in the neck or shoulders, sore throat, hoarseness or laryngitis, earaches or infection, dental issues or TMJ, thyroid issues

Third Eye Chakra

Pituitary, eyes, brow, base of skull, biorhythms

Physical Symptoms of Unbalance:- Vision problems, headaches or migraines, insomnia or sleep disorders, seizures, nightmares (though this isn't a physical symptom per se, it is a common occurrence)

Crown Chakra

Pituitary and pineal glands, brain, hypothalamus, cerebral cortex, central nervous system

Physical Symptoms of Unbalance:- Dizziness, confusion, mental fog, neurological disorders, nerve pain, schizophrenia or other mental disorders

As you can see, a lot of these physical symptoms are not to be taken lightly!

The difficult thing to remember is that the physical and energy body is going to keep sending us its message amping up the intensity if it needs to until we pay attention and engage in physical, mental, emotional and energetic chakra healing.

Chakras and Your Energetic Frequency

The energy of our chakras influences our physical processes via inhibition and stimulation. Remember, chakras are like wheels whose job is not only to keep energy moving, but also to constrict or close as a defense against negative energy. In order to compensate for a constricted, underactive chakra, another chakra will become overactive, sending out your low-frequency vibes at a greater rate, which then requires further balancing in the chakra healing process. That in turn creates and prolongs a low-frequency reality. If your chakras are these energy centers emitting and absorbing energy, then are they the source of your frequency, or are they the result of it? Are your chakras the chicken or the egg? they're both.The dual role of the chakras, in terms of your consciousness and your physical self, really speaks to the relationship between the mind and the body. When you work on the body, the mind comes along for the ride, and vice-versa. It's the same with your frequency and your chakra energy. When you're in ego frequency, it affects the flow of energy within your chakras and your physical and energy body as a whole creating more of a need for energy body and chakra healing, among other things. However, as you clear, clean and heal your chakras by moving energy around, then you are also making a positive change in your frequency. Just remember, if you're operating on a lower frequency, then

(1) you're creating your reality, because your five senses are picking up what you're applying your consciousness to ("This is where we are, find me all the things that reinforce that"), and

(2) your resonant frequency is what you're putting out into the quantum field and what you're drawing into yourself through your chakras, impacting your physical state.

Exercise: Fire Breath Chakra Balancing & Healing

This exercise is a chakra healing and energy body oriented orgasmic meditation named by a Cherokee medicine man, Harley Swiftdeer. You will be breathing into each of your chakras and, as you do so, imagining the colors of that chakra illuminating with bright, healing light. As you continue to breathe, you will move this beautiful energy up your physical and energy body in circles, and by the time it reaches your upper chakras it will feel like it has taken on a life of its own.

Fire Breath is extremely relaxing, rejuvenating and healing for your chakras and energy body, but it can also yield some unexpected discoveries. Big emotions may move through you, often emotions you weren't even aware you were holding. You may want to release tears or express anger. While it can absolutely be done with your partner, I suggest doing it on your own first.

1. Drop any expectations and put yourself in the mind-set and energy state of the feeling you desire. Let go of any attachment or expectation with regard to outcome.
2. Lie on your back with your knees up and feet flat on the floor (or bed). Relax your jaw. Breathe in through your nose and exhale through your mouth.
3. Imagine your breath filling up your belly like a balloon. As you exhale, flatten your lower back to the floor. There should be a gentle rocking in your pelvis as you do this.
4. Squeeze your Kegels as you exhale.
5. As you breathe in, imagine pulling energy from your root chakra—your perineum. You don't have to push or pull the energy. It will follow your thoughts.
6. Next, inhale your energy from your root chakra up to your sacral chakra. Then exhale, circulating the energy back down to the root. Continue moving your energy between the root and sacral chakras by breathing in and feeling it rise, breathing out and letting it go back to the root. Repeat several times and you will notice it feels like the energy is moving easily and almost on its own.
7. Now enlarge the circle by breathing healing energy from your root chakra up to your solar plexus chakra, squeezing your Kegel muscles as you breathe out. Repeat this several times as well. When this feels complete, reduce the circle so that the energy goes between your sacral chakra and your solar plexus.
8. As you continue breathing and squeezing your Kegels, enlarge the circle of energy so that it moves between your sacral chakra and your heart. When this feels complete, reduce the circle so that the energy goes between your solar plexus and your heart center. You are moving your energy from sacral to heart and solar plexus to heart.
9. Next make a circle of energy between the solar plexus and throat, followed by a smaller circle between heart and throat. When you reach the throat, make some sounds if you aren't already doing so, anything from sighs to moans to "aahs." This is liberating and helps move energy and create deeper chakra healing. The energy may start moving up the chakras in circles on its own as the momentum gets building.
10. Breathe in, moving energy from the heart to the third eye, and breathe out and back down to the heart. Do this several times, followed by a smaller circle between the throat and the third eye. When you're sending energy into your third eye, roll your eyes up (keeping them closed) as if you can see out the top of your head. This will help your energy rise and your chakras heal and balance.
11. The next circle is from the throat to the crown followed by a smaller circle between the third eye and the crown chakra.
12. Keep breathing and moving your hips and moving the energy in circles, giving your body the space to go through the full process of chakra healing and energy body rejuvenation.

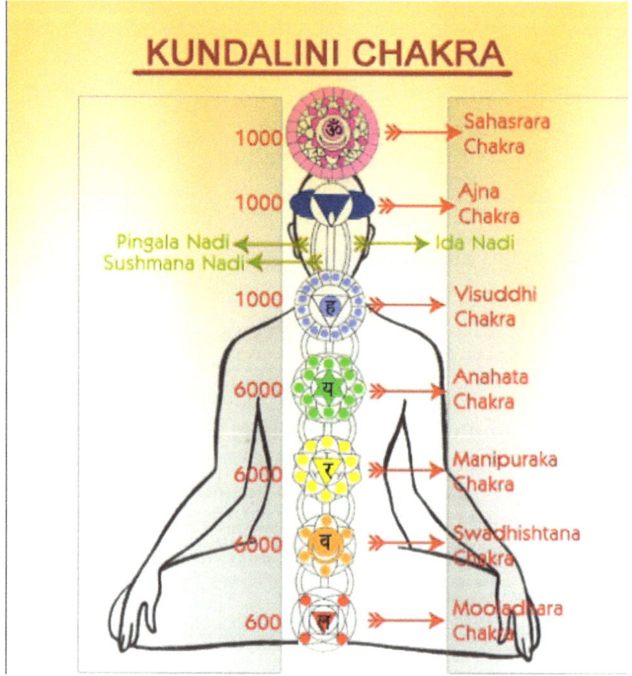

Fig. 27.3: *Illustration showing different Kundalini chakras in the practice of Kundalini yoga*

Sahaja Yoga

In 1970, Shri Mataji Nirmala Devi founded Sahaja Yoga, a dynamic technique for meditation that takes us beyond our limitations. Through the awakening of the spiritual energy, we can experience the integration of whole aspects of our lives.There is a power which is a residual power of Kundalini. It is called as Kundalini because it is coiled as three-and-a-half coil. It is resting in the triangular bone . This is the energy that has to be awakened and when it is awakened it rises through 6 very subtle energy centers and pierces through the fontanelle bone area. And then you feel as if a cool breeze is coming out of your fontanelle bone area. But this is just like a connection with the mains as we have for every instrument With this happening, you become a Self-realized person in the sense that you develop a new dimension in your awareness, in your central nervous system.

Saha means with and ja is born with you. Also Sahaja means spontaneous.Yoga means the union with All-pervading Divine Power. Sahaja Yoga is the right of every human being to achieve that ascent To get to the absolute knowledge, we have to rise higher into new realm, beyond thought and this is the new realm which you achieve after Sahaja Yoga. With the awakening of the Kundalini, so many things also happen. Because it nourishes all your chakras. By the nourishment of your chakras, you find that your health suddenly improves

It is such a remarkable thing that it has to happen to all of us as the last jump or break through into the evolutionary process. Sahaja Yoga is not a new thing. It has been there but it was only transmitted from one master to one disciple… and now it is becoming practical and thousands of people are getting Realization all over the world

How to Practice The Chakra Balancing and Activating Meditation

Because breathing and oxygenation is so vital to the energy system, chakra meditations are very important in the process of Wholeness.

Opening and Closing Chakras

The opening and closing of our chakras works like an energetic defense system. A negative experience (and the low-frequency energy that comes with it) can cause the associated chakra energy to close in order to block that energy out. Similarly, if we are clinging to a low-calibrating feeling like blame, prolonging the emotion because we refuse to deal with or move it, we close off the chakra (the channel through which the energy would otherwise escape), which then requires special chakra healing techniques like the Fire Breath exercise. Any of the emotions that sit at the lower end of the Quantum Lovemap will likely trigger a chakra energy constriction. It is believed that constriction as the tightness that comes into our mind and body when we are stressed.

As we open and heal our chakras, energy is able to flow freely once again and things return to normal. Sometimes it's a matter of moving energy throughout our body, moving our own frequency up the Quantum Lovemap, or tackling and extracting a difficult thorn that is stressing us out. For now, you have to understand how important chakra healing is and that your chakras be open and allow energy to move through you without obstruction. Each chakra's connection to a key endocrine gland and nervous system in your body means that an energy deficiency could lead to serious physical consequences if you ignore it for too long.

Balance is Key in Chakra Healing

No one chakra is better than the others or more important than any other in the process of energy body balancing and chakra healing. You don't want to have extra heart chakra energy and less throat chakra energy; it simply doesn't work like that. Ideally, all seven of your chakras are healed, balanced, open, and humming, allowing energy to flow into and out of your body. The amazing thing is that your body is going to find a way to move energy in and out (unless, of course, your ego self is telling it to hold on to something). If one of your chakras is closed or underactive, there is a very good chance that another chakra will be overactive to make up the difference.

Because your body wants to achieve energetic balance in your chakras, moving too far in either direction (underactive or overactive) in any one chakra can actually yield negative effects in your body and be counterproductive to the energy body and chakra healing process. An underactive chakra kicks another chakra into overdrive, which in turn pulls extra energy away from that part of the body. The descriptions below show how you may act or feel when your chakras get knocked out of balance and need healing. The first one lists the physical systems associated with each chakra and the potential physical *symptoms* that may tell you something's out of whack.

Root Chakra

Step 1: In all meditations find a comfortable position with back straight. Close your eyes and begin deep belly breathing. If you are a beginner in deep breathing, a good way to know that you are doing it correctly is to lie down and breathe in through your nose. Notice that as you inhale the belly fills first and the chest follows. The neat thing about lying down is that you cannot do it incorrectly. When you get the feel for it and have some practice, you may sit up if you prefer.

Breathe deeply through you nose without separation between inhalation and exhalation; feel yourself relaxing. Do this for about five minutes and become aware of your body as you breathe. An easy way to do this is to focus on your breath as it goes in and out. Allow your breathing to become deeper and more rhythmic. With each breath you are relaxing more and more.

Step 2: Now put your attention on your first chakra in your body at the base of your spine.

Imagine you are breathing in and out through your first chakra in the human body. The air goes all the way down to the base of the spine on the inhalation and all the way up through the nose on the exhalation with no separation between breaths. On each exhalation, visualize or sense the energy in the first chakra growing stronger through the chakra meditation. Visualize the chakra as a fiery red ball growing brighter and stronger on each exhalation. Let your consciousness move down into the ball of energy. Become the ball of energy and feel yourself being drawn downward into the earth.

Step 3: As this happens pay attention to how you feel physically, emotionally and mentally. Be aware of what you experience. It is different for everyone. Some people have experienced imagery with the earth or the cycles of the earth, birth and death, or a partnership and belonging associated with Mother Earth and nature. By meditating on this chakra you will get in touch with different aspects of your earth-like nature and connection and your interdependent relationship with the earth.

Do this part for about ten minutes or until you are satisfied. When you are ready to return to the room, say "Every time I reach this relaxed state I learn to use my mind more creatively and become more aware of energy blocks that have kept me a prisoner so that I may heal myself." Release the ball of energy and the imagery and count from one to five feeling refreshed, relaxed and peaceful as you return to the room and open your eyes.

Second Chakra – Sexual Center

Step 1: If you are only doing one chakra, follow step one under the first chakra meditation heading, otherwise continue unabated from the previous.

Step 2: Now put your attention on your second chakra in your body at the base of your spine.

Imagine you are breathing in and out through your second chakra in the human body. The air goes all the way down to your sexual organs on the inhalation and all the way up through the nose on the exhalation with no separation between breaths. On each exhalation, visualize or sense the energy in the second chakra growing stronger. Visualize the chakra as an orange ball growing brighter and stronger on each exhalation. Let your consciousness move down into the ball of energy. Become the ball of energy and feel yourself beginning to radiate outward from that center through your body and then into the outer environment. Feel the sense of magic and wonder that radiates from the second chakra through meditation.

Step 3: As this happens pay attention to how you feel physically, emotionally and mentally. Be aware of what you experience. It is different for everyone. Some people may feel spontaneous bursts of energy running up and down their spine or through their body. They are normal; enjoy them. Some people may feel them as a warm current of energy or vibrations running through their body. Thesesensations represent an increased flow of energy in the body. Pay attention to the changes you experience. Just observe; do not try to influence them. By meditating on this chakra you will get in touch with different aspects of your sexuality as well as the creative process.

Do this part for about ten minutes or until you are satisfied. When you are ready to return to the room, say "Every time I reach this relaxed state, I learn to use my mind more creatively and become more aware of energy blocks that have kept me a prisoner so that I may heal myself." Release the ball of energy and the imagery and count from one to five feeling refreshed, relaxed and peaceful as you return to the room and open your eyes.

Third Chakra – Solar Plexus

This chakra allows you to transcend the conscious mind and "me" concerns and experience selflessness that allows a deep connection with other people.

Step 1: If you are only doing one chakra, follow step one under the first chakra meditation heading, otherwise continue unabated from the previous.

Step 2: Now put your attention on the third chakra in the human body. Imagine you are breathing in and out through your third chakra. The air goes down to your third chakra on the inhalation and all the way up through the nose on the exhalation with no separation between breaths. On each exhalation visualize or sense the energy in the third chakra growing stronger. During third chakra meditation, visualize a golden yellow ball growing brighter and stronger on each exhalation. Let your consciousness move down into the ball of energy. Become the ball of energy and feel yourself begin to radiate outward from that center through your body and then into the outer environment. You will begin to feel as if you are beginning to melt.

Step 3: As this happens pay attention to how you feel physically, emotionally and mentally. Be aware of what you experience. It is different for everyone. You may feel yourself become watery and fluid as your consciousness radiates from this center, and you may feel a profound empathy. This empathy, a product of trust and contentment, will permit you to feel compassion for the pain and suffering of others as well as for yourself. Surrender to these feelings and let them flow through you.

Do this part for about ten minutes or until you are satisfied. When you are ready to return to the room, say "Every time I reach this relaxed state I learn to use of my mind more creatively and become more aware of energy blocks that have kept me a prisoner so that I may heal myself." Release the ball of energy and the imagery and count from one to five feeling more refreshed, relaxed and peaceful than before as you return to the room and open your eyes.

Fourth Chakra – Heart

Step 1: If you are only doing one chakra, follow step one under the first chakra meditation heading, otherwise continue unabated from the previous.

Step 2: Now put your attention on your heart chakra. Imagine you are breathing in and out through your fourth chakra in your body. The air goes down to your heart chakra on the inhalation and all the way up through the nose on the exhalation with no separation between breaths. On each exhalation, visualize or sense the energy in the fourth chakra growing stronger. During fourth chakra meditation, visualize an emerald green ball of light growing brighter and stronger on each exhalation. Let your consciousness move down into the ball of energy. Become the ball of energy and feel yourself begin to radiate outward from that center through your body and then into the outer environment.

Step 3: Feel the transcendent love, which radiates through the heart and into the rest of the 7 chakras, and pay attention to how you feel physically, emotionally and mentally. The more you are centered in the heart, the more you will feel the "mystic heart" of Christ in you, your Christ consciousness. As the rivers of living water radiate through your heart, your entire body will pulsate with energy from the top of your head to the bottoms of your feet. Searing currents of energy will shoot everywhere. You will experience warmth that pulsates from your heart and fills your entire body. By surrendering to the energy radiating through your heart, you will experience compassion and unconditional love for yourself as well as everyone else. You may also experience the condition, which Jesus describes as "the peace that passes all understanding."

Do this part for about ten minutes or until you are satisfied. When you are ready to return to the room, say "Every time I reach this relaxed state I learn to use my mind more creatively and become more aware of energy blocks that have kept me a prisoner so that I may heal myself." Release the ball of energy and the imagery and count from one to five feeling more refreshed, relaxed and peaceful than before as you return to the room and open your eyes.

Fifth Chakra – Throat

Step 1: If you are only doing one chakra, follow step one under the first chakra meditation heading, otherwise continue unabated from the previous.

Step 2: Now put your attention on your throat chakra meditation. Imagine you are breathing in and out through your throat chakra. The air goes in and out your throat with no separation between breaths. On each exhalation, visualize or sense the energy in the throat chakra growing stronger. During this chakra meditation, visualize a glimmering blue ball of light growing brighter and stronger on each exhalation. Let your consciousness move down into the ball of energy. Become the ball of energy and feel yourself begin to radiate outward from that center through your body and then into the outer environment.

Step 3: Feel your character as fearless, noble and full of courage. Experience the integrity of choosing yourself at every moment. Feel your inner affirmation that says "yes" to life at every moment. Being centered in your throat allows you to feel more triumphant. Your life will be victorious at every moment without diminishing anyone else. You may choose to say the affirmation, "At last I am free," over and over to yourself.

As you experience this victory, you may feel streams of energy shooting up your spine. As they pass the throat they become currents of unconditional joy. You will be fulfilling your purpose in life by accepting this victory.

Do this part for about ten minutes or until you are satisfied. When you are ready to return to the room, say "Every time I reach this relaxed state I learn to use my mind more creatively and become more aware of energy blocks that have kept me a prisoner so that I may heal myself." Release the ball of energy and the imagery and count from one to five feeling more refreshed, relaxed and peaceful than before as you return to the room and open your eyes.184

Sixth Chakra – Third Eye

Step 1: If you are only doing one chakra, follow step one under the first chakra meditation heading, otherwise continue unabated from the previous.

Step 2: Now put your attention on the sixth of the 7 chakras in the human body. Imagine you are breathing in and out through your third eye. The air goes in and out with no separation between breaths. On each exhalation, visualize or sense the energy in the third eye growing stronger. During this chakra meditation, visualize an indigo ball of light growing brighter and stronger on each exhalation. Let your consciousness move up into the ball of energy. Become the ball of energy and feel yourself begin to radiate outward from that center through your body and then into the outer environment.

Step 3: Feel yourself as the union of selves. Feel your mind radiate simultaneously in all directions and sense filling the room with your consciousness. Pay attention to how you feel physically, emotionally and mentally. The more you are centered in your third eye the more complete will be your union of the consciousness and the unconsciousness.

This condition will produce an electrical current running through your physical body and your entire head will glow with this center, the third eye.

Do this part for about ten minutes or until you are satisfied. When you are ready to return to the room, say "Every time I reach this relaxed state I learn to use my mind more creatively and become more aware of energy blocks that have kept me a prisoner so that I may heal myself." Release the ball of energy and the imagery and count from one to five feeling more refreshed, relaxed and peaceful than before as you return to the room and open your eyes.

Important note: However you experience each chakra meditation is right for you for where you are now. As you heal and clear your energetic system, your meditations will change also. Remember not to judge yourself. Accept and allow yourself to grow at your own pace. Give the gift of the fourth chakra in your body, unconditional love and compassion, to yourself.

Seventh Chakra – Crown

No meditation is possible with the crown chakra because a person does not exist as a separate being; therefore, the ALL at every moment is meditating through him/her.

By doing the meditations on each of the 7 chakras, you will activate awareness of emotional blocks and feelings. These will come in different ways for different people, depending on the spiritual gifts that you may already have developed. Removing and clearing energy blocks enhances your spiritual gifts by either making you stronger or opening you to new awareness and abilities you were not aware of before. Just remember that whatever occurs, it is perfect for you.

The following is a list of the psychic gifts of the 7 chakras. The root or first chakras gift is unlimited intuition, gut feelings. The sexual or second chakras gift is clairsentience, which is clear feeling, the sensing of ideas, energies, love, etc., through the feeling nature, including smelling of heavenly fragrances. The gift of the third chakra meditation, the solar plexus, is sensitivity to vibrations from other people and places. The gift of the fourth or heart chakra is the ability to be empathetic with people because you have journeyed down the path that you now see others working through. The gift of the thymus is telepathy, the ability to speak or communicate to another through the mind.

The gift of the fifth or throat chakra meditation is clairaudience, which is clear hearing, hearing through the inner ear words and ideas from the higher vibrational levels, music or sounds of the spiritual universe. The gift of the third eye or sixth chakra is clairvoyance, which is clear seeing, seeing into the higher levels of vibration forms which cannot be seen with the physical eyes, such as visions, auras, energies, and higher beings. The gift of the crown or 7th chakra in the human body is Comic Consciousness, Ascension and the I AM. The purpose of this chapter has been to lay a foundation upon which to build your spiritual development. Everyone will be at a different place to start. You cannot begin any journey until you start, and to start you need a roadmap in order to assist you in where you are going. Understanding the bodies comprising your energy field, the chakras in our bodies, their functioning or lack of functioning and the diseases that occur by continuing to ignore or repress our feelings in the human energetic system is a good start. The Rapid Healing Technique is a road map to transform your life and lead you to Wholeness or Ascension, if that is your intention and you are willing to keep yourself focused on your journey. You can make your intention for clearing fears and negative emotions and take it as far as you feel is your soul's contract for this lifetime.

Benefits of Kundalini Yoga

Kundalini yoga is a system of exercises brought to America by Yogi Bhajan, who began practicing them as a boy in India. Previously, Kundalini yoga had been kept secret, and only serious spiritual seekers had access to its teachings, according to 3HO, a Kundalini yoga organization founded by Yogi Bhajan. The practice involves linking the breath with movement and working to heal the body with specific postures and chanting.

Tone the Body

Each active Kundalini yoga movement works a different part of the body to build muscle strength. However, people looking to build large muscles might look elsewhere. Kundalini yoga is more effective at toning the body than making it tightly muscled, according to the New York University Langone Medical Center. Poses to tone the body include Cobra pose, in which you lie on the floor with your hands under your shoulders. Push your hands into the ground as you lift your chest into the air to form a back bend. Cobra pose stretches the entire upper body, including the abdomen, chest and shoulders, and makes the spine stronger. To strengthen the legs, try Frog pose. Begin this pose by squatting on the floor, balanced on the balls of your feet. Touch your heels together, spread your knees apart and place your hands on the floor between your legs. Straighten your legs as you inhale, keeping your head down and fingertips on the floor. Return to the original squatting position, your fingertips never leaving the floor, and repeat this movement for one to two minutes.

Balance Energy

Practitioners of Kundalini yoga believe the body has seven energy centers known as chakras. These energy centers begin at the crown of your head and occur at various places along your spine, such as your heart and belly. The last one lies near the sexual organs. Kundalini yoga practitioners believe the practice's poses, chanting and meditations balance the chakras and remove any energy blocks. In the Kundalini philosophy, the practice of working the body's energy centers is also believed to increase spiritual awareness.

Calm the Mind

Practitioners of Kundalini yoga believe that breath and emotion are intricately linked. For example, short, shallow breaths may create anxiety, while long, deep breaths promote peacefulness. The average person breathes 16 times per minute, according to 3HO Foundation, but when the breath slows to eight times per minute, the mind calms down. A goal of Kundalini yoga is to control the breath by connecting it to the body's movement. Practitioners slow their breathing as they move through each pose. The peacefulness felt can last long after practice ends.

Increase Flexibility

Many Kundalini yoga poses focus on increasing the body's flexibility, especially the spine. In this yoga's philosophy, a flexible spine helps ensure a healthy and youthful body. Exercises such as the spinal flex involve sitting on the floor with your legs folded in, but not crossed. Hold onto your ankles and flex your spine back and forth, allowing the momentum to move your body. Other poses focus on stretching the backs of the legs, sides of the belly, neck and shoulders.

Manage the Emotions

Kundalini yoga techniques may be useful in treating obsessive-compulsive disorder, according to a study conducted by researchers at the University of California, San Diego. The small study analyzed the effects of Kundalini yoga on 12 people with the disorder. Those who practiced Kundalini yoga meditations experienced statistically significant improvements on scales that measure OCD. A paper published in "Journal of Alternative and Complementary Medicine" reports that Kundalini yoga techniques might be helpful for a host of emotional disturbances, including depression, anger, fatigue and grief.

The experiences of some people practicing kundalini yoga has created the impression that it is dangerous. While

Kundalini Yoga Dangers

it is true that students should approach this method of raising kundalini energy with caution, this type of yoga is only risky if the student advances too quickly beyond his physical and emotional capacity to handle the energy. Finding a well-qualified teacher is advised if you want to practice in a safe environment.

An 82-year-old Indian Sadhu (wandering monk, or holy man) Prahlad Jani has claimed that he has been living for 70 years without food or water..He is dead now

Indian Sadhu without food & drink for 70 years?

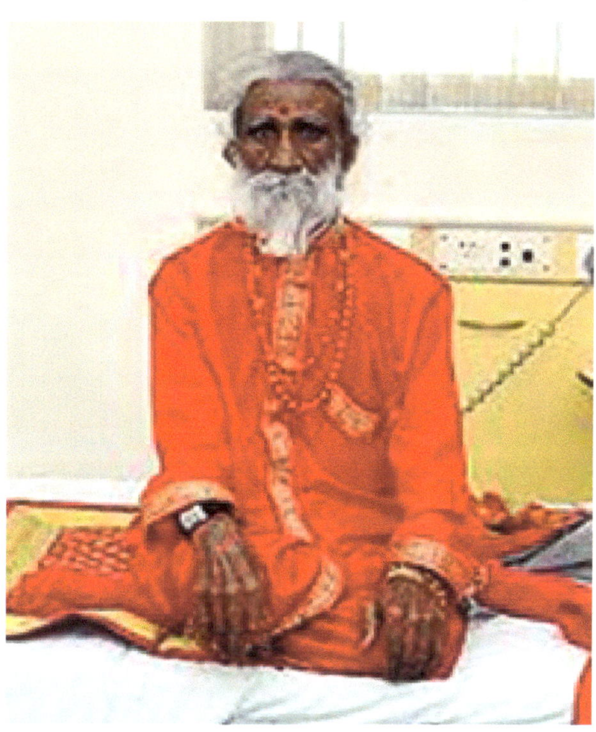

Fig 24.4: *Photograph of An 82-year-old Indian Sadhu (wandering monk, or holy man) Prahlad Jani has claimed that he has been living for 70 years without food or water. If it is true ,he may be getting the energy for his living through awakening of one of the Kundalini Chakras*

"I feel no need for food and water," states Prahlad Jani, a seventy-six year old Indian ascetic who lives in a cave near the Ambaji temple in the state of Gujarat. Mr. Jani claims that he has not had food or fluids to drink for the last sixty-five years. At the age of seven years he left home in search of spiritual unfoldment. Jani states that at the age of eleven years he was blessed by a goddess. He claims that since that blessing he has gained his sustenance from nectar that filters down through a hole in his palate, and has not passed urine or stools since then. Mr. Jani explained, "I get the elixir of life from the hole in my palate, which enables me to go without food and water." Almost daily Mr. Jani enters a state of Samadhi characterized by extreme bliss and enormous light and strength. He says that he has never experienced medical problems. He says that he did not speak for a period of forty-five years

Another similar research study, also headed by Dr. Sudhir V. Shah at Sterling Hospital, was conducted on Hira Ratan Manek. Mr. Manek claimed not to have eaten since 1995. Mr. Manek was kept under scientific observation round-the-clock for 411 continuous days. During this time Mr. Manek subsisted only on boiled water.The two brothers have come to be known as the "solar kids" and their case has completely mystified Pakistani doctors.

Mystery of Pakistans "solar kids;s Baffles Doctors in Pakistan (Fig. 24.5)

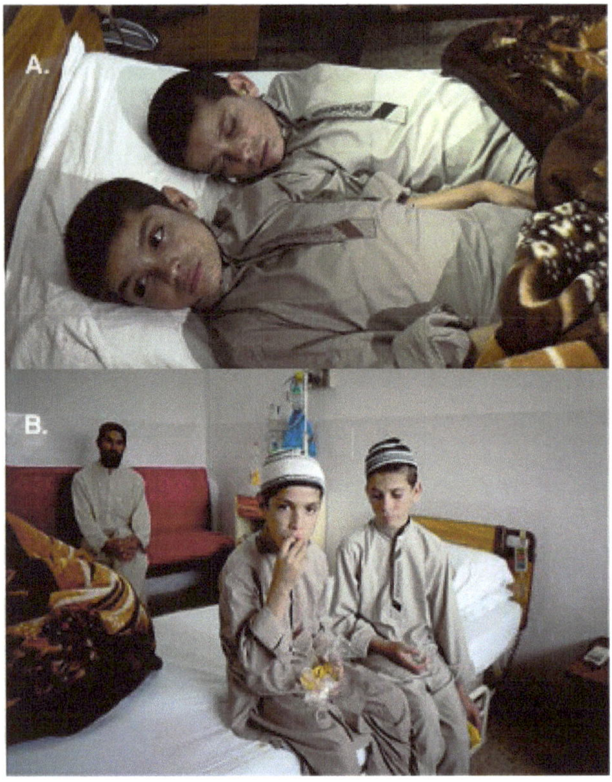

Fig. 27. 5: *Photographs of two brothers Abdul Rasheed, 9, front, and Shoaib Ahmed, 13, lie in a bed during night (top) and sitting comfortabily on the bed during Sunny day (bottom) .These two brothers are residents of Quetta,the capital of southwestern Baluchistan province,Pakistan .These kids are dependant of solar energy through one of the Kundalini Chakras*

Aged nine and 13, the boys are normal active children during the day. But once the sun goes down, they both lapse into a vegetative state -- unable to move or talk. Javed Akram, a professor of medicine at the Pakistan Institute of Medical Sciences, told The Associated Press on Thursday that he had no idea what was causing the symptoms.

"We took this case as a challenge. Our doctors are doing medical tests to determine why these kids remain active in the day but cannot open their eyes, why they cannot talk or eat when sun goes down," he said, as he visited the pair at his hospital. Akram said the government was providing free medical care to the siblings, who come from an impoverished family.

The brothers are undergoing extensive medical testing in the capital, Islamabad, and samples of their blood have been sent to overseas specialists for further examination, he said. Researchers are also collecting soil and air samples from the family's home village.

Mohammad Hashim, the father of the two brothers, comes from a village near Quetta, the capital of southwestern Baluchistan province. He and his wife are first cousins and two of their six children died at an early age. Their other two children have not displayed any unusual symptoms.

His simple theory: "I think my sons get energy from sun." But doctors have already dismissed the idea that sunlight plays a role, noting that the boys can move during the day even when kept in a dark room or during a rainstorm.During the day, 13-year old Shoaib Ahmed and his brother Abdul Rasheed did indeed seem normally active, energetic and cheerful as they emerged from their hospital room on Friday and walked to a nearby canteen to have tea."I will become a teacher," Shoaib Ahmed told the AP, while his younger brother said he wants to be an Islamic scholar

Bibliography and Acknowledgement

- Anonymous. Yoga relieves RA. Pulse of the Montana State Nurses Association 1991; May:2518.
- Anonymous. Yoga, meditation, help teen sex offenders. *J Psychosoc. Nurs. Ment. Health Serv*. 1999; **37**(6):6.
- Bernardi, L., Passino, C., Wilmerding, V., Dallam, G. M., Parker, D. L., Robergs, R. A., and Appenzeller, O. Breathing patterns and cardiovascular autonomic modulation during hypoxia induced by simulated altitude. *J Hypertens*. 2001; **19**(5):947-958.
- Bulavin, V. V., Kliuzhev, V. M., Kliachkin, L. M., Lakshmankumar, Zuikhin, N. D., and Vlasova, T. N. [Elements of yoga therapy in the combined rehabilitation of myocardial infarct patients in the functional recovery period]. *Vopr. Kurortol.Fizioter.Lech.Fiz Kult*. 1993;(4):7-9.
- Devi S, Chansouria JP, Malhotra OP, and *et al*. Certain neuroendocrine responses following the practice of Kundalini yoga. *Alternative Medicine* 1986; **1**(3):247-255.
- Friedell, A. Automatic attentive breathing in angina pectoris. *Minnesota Medicine* 1948; **31**:875-881.

- Jella, S. A. and Shannahoff-Khalsa, D. S. The effects of unilateral forced nostril breathing on cognitive performance. *Int. J Neurosci*. 1993; **73**(1-2):61-68.
- M. E. The effects of unilateral forced nostril breathing on cognition. *Int J Neurosci*. 1991; **57**(3-4):239-249.
- Maevskii, A. A. [A complex of breathing exercises (hatha yoga) to arrest the developing attacks of dyspnea in bronchial asthma*]. Klin Med (Mosk)* 1995; **73**(4):87-88.
- Nespor, K. [Occupational stress in health personnel and its prevention. Possible use of yoga]. Cas.Lek.Cesk. 8-3-1990; **129**(31):961-964
- Nespor, K. and Cs, emy L. [Alcohol and drugs in Central Europe--problems and possible solutions]. Cas.Lek.Cesk. 8-22-1994; **133**(16):483-486.
- Puskarich, C. A., Whitman, S., Dell, J., Hughes, J. R., Rosen, A. J., and Hermann, B. P. Controlled examination of effects of progressive relaxation training on seizure reduction. *Epilepsia* 1992; **33**(4):675-680.
- Reilly, R. Acute and prophylactic treatment of migraine. *Nurs. Times* 7-20-1994; **90**(29):35-36.
- Schumacher J. Rehab for the heart. *Yoga Journal* 1985;(May/June):15-17.
- Shannahoff-Khalsa DS, Ray LE, Levine S, and *et al*. Randomized controlled trial of yogic meditation techniques for patients with obsessive-compulsive disorder. CNS Spectrums 1999; 4(12):34-47.
- Shannahoff-Khalsa, D. Complementary healthcare practices. Stress management for gastrointestinal disorders: the use of kundalini yoga meditation techniques. *Gastroenterol.Nurs*. 2002; **25**(3):126-129.
- Shannahoff-Khalsa, D. S. An introduction to Kundalini yoga meditation techniques that are specific for the treatment of psychiatric disorders. *J Altern.Complement Med* 2004; **10**(1):91-101.
- Shannahoff-Khalsa, D. S. and Beckett, L. R. Clinical case report: efficacy of yogic techniques in the treatment of obsessive compulsive disorders. *Int J Neurosci*. 1996; **85**(1-2):1-17.
- Sharma, I. and Singh, P. Treatment of neurotic illnesses by yogic techniques. *Indian J Med Sci*. 1989; **43**(3):76-79.
- Telles, S. and Naveen, K. V. Yoga for rehabilitation: an overview. *Indian J Med Sci*. 1997; **51**(4):123-127.
- Usman Cheema published in Dawn, Rising and setting with the sun, Pakistan's 'solar kids' puzzle doctors May 13th, 2016
- Winterholler, M., Erbguth, F., and Neundorfer, B. [The use of alternative medicine by multiple sclerosis patients- patient characteristics and patterns of use]. *Fortschr.Neurol.Psychiatr*. 1997; **65**(12):555-561.

Application of Tai Chi & Qi Gong Discipline In Cardiovascular System

Tai Chi and Qi Gong are essential elements of traditional Chinese medicine (TCM). As part of that system of care, these graceful, slow-motion movements and breathing exercises are used extensively for health promotion and disease prevention. In this chapter, we will examine the applicability of these techniques to cardiovascular disease. Both Tai Chi and Qi Gong have been shown to have measurable impacts on the autonomic system, plasma catecholamines, cortisol, lipids, and blood pressure. In addition, measurements of oxygen uptake (maximum) (V°zmax), pulmonary capacity, plasma lactate levels, walking speeds, and muscle strength have all been positively affected. The slow, diaphragmatic breathing used in both Tai Chi and Qi Gong, similar to that used in yogic breathwork, has been found to be a stress mitigator and aid to improved oxygenation in multiple studies in cardiovascular and pulmonary health. Finally, the gentle activity ofTai Chi and Qi Gong have surprisingly been found to impact aerobic and fitness capacity, improve flexibility, reduce falls and fears of falling, and enhance general conditioning. By increasing activity levels, Tai Chi and Qi Gong can be a part of useful approaches to cardiac rehabilitation and heart failure (Fig. 25.1)

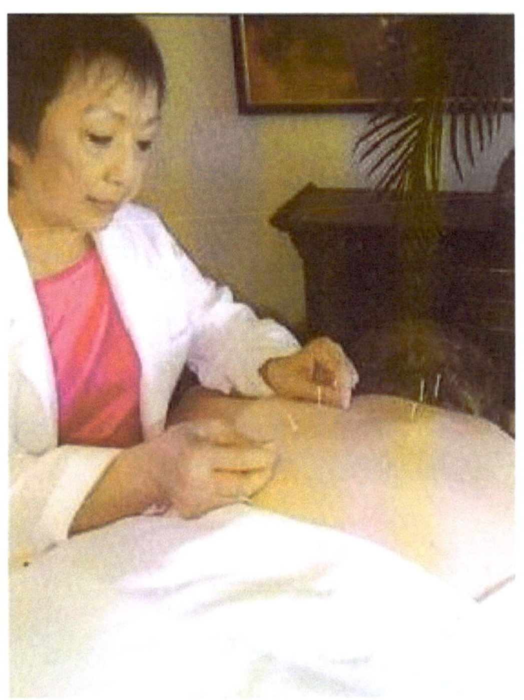

Fig. 25.1: *Photograph of Dr. Effie Chow PHD, She has practiced and taught Chi Gong, Taichi, acupuncture, and the Traditional Chinese Medicine (TCM) training for more than 40 years and trained thousands to be a self-healers or medical professionals to cure others. As an acupuncturist and TCM doctor herself, Dr. Chow has cured thousands of patients with acupuncture and medical Chi Gong. In July 2000, Dr. Chow was appointed by President Bill Clinton to be on the White House Commission on Complementary and Alternative Medicine Policy. She co-authored Miracle Healing From China - Qigong with Charles T McGee, MD. She combined the essence of the traditional Chinese Chi Gong with western medicine and created "Chow Integrated Healing System - Qigong Exercise*

Strengthen The Heart With Qi Gong

A 4,000-year-old technique may do wonders for heart health. From high blood pressure to cardiac rehabilitation, the ancient Chinese practice of Qi Gong has been proven to strengthen and revitalize the heart.

Overview of Qigong and Tai Chi

Qigong is, definitively, more ancient in origin than Tai Chi and it is the over-arching, more original discipline incorporating widely diverse practices designed to cultivate functional integrity and the enhancement of the life essence that the Chinese call Qi.

Both Qigong and Tai Chi sessions incorporate a wide range of physical movements, including slow, meditative, flowing, dance-like motions. In addition, they both can include sitting or standing meditation postures as well as either gentle or vigorous body shaking. Most importantly, both incorporate the purposeful regulation of both breath and mind coordinated with the regulation of the body. Qigong and Tai Chi are both based on theoretical principles that are inherent to traditional Chinese medicine (TCM) In the ancient teachings of health-oriented Qigong and Tai Chi, the instructions for attaining the state of enhanced Qi capacity and function point to the purposeful coordination of body, breath and mind (paraphrased here): "Mind the body and the breath, and then clear the mind to distill the Heavenly elixir within." This combination of self-awareness with self-correction of the posture and movement of the body, the flow of breath, and stilling of the mind, are thought to comprise a state which activates the natural self-regulatory (self-healing) capacity, stimulating the balanced release of endogenous neurohormones and a wide array of natural health recovery mechanisms which are evoked by the intentful integration of body and mind.

Despite variations among the myriad forms, we assert that health oriented Tai Chi and Qigong emphasize the same principles and practice elements. Given these similar foundations and the fashion in which Tai Chi has typically been modified for implementation in clinical research, we suggest that the research literature for these two forms of meditative movement should be considered as one body of evidence.

Qigong

Qigong translates from Chinese to mean, roughly, to cultivate or enhance the inherent functional (energetic) essence of the human being. It is considered to be the contemporary offspring of some of the most ancient (before recorded history) healing and medical practices of Asia. Earliest forms of Qigong make up one of the historic roots of contemporary Traditional Chinese Medicine (TCM) theory and practice. Many branches of Qigong have a health and medical focus and have been refined for well over 5000 years. Qigong purportedly allows individuals to cultivate the natural force or energy ("Qi") in TCM that is associated with physiological and psychological functionality. Qi is the conceptual foundation of TCM in acupuncture, herbal medicine and Chinese physical therapy. It is considered to be a ubiquitous resource of nature that sustains human well-being and assists in healing disease as well as (according to TCM theory) having fundamental influence on all life and even the orderly function of celestial mechanics and the laws of physics. Qigong exercises consist of a series of orchestrated practices including body posture/movement, breath practice, and meditation, all designed to enhance Qi function (that is, drawing upon natural forces to optimize and balance energy within) through the attainment of deeply focused and relaxed states. From the perspective of Western thought and science, Qigong practices activate naturally occurring physiological and psychological mechanisms of self-repair and health recovery.

Also considered part of the overall domain of Qigong is "external Qigong" wherein a trained medical Qigong therapist diagnoses patients according to the principles of TCM and uses "emitted Qi" to foster healing. Both internal Qigong (personal practice) and external Qigong (clinician emitted Qi) are seen as affecting the balance and flow of energy and enhancing functionality in the body and the mind. For the purposes of our review, we are focused only on the individual, internal Qigong practice of exercises performed with the intent of cultivating enhanced function, inner Qi that is ample and unrestrained. This is the aspect of Qigong that parallels what is typically investigated in Tai Chi research.

There are thousands of forms of Qigong practice that have developed in different regions of China during various historic periods and that have been created by many specific teachers and schools. Some of these forms were designed for general health enhancement purposes and some for specific TCM diagnostic categories. Some were originally developed as rituals for spiritual practice, and others to empower greater skill in the martial arts. An overview of the research literature pertaining to internal Qigong yields more than a dozen forms that have been studied as they relate to health outcomes (e.g., Guo-lin, ChunDoSunBup, Vitality or Bu Zheng Qigong, Eight Brocade, Medical Qigong)

The internal Qigong practices generally tested in health research (and that are addressed in this review), incorporate a range of simple movements (repeated and often flowing in nature), or postures (standing or sitting) and include a focused state of relaxed awareness and a variety of breathing techniques that accompany the movements or postures. A key underlying philosophy of the practice is that any form of Qigong has an effect on the cultivation of balance and harmony of Qi, positively influencing the human energy complex (Qi channels/pathways) which functions as a holistic, coherent and mutually interactive system.

Tai Chi

Tai Chi translates to mean, "Grand Ultimate", and in the Chinese culture, it represents an expansive philosophical and theoretical notion which describes the natural world (i.e., the universe) in the spontaneous state of dynamic balance between mutually interactive phenomena including the balance of light and dark, movement and stillness, waves and particles. Tai Chi, the exercise, is named after this concept and was originally developed both as a martial art (Tai Chi Chuan or taijiquan) and as a form of meditative movement. The practice of Tai Chi as meditative movement is expected to elicit functional balance internally for healing, stress neutralization, longevity, and personal tranquility. This form of Tai Chi is the focus of this review.

For numerous, complex sociological and political reasons, Tai Chi has become one of the best known forms of exercise or practice for refining Qi and is purported to enhance physiological and psychological function. The one factor that appears to differentiate Tai Chi from Qigong is that traditional Tai Chi is typically performed as a highly choreographed, lengthy, and complex series of movements, while health enhancement Qigong is typically a simpler, easy to learn, more repetitive practice. However, even the longer forms of Tai Chi incorporate many movements that are similar to Qigong exercises. Usually, the more complex Tai Chi routines include Qigong exercises as a warm-up, and emphasize the same basic principles for practice, that is, the three regulations of body focus, breath focus and mind focus. Therefore Qigong and Tai Chi, in the health promotion and wellness context, are operationally equivalent.

Tai Chi as Defined in the Research Literature

It is especially important to note that many of the RCTs investigating what is described as Tai Chi (for health enhancement), are actually not the traditional, lengthy, complex practices that match the formal definition of traditional Tai Chi. The Tai Chi used in research of both disease prevention and as a complement to medical intervention is often a "modified" Tai Chi (e.g., Tai Chi Easy, Tai Chi Chih, or "short forms" that greatly reduce the number of movements to be learned). The modifications generally simplify the practice, making the movements more like most health oriented Qigong exercises that are simple and repetitive, rather than a lengthy choreographed series of Tai Chi movements that take much longer to learn (and, for many participants, reportedly delay the experience of "settling" into the relaxation response). A partial list of examples of modified Tai Chi forms from the RCTs in the review are : balance exercises inspired by Tai Chi, Tai Chi for arthritis, 5 movements from Sun Tai ChiTai Chi Six Form, Yang Eight Form Easy, and Yang Five Core Movements.,

In 2003, a panel of Qigong and Tai Chi experts was convened by the University of Illinois and the Blueprint for Physical Activity to explore this very point. The expert panel agreed that it is appropriate to modify (simplify) Tai Chi to more efficiently disseminate the benefits to populations in need of cost effective, safe and gentle methods of physical activity and stress reduction. These simplified forms of Tai Chi are very similar to the forms of Qigong used in health research. For this reason, it is not only reasonable, but a critical contribution to the emerging research dialogue to review the RCTs that explore the health benefits resulting from both of these practices together, as one comprehensive evidence base for the meditative movement practices originating from China.

Fundamentals of Tai Chi and QiGong in TCM (Fig. 25.2)

A meaningful discussion of Tai Chi and Qi Gong must first begin with an overview of the foundations of TCM. Many different models and approaches, ranging from a metaphysical paradigm to strictly neurophysiologic explanations, have been used to describe the mechanisms underlying TCM. This chapter, will attempt to integrate biomedical and basic metaphysical perspective

A complete system of health care that has been practiced in China for thousands of years, TCM is based on the fundamental concept that an animating life-force or energy exists giving us the power to walk, talk, think, and achieve our goals. In India, this life-force is called Prana. InJapan, it is called Ki. In China, it is called Chi or Qi (pronounced chee). Along with acupuncture, herbs, food therapy, and Tui Na (Chinese bodywork), Tai Chi and Qi Qong are primary components of TCM. The concept of Qi has been discussed by Chinese philosophers throughout time. The term "Qi" may be defined narrowly (i.e., bioelectromagnetic energy existing within the human body) or broadly (i.e., universal energy existing within and between all things). In the Chinese language, the symbol representing Qi indicates something that is simultaneously material and immaterial, and some authors have described Qi as "matter + energy" or "mattergy." Another defini tion of Qi is that it is "matter on the verge of becoming energy; energy at the point of materializing." Note the dynamic, operational descriptions of Qi.

In ancient Chinese thought, Qi was believed to be a fundamental, vital sub stance of the universe and necessary for the human body to function. It was believed that all phenomena were produced by its changes.

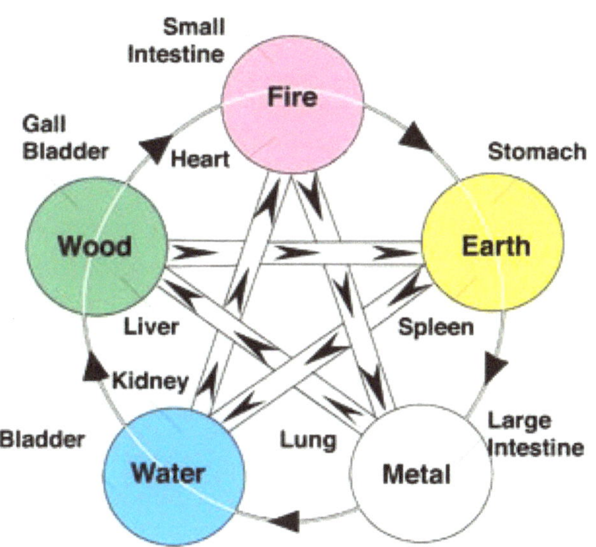

Fig. 25.2: *Showing KO Cycle balancing the functions of various systemic organs and five elements of the body such as Fire,Wood,Earth,Water and Metal . Acupuncture, herbal medicine, and Tai Chi/QiGong use the Zang Fu system to understand how the body, mind, and emotions integrate. A problem with a particular organ may have emotional symptoms. Likewise, a chronic emotional state may have a physical impact on the organs. The following list explains the Zang Fu connection between organs and emotions commonly related to imbalances with those organs or their energy channels : Liver = Depression, anger Heart = Excess joy (such as manic behavior), excess mental function Spleen = Obsession Lung = Anguish, grief, melancholy, Kidney = Fear, fright*

There are many different types of Qi that help maintain normal activities. They are categorized according to source, function, and distribution. According to classical TCM theory, Qi flows along organized pathways known as channels or meridians, and balanced, unobstructed flow throughout the system is necessary for a state of good health.

Ancient Chinese scholars viewed humans as a microcosmic reflection of the universe. A state of mental, physical, emotional, and spiritual good health, known as Wu Chi, is achieved when one becomes aware that all things are connected and that not only do we exist within the world, but the world exists within us. Daily practice of Qi Gong and/ or Tai Chi over a number of years can lead one to achieve a state of Wu Chi. Also fundamental to TCM is yin-yang theory. Yin and yang are relative opposing, positive and negative forces that can be applied to all things, including the human body. Hot/cold, internal/external, malelfemale are examples of yin and yang. Yin always possesses some characteristics or seeds of yang, and yang always possesses characteristics or seeds of yin. Yin and yang forces are interdependent, support each other, and may be simultaneously opposite and yet complementary. Yin and yang also consume each other and may, under certain circumstances, transform into each other. According to TCM, health problems develop when there is an imbalance in yin and yang forces.

Yin conditions result when there is a Qi deficiency, and yang conditions result when there is excess Qi that needs to be reduced . In TCM, it is said that, "The Heart governs Blood and the Lungs govern Qi."* The relationship between Heart and Lungs is thus the relationship between Blood and Qi. Blood is considered yin in comparison *to* Qi (i.e., denser and more material). Qi has more yang characteristics than blood and is the energetic force behind blood circulation (i.e., relatively immaterial *to* Blood). It is important *to* note that the terms Heart, Lung, and Blood have broader meanings in TCM than in Western biomedicine. "Heart" not only refers *to* the organ, but to additional functional relationships as well. For example, it is said in TCM that "the Heart houses the mind." Interestingly, recent research! has confirmed the link between cardiovascular risk factors and Alzheimer's disease.

Similarly, the concept of Blood is much broader in TCM than in biomedicine. Blood is more dense and therefore considered a yin form of Qi. It circulates continuously through blood vessels as well as the meridian pathways, although the latter carries relatively more Qi while the former carries relatively more Blood. The major functions of Blood in TCM are to nourish, maintain, and moisten various parts of the body and to provide the material foundation for mental, emotional, and spiritual activities. Qi and Blood are inseparable. Without Qi, Blood would merely be an inert fluid.

Powerful Ancient Qigong Exercises for Cultivating Healing Energy in the Body

What is Qigong and Why is it Essential?

Qigong (pronounced:chee-gun), which combines meditative and physically active elements, is the basic exercise system within Chinese medicine. Qigong exercises are designed to help you preserve your Jing, strengthen and balance the flow of Qi energy, and enlighten your Shen.

This is a sequence of 8 exercises which, aside from moving our whole body, have therapeutic qualities, like all of the Qigong exercises. They are called BA Di M GUM *(eight jewelry pieces)* and their name is indicative of their importance for improving the physical and mental health of those who practice them.

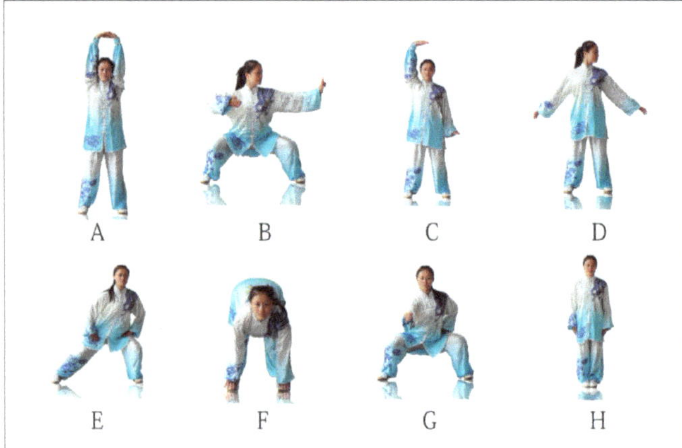

Fig. 25.3: *Ba Duan Jin exercise program. (A) Prop up the sky with hands to regulate the triple energizer. (B) Draw a bow on both sides, like shooting a vulture. (C) Raise single arm to regulate spleen (Pi) and stomach (Wei). (D) Look back to treat five strains and seven impairments. (E) Sway head and buttocks to expel heart (Xin)-fire. (F) Pull toes with both hands to reinforce the kidney (Shen) and waist. (G) Clench fists and look with eyes wide open to enhance strength and stamina. (H) Rise and fall on tip toes to prevent all diseases.*

A. First exercise:

Triple Heater is a term used in traditional Chinese Medicine to describe the upper, middle and lower portions of the body. So the first exercise acts beneficially on the eyes, ears, face and respiratory functions of the upper heater. The internal organs and digestive functions of the middle heater strengthen the kidneys and reproductive organs of the lower heater.

1. This exercise is performed standing.
2. The fingers of both hands are intertwined at the height of the abdomen, and then arms are moved up until hands are above the head while rising on ones tiptoes.
3. When arms are moved up, one inhales, and when returning to the original position one exhales.

B. Second exercise

This exercise fortifies the muscles and tendons of shoulders and arms and when lungs expand, the capacity of the practitioner's lungs increases. The practitioner takes a side step to stand in the horse position with 70% of his body weight on his front foot. The arms must move as ifthey were opening a bow, while the eyes always follow the arrow.

C. Third exercise:

The objective of this exercise is to promote harmony between the spleen (a Yin organ) and the stomach (a complementary Yan organ) and to promote the circulation of energy throughout internal organs.

The person stands with one arm stretched up in a vertical position.

D. Fourth exercise:

This exercise strengthens the neck and chest muscles as well as the lungs, thus preventing respiratory disorders. In a standing position, keeping his/her back straight, the practitioner turns to one side and then to the other one trying to look back, but without moving his waist.

E. Fifth exercise:

In this exercise, movements are firm, they increase the CHI and strengthen the body metabolism.

In the square horse position, the practitioner firmly holds his fists against his waist with his elbows turned in. Then he moves one of his fists to the front, and then the other one keeping his muscles firm and a serious and angry look.

F. Sixth exercise:

This exercise acts on digestion and circulation; it prevents and cures heart diseases and blood pressure disorders. With legs slightly bent, like in the square horse position, and with hands resting on the knees, the practitioner moves his body describing circular movements as wide as possible.

G. Seventh exercise.

This exercise helps you keep your body in shape and your nervous system strong and young.

Stand on the tip of your toes and bounce seven times. Do ten sets.

H. Eighth and last exercise:

This exercise keeps your waist flexible, stimulates your kidneys and straightens your backbone.

In a standing position, bend down at the level of your waist and touch the tips of your toes.Do not bend your knees

Table 25.1: *Tai Chi Protocol outline of exercises and duration*

Week	Activities	Approximate Duration (min)
1–2*	Check-in	2
	Tai Chi Warm-up Exercises—Standing	
	Shaking to Awaken the Body	
	Tai Chi Swinging and Drumming the Body	
	Swinging Up and Down	
	Spiraling the Waist	
	Tai Chi Warm-up Exercises—	
	Seated Mindful stretching	
	Lower Extremities (feet, ankles, knees)	38
	Upper Extremities (hands, arms, shoulders)	
	Spinal Cord Breathing	
	Washing with Qi from the Heaven	
	Tan Tien Breathing	
	Introduction to Tai Chi Movement #1:	15
	Raising the Power	
	Tai Chi Cool-Down Exercises	5
	Self-massage and meridian tapping	
	Washing with chi from heavens	
3–8	Check-in	2
	Tai Chi Warm-up Exercises	18
	Breathing Exercises	10
	Review and practice Tai Chi Movement #1	5
	Learn and practice Tai Chi Movements #2 and #3	20
	Push and Withdraw	
	Wave Hands Like Clouds	
	Tai Chi Cool-Down Exercises	5
9–12	Check-in	2
	Tai Chi Warm-up Exercises	13
	Breathing Exercises	10
	Review and practice Tai Chi Movements #1–3	10
	Learn and practice Tai Chi Movements # 4–6	20
	Brush Knee Twist Step	
	Cross hands	
	Tai Chi Cool-Down Exercises	5
Plus Group only:		
13–24	Check-in	2
	Tai Chi Warm-up Exercises	13
	Breathing Exercises	10
	Review and practice Tai Chi Movements #1–5	30
	Tai Chi Cool-Down Exercises	5

***Note:** A 10-minute introductory lecture will be given in the first class outlining the goals and structure of the intervention, as well as participant responsibilities

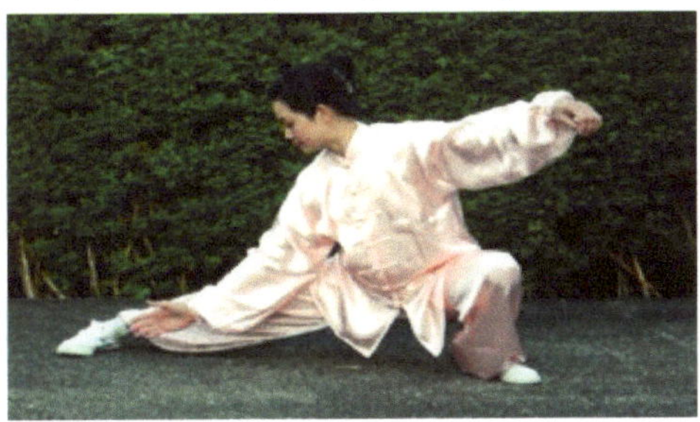

Fig. 25.4: *Tai Chi and Qigong are forms of low impact exercise and suitable for all ages, a form of exercise to increases stamina, and improves the body's flexibility, balance and coordination , as well as teaches you to relax and improves the flow of your inner energy, (Chi) Tai Chi consists of a series of slow, balanced movements. Tai Chi is the most widely known and is practiced by one in five of the world's population*

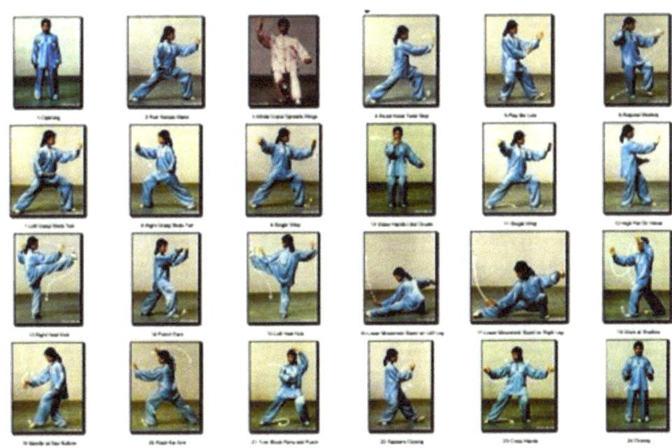

Fig. 25.5: *Illustrations showing 24 Forms of Tai Chi chuan exercises*

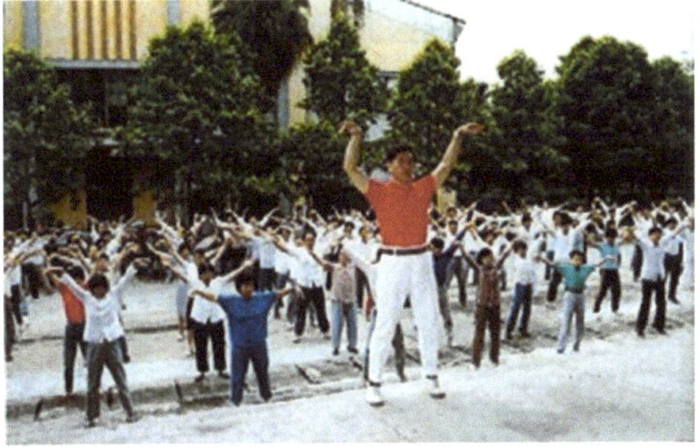

Fig 25.6: *Photograph showing People practicing Tai Chi Qigong Shibashi in China*

Its dynamic exercises and meditations have Yin and Yang aspects : The Yin is being it; the Yang is doing it. Yin qigong exercises are expressed through relaxed stretching, visualization, and breathing.

Yang qigong exercises are expressed in a more aerobic or dynamic way. They are particularly effective for supporting the immune system. In China, Qigong is used extensively for people with cancer. Qigong's physical and spiritual routines move Qi energy through the Twelve Primary Channels and Eight Extra Channels, balancing it, smoothing the flow, and strengthening it. Chinese medicine uses Qigong exercises to maintain health, prevent illness, and extend longevity because it is a powerful tool for maintaining and restoring harmony to the Organ Systems, Essential Substances, and Channels. Qigong is also used for non-medical purposes, such as for fighting and for pursuing enlightenment.

Anyone of any age or physical condition can do Qigong. You don't have to be able to run a marathon or bench press a car to pursue healthfulness and enjoy the benefits.

When you design your qigong exercise / meditation practice, you will pick what suits your individual constitution. Some of us are born with one type of constitution; some with another. We each have inherited imbalances that we cannot control but with which we must work. That's why for some people it is easier to achieve balance and strength than it is for others. But whatever your nature, Qigong can help you become the most balanced you can be.

Qigong is truly a system for a lifetime. That's why so many people over age sixty in China practice Qigong and Tai Chi. The effects may be powerful, but the routines themselves are usually gentle. Even the dynamic exercises-some of which explode the Qi energy- use forcefulness in different ways than in the West. The following are some effects of Qigong exercises practiced regularly.

The Benefits of Regular Practice

Maintaining Health

Qigong exercises help maintain health by creating a state of mental and physical calmness, which indicates that the Qi energy is balanced and harmonious. This allows the mind/body/spirit to function most efficiently, with the least amount of stress.

When you start practicing Qigong exercises, the primary goal is to concentrate on letting go, letting go, letting go. That's because most imbalance comes from holding on to too much for too long. Most of us are familiar with physical strength of muscles, and when we think about exercising, we think in terms of tensing muscles. Qi energy is different. Qi strength is revealed by a smooth, calm, concentrated effort that is free of stress and does not pit one part of the body against another.

qigong exercises are often used to develop and strengthen the energy body in preparation for higher states and stages of consciousness. photo : lerina winter

Managing Illness

It's harder to remedy an illness than to prevent it, and Qigong has powerful preventive effects. However, when disharmony becomes apparent, Qigong exercises also can play a crucial role in restoring harmony.

Qigong movement and postures are shaped by the principle of Yin/Yang : the complementary interrelationship of qualities such as fast and slow, hard and soft, Excess or Deficiency, and External and Internal. Qigong exercises use these contrasting and complementary qualities to restore harmony to the Essential Substances, Organ Systems, and Channels.

Extending Longevity

In China, the use of Qigong exercises for maintaining health and curing illness did not satisfy those Buddhists and Daoists who engaged in more rigorous self-discipline. They wanted to be able to amplify the power of Qi energy and make the internal Organ Systems even stronger. This arcane use of Qigong was confined mostly to monasteries and the techniques have not been much publicized. One of the most difficult and profoundly effective techniques is called Marrow Washing Qigong. Practitioners learn to master the intricate manipulation of Qi—infusing the Eight Extraordinary Channels with Qi, and then guiding the Qi energy through the Channels to the bone marrow to cleanse and energize it. The result, according to religious tradition, is that monks can extend their life span to 150 years or more. The Daoists have a saying, "One hundred and twenty years means dying young."

Although few if any of us can devote our lives to the stern practices of the monks, the health benefits of Qigong exercises certainly do improve the quality of life of everyone who practices it.

Waging Combat

Around 500 CE, in the Liang Dynasty, Qigong was adopted by various martial artists to increase stamina and power. For the most part, the breathing, concentration, and agility were assets to the warriors and improved their well-being.

Attaining Enlightenment

Buddhist monks who use Qigong exercises in their pursuit for higher consciousness and enlightenment concentrate on the Qigong's ability to influence their Shen. Mastering Marrow Washing allows the practitioner to gain so much control over the flow of Qi energy that he or she can direct it into the forehead and elevate consciousness. The rest of us can enjoy the influence of Qigong on our Shen (spiritual body/energy), but at a lower level.

Whatever reason you use Qigong, the practice should raise your Qi to a higher state if you increase concentration, practice controlled breathing, and execute the Qigong routines.

The Foundational Techniques

Here are the basic Qigong exercise techniques.

Concentration

Concentration leads to and results from Qi energy awareness, breathing techniques, and Qigong exercises. It is a process of focusing in and letting go at the same time. Focusing does not mean that you wrinkle up your forehead and strain to pay attention.

Instead, through deep relaxation and expanding your consciousness, you are able to create a frame of mind that is large enough to encompass your entire mind – body – spirit's functions, yet focused enough to allow outside distractions, worries, and everyday hassles to drift away.

This inward focus that expands outward to join you with the rhythms of the universe epitomizes Yin/Yang. Yin energy tends to be more expansive, and Yang energy more concentrated. You discover your Yin/Yang balance by treating Yin and Yang as ingredients in a recipe : Add a bit more Yin, toss in a dash of Yang to make the mixture suit your constitution or circumstances.

Some people need more or less Yin or Yang, depending upon the situation. 'Extending the Qi exercise' outlined below provides a clear demonstration of how you can practice establishing your balanced blend of Yin and Yang.

You will find that as you do qigong exercise and meditation you become more adept at this form of concentration, because it is the natural expression of the practice. As you learn to concentrate more effectively, you will find you have greater power to affect Qi energy through the various Qigong exercises in this chapter or through the use of other focused meditations and Tai Chi.

Breathing

In the sixth century BCE, Lao Tzu first described breathing techniques as a way to stimulate Qi energy. From there, two types of Qigong breathing exercises evolved : Buddha's Breath and Daoist's Breath. Both methods infuse the body with Qi and help focus meditation.

Buddha's Breath: (Fig. 25.7)

When you inhale, extend your abdomen, filling it with air. When you exhale, contract you abdomen, expelling the air from the bottom of your lungs first and then pushing it up and out until your abdomen and chest are deflated. You may want to practice inhaling for a slow count of eight and exhaling for a count of sixteen. As you breathe in and out, imagine inviting your Qi energy to flow through the Channels. Use your mind to invite the Qi to flow; you want to guide the flow, not tug at it or push it.

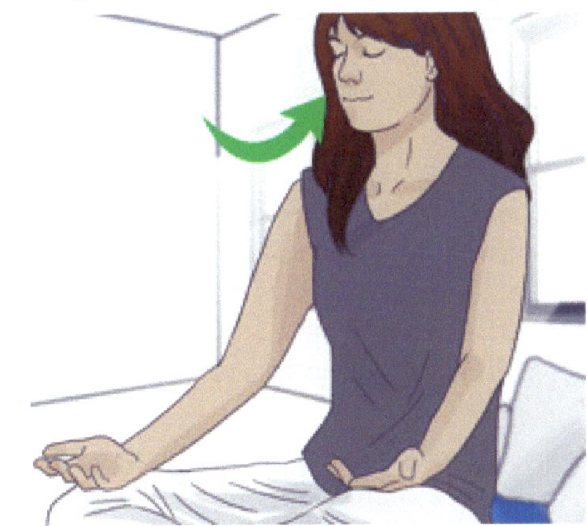

Fig. 25.7: *showing breath Meditation (Anapanasati)*

Daoist's Breath: (Fig. 29.8) The pattern is the opposite of above. When you breathe in, you contract your abdominal muscles. When you exhale, you relax the torso and lungs.

As you travel through these steps, remember that Qigong is a process of building awareness. However you are comfortable doing the routines is what's right for you at that time.

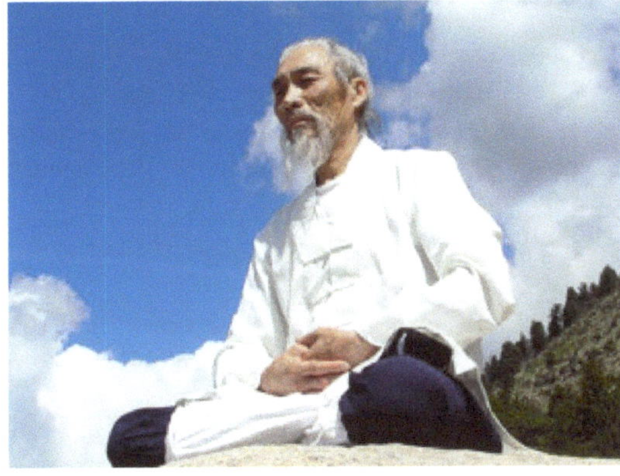

Fig. 25.8: *Breathing (Shun Hu Xi) is the best place to start.*

Effective meditation and qigong both require good breathing skills; this lesson will give you a method that you can use every time you start your practice. This exercise takes about 5 or 6 minutes to learn, and after a few times you can tune up in about 2 minutes.

Advanced Qigong Breathing Exercise

Breathing can direct Qi energy through the body like the wind filling the sails of a ship. Qigong breathing exercises can invigorate or sedate, depending on how you use them.

On alternate days, practice the following routine, using Buddha's Breath and Daoist's Breath breathing techniques.

1. Sit on the floor with your legs crossed in lotus or cross-legged style. This is important so that Qi energy does not enter and become Stagnant in the lower body, but follows the breathing path through your torso and your head.
2. Inhale to a count of four to eight, depending on what you are comfortable with. For Buddha's Breath, extend your belly, filling it up from the bottom. For Taoist's Breath, inhale, contracting your abdomen, and exhale, letting your abdomen relax outward.
3. As you inhale, turn your attention to your nose. Guide the Qi energy downward from your nose toward the Dantian, 1 to 2 inches (2.5 to 5 cm) below the navel. Women should not concentrate on the Dantian during their periods. Concentrate on your solar plexus instead.
4. Exhale to a count of eight to sixteen and move the Qi energy down the torso, around your pelvic region, and up to your tailbone.
5. Inhale and move the Qi up the back to the top of your shoulders.
6. Exhale and move the Qi up the back of your head and back to your nose.
7. If you cannot feel the Qi clearly, patience and practice will make it more apparent.
8. Once you are comfortable with this Qigong practice, you may increase the pace by completing the cycle in one inhalation and one exhalation.
9. On the inhalation, move Qi energy from your nose to your tailbone. On the exhalation, move Qi from your tailbone back to your nose.

Tai Chi Exercise for Patients with Cardio-vascular Conditions and Risk Factors:

A Systematic Review

The available studies suggest that tai chi exercise may have beneficial effects for patients with cardiovascular conditions and some cardiovascular risk factors, although the literature to date is limited. Very few studies specifically examine patients with coronary artery disease or heart failure, although the available studies report positive results in both functional and physiological parameters. In investigations of patients with cardiovascular risk factors, most information is available on blood pressure effects and hypertension. The data on tai chi's effect on lipids and glucose metabolism are unclear. More than half of the studies in this review were published in Chinese and offer data that have historically been excluded from other reviews.

Clinical Implications and Advantages of Tai Chi

Table 25.2: *Current Indications for Including Tai Chi Qi Cong Practice as Part of a Cardiovascular Fitness Prescription*

Primary Prevention/Health and Wellness Promotion	Treatment of Early and Mild Cardiovascular Diseas	Cardiac Rehabilitation and Secondary Prevention	Treatment for Advanced Cardiac Disease
Stress reduction, cognitive enhancement, self-efficacy	Hypertension, dyslipidemia, anxiety, depression, stress reduction	post-myocardial infarction, post coronary bypass, angioplasty/ stene-adjunective to erobic training	Chronic heart failure-adjunctive to standard medical treatment and fitness prescription
Body awareness	Falling and fear of falling	Improved blood pressure and lipid profile, stress reduction	Low-intensity easily achievable cardiac demand
Improved lipid profile, general conditioning	Improved general conditioning	Improved cordiopulmonary funtion and musculoskeletal conditioning	Treatment of cardiopulmonary and musculoskeletal deconditioning
Flexibiligy, balance, leg strength	Reduction in epinephrine, norepinephirine, cortisol	Increased confidence in physical funtion,Self-efficincy and acceptable for sustained physical activity.	Increased sense of self efficancy physical capability, balance, leg strengh

Given the existing evidence, tai chi exercise may be a reasonable adjunct to conventional care. It may be appropriate for those unable or unwilling to engage in other forms of physical activity, or as a bridge to more rigorous exercise programs in frail or de-conditioned patients. Patients with early detection of cardiovascular risk factors (eg, borderline hypertension) may be reluctant to begin drug therapy and non-pharmacological approaches are often welcomed. These lifestyle interventions have been recognized as important and effective strategies for primary prevention.42 In addition, patients with either pre-hypertension or established hypertension, who otherwise feel well, may be less motivated and find it difficult to engage in and maintain a regular exercise regimen. Finding an appropriate, non-threatening, easy-to-perform activity that patients will maintain is critical to therapeutic success. Clinical trials have reported excellent compliance with tai chi interventions, and suggest that tai chi may promote exercise self-efficacy.43,44 Likewise, exercise is a well-recognized and effective strategy for secondary prevention in patients with established cardiovascular disease. Unfortunately, studies have continued to show that conventional cardiac rehabilitation programs are underutilized.45 Therapies such as tai chi may offer patients additional options, whether as an adjunct to formal cardiac rehabilitation, as a part of maintenance therapy, or as an exercise alternative at any point along this continuum.

Specific Cardiovascular disorders which can be managed with Tai Chi/ Q i Gong

Hypertension

Although blood pressure is a commonly measured outcome in many Tai Chi/ Qi Gong studies, few published studies examine patients with hypertension.

An older, frequently cited study by Young compared a 12-week Tai Chi intervention to a moderate-intensity conventional exercise program (walking and aerobic dance) in patients with Stage I hypertension. Investigators reported decreases in blood pressure in both groups (systolic/diastolic : change of -7.0/-2.4 with Tai Chi versus -8.4/-3.2 mm Hg with conventional exercise). There were no significant differences between groups, suggesting comparable effects of each intervention. Although class attendance was comparable among the two groups, the home exercise frequency was greater in the Tai Chi grou

A few studies in patients with hypertension also measured lipid profile. Tsai et al randomized 76 individuals with Stage I hypertension to either 12 weeks ofTai Chi or to usual care. In addition to decreases in systolic blood pressure (-15 vs. +6 mm *Hg,p* <.001) and diastolic blood pressure (-9vs. +3 mm *Hg,p* <.05), investigators reported decrease in total cholesterol (-15 vs. +4 mg/dL, *p* <.01), triglyceride (TG) (-24vs. +9 mg/dL,p <.001), and low-density lipoprotein (LDL) (-20 vs. +3 mg/dL, *p* ~.01), and increases in high-density lipoprotein (llDL) (+4 vs. -1 mg/dL, *p* <.05) compared to controls. In addition, authors reported improvements in anxiety scores in those who practiced Tai Chi. Similarly, Lee studied the effects of Shuxinpingxuegong, a particular style of Qi Gong developed in China specifically for circulatory system disease. About 36 individuals with essential bypertension (mean age 53, mean BP approximately 150/95, mean total cholesterol approximately 190 mg/dL) were randomized to either 8 weeks of Qi Gong or to usual care. Investigators reported significant decreases in blood pressure (-15/-12 mm Hg with Qi Gong vs. *+11+2* mm Hg with usual care, *p* <.01), decreases in total cholest- (-10 vs. +1 mg/dL, *p* <.05), increases in HDL (+4 vs. 0 mg/dL, *p* <.01) and increases in apolipoprotein 1 (Apo-AI) (+27 vs. +2 mg/dL, *p* <.05).20

In a review article of Qi Gong and hypertension by Mayer, 70 studies were found examining Qi Gong for hypertension. Most, as mentioned above, came from conference proceedings, book excerpts, or informal reports. Many studies were incompletely described with varied levels of methodological detail, and most were not subject to peer-review. Of the 30 "representative" articles reviewed, 5 did report a randomized design. Reported improvements included blood pressure, microcirculation, blood flow, blood viscosity, platelet aggregation, left ventricular function, and lipid profile.

Coronary heart disease

As with hypertension, relatively few studies are available specifically in patients with known coronary disease. However, the existing literature suggests that Tai Chi/Qi Gong may be a viable option for cardiac rehabilitation. Two older, yet classic studies investigated patients after cardiac ischemic events. Channer randomized 126 patients 3 weeks after discharge following an acute myocardial infarction to one of three groups : Tai Chi/Qi Gong, a conventional aerobic "exercise to music" group, or a nonexercise cardiac support group. Patients attended Tai Chi/Qi Gong class twice a week for 3 weeks, then once a week for the remaining 5 weeks. Mean baseline blood pressure was approximately 133/84. At the end of 8 weeks, investigators reported significant within group decreases in systolic blood pressure similarly in both exercise groups, and decreases in diastolic blood pressure only with Tai Chi (each *p* <.01). In addition, the Tai Chi group showed a trend in decreasing resting HR. Compliance was higher with Tai Chi compared to aerobic exercise (82% vs. 73%), while attendance at support groups was poor (8%).

In a smaller study of 20 patients, Lan examined individuals after coronary artery bypass graft surgery that had completed a postoperative Phase II conventional cardiac rehabilitation program. They were then assigned to either a I-year Tai Chi program or a home-based exercise program that included walking at a nearby park. After 1 year of training, the Tai Chi group showed significant improvements in cardiorespiratory function, with 10.3% increase in peak V02 ($p < .05$), 11 % increase in peak Work rate ($p < .05$), while the control group had no change or slight decreases in function. Compliance was greater with Tai Chi.

More recently, in Stenlund's study, 95 elder patients with documented coronary artery disease were randomized to either a 12-week Qi Gong and group education class or to usual care. Classes consisted of 1 hour Qi Gong and 2 hours of group discussion on various topics related to cardiac disease in the elderly. At the end of 12 weeks, patients increased their self-reported activity levels (p =.01) and showed improvements in the right-sided one leg stance (p = .03), box climb test (p = .04), stand and flex tests (p = .02), as measures of balance and coordination. Fear of falling did not change, although most reported

Safety

Collectively, these studies suggest that tai chi may be safe for patients with cardiovascular disease. The three studies with higher-risk coronary patients reported no adverse effects.13–15 In addition, exercise intensity of tai chi can be easily modified. Many studies have reported metabolic equivalents of 1.5–4.0 (approximately low-moderate intensity aerobic exercise), which may be a reasonable exercise level for even the more deconditioned cardiac patient.

Heart-Boosting Qigong Exercises

There are three heart-boosting qigong exercises that only take few minutes to perform. These qigong techniques are specifically effective in relieving constriction and compression that occur in blood vessels.

Proper Posture

It begins with proper postural alignments (in standing Qigong exercise). Later on, this can be applied on every daily activity such as when sitting in front of your work desk. By standing properly, with focus on the spine, you get rid of the kinks out of your blood vessels. The blood vessel will return to its ideal position, letting blood to flow freely and unimpeded.

Lengthening Routine

When the body is properly aligned, lengthening the spine, going to the fingers, head and toes will further aid blood flow, release any blocked arteries and take off excess pressure to the heart.

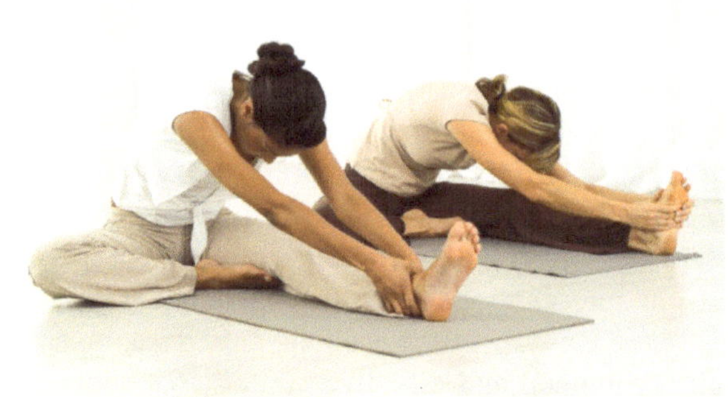

Fig. 25.9: *Photographs of two young ladies performing stretching exercises*

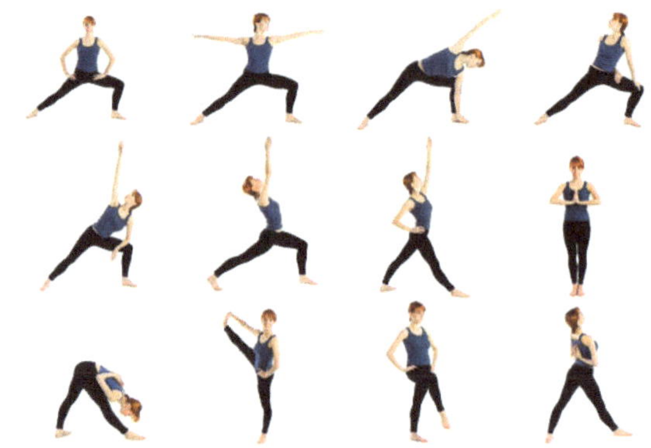

Fig. 25.10: *showing 12 body stretching exercises in different poses as directed by a trainer*

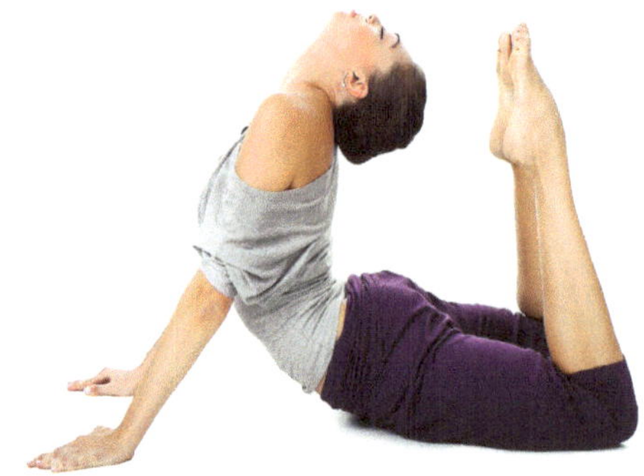

Fig. 25.11: *Illustrations of spinal stretching exercise to lengthen and alleviate compression of the spine.*

Qigong healing key point: Stretch the vertebrae by bowing and arching the spine along with deep diaphragmatic breathing.

Deep Diaphragmatic Breathing: When proper posture and lengthening exercise are applied into daily practice, the next and last step part to focus on is the breathing. Deep qigong breathing is very important to increase blood flow to the arteries. Once the blood circulates all over the body, it also takes burden off the heart. This lowers the stress and tension that build up in the heart.

Qigong Exercises for Life

There are seemingly plenty of Qigong exercises to improve circulation and protect the heart, and the best way to start is to practice proper body alignment at all times to prevent kinks in your veins and arteries. Lengthening exercises will stretch the 'tubes' or blood vessels so blood and Qi can flow freely and unimpeded. Along with deep breathing, your blood will deliver nutrients and oxygen that is necessary for every cell of the body.

Blood pressure and heart rate

A few studies have measured the longitudinal effects of Tai Chi/Qi Gong on blood pressure in normotensive individuals. For example, Thornton studied 34 relatively inactive middle-aged Chinese women assigned to either 12 weeks of Tai Chi or to usual activity, reporting decreases in both systolic and diastolic blood pressure (-9.7 and 7.5 mm Hg, respectively) and improvements in functional reach and flexibility. Baseline blood pressure in these women was in the normal range (mean *122/80* mm Hg). Authors suggest that Tai Chi may be a viable option for healthy aging, given prognostic significance of elevated blood pressure in later life.26 The immediate clinical significance of the blood pressure changes in normotensive individuals, however, is unclear.

Other studies have examined the acute effects ofTai Chi on blood pressure and heart rate. Perhaps not surprisingly, most effects reported are what one would expect with conventional exercise. Heart rate increases steadily with Tai Chi until a "maximal" steady state is achieved (usually 50-74% of maximal heart rate on bicycle or treadmill stress test). Blood pressure also may increase acutely in response to the physical aerobic activity. A few studies have reported that Tai Chi practitioners have a more rapid return to baseline resting values after exercise.

On the other hand, Lee has reported acute effects of Qi Gong training that is more similar to what one would expect with quiet, motionless meditation. In a small observational trial, 12 healthy volunteers were studied during Korean Qi-training (ChunDoSunBup). The session involved 10 minutes of sound exercise (reciting "meaningless words"), 10 minutes of movement, and 40 minutes of sitting meditation. Investigators reported significant decreases in blood pressure, heart rate, and respiratory rate during training and 10 minutes after training..

Heart rate variability.

Recently, power spectral analysis of heart rate variabilityhas emerged as a primaryoutcome measure in several studies, with growing interest in modulation of autonomic tone as a potential mechanism of mind-body therapies. As dis cussed previously, healthy states are associated with sympathovagal balance, whereas states of stress trigger sympathetic overactivation and dominance. In cardiac conditions, such as heart failure, this sympathetic overdrive is at the root of disease. Increased heart rate variability suggests an increase in vagal (or parasympathetic) tone, and shift toward a more healthy autonomic balance. In an observational trial by Vaananen, electrocardiographic recordings were taken while older and younger Tai Chi practitioners performed two ses sions of Tai Chi. Acute increases in time domain measures of heart rate vari ability were seen in both groups (5% increase in R-R interval [RRI] in older group, $p < .01$; 61 % increase in standard deviation of N-N intervals (SDNN) in younger group, $p < .001$; 143% increase in total variance ofN-N intervals (TV) in younger group, $p < .001$). More prominent changes were seen in the young.

In Lee's trial, both Qi Gong practitioners and non-Qi Gong practitioners performed "Qi training" (meditation with frequency-controlled respiration of 7.5 breaths/minute). Frequency domain measures of heart rate variability acutely increased in both groups (increase in high-frequency (HF) component, $p < .01$; decrease in low-frequency/high-frequency (LF/HF) ratio, $p < .001$), although effects in Qi Gong practitioners were enhanced. The results in non Qi Gong practitioners suggest that certain Qi Gong techniques may have pow erful and immediate effects even in those with minimal training.

Balance. strength. Flexibility (Fig. 25.12)

Much evidence is available for Tai Chi's beneficial effects on measures of balance, strength, and flexibility. Several trials have examined risk and frequency of falls and fear of falling in community elders. In one of the largest and classic Tai Chi studies by Wolf, 200 seniors >70 years of age were randomized to receive either Tai Chi classes, a computerized balance training program, or education classes. At the end of 15 weeks, investigators reported lowered systolic blood pressure, improvements in grip strength and lower extremity range of motion, increased psychosocial well-being, decreased fear of falling, and decreased risk of multiple falls by 48% ($p = .01$). Interestingly, many Tai Chi participants provided anecdotal testimony ot aborted fall events, citing newly acquired awareness of environment and compensatory body maneuvers during unexpected disturbances.

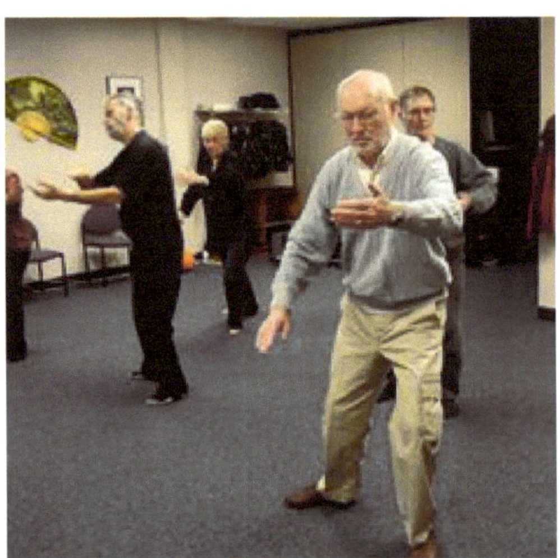

Fig. 25.12: *Elderly people with Parkinson's disease can be helped with Tai chi for better Balance. strength. flexibility*

A more recent trial by Li compared Tai Chi to non-meditative stretching exercises in 256 older adults >70 years of age. Participaats attended class three times a week. At the end of 6 months, investigators, as in the Wolf study, reported fewer falls (38 vs. 73, $P = .007$), reduced fear of falling ($p < .001$), and decreased risk of multiple falls by 55% (RR = .45, 95% CI 0.3—0.7) in the Tai Chi group as compared to conn-ol. Investigators also reported Tai Chi-related improve ments in functional balance (Berg Balance Scale, Dynamic Gait Index, functional reach, single-leg stand, each $p < .001$) and physical performance (50-foot speed walk, Up and Go test, each $p < .001$)

Role of Acupuncture in Tal Chi and Qigong Discipline

Acupuncture is an ancient healing art that has been practiced for thousands of years. It has it's roots deeply planted in China and Taoism. More people have been treated with acupuncture than any other form of treatment in the time of history. Acupuncture is a very safe and effective treatment that is used to treat illness, prevent disease, and improve health/well-being. Very small, hair-thin needles are inserted into specific points in the body, where they are gently stimulated to elicit the body's natural healing response. Acupuncture is effective for controlling pain and can regulate the body's physiological functions to treat various internal dysfunction and disorders.

According to traditional acupuncture theory, there are twelve energy channels called "meridians" running vertically along the length of the human body, each one linking to a specific organ. Illness is caused by obstructed energy flow at certain points along the meridians. Acupuncture therapy stimulates meridian flow and harmonizes the body's energy to influence the health of both body and mind. Researchers have begun to examine in Western medical terms the mechanisms by which acupuncture brings about physiological change. Studies have shown that acupuncture influences both the central and peripheral nervous systems. Further evidence indicates that acupuncture stimulates the release of brain chemicals such as endorphins, which function to relieve pain. Research also suggests that acupuncture increases immune system functioning, improves the circulatory system, decreases muscle tightness, and increases joint flexibility. Clinical trials lend credence to these results : acupuncture has been shown to bring about significant improvement for a variety of diseases.

In countries such as Japan and China, which make up about a fifth of the world's population, acupuncture has been established as a primary form of health care for thousands of years, where the acupuncturist's role was comparable to that of the physician. Today in such countries, acupuncture treatment remains an integral component of the health care system, offered in conjunction with Western medicine. In North America, acupuncture has drawn growing public attention in recent years. The flood of headlines in the mass media describe this expanding interest and acceptance : The Washington Post, for example, reported in 1994 that an estimated 15 million Americans, or about 6 percent of the population, have tried acupuncture for various ailments that include chronic pain, fatigue, nausea, arthritis, and digestive problems.

In 1995, the US Food and Drug Administration (FDA) reclassified acupuncture needles from the Class III (investigational device) category to the Class II (safe and effective but requiring restrictions) category. In November 1997, the US National Institute of Health held a major conference to discuss the use, efficacy, and safety of acupuncture. Based on their conclusions, the NIH issued a report entitled "Acupuncture : The NIH stated that acupuncture is a useful method for the treatment of a variety of conditions such as post-operative pain, nausea, migraines, arthritis, menstrual cramps, low back pain, and tennis elbow. Furthermore, the NIH acknowledged that the side-effects of acupuncture are considerably less compared with other medical procedures such as drugs and surgery. In addition, the NIH made a recommendation to US insurance companies to provide coverage of acupuncture treatments for certain conditions. This expanding paradigm is changing the face of medicine as we know it. Acupuncture has already been accepted as one of the more common forms of pain management therapy in many pain clinics in US and Canadian hospitals. As a result, acupuncture is becoming accessible for more and more Canadians. Doctors are recommending acupuncture for their patients for various conditions and insurance plans are beginning to include acupuncture treatments.

Different styles of acupuncture?

Acupuncture originated in China but has spread to Korea, Japan, Vietnam, Europe, and America. Different styles have developed over the centuries based on different opinions as to theory and technique. While the basic theoretical principles of acupuncture remain the same, different styles of acupuncture differ greatly in technique and diagnosis. There is no evidence that one particular style is more effective than another. At the Acupuncture Center, Traditional Chinese techniques are used as well as auricular acupuncture and some medical acupuncture for pain management.

Traditional Chinese Acupuncture (TCM)

Traditional Chinese Medicine (TCM) is the most common form of acupuncture studied and practiced in the United States. At the Acupuncture Center, we embrace all aspects of TCM. The main focus in this style is to promote balance to the body, no matter what the condition is. If one is balanced, then their physical, mental, emotional, and even spiritual well-being is optimally functioning.

Japanese Style Acupuncture

Japanese style acupuncture takes a more subtle route than TCM. Fewer and thinner needles are used with less stimulation. Japanese acupuncture is also called Classical Acupuncture. It really focuses on applying laws of the Five Element Theory.

Korean Acupuncture

Korean acupuncture shares the same Classical acupuncture approach that Japanese style embraces. One difference between the two is in Korean acupuncture a lot of needles are used in treatments. It is not uncommon to have close to a hundred needles in one session!

Korean Hand Acupuncture

Points in the hand correspond to areas of the body and to certain disharmonies. This is a microsystem category of acupuncture. This means only the hand is used to treat the entire body.

Auricular Acupuncture

Points in the ear correspond to areas of the body and to certain disharmonies. This system is commonly used for pain control and drug, alcohol, and nicotine addictions. This is a microsystem category of acupuncture. This means only the ear is used to treat the entire body.

Acupuncture and Medical Qigong: A Cutting-Edge Combination:- When a Western Doctors performs Acupuncture; it is defined as Medical Acupuncture. Medical Acupuncture's main goal is the cessation of pain, or pain management. Acupuncture points are selected to yield neurological responses to block pain. Many times electric stimulation is added to the needles at a specific setting to act as a nerve block.

Qigong practice is on the rise here in the U.S. and has the potential to soon be as popular as yoga. Qigong literally means "energy practice." The theory behind qigong is that the imbalance of mind, body and spirit is behind all physical and emotional disease.

The practice of medical qigong also is on the rise and might soon be as popular as massage therapy. Along with herbs, medical qigong is the most ancient form of Chinese medicine and is the forefather of acupuncture. Many acupuncture students are required to take qigong and/or tai chi classes, and some are delving into the practice of medical qigong.

It's a wonderful thing to see these practices entering our fields of consciousness. The question is how does the average practitioner understand and apply the incredible power of something so subtle and so intangible? How do we go from intellectually understanding qi to actually making this universal life force tangible to us?

Practitioners of TCM, as well as practitioners of the Five-Element Theory here in the U.S., spend a lot of time in the classroom learning about qi theory. That is most appropriate. You'll find the practice as part of the curriculum at the Hai Dian University in China, for example, or in less formal settings such as with a master teacher high in the mountains of Tibet. American students may need a greater emphasis on practicing the actual cultivation of qi itself.

Veterinary Acupuncture

Today, veterinary acupuncture is an acknowledged and respected field of medicine which requires formal training and certification in order to practice. In most States, provinces and countries, veterinary acupuncture is considered a surgical procedure that, legally, may ONLY be performed by a licensed doctor of veterinary medicine. Look for a veterinarian with formal training in the practice of animal acupuncture. Acupuncture and Oriental medicine is an art and a science that takes years to master. While any licensed vet can stick needles into an animal, for a positive experience and results, find a veterinary acupuncturist with experience treating a similar condition (with acupuncture) to what your animal has.

The Meridian System and Acupuncture

According to traditional Chinese medicine theory, our body consists of a giant web called the meridian system linking different parts together; its channels making up a comprehensive yet complex body map that supplies qi (vital energy) to every part of the body, assists the distribution of blood and body fluids, maintains the balance between yin and yang elements, and protects the body against disease. Along these channels, acupoints are the sites through which the qi of the organs and meridiansis transported to the body surface. It is generally believed that diseases can be treated when the affected meridians or the affected organs are cleared. Acupuncturists work on these points to regulate corresponding organs or meridians so that the body can return to a state of balance and health.

The meridian system is made up by a series of channels, which are sequential to each other in the circulation of qi (vital energy). In the system, the twelve regular meridians form the major structure; they branch out twelve large collaterals to enter the chest, abdomen and head for connecting the internal organs; fifteen external collaterals to run along the limbs and on the trunk. There are also twelve small collaterals for controlling the muscles and tendons, and smaller collaterals disturbed on the skin surface, and the eight extra meridians to enhance the communications and functions within the system. They work closely with each other, with a dysfunction in one usually affecting another. In Chinese medicine, to be knowledgeable about the meridian system is as important as anatomy and physiology in Western medicine.

Twelve Regular Meridians

The twelve regular meridians make up the main part of the meridian system. They are distributed symmetrically on both sides of the body and are paired with their corresponding internal organs. TCM groups the meridians under arm, leg, yin and yang.

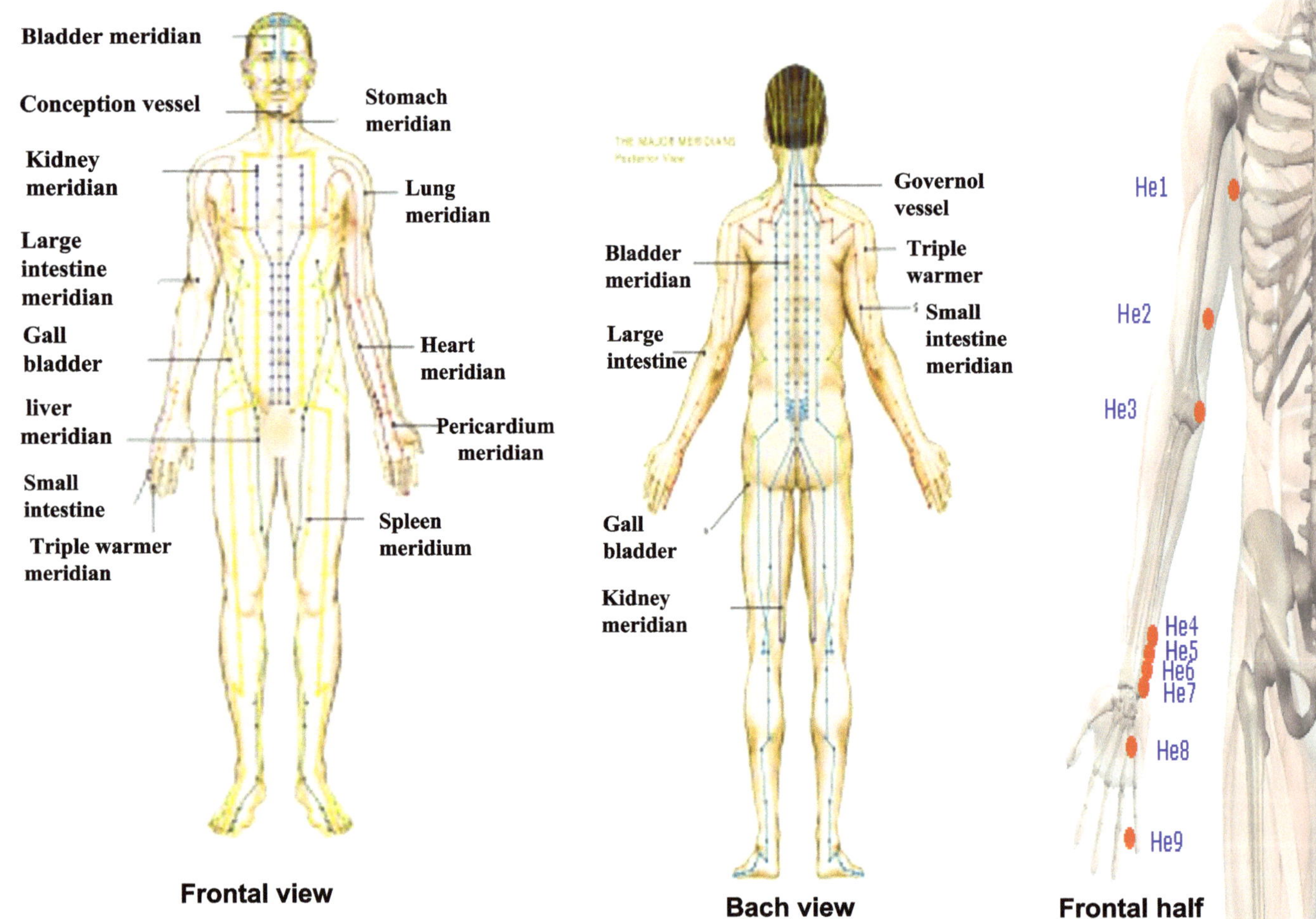

Fig. 25.13: *Illustrations showing (left) body meridians and heart meridian (right)*

Table 25.3: *showing the Order and Arrangement of the 12 Regular Meridians*

Arm / Leg	Distribution	Yang / Yin	The Twelve Regular Meridians	Order of flow
Arm	Yin aspect of the body: starts from the chest, runs along the front arm to the hand	Greater Yin (tai yin)	Lung Meridian(Lu)	1
		Absolute Yin (jue yin)	Pericardium Meridian(Pc)	9
		Lesser Yin (shao yin)	Heart Meridian (Ht)	5
	Yang aspect of the body: starts from the hand, run along the back arm to the head	Brightness Yang (yang ming)	Large Intestine Meridian (Li)	2
		Lesser Yang (shao yang)	Triple Burner Meridian (Sj)	10
		Greater Yang (tai yang)	Small Intestine Meridian (Si)	6
Leg	Yang aspect of the body: starts from head, runs across the trunk, and along the front, lateral and back sides of leg to the foot	Brightness Yang (yang ming)	Stomach Meridian (St)	3
		Lesser Yang (shao yang)	Gallbladder Meridian(Gb)	11
		Greater Yang (tai yang)	Bladder Meridian (Bl)	7
	Yin aspect of the body: starts from the foot, runs along the inner side of leg, cross the front chest and abdomen to the head	Greater Yin (tai yin)	Spleen Meridian(Sp)	4
		Absolute Yin (jue yin)	Liver Meridian (Lr)	12
		Lesser Yin (shao yin)	Kidney Meridian (Ki)	8

The order and arrangement of the twelve regular meridians result in particular ways of communication inside the body, TCM uses Yin/Yang characteristics to distinguish and understand the pattern of meridian flow. All the twelve meridians run through the limbs, with certain meridians and their corresponding organs creating an interior and exterior relationship. For example, the lung meridian (greater yin of arm) and the large intestine meridian (brightness yang of arm) are paired based on their pathways, and clinically they are closely related; problems in the lung or its meridian can also be treated by using various points on the larger intestine meridian. Furthermore, the arm and leg meridians of the same yin/ yang names are also related. For example, problems in the lung or its meridian (greater yin of arm) can be treated by using various points on its communication partner the spleen meridian (greater yin of leg), besides the ones on the lung meridian.

Summary

As we have seen, there is a growing body of literature on Tai Chi and Qi Gong in cardiovascular health. The best support for its cardiovascular effects has been found on blood pressure, heart rate, heart rate variability and autonomic tone, exercise physiology, and lipids. Additionally, benefits on balance, strength, and flexibility are all relevant to cardiac rehabilitation.

There is also a more limited but growing literature on Tai Chi use in specific cardiac populations such as chronic heart failure (CHF) examining not only cardiac parameters, but also disease-specific quality of life measures such as mood. Furthermore, the benefits of compliance and exercise self-efficacy are important as studies have consistently shown that maintenance of an exercise program is essential to maintaining beneficial effects. Tai Chi and Qi Gong appear to be enjoyable activities that people will continue to do.

The mechanisms of action are increasingly. better understood and plausible. Afferent effects on the hypothalamic-pituitary-adrenal axis by mediation of stress through the mind-body, relaxation component are clearly a factor. Efferent effects on sympathovagal tone are demonstrated by changes in blood pressure and heart rate variability. Improvement in oxygen consumption and respiratory efficiency through breathing exercises and general conditioning through Tai Chi movements parallel benefits in other forms of mild to moderate aerobic exercise.

Tai Chi and Qi Gong have promising benefits across the spectrum of cardiovascular disease from primary prevention to rehabilitation. They should be considered by physicians and other providers who are informed of the scientific support as presented here. Such referrals must be coupled with the usually high degree of patient acceptability. They are most likely to be beneficial when Tai Chi/Qi Gong methods are taught by well-trained teachers.

Bibliography and Acknowledgement

- 122. Jones BM. Changes in cytokine production in healthy subjects practicing guolin qigong: A pilot study. BMC Complementary and Alternative Medicine. 2008 September **29**; 2001:1.
- Baranowski T, Perry CL, Parcel GS. How individuals, environments, and health behavior interact: Social cognitive theory. In: Glanz K, Rimer BK, Lewis FM, editors. Health Behavior and Health Education: Theory, Research, and Practice. 3. San Francisco: John Wiley & Sons; 2002. p. 8.

- Brismee J, Paige RL, Chyu M, *et al.* Group and home-based tai chi in elderly subjects with knee osteoarthritis: A randomized controlled trial. Clinical Rehabilitation. 2007; **21**:99–111
- Chao YF, Chen SY, Lan C, Lai JS. The cardiorespiratory response and energy expenditure of Tai-Chi-Qui-Gong. *Am J Chin Med.* 2002; **30**:451–461.
- Chou K, Lee PWH, Yu ECS, *et al.* Effect of tai chi on depressive symptoms amongst Chinese older patients with depressive disorders: A randomized clinical trial. *International Journal of Geriatric Psychiatry*. 2004;19:1105–7. Irwin MR, Olmstead R, Oxman MN. Augmenting immune responses to varicella zoster virus in older adults: A randomized, controlled trial of tai chi. *Journal of the American Geriatrics Society*. 2007; **55:**511–7.
- Fang Z, Wang ZY. Clinical comparison of simplified Taichiquan, breathing exercise, tab, hypotensor co, and simple convalescence in treatment of hypertension. *J Chin Phys.* 1985; **2**:96–97.
- Fontana JA, Colella C, Wilson BR, Baas L. The energy costs of a modified form of T'ai Chi exercise. *Nurs Res*. 2000; **49**:91–96.
- Gong LS, Qian JA, Zhang JS, *et al.* Changes in heart rate and electrocardiogram during taijiquan exercise: analysis by telemetry in 100 subjects. *Chin Med J* (Engl) 1981**;** **94**:589–592.
- Greenspan AI, Wolf SL, Kelley ME, *et al.* Tai chi and perceived health status in older adults who are transitionally frail: A randomized controlled trial. *Physical Therapy*. 2007; **87**:525–35.
- Hammond A, Freeman K. Community patient education and exercise for people with fibromyalgia: A parallel group randomized controlled trial. Clinical Rehabilitation. 2006; **20:**835–46.
- Hui PN*, et al.* An evaluation of two behavioral rehabilitation programs, quigong versus progressive relaxation, in improving the quality of life in cardiac patients.Journal of Alternative and Complementary Medicine. 2006 May; **12**(4):373-8.
- Jackson L, Leclerc J, Erskine Y, Linden W. Getting the most out of cardiac rehabilitation: a review of referral and adherence predictors. Heart. 2005; **91**:10–14.
- Jones AY, Dean E, Scudds RJ. Effectiveness of a community-based tai chi proram and implications for public initiatives. *Arch Phys Med Rehabil*. 2005; **86**:619–625.
- Joseph C.N., Porta C., *et al.* Slow breathing improves arterial baroreflex sensitivity and decreases blood pressure in essential hypertension. Hypertension. 2005 Oct; **46**(4):714-8. Epub 2005 Aug 29.
- Kaushik RM, *et al.* Effects of mental relaxation and slow breathing in essential hypertension. Complementary & Teoretical Medicine. 2006 Jun; **14**(2):120-6. Epub 2006 Jan 10.
- Kui RQ, Lin YH, Sun YX, Zhou N. The effect of Qigong and Taijiquan on pulmonary function in the elderly. *Chin J Rehabil.* 1990; **5**:115–117.
- Kutner NG, Barnhart H, Wolf SL, McNeely E, Xu T. Self-report benefits of Tai Chi practice by older adults. *J Gerontol B* Psychol Sci Soc Sci. 1997; 52:P242–P246.
- Kutner NG, Barnhart H, Wolf SL, McNeely E, Xu T. Self-report benefits of tai chi practice by older adults. *J Gerontol B Psychol Sci Soc Sci*. 1997; **52**B:P242–6.
- Lan C, Chou SW, Chen SY, Lai JS, Wong MK. The aerobic capacity and ventilatory efficiency during exercise in Qigong and Tai Chi Chuan practitioners. *Am J Chin Med.* 2004; **32:**141–150.
- Lee M, Soo Lee M, Kim H, Moon S. Qigong reduced blood pressure and catecholamine levels of patients with essential hypertension. *International Journal of Neuroscience*. 2003; **113:**1691.]
- Lee MS, Lim HJ, Lee MS. Impact of qigong exercise on self-efficacy and other cognitive perceptual variables in patients with essential hypertension. *The J Alternative and Complimentary Medicine*. 2004; **10**:675–680.
- Li F, Fisher KJ, Harmer P, Irbe D, Tearse RG, Weimer C. Tai chi and self-rated quality of sleep and daytime sleepiness in older adults: A randomized controlled trial. *Journal of the American Geriatrics Society*. 2004; **52:**892–900
- Li F, Fisher KJ, Harmer P, McAuley E. Falls self-efficacy as a mediator of fear of falling in an exercise intervention for older adults. *J Gerontol B Psychol Sci Soc Sci.* 2005; **60B**:P34–40.
- Li F, Harmer P, Chaumeton NR, Duncan T, Duncan S. Tai chi as a means to enhance self- esteem: A randomized controlled trial. *Journal of Applied Gerontology*. 2002; **21**:70–89.
- Li F. 145.Myeong Soo Lee, Byung Gi Kim, *et al.* "Effect of Qi-training on blood pressure, heart rate, and respiration rate. *Clinical Psychology* 2000: **20**(3),173-176
- Li ZQ, Shen Q. The impact of the performance of wu's tai chi chuan on the activity of natural killer cells in peripheral blood in the elderly. *Chinese Journal of Sports Medicine*. 1995: 53–56.
- Li, F., et al. "An evaluation of the effects of Tai Chi exercise on physical function among older persons: a randomized control trial*." Annuals of Behavioral Medicine*., 2001 Spring; **23(2)**:139-46.
- Liu JS, Ren HY, Pong LL, Liu ZJ, Liu YF. Effect of Tai Chi on cardiorespiratory function. *Chin J Rehabil*. 1993; **1**:20–21.
- Liu TM, Li SX. Effect of shadow boxing on the cardiovascular excitability, adaptability and endurance in middle-aged and elderly patients with hypertension. *Chin J Clin Rehabil.* 2004; **8**:7508–7509.
- Liu YP, Yang BL, Bai XL. Effects of continuously 24-Form Taijiquan exercise one to three times on cardiovascular functions for elderly. *J Beijing University Physical Education*. 1996; **19**:41–46.
- Lu JB, Wang YF, Hu M, Cha ZB. A Preliminary observation on the therapeutic effect of breathing exercise and shadow boxing training on hypertension in the elderly. *J WCUMS.* 1987; **18**:37–39.
- Manzaneque JM, Vera FM, Maldonado EF, *et al.* Assessment of immunological parameters following a qigong training program. *Medical Science Monitor.* 2004; **10**:CR264–70.

- Morris Docker S. Tai Chi and older people in the community: a preliminary study. Complement *Ther Clin Pract.* 2006; **12**:111–118.
- Myeong Soo Lee, Byung Gi Kim, *et al.* "Effect of Qi-training on blood pressure, heart rate, and respiration rate. *Clinical Psychology* 2000: **20**(3),173-176.
- Orr R, Tsang T, Lam P, Comino E, Singh MF. Mobility impairment in type 2 diabetes: association with muscle power and effect of Tai Chi intervention. *Diabetes Care.* 2006; **29**:2120–2122.
- Rogers CE, Larkey LK, Keller C. A review of clinical trials of tai chi and qigong in older adults. [Accessed 1/30/2009];Western *Journal of Nursing Research.* 2009 **31**:245–279
- Ryu H, Jun CD, Lee BS, Choi BM, Kim HM, Chung HT. Effects of qigong training on proportions of T lymphocyte subsets in human peripheral blood. *American J Chinese* Medicine. 1995; **23:27**–36.
- Sattin RW. Falls among older persons: A public health perspective. *Annual Review of Public Health.* 1992; **13**:489–508.
- Sheng ZS, Su XH. The effect of Tai Chi Qigong form 18 on hypertension. Modern Rehabil. 2000; **4**:33–34.
- Song R, Lee E, Lam P, Bae S. Effects of a sun-style tai chi exercise on arthritic symptoms, motivation and the performance of health behaviors in women with osteoarthritis. Daehan Ganho Haghoeji. 2007; **37**:249–56.
- Sun XS, Xu YG, Xia YJ. Determination of e-rosette-forming lymphocyte in aged subjects with tai ji quan exercise. *International Journal of Sports Medicine.* 1989; **10**:217–219.
- Sun YX, Zhou N, Wang XP, Y XZ, Kui RQ, Lin YH. The effect of Qigong and Tai Chi Quan on pulmonary function in respiratory rehabilitation. *J Chin Rehabil Med.* 1988; **3**:168–171.
- Taylor-Piliae RE, Haskell WL, Froelicher ES. Hemodynamic responses to a community-based tai chi exercise intervention in ethnic Chinese adults with cardiovascular disease risk factors. *Eur J Cardiovasc Nurs.* 2006; **5**:165–174.
- Tejada T, Fornoni A, Lenz O, Materson BJ. Nonpharmacological therapy for hypertension: does it really work? *Curr Cardiol Rep.* 2006; **8**:418–424.
- Thomas GN, Hong AWL, Tomlinson B, *et al.* Effects of tai chi and resistance training on cardiovascular risk factors in elderly Chinese subjects: a 12-month longitudinal, randomized, controlled, intervention study. Clin Endocrinol. 2005; 63:663–669.
- Tsai JC, Wang WH, Chan P, et al. The beneficial effects of Tai Chi Chuan on blood pressure and lipid profile and anxiety status in a randomized controlled trial. J Altern Complement Med. 2003; 9:747–754.
- Tsang T, Orr R, Lam P, Comino E, Singh MF. Effects of Tai Chi on glucose homeostasis and insulin sensitivity in older adults with type 2 diabetes: a randomized double-blind sham-exercise-controlled trial. Age Aging. 2007 Oct 25; [Epub ahead of print] [PubMed]
- Wang ZY, Liu DN, Kong DZ. The effect of Tai Chi on lowering blood pressure. Chinese Chi Gong. 2000; **10**:4–5.
- Wayne PM, Kaptchuk TK. Challenges inherent to t'ai chi research: part 1- t'ai chi as a complex multicomponent intervention. *J Altern Complement Med.* 2008; **14**:95–102
- Winsmann F. Dissertation. Santa Barbara, CA: Fielding Graduate University; 2005. The effect of tai chi chuan meditation on dissociation in a group of veterans.
- Xu SW, Wang WJ. A study of the effects of tai ji quan on endocrinology. *Chinese Journal of* Sports Medicine. 1986; **5**:150–151.
- Yang Y, Verkuilen J, Rosengren KS, *et al.* Effects of a taiji and qigong intervention on the antibody response to influenza vaccine in older adults. *American Journal of Chinese Medicine.* 2007; **35:**597–607
- Yao FT, Zhang T, Yao SX. The effect of Tai Chi Quan and Tai Chi Sword on cardiac rhythm and heart rate in elderly. *J HeNan Prev Med.* 1996:2–3.
- Yeh SH, Chuang H, Lin LW, Hsiao CY, Wang PW, Yang KD. Tai chi chuan exercise decreases A1C levels along with increase of regulatory T-cells and decrease of cytotoxic T-cell population in type 2 diabetic patients. *Diabetes Care.* 2007; **30**:716–718.
- Young DR, Appel LJ, Lee SH. The effects of aerobic exercise and T'ai Chi on blood pressure in older people: results of a randomized trial. *J Am Geriatr Soc.* 1999; **47:**277–284.
- Zhang GD. The impacts of 48-form tai chi chuan and yi qi yang fei gong on the serum levels of IgG, gM, IgA, and IgE in human. *Journal of Beijing Institute of Physical Education.* 1990; **4**:12–14.
- Zhang HL, Gao HH. The effect of performing form 15 Qigong and Tai Chi on cardiovascular function. J Chin Traditional *Chin Med Pharm.* 1988; **1:16**–18.

Management of Coronary Heart Disease with Acupuncture

Coronary artery disease develops when your coronary arteries - the major blood vessels that supply your heart with blood, oxygen and nutrients - become damaged or diseased. Cholesterol-containing deposits (plaque) on your arteries are usually to blame for coronary artery disease.When plaques build up, they narrow your coronary arteries, causing your heart to receive less blood. Eventually, the decreased blood flow may cause chest pain (angina), shortness of breath, or other coronary artery disease signs and symptoms. A complete blockage can cause a heart attack.Because coronary artery disease often develops over decades, it can go virtually unnoticed until you have a heart attack. But there's plenty you can do to prevent and treat coronary artery disease. Start by committing to a healthy lifestyle. **(Fig. 26.1)**

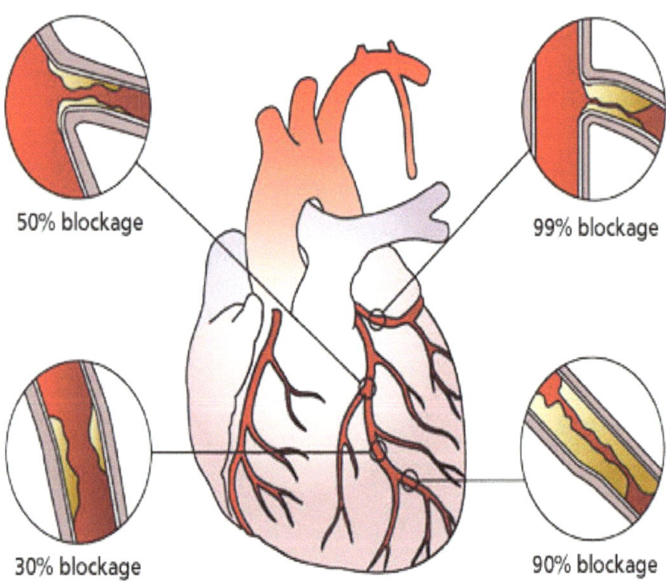

Fig. 26.1: *Diagram showing different percentage of obstruction in atherosclerotic coronary artery disease*

Syndromic Presentation of Heart Disease

- Cold coagulation in the heart vessels
- Attack of angina pectoris due to cold, pain in the heart radiating to the back, cold sensation in the body and aversion to cold, cold sweating, palpitation and shortness of breath, light-colored tongue with thin and white fur, taut and tense pulse.
- Obstruction of phlegm
- Pain and oppression in the chest, heaviness of limbs, shortness of breath and dyspnea,obesity, profuse phlegm, light-colored tongue with thick, white and greasy fur, taut and slippery pulse.
- Stagnation of blood stasis in the collaterals
- Fixed stabbing pain in the chest, aggravation of pain in the night, chest oppression and shortness of breath, palpitation, purplish tongue or tongue with ecchymoses, thin and unsmooth pulse.
- Asthenia of both the heart and spleen
- Oppression and dull pain in the chest, dizziness, am-nesia and insomnia, poor appetite, lassitude, lusterless complexion, light-colored tongue with thin and white fur, thin and weak pulse or slow pulse with irregular intervals and slow regular intermittent pulse.
- Asthenia of heart and kidney yang
- Oppression in the chest, palpitation and shortness of breath, spontaneous sweating, scanty urine and edema, light-colored tongue with thin and white fur, weak and thin pulse or slow pulse with irregular intervals and slow regular intermittent pulse.
- (Semen Vaccariae) is used for ear pressure

Modern Imaging Studies in Diagnosis of Coronary Heart Disease

Chest Radiography:-(**Fig. 26..2**) Chest radiography helps in assessing cardiomegaly and pulmonary edema, or it may reveal complications of ischemia, such as pulmonary edema. It may also provide clues to alternative causes of symptoms, such as thoracic aneurysm or pneumonia (which can be a precipitating cause of ACS)

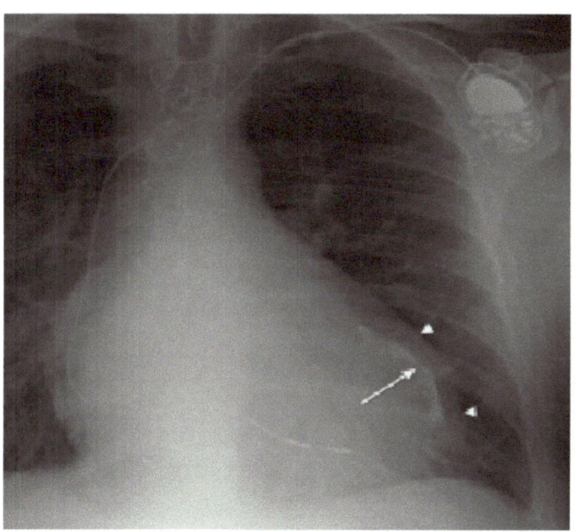

Fig. 26.2: *Myocardial calcification in a 52-year-old male with a history of a large myocardial infarction 16 years earlier, necessitating treatment with coronary artery bypass graft and pacemaker. Frontal radiograph shows focal curvilinear calcification over the left side of the heart (white arrow), a location that is more typical of myocardial rather than pericardial calcification. Note the peripheral shadow of myocardial tissue extending beyond the calcification (white arrowheads), which also aids in distinguishing myocardial from pericardial calcification.*

Electrocardiography:- (**Figs. 26.3—26.4**) ECGs should be reviewed promptly. Involve a cardiologist when in doubt. Recording an ECG during an episode of the presenting symptoms is valuable.

Transient ST-segment changes (>0.05 mV) that develop during a symptomatic period and that resolve when the symptoms do are strongly predictive of underlying CAD and have prognostic value. Comparison with previous ECGs is often helpful.Alternative causes of ST-segment and T-wave changes are left ventricular aneurysm, pericarditis, Prinzmetal angina, early repolarization, Wolff-Parkinson-White syndrome, and drug therapy (eg, with tricyclic antidepressants, phenothiazines). In the emergency setting, ECG is the most important ED diagnostic test for angina. It may show changes during

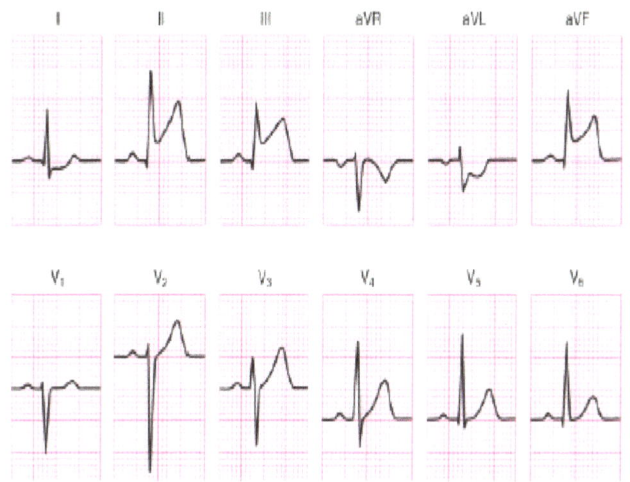

Fig. 26.3: *ECG showing Q waves and ST elevation in leads 11,111 and aVF due to acute inferior wall myocardial infarction*

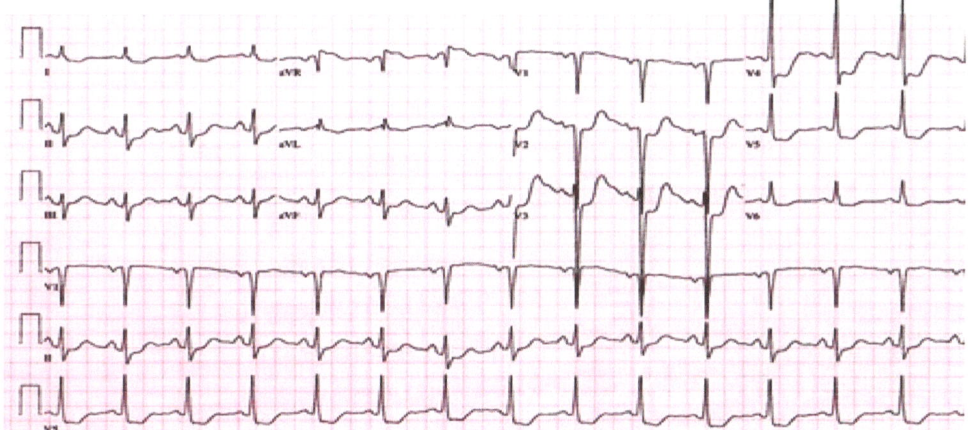

Fig. 26.4: *A 12-lead electrocardiograph of ischemic anterolateral ST-segment depression in a patient with known coronary artery disease*

symptoms and in response to treatment, confirm a cardiac basis for symptoms. It also may demonstrate preexisting structural or ischemic heart disease (left ventricular hypertrophy, Q waves). A normal ECG or one that remains unchanged from the baseline does not exclude the possibility that chest pain is ischemic in origin. Changes that may be seen during anginal episodes include the following:

- Transient ST-segment elevations
- Dynamic T-wave changes - Inversions, normalizations, or hyperacute changes
- ST depressions - May be junctional, downsloping, or horizontal

In patients with transient ST-segment elevations, consider LV aneurysm, pericarditis, Prinzmetal angina, early repolarization, and Wolff-Parkinson-White syndrome as possible diagnoses. Fixed changes suggest acute myocardial infarction. When deep T-wave inversions are present, consider the possibility of central nervous system (CNS) events or drug therapy with tricyclic antidepressants or phenothiazines as the cause.Diagnostic sensitivity may be increased by performing right-sided leads (V4 R), posterior leads (V8, V9), and serial recordings.

Echocardiogram:- **(Fig.26.5)** An echocardiogram uses sound waves to produce images of your heart. During an echocardiogram, your doctor can determine whether all parts of the heart wall are contributing normally to your heart's pumping activity. Parts that move weakly may have been damaged during a heart attack or be receiving too little oxygen. This may indicate coronary artery disease or various other conditions.

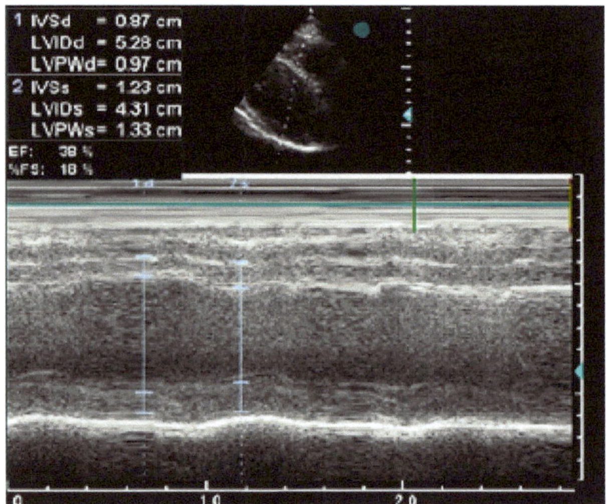

Fig.26.5: *Echocardiogram showed an akinesia with thinning of the basal and mid 1/3 of the inferior and posterior walls, no MR, LVEF 55%*

Stress test: If your signs and symptoms occur most often during exercise, your doctor may ask you to walk on a treadmill or ride a stationary bike during an ECG. This is known as an exercise stress test. In some cases, medication to stimulate your heart may be used instead of exercise.

Some stress tests are done using an echocardiogram. For example, your doctor may do an ultrasound before and after you exercise on a treadmill or bike. Or your doctor may use medication to stimulate your heart during an echocardiogram.

Nuclear stress test: **(Fig. 26.6)** Another stress test known as a nuclear stress test helps measure blood flow to your heart muscle at rest and during stress. It's similar to a routine exercise stress test but with images in addition to an ECG. Trace amounts of radioactive material - such as thallium or a compound known as sestamibi (Cardiolite) – are injected into your bloodstream. Special cameras can detect areas in your heart that receive less blood flow.

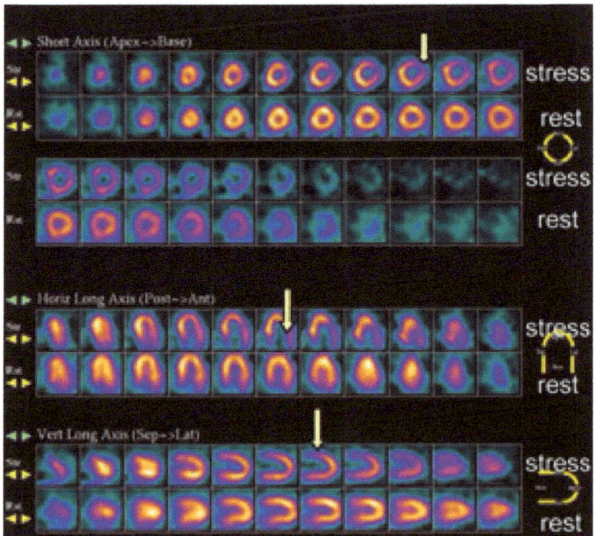

Fig. 26.6: *Myocardial perfusion scan. Stress images (arrows) demonstrate inferolateral and anterolateral (left circumflex) ischemia*

Cardiac catheterization or angiogram:-**(Fig 26.7)** To view blood flow through your heart, your doctor may inject a special dye into your arteries (intravenously). This is known as an angiogram. The dye is injected into the arteries of the heart through a long, thin, flexible tube (catheter) that is threaded through an artery, usually in the leg, to the arteries in the heart. This procedure is called cardiac catheterization. The dye outlines narrow spots and blockages on the X-ray images. If you have a blockage that requires treatment, a balloon can be pushed through the catheter and inflated to improve the blood flow in your coronary arteries. A mesh tube (stent) may then be used to keep the dilated artery open.

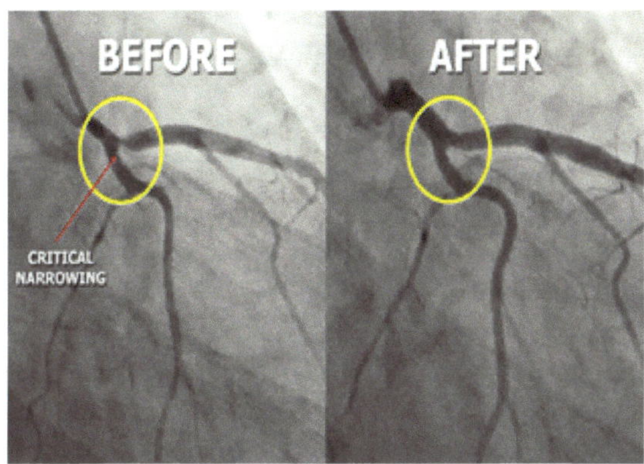

Fig.26.7: *Angiogram showing obstructed coronary artery(left) and complete opening of the artery after stentoplasty (right)*

Computerized tomography (CT) and Perfusion Scans:- **(Fig.30.8)** Technologies, such as electron beam computerized tomography (EBCT) or a CT coronary angiogram, can help your doctor visualize your arteries. EBCT, also called an ultrafast CT scan, can detect calcium within fatty deposits that narrow coronary arteries. If a substantial amount of calcium is discovered, coronary artery disease may be likely. A CT coronary angiogram, in which you receive a contrast dye injected intravenously during a CT scan, also can generate images of your heart arteries.

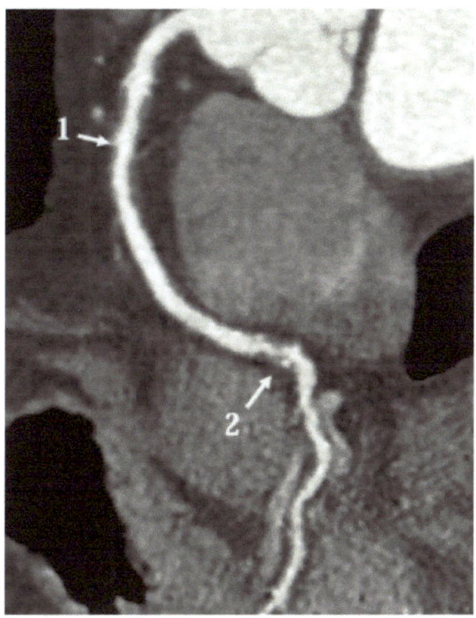

Fig. 26.8: *Computed tomography angiogram of the right coronary artery. (1, Mild proximal stenosis with expansive remodelling and predominantly nonexpansive plaque; 2, Partially calcified advanced mid to distal stenosis.)*

Magnetic resonance angiography (MRA):- This procedure uses MRI technology, often combined with an injected contrast dye, to check for areas of narrowing or blockages - although the details may not be as clear as those provided by coronary catheterization.

Acupuncture is a treatment based on Chinese medicine

A system of healing that dates back thousands of years. At the core of Chinese medicine is the notion that a type of life force, or energy, known as qi (pronounced "chee") flows through energy pathways (meridians) in the body. Each meridian corresponds to one organ, or group of organs, that governs particular bodily functions. Achieving the proper flow of qi is thought to create health and wellness. Qi maintains the dynamic balance of yin and yang, which are complementary opposites. According to Chinese medicine, everything in nature has both yin and yang. An imbalance of qi (too much, too little, or blocked flow) causes disease. To restore balance to the qi, an acupuncturist inserts needles at points along the meridians. These acupuncture points are places where the energy pathway is close to the surface of the skin.

Historical background of acupuncture

The earliest recorded use of acupuncture dates from 200 BCE. Knowledge of acupuncture spread from China along Arab trade routes towards the West. Most Americans first heard of acupuncture in the early 1970s.

Acupuncture gained attention in the United States after President Nixon visited China in 1972. Traveling with Nixon was *New York Times* reporter James Reston, who received acupuncture in China after undergoing an emergency appendectomy. Reston was so impressed with the post-operative pain relief the procedure providedÂ that he wrote about acupuncture upon returning to the United States.

In 1997, the U.S. National Institutes of Health (NIH) formally recognized acupuncture as a mainstream medicine healing option with a statement documenting the procedure' s safety and efficacy for treating a range of health conditions. While awareness of acupuncture is growing, many conventional physicians are still unfamiliar with both the theory and practice of acupuncture.

There are hundreds of clinical studies on the benefits of acupuncture now. Many of these clinical studies are performed in China. Acupuncture has been used successfully in the treatment of conditions ranging from musculoskeletal problems (back pain, neck pain, and others) toÂ nausea, migraine headache, anxiety, and insomnia.

Mechanism of action in acupuncture

The effects of acupuncture are complex. How it works is not entirely clear. Research suggests that the needling process, and other techniques used in acupuncture, may produce a variety of effects in the body and the brain. One theory is that stimulated nerve fibers transmit signals to the spinal cord and brain, activating the body' s central nervous system. The spinal cord and brain then release hormones responsible for making us feel less pain while improving overall health. In fact, a study using images of the brain confirmed that acupuncture increases our pain threshold, which may explain why it produces long-term pain relief. Acupuncture may also increase blood circulation and body temperature, affect white blood cell activity (responsible for our immune function), reduce cholesterol and triglyceride levels, and regulate blood sugar levels.

Dynamic Effects of Acupuncturist on the Body

In addition to asking questions, the acupuncturist may take your pulse at several points along the wrist and look at the shape, color, and coating of your tongue. The acupuncturist may also look at the color and texture of your skin, your posture, and other physical characteristics that offer clues to your health. You will lie down on a padded examining table, and the acupuncturist will insert the needles, twirling or gently jiggling each as it goes in. You may not feel the needles at all, or you may feel a twitch or a quick twinge of pain that disappears when the needle is completely inserted. Once the needles are all in place, you rest for 15 - 60 minutes. During this time, you'll probably feel relaxed and sleepy and may even doze off. At the end of the session, the acupuncturist quickly and painlessly removes the needles.

For certain conditions, acupuncture is more effective when the needles are heated, using a technique known as "moxibustion." The acupuncturist lights a small bunch of the dried herb moxa (mugwort) and holds it above the needles. The herb, which burns slowly and gives off a little smoke and a pleasant, incense like smell, never touches the body. Another variation is electrical acupuncture. This technique consists of hooking up electrical wires to the needles and running a weak current through them. In this procedure, you may feel a mild tingling, or nothing at all. Acupuncturists trained in Chinese herbal preparations may prescribe herbs along with acupuncture.

Different Methodologies in Acupuncture

There are several different approaches to acupuncture. Among the most common in the United States today are:

1. **Traditional Chinese Medicine (TCM) based acupuncture :** The most commonly practiced in the United States, it bases a diagnosis on eight principles of complementary opposites (yin/yang, internal/external, excess/deficiency, hot/cold).
2. **French energetic acupuncture :** Mostly used by MD acupuncturists, it emphasizes meridian patterns, in particular the yin/yang pairs of primary meridians.
3. **Korean hand acupuncture :** Based on the principle that the hands and feet have concentrations of qi, and that applying acupuncture needles to these areas is effective for the entire body.
4. **Auricular acupuncture :** This technique is widely used in treating addiction disorders. It is based on the idea that the ear is a reflection of the body and that applying acupuncture needles to certain points on the ear affects corresponding organs.
5. **Myofascially based acupuncture :** Often practiced by physical therapists, it involves feeling the meridian lines in search of tender points, then applying needles. Tender points indicate areas of abnormal energy flow.
6. **Japanese styles of acupuncture :** Sometimes referred to as "meridian therapy," it emphasizes needling technique and feeling meridians in diagnosis.

Number of treatments needed for completion of Acupuncture therapy

The number of acupuncture treatments you need depends on the complexity of your illness, whether it's a chronic or recent condition, and your general health. For example, you may need only one treatment for a recent wrist sprain, while a long-term illness may require treatments for several months to achieve good results.

Acupuncture Helps Patients With Heart Disease To Exercise

For people who suffer from heart disease, the road to recovery can involve a number of changes in their lifestyle. In many cases, this includes a modified diet and some level of activity to help strengthen the heart. However, patients should only partake in exercise under the strict guidance of their doctor, for too much exertion can place undue stress on the heart.

Now, researchers have found that acupuncture can help heart disease patients to better tolerate exercise. While acupuncture does not seem to aid the heart's ability to pump, it appears to have an effect on the strength of the skeletal muscles. Consequently, stamina improves and allowable walking distances thereby increase.

The findings, published in the journal Heart, come from a study that looked at heart disease patients who had been stabilized with conventional treatments. The patients were divided into two groups : one who took part in 10 acupuncture sessions and a control group who received simulated needle pricks (placebo) that did not break the skin. The acupuncture in question targeted acupuncture points that, according to Traditional Chinese Medicine (TCM), are believed to increase general strength.

What the researchers found was that after the TCM therapy, the acupuncture group was able to cover a greater walking distance than the control (placebo) group. The test group subjects were also able to recover more quickly and reported feeling less exhaustion. Tests indicated, however, that the working capacity of their hearts had not changed.

It is known in medical circles that when a patient suffers from heart disease, their ability to endure exercise is often independent of their heart's ability to pump. Fatigue seems to instead stem from the functioning of the muscles. More specifically, inflammation signals that activate certain receptors are elevated in heart disease patients make the muscle tired. As a result, the body's muscles can no longer endure work loads.

Acupuncture, in turn, appears to decrease the level of a specific messenger, tumor necrosis factor alpha (TNF alpha), which can lead to a decrease in muscle mass, strength, and function.

Chronic weakness of the heart is one of the most prevalent diseases to affect people, and one of the leading causes of death worldwide. One of the hallmarks of the disease is a significant reduction in work capacity, manifested by a shortness of breath and fatigue that results from exercise.

Previously, it was assumed that the problems with endurance were rooted in the weakening of the heart muscles, but now doctors are beginning to understand that the problem is much more complex than that and includes an imbalance in the autonomic nervous system. The goal of acupuncture is to restore that balance.

If you have questions or concerns about heart disease, speak with your doctor. For more information about acupuncture, visit Medline, a service of the National Library of Medicine, a division of the National Institutes of Health (NIH)

Coronary heart disease (Fig. 26.9)

Coronary heart disease is a kind of heart disease due to myocardial ischemia and hypoxia resulting from coro-nary atherosclerosis. The clinical manifestations are angi-na pectoris, myocardiac infarction, arrhythmia, heart failure and cardiectasis. The electrocardiogram may indi-cate myocardial ischemia or corresponding changes. Coro-nary heart disease is one of the commonly encountered heart vessel diseases among the middle aged and old people. It is similar to chest obstructive syndrome, angina pectoris and precordial pain in TCM. The occurrence of coronary heart disease is usually related to aging, weak-ness, improper diet and emotional factors that often lead to inactivation of chest yang, stagnation of cold and phlegm in the collaterals as well as qi stagnation and blood stasis.

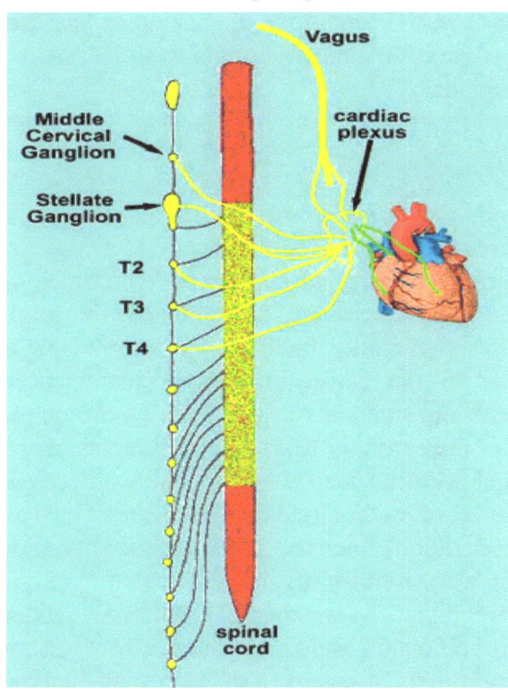

Fig. 26.9: *showing innervation of the heart*

Selection of acupoints

During treatment of coronary heart disease, we Selected "shu" and" mu" points of the yin-and yang-meridian, exterior and interior meridians in combination. Jueyinshu (BL 14) the " shu-point" of the pericardium, was used in combination with Tanzhong (CV 17), the" mu-point" of the pericardium and a converging point of qi, to promote circulation of qi and blood; Xinshu (BL 15), the" shu-point" of the heart was employed in combination with Juque (CV14), the "mu-pointýÿÿÿ?of the heart, to dredge meridian qi. The above-mentioned four acupoints were used together for nourishing the kidney, invigorating qi and blood, replenishing yin and restoring normal function of the body to consolidate the constitution. Zusanli (ST 36) can function in tonifying the kidney, reinforcing qi and blood, and removing pathogenic dampness. Sanyinjiao (SP 6) can function in dredge meridians, eliminating blood stasis and dampness. In addition, Sanyinjiao(SP 6) serves as a converging point of the Liver, Spleen and Kidney. Meridians and thus is capable of reinforcing the spleen, liver-yin and kidney-yang. Neiguan (PC 6) can get rid of pathogenic heat in the chest, promote diuresis and remove dampness to accelerate free flow of qi. These three acupoints were employed together could treat the secondary aspects of the coronary heart disease including sputum-dampness, blood stasis, etc. The aforementioned 7 acupoints of yin- and yang, exterior- and interior- meridians were used in combination and could treat the symptoms and causes at the same time, balancing qi and blood by way of connection among yin- and yang meridians, Zang and fu-organs

Acupuncture Treatment of Coronary Heart Disease

Differentiation of syndromes and treatment of coronary heart disease According to the theory of TCM, coronary heart disease belongs to the mixed syndromes of both deficiency and excess, i. e., deficiency in origin and excess in superficiality. In clinic, it was found that despite variances in the cause of disease, pathogenesis and symptoms and signs, the blood stasis syndrome exists in nearly all the coronary heart disease patients, manifested by angina pectoris, deep purple tongue with ecchymoses, disturbance of microcirculation (indicated by nail fold microcircu1ation), increase in blood viscosity and blood lipid, as well as lowering in RBC electrophoretic rate. In differentiation of syndromes, deficiency and excess of the superficiality and origin of this disease should be understood first. In regard to the excess in superficiality, we should identify sputum syndrome or blood stasis syndrome, while concerning deficiency in origin, we need to distinguish yin-or yang, qi-or blood-deficiency type. When it is treated, the excess of superficiality should be considered first, then it is followed by treatment of the origin. If needed, both the symptoms and cause of angina pectoris are treated at the same time. For eliminating pathogens to treat superficiality, therapeutic principles of promoting blood circulation and removing blood stasis, warming and activating chest-yang, dispelling pathogenic sputum are adopted predominantly; and for strengthening body resistance to consolidate the constitution, principles of warming yang, reinforcing qi, nourishing yin or tonifying the kidney are used.

Mechanisms of the effect of acupuncture in treatment of coronary heart disease

It is wel1 known that angina pectoris results from decrease of coronary blood flow and myocardial ischemia. The above-mentioned results indicated that after acupuncture treatment, the amplitude of vibration of the back wall of the left ventricle and the cardiac output increased significantly, vascular resistance and blood viscosity lowered, thus, improving coronary circulation, lessening cardiac pre- and post-1oad, and lowering myocardial oxygen consumption. As a resu1t, angina pectoris was relieved at last. In a word, from long-term clinical experience, I realize that acupuncture therapy is a good method for coronary heart disease both in treating the superficiality and origin and in emergency treatment. Therefore, it is well received by the coronary heart disease patients.

The Effect of Acupuncture Therapy for Emergency Treatment of Acute Myocardial Infarction

Regarding treatment of acute myocardial infarction, clinical practice demonstrates that when administration of drugs could not achieve satisfactory results in suppressing violent colic induced by myocardial ischemia, acupuncture stimulation often works well. In addition, acupuncture can relieve patient fright feeling, and lower sympathetic excitability to slow down the heart rate, hence, reducing the possibility of arrhythmia. It can also lighten the degree of myocardial injury and reduce the range of myocardial infarction and the occurrence of complications.

Acupuncture Prevents Heart Attacks?

New Research ((Figs. 26.10 - 26.12)

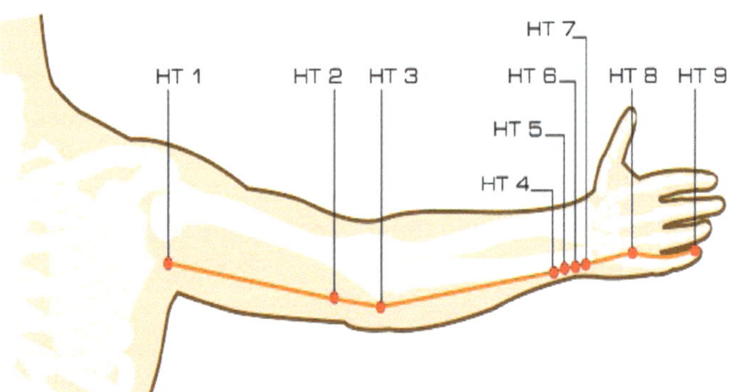

Fig. 26.10: *Illustration showing heart meridian points:*

Heart Meridian Points:

HT 1:- ji quan / Highest Spring

Function: Nourishes Heart yin, clears empty heat.

Indications: Pain in the costal and cardiac regions, scrofula, cold pain of the elbow and arm, dryness of the throat.

HT 2:- qing ling / Cyan Spirit

Function: Frees the channels and quickens the connecting vessel, regulates Qi and blood.

Indications: Pain in the cardiac and hypochondriac regions, shoulder and arm.

HT 3:- shao hai / Lesser Sea

Function: Removes obstructions from the channel, calms the mind, clears heat.

Indications: Cardiac pain, spasmodic pain and numbness of the hand and arm, tremor of the hand, scrofula, pain in the axilla and hypochondriac region.

HT 4:- ling dao / Spirit Pathway

Function: Removes obstructions from the channel.

Indications: Cardiac pain, spasmodic pain of the elbow and arm, sudden loss of voice.

HT 5:- tong li / Penetrating the Interior

Function: Calms the mind, tonifies Heart Qi, benefits the tongue, benefits the Bladder.

Indications: Palpitations, dizziness, blurring of vision, sore throat, sudden loss of voice, aphasia with stiffness of the tongue, stuttering, pain in the wrist and elbow.

HT 6:- yin xi / Yin Cleft

Function: Nourishes Heart yin, clears heat, stops sweating, calms the mind.

Indications: Cardiac pain, hysteria, night sweating, hemoptysis, epistaxis, sudden loss of voice.

HT 7:- shen men / Spirit Gate

Function: Calms the mind, nourishes Heart blood, opens orifices.

Indications: Cardiac pain, irritability, palpiation hysteria, amnesia, insomnia, mania, epilepsy, dementia, pain in the hypochondriac region, feverish sensation in the palm, yellowish sclera.

HT 8:- shao fu / Lesser Mansion

Function: Clears Heart fire, Heart empty heat, Heart phlegm fire, calms the mind.

Indications: Palpitations, pain in the chest, spasmodic pain of the little finger, feverish sensation in the palm, enuresis, dysuria, pruritus of the external genitalia.

HT 9:- shao chong / Lesser Surge

Function: Clears heat, subdues wind, opens the Heart orifices, relieves fullness, restores consciousness.

Indications: Palpitations, cardiac pain, pain in the chest and hypochondriac regions, mania, febrile diseases, loss of consciousness.

Primary Functions

1. The Heart meridian has the primary function of governing the blood and blood vessels of the body.
2. It also governs the sweating function of the body, and strongly affects the performance of the tongue due to the secondary Heart energy channels which connect the Heart meridian itself with the base of the tongue.
3. The healthiness of the Heart meridian manifests in the complexion of the skin.
4. The Heart meridian is also said to house the spirit of the human soul, which correlates with the idea that a person "has lots of heart" if they have a strong spirit.

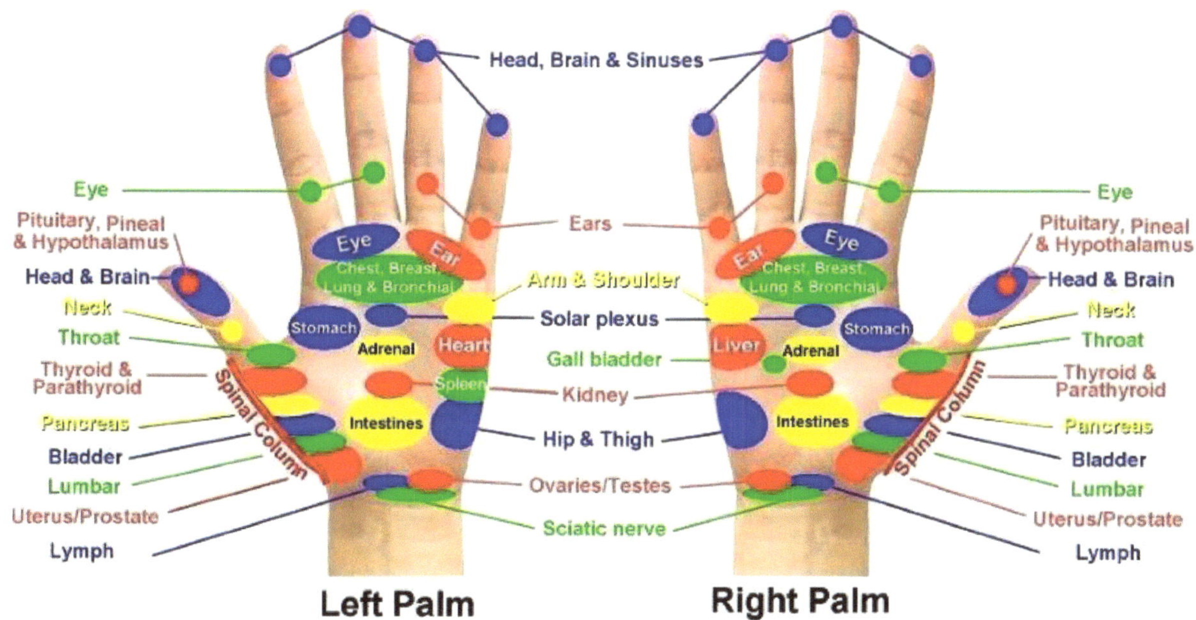

Fig. 26.11: *showing vita -Flex acupoints on hands of different organs of the body including heart point*

Common Uses

- Treats chest pain and disorders related to the rhythm of the physical heart.
- Improves circulation and performance of the blood vessels throughout the entire body.
- Calms the spirit and improves emotional wellbeing.
- Heals disorders of the tongue and speech disorders. This is because the Heart meridian is connected to the tongue via the secondary energy channels.
- Treating throat problems such as pain, swelling, and congestion. The Heart meridian is connected to the throat via the secondary channels.
- Treating eye problems such as redness, pain, or swelling. This is because the secondary Heart channels connect with the eyes.
- Improving problems with the complexion of the skin, especially on the face where the Heart secondary channels reach.

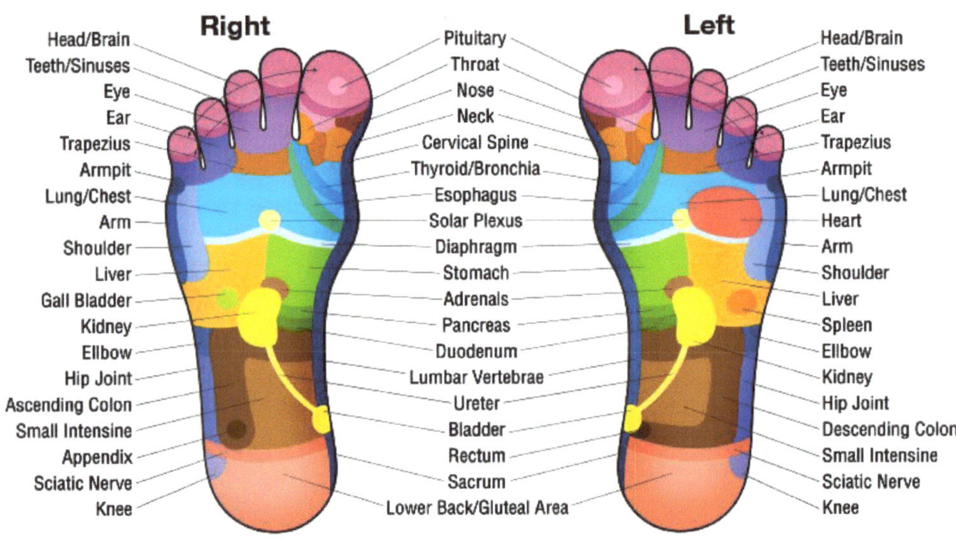

Fig. 26.12: *Acupoints on feet showing different organs of the body including heart point*

Heart disease is the number one cause of death worldwide. These findings demonstrate that acupuncture is a successful tool in benefitting the heart. Acupuncture has been proven to prevent heart tissue damage, reduce arrhythmias such as atrial fibrillation and acupuncture has been shown to reduce high blood pressure.

Method of Performance

Juque (CV 14) is needled obliquely downward 0.5- 1 cun. Tanzhong (CV 17) is needled 1 curl obliquely toward the left breast root. The needles are retained for 30 minutes and manipulated at intervals. For severe cases, the retention of needles may be pro-longed for one or several hours. Back-Shu, Front-Mu acu-points and Qihai (CV 6), Guanyuan(CV 4), Shenque (CV 8) and Zusanli (ST 36) can be moxibusted after needling.

2. Ear acupuncture (Fig. 26.13)

Prescription: Heart (C015), Kidney (CO10), Spleen (C013), Sympathetic (AH6a), Endocrine (CO18), Sub-cortical (AT4) and Ear Shenmen (TF4).

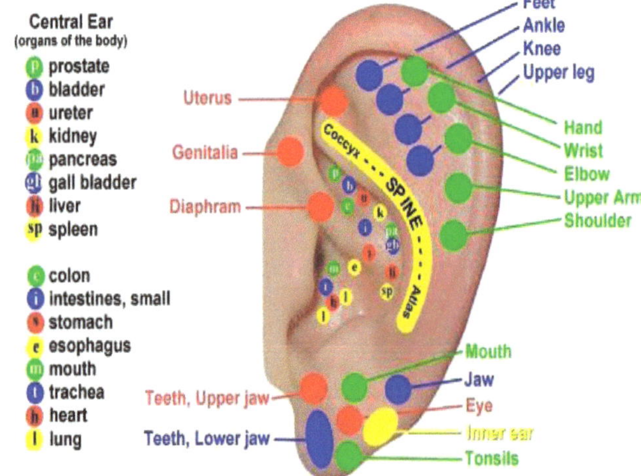

Fig.26.13 *Acupoints on ear of a person showing different organs of the body including heart point*

Performance: Each time 3 - 5 acupoints are selected. In the stage of attack, filiform needles are used with strong stimulation and retained for 30 60 minutes. The needles are manipulated once every 5 - 10 minutes. In the remission stage, filiform needles are used with mild stimulation, retained for 30 minutes and manipulated once every 10 minutes. Or Wangbuliuxingzi.

Contraindications of Acupuncture

In general, acupuncture is safe and well tolerated. One large study found only 43 minor adverse events associated with 34,407 acupuncture treatments. No serious adverse effects were reported. Some health care providers may avoid treatment during pregnancy. Others may be very competent in treating patients who are pregnant. There are certain points that are contraindicated during pregnancy, however other points are thought to benefit pregnancy. Make sure your acupuncture practitioner is competent in addressing the question of risks and benefits of acupuncture during pregnancy before you receive treatment. Tell your acupuncturist about any treatments or medications you are taking and all medical conditions you have. According to some theories, acupuncture is not recommended during menstruation.

Follow up of patients after Acupuncture Therapy

Be sure your acupuncturist uses only disposable needles. If your acupuncturist prescribes herbs and would like you to take them as part of your treatment, talk to your doctor. Herbs are potent substances that can be harmful if you suffer from certain conditions. They can also interact with drugs you may be taking and cause side effects. It is best to avoid strenuous physical activity, heavy meals, alcohol intake, or sexual activity for up to 8 hours after a treatment.

Bibliography and Acknowledgement

- Benzon: Raj's Practical Management of Pain, 4th ed. Philadelphia, PA: Mosby Elsevier, Inc. 2008.
- Chen D, *et al*. Clinical study on needle-pricking therapy for treatment of polycystic ovarial syndrome. *Zhongguo Zhen Jiu.* 2007; **27**(2):99-102.
- Cheuk DK, Yeung WF, Chung KF, Wong V. Acupuncture for insomnia. Cochrane Database *Syst Rev.* 2007;(3):CD005472.
- de Leon: Cancer Pain, 1st ed. Philadelphia, PA: Saunders Elsevier Inc., 2006.
- Dickman R, Schiff E, Holland A, Wright C, Sarela SR, Han B, Fass R. Acupuncture vs. doubling the PPI dose in refractory heartburn. *Aliment Pharmacol Ther.* 2007; [Epub ahead of print].
- Facco E, Liguori A, Petti F, et al. Traditional Acupuncture in Migraine: A Controlled, Randomized Study. Headache. 2007;[Epub ahead of print].
- Flachskampf FA, Gallasch J, Gefeller O, *et al*. Randomized trial of acupuncture to lower blood pressure. *Circulation*. 2007; **115**(24):3121-9.
- Haake M, Muller HH, Schade-Brittinger C, *et al*. German Acupuncture Trials (GERAC) for chronic low back pain: randomized, multicenter, blinded, parallel-group trial with 3 groups. *Arch Intern Med.* 2007; **167**(17):1892-8.
- Hollifield M, Sinclair-Lian N, Warner TD, Hammerschlag R. Acupuncture for posttraumatic stress disorder: a randomized controlled pilot trial. *J Nerv Ment Dis.* 2007; **195**(6):504-13.
- Itoh K, Katsumi Y, Hirota S, Kitakoji H. Randomised trial of trigger point acupuncture compared with other acupuncture for treatment of chronic neck pain. *Complement Ther Med.* 2007; **15**(3):172-9.
- Kelly R. Acupuncture for Pain. *American Family Physician.* 2009; **80**(5).
- Law S, Li T. Acupuncture for glaucoma. *Cochrane Database Syst Rev*. 2007; (4):CD006030.
- Linde K, Allais G, Brinkhaus B, Manheimer E, Vickers A, White AR. Acupuncture for migraine prophylaxis. *Cochrane Database Syst Rev*. 2009;(1).
- Lu W, Dean-Clower E, Doherty-Gilman A, Rosenthal D. The value of acupuncture in cancer care. Hematology/*Oncology Clinics of North America*. 2008; **22**(4).
- Manheimer E, Linde K, Lao L, Bouter LM, Berman BM. Meta-analysis: acupuncture for osteoarthritis of the knee. *Ann Intern Med.* 2007; **146**(12):868-77.
- Pilkington K, Kirkwood G, Rampes H, Cummings M, Richardson J. Acupuncture for anxiety and anxiety disorders — a systematic literature review. *Acupunct Med.* 2007; **25**(1-2):1-10.
- Price S, Lewith G, Thomas K. Acupuncture care for breast cancer patients during chemotherapy: a feasibility study. *Integr Cancer Ther.* 2006; **5**(4):308-14.
- Schneider A, Streitberger K, Joos S. Acupuncture treatment in gastrointestinal diseases: a systematic review. *World J Gastroenterol.* 2007; **13**(25):3417-24.
- Sierpina V, Frenkel, M. Acupunture: A Clinical Review. *Southern Medical Journal,* 2005; **98**(3):330-337.
- Steven D. Ehrlich, NMD, Solutions Acupuncture, a private practice specializing in complementary and alternative medicine, Phoenix, AZ. Review provided by VeriMed Healthcare Network.
- Wu TP, Chen FP, Liu JY, Lin MH, Hwang SJ. A randomized controlled clinical trial of auricular acupuncture in smoking cessation. *J Chin Med Assoc.* 2007; **70**(8):331-8.

Music Therapy In Medical Care System

The understanding of music's role and function in therapy and medicine is undergoing a rapid transformation, based on neuroscientific research showing the reciprocal relationship between studying the neurobiological foundations of music in the brain and how musical behavior through learning and experience changes brain and behavior function. Through this research the theory and clinical practice of music therapy is changing more and more from a social science model, based on cultural roles and general well-being concepts, to a neuroscience-guided model based on brain function and music perception. This paradigm shift has the potential to move music therapy from an adjunct modality to a central treatment modality in rehabilitation and therapy. (Figs. 27.1 - 27.3)

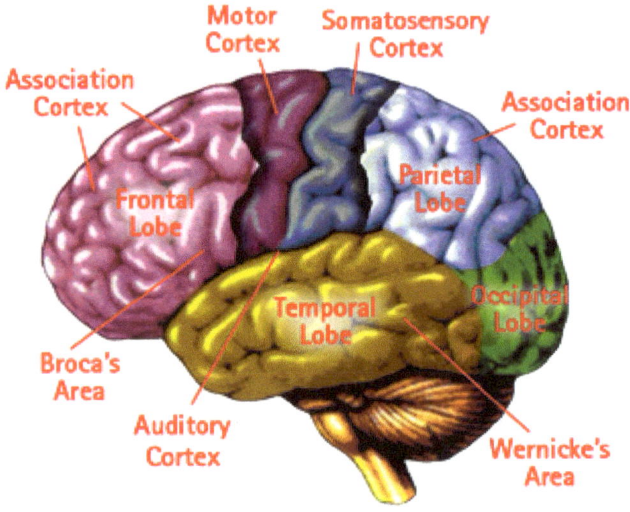

Fig. 27.1: *Brain anatomy showing Several brain regions and areas working in perfect coardination for performing various functions of the body*

History of Music Therapy

Music has been used as a healing force for centuries. Apollo is god of music and of medicine. Aesculapius was said to cure diseases of the mind by using song and music, and music therapy was used in Egyptian temples.

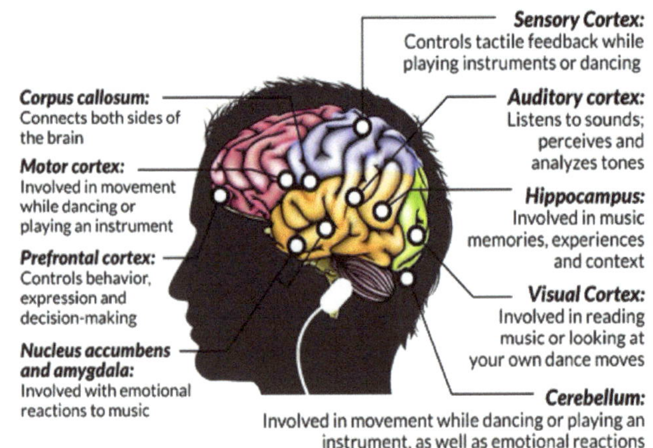

Fig.27.2: *Mind boosting benefits Of music therapy, in preventing different types of heart ailments, such as hypertension, angina, heart attack and brain stroke*

Plato said that music affected the emotions and could influence the character of an individual. Aristotle taught that music affects the soul and described music as a force that purified the emotions. Aulus Cornelius Celsus advocated the sound of cymbals and running water for the treatment of mental disorders. Music therapy goes back to biblical times, when David played the harp to rid King Saul of a bad spirit. As early as 400 B.C., Hippocrates, played music for his mental patients. In the thirteenth century, Arab hospitals contained music-rooms for the benefit of the patients. In the United States,

Native American medicine men often employed chants and dances as a method of healing patients. The Turco-Persian psychologist and music theorist al-Farabi (872–950), known as "Alpharabius" in Europe, dealt with music therapy in his treatise Meanings of the Intellect, where he discussed the therapeutic effects of music on the soul. Robert Burton wrote in the 17th century in his classic work, The Anatomy of Melancholy, that music and dance were critical in treating mental illness, especially melancholia. Music therapy as we know it began in the aftermath of World Wars I and II. Musicians would travel to hospitals, particularly in the United Kingdom, and play music for soldiers suffering from war-related emotional and physical trauma.

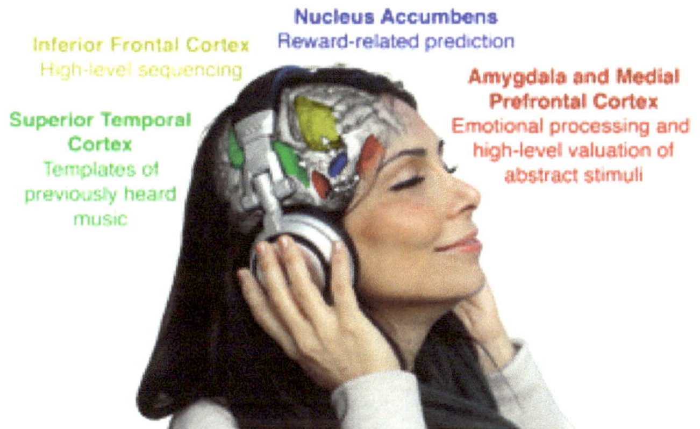

Fig. 27.3 *Neural harmony. Several brain regions work together to produce good vibrations when listening to favorite music.*

Types of Music Therapy

There are 2 types of Music therapy

- Active
- Passive.

The active form of therapy is good to enhance speech, improve concentration level in children, to control hyperactive kids etc, where as Passive form is beneficial in almost all kinds of ailments.icIndian classical ragas, have been found to have healing effects.The basic 7 swaras of the musical octave have correspondence with the chakras.

The lowermost chakra, Mooladhara is associated with the swara,"Sa", which means that chanting this particular note will have an impact on awakening or activation of this chakra.All ragas donot have the same effect on the every human being, it depends on the emotional setup of the individual.So the correct selection of the raga is very important. Research has shown that music has a profound effect on your body and psyche, it refreshes our mind and soul thereby releasing us from stress.

Music has also beenfound to bring many other benefits, such as lowering blood pressure (which can also reduce the risk of stroke and other health problems over time), boost immunity, ease muscle tension, stabilise heart rate, relieve depression, reduce pre-treatment anxiety, help manage pain, reduce nausea after chemotherapy, also improves stability of people with Parkinson's disease. With so many benefits and such profound physical effects, it's no surprise that so many are seeing music as an important tool to help the body in staying (or becoming) healthy. One obvious use of music is that of a sedative. It can replace the administration of tranquillizers , or at least reduce the dosage of tranquillizers

Music therapy interventions can be designed to (Fig. 27.4)

- Promote Wellness
- Manage stress
- Alleviate pain,
- Express feelings,
- Enhance memory,
- Improve communication,
- Promote physical rehabilitation

- Music is the best means of expressing the inner feelings, and good music is often described as the "voice of the heart".
- Music therapy can be used as supportive and complementary therapy with the other systems of medicine.

Approaches used in music therapy that have emerged from the field of education include Orff-Schulwerk (Orff), Dalcroze Eurhythmics, and Kodaly. Two models that developed directly out of music therapy are Nordoff-Robbins and the Bonny Method of Guided Imagery and Music.

Music therapists may work with individuals who have behavioral-emotional disorders. To meet the needs of this population, music therapists have taken current psychological theories and used them as a basis for different types of music therapy. Different models include behavioral therapy, cognitive behavioral therapy, and psychodynamic therapy.

One therapy model based on neuroscience, called "neurological music therapy" (NMT), is "based on a neuroscience model of music perception and production, and the influence of music on functional changes in non-musical brain and behavior functions."

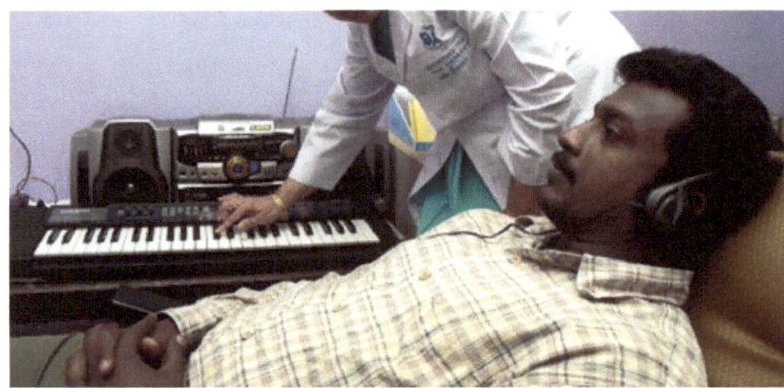

Fig. 27.4: *One of the music techniques practiced in medical therapy*

In other words, NMT studies how the brain is without music, how the brain is with music, measures the differences, and uses these differences to cause changes in the brain through music that will eventually affect the client non-musically. As one researcher, Dr. Thaut, said : "The brain that engages in music is changed by engaging in music. NMT trains motor responses (i.e. tapping foot or fingers, head movement, etc.) to better help clients develop motor skills that help "entrain the timing of muscle activation patterns".

Tune in to sacred music (Fig. 27.5)

Music has been regarded as a sacred art. In the Vedic age, religious songs were sung in India in simple chants. Later on, Gandharva music "was seen by the Creator in His contemplation and afterwards performed by seers and saints", and was considered as the surest means of attaining liberation.

Sacred music was known as Marga Sangeet, while secular music was calledDesi Sangeet.In medieval Europe, hymnswere popularin churches. Chateaurbri and regarded music as "the child of prayer and the companion of religion". In England, church choirs and children's groups were established. Addison valued music as a spiritual aid because it "wakes the soul and lifts it high and wings it with sublime desires and fits it to bespeak the deity".

In India, saints and seers have contributed greatly to the development of classical music with their devotional songs. Jayadev Goswami was one of the first mystical singers of Vaishnavite Bhakti. His Geet Govinda is regarded as a classic of devotional music. He sang of the love of Krishna and Radha with great emotion and sincerity. Chaitanya of Bengal too sang of the mystic love of Krishna and Radha. Swami Haridas, Tansen's teacher, was an expert in the dhrupad style of devotional music.

The first five Sikh gurus were also great musicians. They encouraged professional singers for the benefit of their congregations. In 1604, that for the first time, the largest ever collection of sacred hymns of the first five gurus, 15 saints and 15 bards was compiled and named Adi Granth. Guru Arjan Dev said : "Union with God is attained through kirtan".

The gurus regarded sacred music as a means of spiritual sadhana. They affirmed that the singing of the praises of God stabilised the mind. In Bengal, Rabindranath Tagore evolved the Rabindra Sangeet style. He wrote : "When Thou commandest me to sing, it seems that my heart would break in pride, and I look to Thy face and tears come to my eyes. Drunk with the joy of singing, I forget myself and call. Thee friend who art my lord."

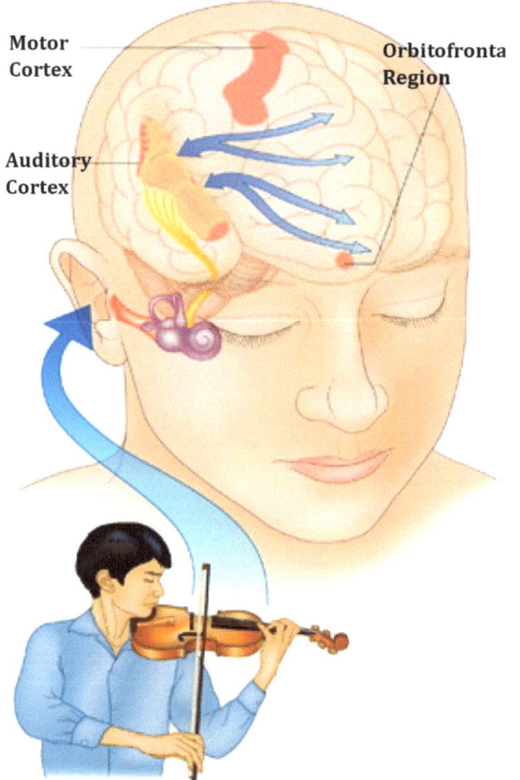

Fig 27.5: *The processing of sound waves from a musical instrument. After being transduced into neural impuls-es by the inner ear, information travels through several waystations in the brainstem and midbrain to reach the auditory cortex. The auditory cortex contains distinct sub-regions that are important for decoding and representing the various aspects of the complex sound. In turn, infor-mation from the auditory cortex interacts with many other brain areas, especially the frontal lobe, for memory for-mation and interpretation. The orbitofrontal region is one of many involved in emotional evaluation. The motor cor-tex is involved in sensory-motor feedback circuits, and in controlling the movements needed to produce music using an instrument.*

Music is an integral part of Sufi devotion. They call it Samai Hakani or spiritual trance. The Chisti mystics of northern India encouraged the qawwals or musicians to sing the praise of God and then got into a situation of rapture when all danced together in a sort of mystic trance. In India, the bhakti movement gave an impetus to sacred music.

There are nine traditional stages of bhakti according to scriptures:

1. Sunan or hearing the holy word,
2. Kirtan or singing the praise of God,
3. Simaran or remembrance of the Lord,
4. Puja or loveworship of God,
5. Pad-sevan or surrender of the self at the Lord's fee
6. t6) Vandana or supplication to the Lord,
7. Dasa-bhava or service to the Lord,
8. Maitri Bhava or friendship with the Lord and total dependence on Him, and
9. Atmanivedan or surrendering oneself to the Lord as an act of total dedication and surrender.

The above leads to the merger of the individual soul with the universal soul. Though kirtan is regarded as the second stage, Sikh gurus gave it supremacy over other forms of devotion and valued it as the chief mode of Sikh worship. Guru Arjan Dev says in this connection : "Gurbani is the treasure of the jewels of Bhakti. By singing, hearing and acting up to it, one is enraptured".

Music as a medical therapy

Definition

Music therapy is a technique of complementary medicine that uses music prescribed in a skilled manner by trained therapists. Programs are designed to help patients overcome physical, emotional, intellectual, and social challenges. Applications range from improving the well being of geriatric patients in nursing homes to lowering the stress level and pain of women in labor. Music therapy is used in many settings, including schools, rehabilitation centers, hospitals, hospice, nursing homes, community centers, and sometimes even in the home.

Origins

Music has been used throughout human history to express and affect human emotion. In biblical accounts King Saul was reportedly soothed by David's harp music, and the ancient Greeks expressed thoughts about music having healing effects as well. Many cultures are steeped in musical traditions. It can change mood, have stimulant or sedative effects, and alter physiologic processes such as heart rate and breathing. The apparent health benefits of music to patients in Veterans Administration hospitals following World War II lead to it being studied and formalized as a complementary healing practice. Musicians were hired to continue working in the hospitals. Degrees in music therapy became available in the late 1940s, and in 1950, the first professional association of music therapists was formed in the United States. The National Association of Music Therapy merged with the American Association of Music Therapy in 1998 to become the American Music Therapy Association.

Benefits

Music can be beneficial for anyone. Although it can be used therapeutically for people who have physical, emotional, social, or cognitive deficits, even those who are healthy can use music to relax, reduce stress, improve mood, or to accompany exercise. There are no potentially harmful or toxic effects. Music therapists help their patients achieve a number of goals through music, including improvement of communication, academic strengths, attention span, and motor skills. They may also assist with behavioral therapy and pain management.

Research & general acceptance (Fig. 27.6-27.7)

There is little disagreement among physicians that music can be of some benefit for patients, although the extent to which it can have physical effects is not as well acknowledged in the medical community.

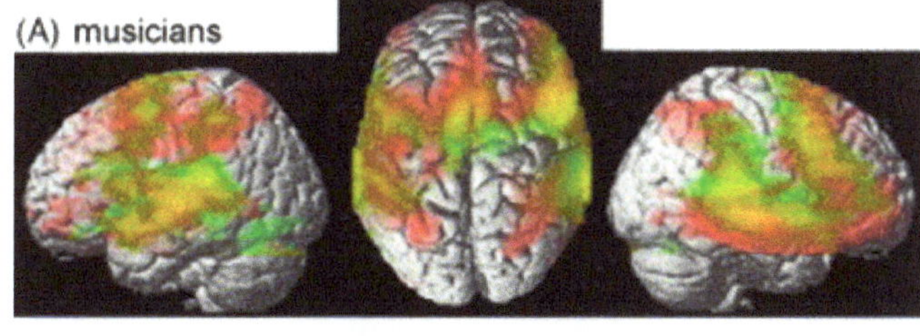

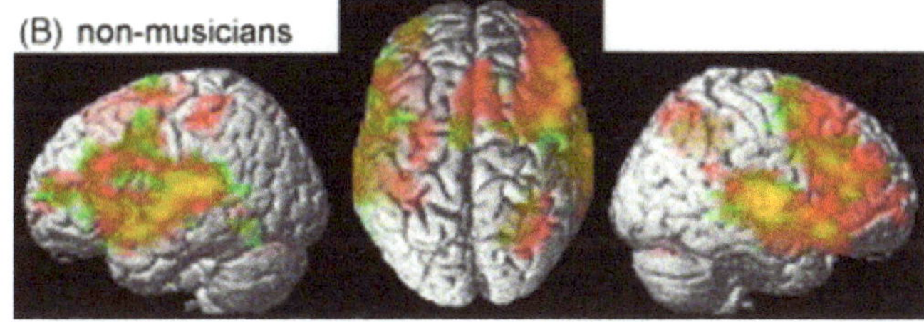

Fig. 27.6: *Brain areas that showed a significant signal increase in the task conditions compared to the baseline are shown for the musician group (A) and for non-musicians (B) ($p < 0.01$, corrected for multiple comparison, with a cluster size threshold of 30 voxels). Voxels with the LIS activation are colored green, while those with the DTT activation red. The overlap is shown in yellow, indicating an activation for both tasks. The base image is a template T1-image provided in SPM99*

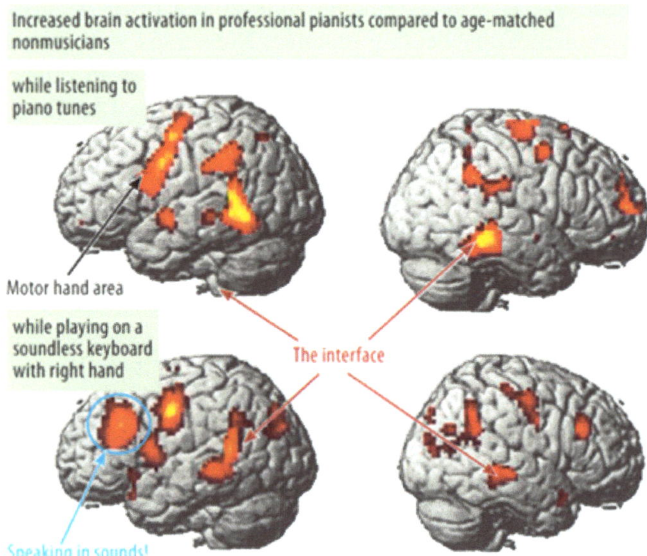

Fig. 27.7: *Additional brain activity (yellow-red zones) in skilled pianists compared to nonpianists when listening to piano tunes without moving their fingers (upper row), or when moving their fingers on a mute keyboard (lower row). When listening, the primary hand area of the precentral area is active (black arrow), revealing an unconscious corepresentation of heard tunes as movement patterns. Furthermore, an auditory association area between the temporal and the parietal lobe lights up (red arrows). This region is also active when the pianists move their fingers on the mute keyboard, and thus seems to be an auditory-motor interface, translating the sounds into fingerings and vice versa. Moving the fingers on a mute keyboard additionally produces activity in Broca's area (blue arrow). This area, therefore, is not confined to language functions as has been traditionally believed but also contributes in a more general manner to complex movement patterns which code symbolic communication. It impressively demonstrates that music 'speaks' to our souls*

Research has shown that listening to music can decrease anxiety, pain, and recovery time. There is also good data for the specific subpopulations discussed. A therapist referral can be made through the AMTA.

Physical effects of music therapy on cardiovascular system

- Blood flow and respiratory rates can synch with music, indicating that music could one day be a therapeutic tool for blood pressure control and rehabilitation, according to a study by Italian researchers published in Circulation: Journal of the American Heart Association.
- The researchers found in an earlier study that music with faster tempos resulted in increased breathing, heart rate and blood pressure. When the music was paused, breathing, heart rate and blood pressure decreased, sometimes below the beginning rate.
- Slower music caused declines in heart rates.
- In an extension of those findings, researchers recently discovered swelling crescendos appear to induce moderate arousal while decrescendos induce relaxation. In music, a crescendo is a gradual volume increase, and a decrescendo is a gradual volume decrease.
- "Music induces a continuous, dynamic - and to some extent predictable - change in the cardiovascular system," said Luciano Bernardi, M.D., lead researcher of the study and professor of Internal Medicine at Pavia University in Pavia, Italy. "It is not only the emotion that creates the cardiovascular changes, but this study suggests that also the opposite might be possible, that cardiovascular changes may be the substrate for emotions, likely in a bi-directional way."
- Researchers studied 24 healthy Caucasians matched for age and sex - 24 to 26 years old with 12 experienced singers (nine women) and 12 participants (seven women) who had no previous musical training. Study participants were fitted with headphones and were attached to electrocardiogram (ECG) and monitors to measure blood pressure, cerebral artery flow, respiration and narrowing of blood vessels on the skin.
- Five random tracks of classical music were played - including selections from Beethoven's Ninth Symphony; an aria from Puccini's Turandot; a Bach cantata (BMW 169); Va Pensiero from Nabucco; Libiam Nei Lieti Calici from La Traviata - as well as two minutes of silence.
- Every crescendo led to increased narrowing of blood vessels under the skin, increased blood pressure and heart rate and increased respiration amplitude. In each music track the extent of the effect was proportional to the change in music profile.
- During the silent pause, changes decreased, with blood vessels under the skin dilating and marked reductions in heart rate and blood pressure. Unlike with music, silence reduced heart rate and other variables, indicating relaxation.
- Music phrases around 10 seconds long, like those used in "Va Pensiero" and "Libiam Nei Lieti Calici," synchronized inherent cardiovascular rhythm, thus modulating cardiovascular control.
- "The profile of music (crescendo or decrescendo) is continuously tracked by the cardiovascular

and respiratory systems," Bernardi said. "This is particularly evident when music is rich in emphasis, like in operatic music. These findings increase our understanding of how music could be used in rehabilitative medicine."

Mental effects (Fig. 27.8)

Depending on the type and style of sound, music can either sharpen mental acuity or assist in relaxation. Memory and learning can be enhanced, and this used with good results in children with learning disabilities. This effect may also be partially due to increased concentration that many people have while listening to music. Better productivity is another outcome of an improved ability to concentrate. The term "Mozart effect" was coined after a study showed that college students performed better on math problems when listening to classical music

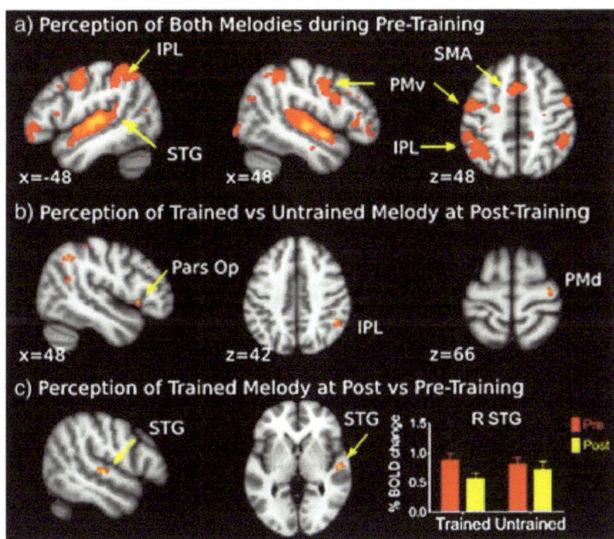

Fig. 27.8: *Listening to melodies. a : images represent re-gions of brain activity when listening to the melodies dur-ing pre-training. b : images represent regions of increased brain activity when listening to the trained compared to the untrained melody, at post-training. c : brain images showing reduced brain activity in the right superior tem-poral gyrus (STG) during perception of the trained melo-dy at post compared to pre-training. Graph shows the % blood oxygenation level dependent (BOLD) signal change (y-axis) in the peak coordinate of the right (R) STG plotted across conditions (x-axis). For all brain images, function-al data are overlaid on the MNI152 standard brain, and thresholded at $z > 3.1$, $p < 0.001$ uncorrected. Abbrevia-tions : inferior parietal lobule (IPL), superior temporal gyrus (STG), ventral premotor cortex (PMv), dorsal pre-motor cortex (PMd), supplementary motor area (SMA), pars opercularis (Pars Op).*

Emotional effects

The ability of music to influence human emotion is well known, and is used extensively by moviemakers. A variety of musical moods may be used to create feelings of calmness, tension, excitement, or romance. Lullabies have long been popular for soothing babies to sleep. Music can also be used to express emotion nonverbally, which can be a very valuable therapeutic tool in some settings.

Objectives of music therapy

Music is used to form a relationship with the patient. The music therapist sets goals on an individual basis, depending on the reasons for treatment, and selects specific activities and exercises to help the patient progress. Objectives may include development of communication, cognitive, motor, emotional, and social skills. Some of the techniques used to achieve this are singing, listening, instrumental music, composition, creative movement, guided imagery , and other methods as appropriate. Other disciplines may be integrated as well, such as dance, art, and psychology. Patients may develop musical abilities as a result of therapy, but this is not a major concern. The primary aim is to improve the patient's ability to function.

Techniques in Music Therapy

Music therapists have numerous interventions and techniques available to help others heal, restore balance in their lives, and live with disabilities and life-threatening illnesses. This page lists some of the more well known or recent interventions developed for music therapy professionals.

1. Creative Interventions

Using creative music therapy interventions, clients take an active role in the music therapy sessions. They create music, compose a song, drum, improvise on instruments, or sing.

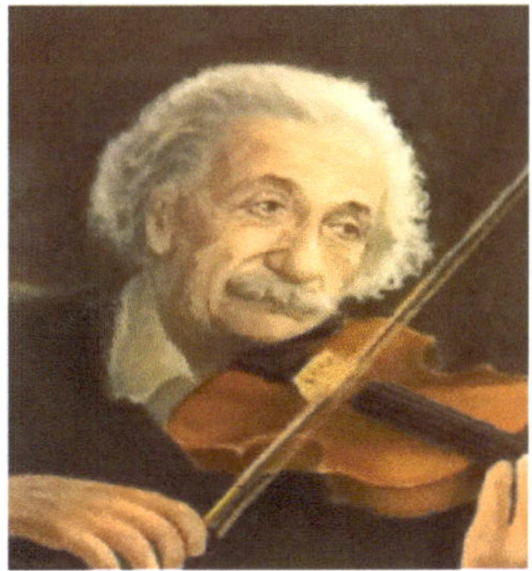

Fig 27.9: *Albert Einstein.. The most incredible story I have heard recently is that of Albert Einstein. At school*

his teachers said he was "too stupid to learn". His mother was told to take him out of school and place him into factory employment. But his mother had more faith than that. She encouraged him to play the violin, and so he did. This is the true legacy behind his success and intelligence. When he was struggling to find an answer, he would turn to the violin and improvise to figure out the equations. You see, the music of the violin exercised his right brain (used for art and creativity). And by doing this, his left brain was able to relax, allowing him access to extraneous, groundbreaking knowledge that changed the world forever! Well, the music and an apple falling from a tree

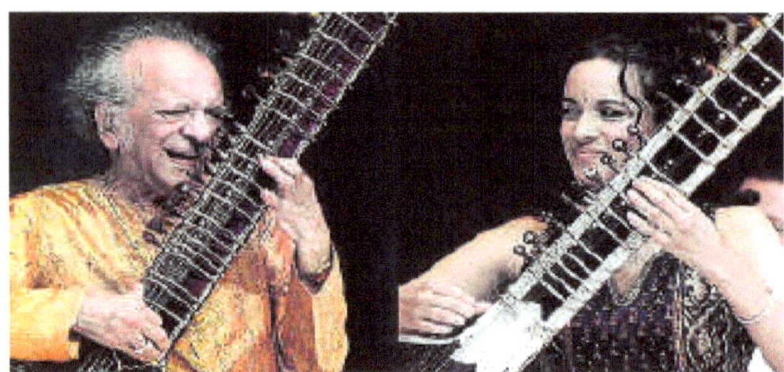

Fig. 27.10: *Sitar vadan;- Showing Pandit Ravi Shankar with his daughter Anouskha performing at one of their concerts*

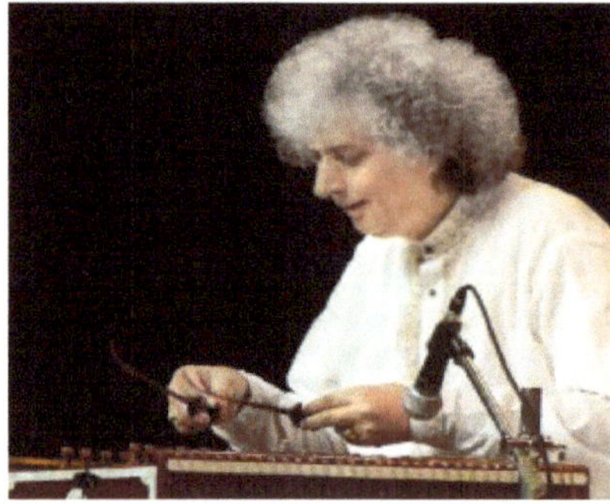

Fig. 27.11: (A) *Santoor Vadan ;-Riding on the waves of rhythm late Pandit Shiv Kumar Sharma atone at his*

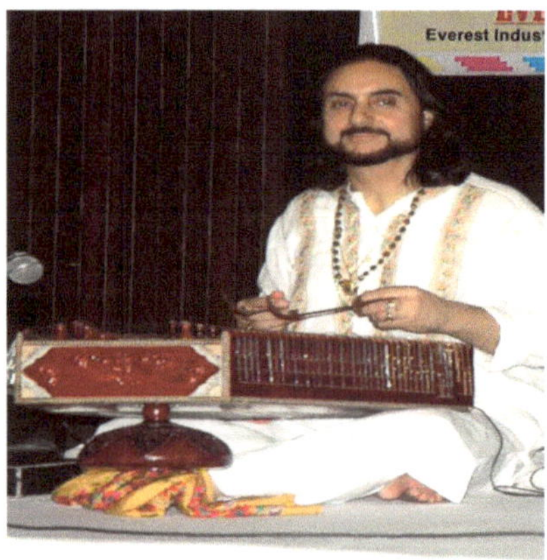

Fig. 27.11: (B) *Santoor Vadan ;-Riding on the waves of rhythm Late Pandit Bhajan Lal Sopori*

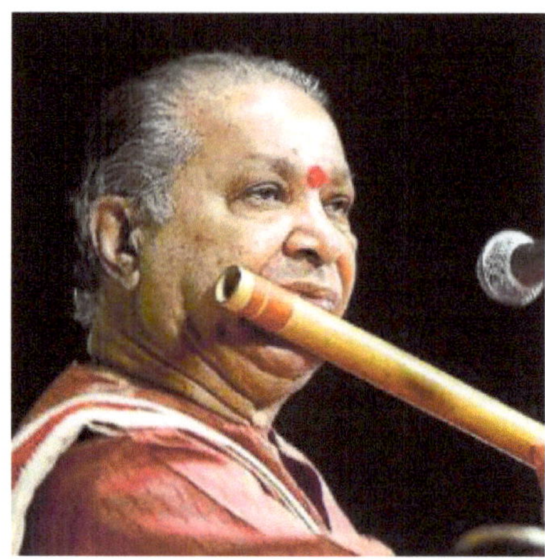

Fig. 27.12: *Flute Vadan ;- Showing Flautist Hari Prasad Chaurasia Ras in Benarasn concert*

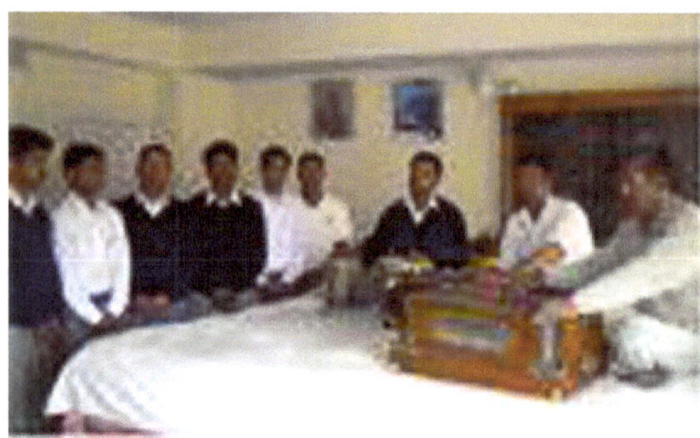

Fig. 27.13: *Harmonium vadan ;- Showing musician per-forming in one of his concerts in front of group of students of music*

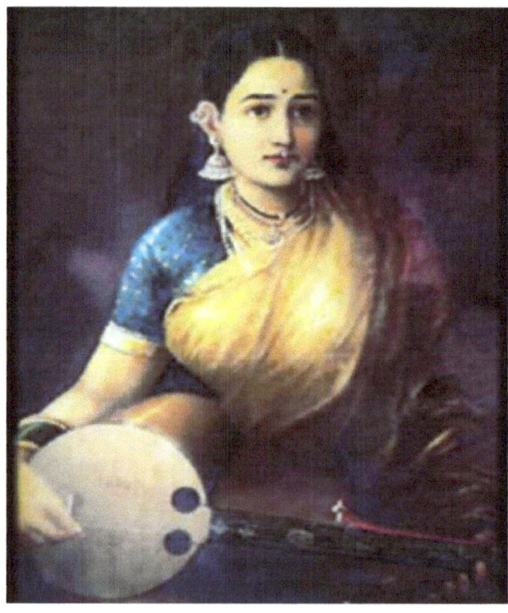

Fig. 27.14: *Showing lady with music instument in Raja Ravi verma's painting*

Drumming and Music Therapy (Fig. 27.15)

Drumming and drumming circles have become increasingly popular in recent years, thanks partly to the researchers and music therapists identifying the emotional, physiological, and social benefits of this musical intervention. Barry Bittman, M.D., and CEO of the Meadville Medical Center's Mind-Body Wellness Center in Pennsylvania, led one of the first clinical research projects measuring the number of infection-fighting immune cells in the bloodstream of drumming group participants. The drummers had increased cell activity related to beneficial immune function, which the researchers said were important agents for fighting neuroendocrine and immunological disorders.

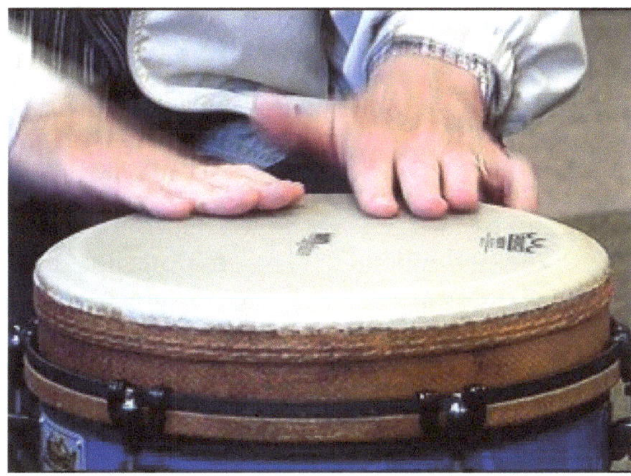

Fig. 27.15: *Music, speciically drumming, may help patients with Parkinson's disease*

Music therapists also point to drummings' benefits of helping those cope with emotional trauma, as well as those seeking self-exploration and realization. According to the Raven Drum Foundation, founded by drummer Rick Allen of Def Leppard and Lauren Monroe, drumming has shown the following benefits:

- Reduces tension, anxiety and stress
- Helps control chronic pain
- Boosts the immune system
- Creates a sense of connectedness with self and others
- Helps us experience being in resonance with the natural rhythms of life
- Releases negative feelings, blockages and emotional trauma
- Provides a medium for individual self-realization

Participants don't need any drumming experience to participate. It's a user-friendly instrument that anyone can play, immediately, and its catchy rhythms are addictive. Its benefits also include a nonthreatening environment that develops camaraderie, group participation, and light-hearted fun.

Drumming and Asthma

At the Meadville Medical Center's Mind-Body Wellness Center, Dr. Bittman leads a group of eight children with asthma in a drumming group, a fun way to teach kids better breathing skills.

He has the kids hang the drums around their necks so they fall on their chests, placing one hand on the drum and the other hand on their stomachs. Now he has them breathe with their diaphragms, watching the movement of the drums.

Soon the kids replace the breathing exercises with free-form drumming, laughing and creating rhythms and beats that pleasantly sync together. The drums teach important breathing skills to kids with a life-threatening condition while also providing relaxation and a way to bond with others.

Singing Therapy (Fig. 27.16)

Stroke, dementia, multiple sclerosis, cancer, and Parkinson's disease are examples of illnesses or conditions that leave people unable to speak - yet, somehow, they are still able to sing.

Scientists have long noted this unusual ability for those who can't talk, belting out songs in their entirety. But only recently have they started to understand the science behind this phenomena.

Wendy Magee told CNN.com that music is a "mega-vitamin for the brain." Magee, an M.D. and International Fellow in Music Therapy at London's Institute of Neuropalliative Rehabilitation, said that music is a useful tool in helping people with brain damage.

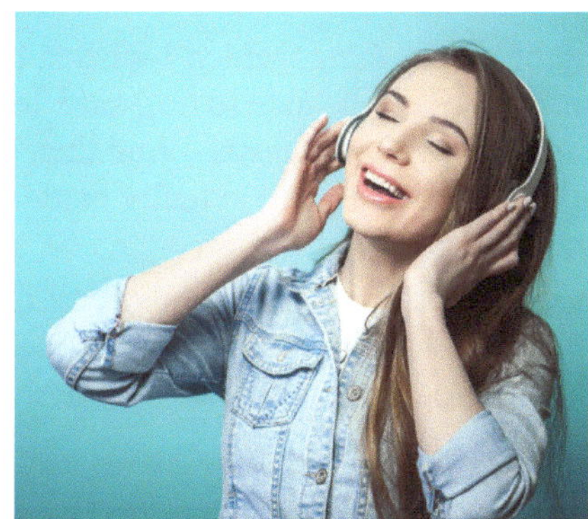

Fig.27.16: *Singing therapy works for left-hemisphere stroke survivors because singing is actually a function of the right brain. Survivors who ind themselves unable to speak might be surprised to ind that they can sing their words instead. During singing therapy (or melodic into-nation therapy), the singing part of your brain can be re-trained to help you speak*

"When neural pathways are damaged for one particular function such as language, musical neural pathways are actually much more complex, and much more widespread in the brain," Magee said.

According to Gottfried Schlaug, M.D., and associate professor of neurology at Beth Israel and Harvard University, when damage occurs to one part of the brain, such as the left side of the brain, or the control center for speech and language abilities, the right side of the brain has the ability to change in structure to compensate.

Also reported on CNN.com, Schlaug credits music-making as a highly effective intervention. He points to Melodic Intonation Therapy that has patients sing tones, then words to those tones. This exercise allows patients to transfer these sound-making skills to spoken words on which they have not been trained.

And it's enjoyable as well for these patients, providing them with a release from the stress and discomfort caused by the illness.

"There's rarely any other activity that could really activate or engage this many regions of the brain that is experienced as being a joyous activity," Schlaug said.

Sing for Joy

In 2003, Nina Temple, diagnosed at age 44 with Parkinson's disease, cofounded with a friend the group "Sing for Joy."

The choir, now numbering around 24 fellow sufferers of Parkinson's and related disorders, has acclaimed jazz singer Carol Grimes as their singing teacher, and the inventive jazz musician Dorian Ford as their pianist. They now perform publicly, ranging from Cole Porter classics to punk songs.

"I was thinking of all the things which I wished I'd done with my life and I wouldn't be able to do," said Temple to CNN about her Parkinson's diagnosis. "And then I started thinking about all the things I still actually could do, and singing was one of those."

For those struggling with chronic, debilitating illnesses, the choir takes "debilitating" out of part of their lives, provides therapeutic vocal exercises, and a cohesive sense of community and belonging.

11. Receptive Interventions

Using receptive interventions, clients listen to music, becoming recipients of the musical experience rather than active music makers. During or after the listening experience, clients discuss evoked thoughts, feelings, and emotions. Or they use receptive music therapy for reaching states of deep relaxation and meditation.

The Bonny Method of Guided Imagery and Music

The most internationally known method of a receptive form of music therapy, the Bonny Method of Guided Imagery and Music, uses western classical music to stimulate a client's unfolding of imagery experiences. Developed by Helen L. Bonny, Ph.D., in the early 1970s, Bonny had a mystical experience with music while playing the violin, revealing to her the healing power of music. She combined her unique understanding of music, her extensive therapeutic training, and her spiritual insight, to research and develop this method.

The Association for Music and Imagery provides detailed information on this music-oriented exploration of consciousness. The website states : "It offers persons the opportunity to integrate mental, emotional, physical and spiritual aspects of well-being, as well as awaken to a greater transcendent identification."

A music therapist trained in the Bonny Method facilitates the sessions, some of which last up to two hours Assessing the reasons for the client's visit, the music therapist discusses the client's current life situation, and establishes a focus for the sessions, also setting specific goals. The therapist uses a guided relaxation technique, and then plays the selected music, allowing it to become a vehicle for exploring deeper states of consciousness. The client verbalizes images, feelings, sensations, memories, and other types of awareness evoked by the music.

During the musical exploration, the music therapist asks questions to help clients further develop the imagery. At the close of the session, the therapist assists the client in returning from the deepened state, reinforcing any insights developed by the exploration. This type of music therapy intervention awakens creativity, and provides reflections on personal relationships, feelings, and personality.

Vibro Acoustic Therapy (Fig. 27.17)

VibroAcoustic therapy (VAT) combines the vibrations of relaxing music with low frequency vibrations. During a VAT session, sound is transferred directly to the body's surface from a specialized table or chair that provides low frequency vibrations, along with speakers or a headset that delivers relaxing music to the client. According to the International Society for VibroAcoustic Therapy,(http://isva.info)"sound waves transfer movement energy to the surface of the body, but it also means that matter inside the body receives vibrations. All molecules inside the body have been put in motion. All cells inside the body have been vibrated by the sound waves which move through the body. We can look upon it this way : The body has received internal massage. Thus organs in the body which we cannot reach by traditional methods - nerves, glands, lungs, heart, deep-lying blood vessels, and brain tissue - will react when being exposed to sound vibrations."

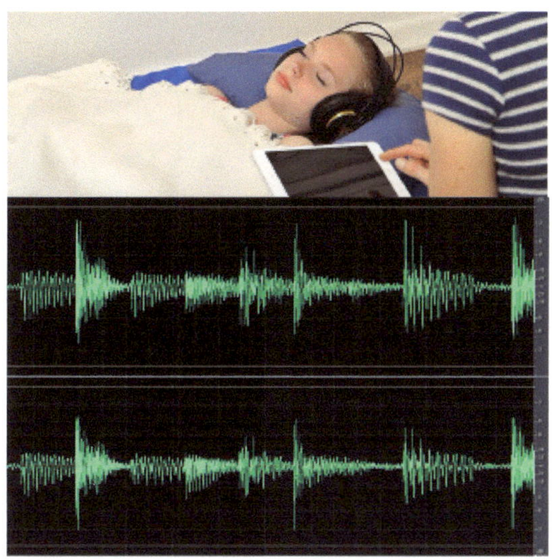

Fig.27.17: *VibroAcoustic therapy (VAT) combines the vibrations of relaxing music with low frequency vibrations*

Developed in the 1980s by Olav Skille, he used vibroacoustic stimulation for severely disabled children, playing them music through large speakers pressed against beanbags that the children were lying on. The vibrations relaxed and stimulated the children, and through the years, he discovered that this therapy helped children with asthma, autism, cystic ibrosis, Parkinson's disease, and a number of other conditions.

VAT is now used by music therapists across the world, thanks to empirical research studies done over the past 30 years, studies showing the most effective frequencies that have a positive in luence on certain de ined health-related conditions.

Music in heart disease (Fig. 27.18)

According to a 2009 Cochrane review of 23 clinical trials, it was found that some music may reduce heart rate, respiratory rate, and blood pressure in patients with coronary heart disease. Benefits included a decrease in blood pressure, heart rate, and levels of anxiety in heart patients. However, the effect was not consistent across studies, according to Joke Bradt, PhD, and Cheryl Dileo, PhD, both of Temple University in Philadelphia. Music did not appear to have much effect on patients' psychological distress. "The quality of the evidence is not strong and the clinical significance unclear", the reviewers cautioned. In 11 studies patients were having cardiac surgery and procedures, in nine they were MI patients, and in three cardiac rehabilitation patients. The 1,461 participants were largely white (average 85%) and male (67%). In most studies, patients listened to one 30-minute music session. Only two used a trained music therapist instead of prerecorded music

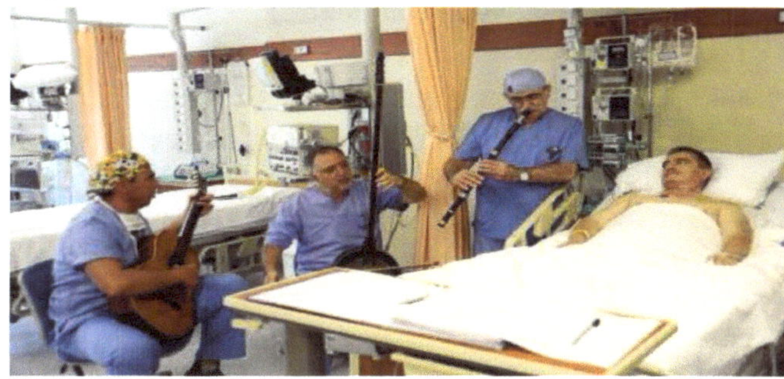

Fig 27.18: *Music therapy cure illnesses. like heart diseases.with release of stress*

Why teach Music in Early Childhood?

Musical activities teach more than just music. Activities that require children to use their whole bodies and interact with others, while also developing musical abilities, have positive effects on a variety of learning. The Kids Music Company early childhood collections are written for whole body and whole brain learning. Using music as a tool, children develop coordination of large and small muscles as they learn how to drive their bodies.

Personal Growth:
Through the development of
• Language
• Listening
• Coordination
• Concentration
• Self Confidence
• Memory
Brain Growth:
Multi-sensory stimulation causes the brain to grow connections across the sections. More connections means faster thinking.
Learning:
Movement, pitch and rhythm can be used to reinforce learning of other important information.
Musical Activities develop the Whole Child
Interpersonal Growth:
• Social Skills
• Respecting others
• Sharing
Musicality:
• Listening
• Moving
• Singing
• Playing
Fun:
If a child is happy the brain is open to learning
Creativity:
Through opportunities to extend ideas

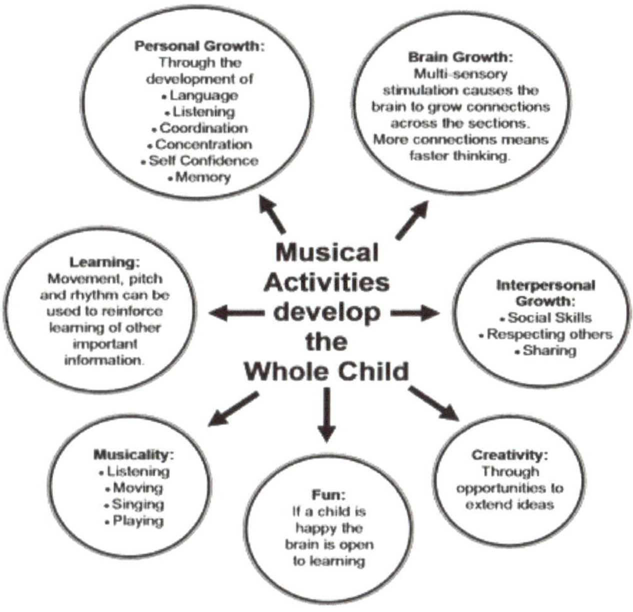

Fig. 2.19: *Illustration depicts the various benefits of music therapy in children*

They develop space perception, listening skills, memory and language as well as social confidence as they interact with others. Children learn to sing, move, and play instruments, and have fun sharing these activities together. This is whole-brain and whole-body learning. What a head start it gives the child as they embark on a life. The years between 0 and 7 are the most critical for brain development. Brain connections are created at their fastest rate.

Whole-brain and whole-body activities undertaken during this time create a network of connections across the brain that can last a lifetime. By their very nature, whole-body activities involve many senses (hearing, vision, vocalizing, touch, and the kinaesthetic sense of muscle movement). They therefore encourage growth across the different areas of the brain involved in the learning. The more connections a child has in their brain, the faster they are able to process information, the faster they can think. Therefore by engaging children in whole-body, whole-brain learning we are setting them up for a lifetime of success.

Music and children (Fig. 27.20-27.22)

Two common approaches are used when conducting music therapy with children : either as a one-on-one session or in a group setting. When a therapist meets with a child for the first time, customarily the therapist and child develop goals to be met during the duration of their sessions. Music therapy can help children with communication, attention, motivation, and behavioral problems.

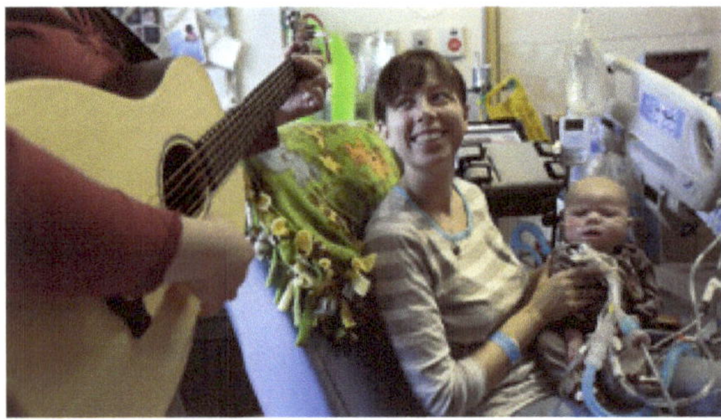

Fig. 27.20: *Klinger plays and sings for Henry Buchert and his mother Stacy Bjorkman. Recent studies suggest the vibrations and soothing rhythms of music, especially performed live in the hospital, might benefit preemies and other sick babies.*

Therapy rooms should have a wide range of different instruments from different places. They should also be colorful, and have different textures. The therapist should either play a piano or guitar to keep everything grounded and in rhythm. The most important thing, though, is to have high quality and well-maintained instruments. As some children will be able to handle an instrument while others cannot, the child should be given an instrument adapted to them. All these elements help the experience and outcome of the music therapy go better and have more successes for the child.

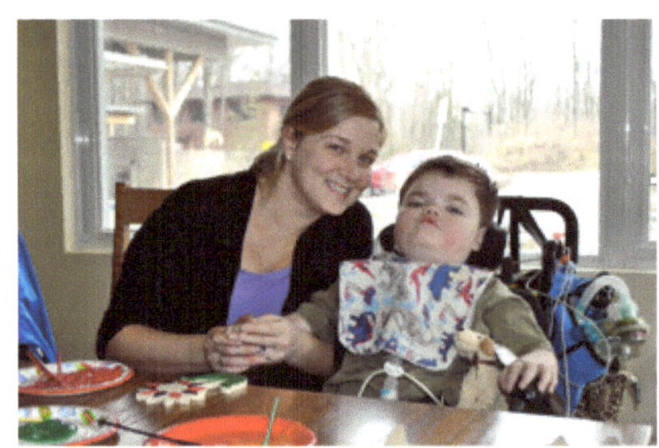

Fig.27.21: *Recreation Therapy is designed to treat and maintain children's physical, mental and emotional well-being. Recreation Therapy provides an enriching experience for the children during their stay as it aids in improving and maintaining physical, cognitive, emotional, and social functioning, preventing secondary health conditions, enhancing independent living skills and overall quality of life. Recreation Therapy includes activities such as arts and crafts, sensory activities, games, baking and nature walks. This type of programming provides an enriching experience for the children during their stay at The Darling Home for Kids*

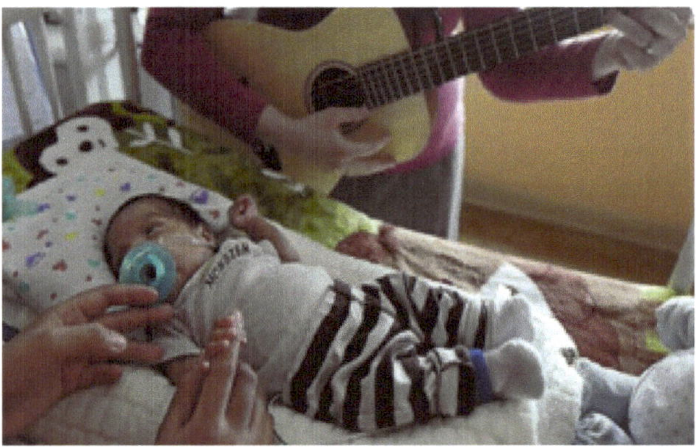

Fig. 27.22: *Music therapist Elizabeth Klinger quietly plays guitar and sings for Augustin Morales as he grips the hand of his mother Lucy Morales, in the newborn intensive care unit at Ann & Robert H. Lurie Children's Hospital in Chicago.*

In fact according to Daniel Levitin, it started inside the womb, surrounded by amniotic fluid, the etus hears sounds. It hears the mother's heartbeat, at times speed up, at other times slow down, not only that but other music, conversations, and environmental noises. Alexandra

Lamont of Keele University in the UK discovered the fetus hears music. She found that, a year after they are born, children recognize and prefer music they were exposed to in the womb. The auditory system of the fetus is fully functional about twenty weeks after conception.

Music and rehabilitation (Fig. 27.23)

Patients with brain damage from stroke, traumatic brain injury, or other neurologic conditions have been shown to exhibit significant improvement as a result of music therapy.

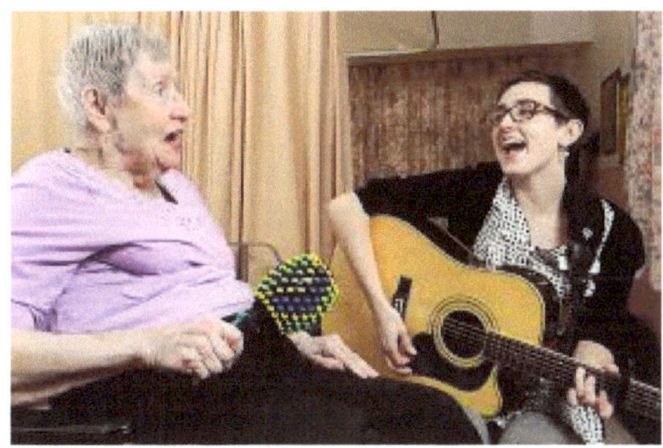

Fig.27.23: *Expressive and receptive communication, choice-making, oral motor, sequencing, motor planning, answering questions, phonemic awareness during rehabilitation with Music therapy*

This is theorized to be partially the result of entrainment, which is the synchronization of movement with the rhythm of the music. Consistent practice leads to gains in motor skill ability and efficiency. Cognitive processes and language skills often benefit from appropriate musical intervention.

Music and the elderly (Fig. 27.24)

The geriatric population can be particularly prone to anxiety and depression, particularly in nursing home residents.

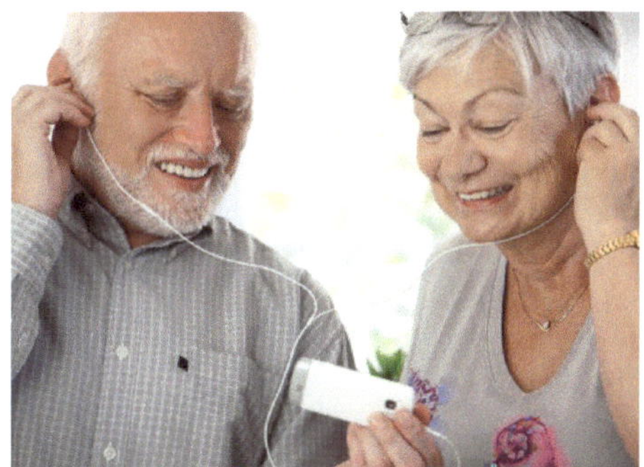

Fig. 27.24: *Music to the ears reaches far beyond the years*

Chronic diseases causing pain are also not uncommon in this setting. Music is an excellent outlet to provide enjoyment, relaxation, relief from pain, and an opportunity to socialize and reminisce about music that has had special importance to the individual. It can have a striking effect on patients with Alzheimer's disease, even sometimes allowing them to focus and become responsive for a time. Music has also been observed to decrease the agitation that is so common with this disease. One study shows that elderly people who play a musical instrument are more physically and emotionally fit as they age than their nonmusical peers are.

Music and the mentally ill (Fig. 27.25 and 27.26)

Music can be an effective tool for the mentally or emotionally ill. Autism is one disorder that has been particularly researched. Music therapy has enabled some autistic children to relate to others and have improved learning skills.

Substance abuse, schizophrenia, paranoia, and disorders of personality, anxiety, and affect are all conditions that may be benefited by music therapy. In these groups, participation and social interaction are promoted through music. Reality orientation is improved. Patients are helped to develop coping skills, reduce stress, and express their feelings.

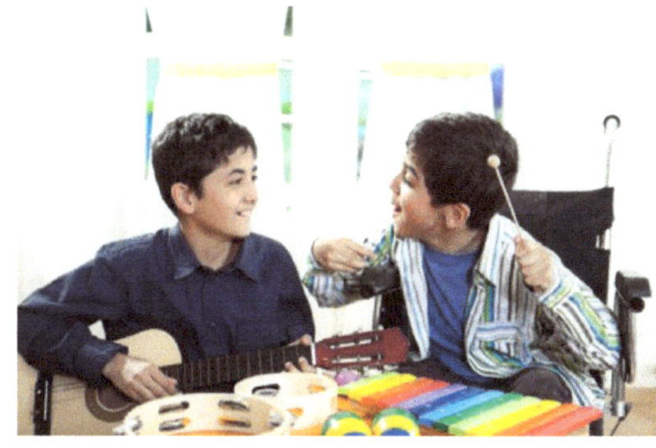

Fig. 27.25: *Musician fellow child is imparting music therapy for the mentally or emotionally ill.*

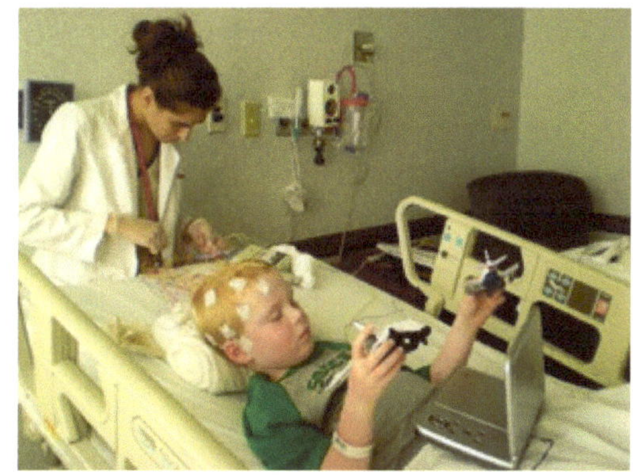

Fig. 27.26: *Music therapy in a child with Autism*

Music therapy in a hopitalised patients (Fig. 27.27)

Pain, anxiety, and depression are major concerns with patients who are terminally ill, whether they are in hospice or not. Music can provide some relief from pain, through release of endorphins and promotion of relaxation.

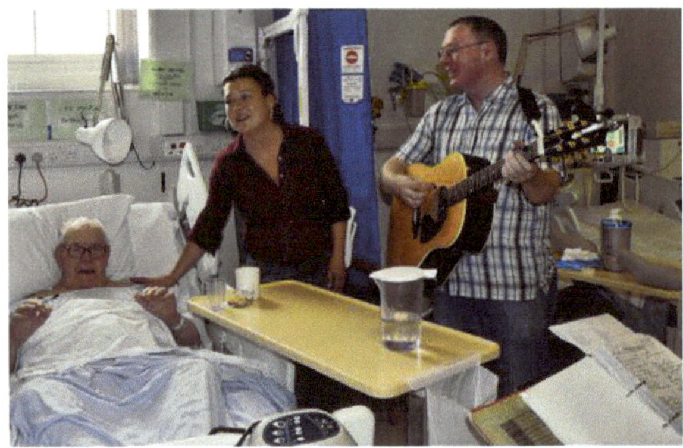

Fig. 27.27: *photograph showing music therapist playing tones to benefit elderly patient admitted in the hospital*

It can also provide an opportunity for the patient to reminisce and talk about the fears that are associated with death and dying. Music may help regulate the rapid breathing of a patient who is anxious, and soothe the mind.

Music therapy during Labor (Fig. 27.28)

Research has proven that mothers require less pharmaceutical pain relief during labor if they make use of music. Using music that is familiar and associated with positive imagery is the most helpful. During early labor, this will promote relaxation. Maternal movement is helpful to get the baby into a proper birthing position and dilate the cervix.

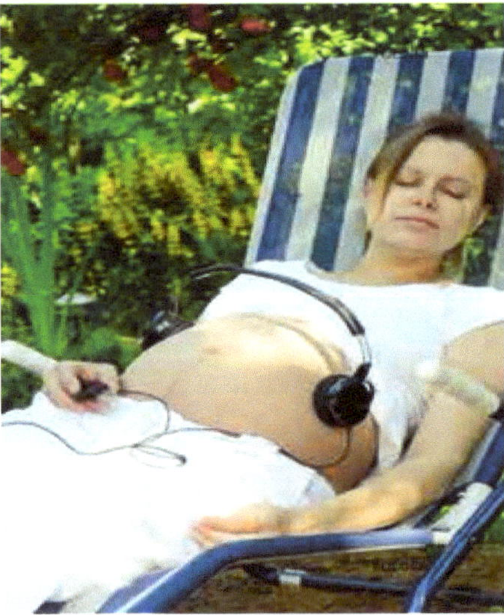

Fig. 27.28: *A pregnant woman undergoing Music therapy*

Enjoying some "music to move by" can encourage the mother to stay active for as long as possible during labor. The rhythmic auditory stimulation may also prompt the body to release endorphins, which are a natural form of pain relief. Many women select different styles of music for each stage of labor, with a more intense, or faster piece feeling like a natural accompaniment to the more difficult parts of labor. Instrumental music is often preferred.

Precautions

Patients making use of music therapy should not discontinue medications or therapies prescribed by other health providers without prior consultation.

Bibliography and Acknowledgement

- Vollert JO, Stork T, ~ose M, Rocker L, Klapp BF, Heller G, *et al.* Reception of music in patients with systemic arterial hypertension and coronary artery disease: endocrine changes, hemodynamics and actual mood. *Perfusion*. 2002; **15**:142-52.
- Campbell, Don. The Mozart Effect. Avon Books, 1997.
- Cassileth, Barrie. The Alternative Medicine Handbook. W. W. Norton & Co., Inc., 1998.
- American Music Therapy Association, Inc. 8455 Colesville Road, Suite 1000 Silver Spring, ML 20910. (301) 589-3300. http://www.musictherapy.org. 36. Almerud S, Petersson K Music therapy—complementary treatment for mechanically ventilated intensive care patients. *Int Crit Care Nurs*. 2003; **19**:21-30.
- Bally K, Campbell D, Chesnick K, Tranmer JE. Effects of patient-controlled music therapy during coronary angiography on procedural pain and anxiety distress syndrome. *Crit Care Nurse*. 2003; **23**:50-8.
- Bally K, Campbell D, Chesnick K, Tranmer JE. Effects of patient-controlled music therapy during coronary angiography on procedural pain and anxiety distress syndrome. *Crit Care Nurse*. 2003; **23**:50-8.
- Bernardi L, Sleight P, Bandinelli G, Cencetti S, Fattorini L, Wdowczyc-Szulc Lagi A. Effect of rosary prayer and yoga mantras on autonomic cardiovascular rhythms: a omparative study. *BMJ.* 2001; **22**:1446-9.
- Cadigan ME, Caruso NE, Haldeman SM, McNamara ME, Noyes DA, Spadafora MA, *et al.* The effects of music on cardiac patients on bed rest. *Prog Cardiovasc Nurs*. 2001 Winter; 5-13.
- Carmichael JM, Agre P. Preferences in surgical waiting area amenities. *Aolt\ J.* 2002; **75:**1077-83.
- Chafin S, Roy M, Gerin W, Christenfeld N. Music can facilitate blood pressure recovery from stress. *BritJ Health Psychol.* 2004; **9:**393-403.
- Chlan LL, Tracy M. Music therapy in critical care: indications and guidelines for intervention. *Crit Care Nurs*. 1999; **19:**3 5-41.
- Chlan LL, Tracy MF, Nelson B, Walker J. Feasibility if a music intervention protocol for patients receiving ventilatory support. *Altern Ther*. 2001; **7**:80—3.

- Chlan LL. Effectiveness of a music therapy intervention on relaxation and anxiety for patients receiving ventilatory assistance. *Heart Lung*. 1998; **27**:160—76.
- Chlan LL. Integrating nonpharmacological, adjunctive interventions into critical care practice: a means to humanize care? *Am J Crit Care*. 2002; **II:** 14-6.
- Chlan LL. Music therapy as a nursing intervention for patients supported by mechanical ventilation. *AACN Clin Issues*. 2000; **11**:128-38.
- Chlan LL. Psychophysiologic responses of mechanically ventilated patients to music: a pilot study. *Am Crit Care*. 1995; **4**:233-8.
- Crowe B. Music and soul-making: toward a new theory of music therapy. Oxford, England: Scarecrow Press; 2004.
- Dileo C, Loewy J, editors. Music therapy at the end of life. Cherry Hill (NJ): Jeffrey Books. p. 2005
- Dileo C, Zanders M.In-between: music therapy with patients awaiting a heart transplant. In: Dileo C, Loewy J, editors. Music therapy at the end of life. Cherry Hill (NJ):Jeffrey Books; 2005. p. 65-76.
- Dileo C. Bradt J. Medical music therapy: a meta-analysis and agenda for future research. Cherry Hill (NJ): Jeffrey Books; 2005.
- Dileo C. Introduction. In: Dileo C, editor. Music therapy and medicine: theoretical and clinical applications. Silver Spring (MD): American Music Therapy Association; 1999. p. 1-10. 5. Wigram T, Dileo C. Music vibration and health. Cherry Hill (NJ): Jeffrey Books; 1997. 6. Dileo C, Bradt J. Entrainment, resonance and pain-related suffering. In: Dileo C, editor. Music therapy and medicine: theoretical and clinical applications. Silver Spring (MD): American Music Therapy Association. 1999. p. 181-8.
- Dillard, James, and Terra Ziporyn. Alternative Medicine for Dummies. IDG Books Worldwide, Inc., 1998.
- Emery CF, Hsiao ET, Hill SM, Frid DJ. Short-term effects of exercise and music on cognitive performance among participants in a cardiac rehabilitation program. *Heart Lung*. 2003; **32**:368-73.
- Gagner-Tjellesen D, Yurkovich EE, Gragert ~. Use of music therapy and other ITNIs in acute care. *Psychosocial Nurs*. 2001; **39**:27-37.
- Halpin LS, Speir AM, CapoBIanco P, Barnett SD. Guided imagery in cardiac surgery. *Outcomes Management.* 2002; **6:**132-7.
- Hamel RJ. The effects of music interventions on anxiety in the patient waiting for cardiac catheterization. Intensive *Crit Care Nurs*. 2001; **17**:279-85.
- Healing Therapies. D K Publishing, Inc., 1997. Organizations
- Hyde R, Bryden F, Asbury AJ. How would patients prefer to spend the waiting time before their operations? *Anaesthesia.* 1998; **53**: 192-200.
- Macnay SK The influence of preferred music on the perceived exertion, mood and time estimation scores of patients participating in a cardiac rehabilitation exercise program. Music Ther Perspect. 1995; 13:91-6.
- Metzger K Assessment of use of music by patients participating in cardiac rehabilitation. *J Music Ther.* 2004; **41:**55-69.
- O'Callaghan C. Song writing in threatened lives. In: Dileo C, Loewy J, editors. Music therapy at the end of life. Cherry Hill (NJ): Jeffrey Books; 2005. p. 117-28.
- Routhieaux RL, Tansik D. The benefits of music in hospital waiting rooms. *Health Care Superv*. 1997; **16**:31-40.
- Salamon E, Bernstein SR, Kim SA, *et al*. The effects of auditory perception and musical preference on anxiety in naIve human subjects. *Med Sci Monit*. 2003;9:
- Schwartz FJ, Ramey GA, Pawli S. Benefits of headphone music on the ICU postoperative recovery of CABG patients, 2001. Paper presented at the Conference of the International Society for Music in Medicine, Hamburg, Germany, June.
- Sears, William, and Martha Sears. The Birth Book. Little, Brown & Co., 1994.
- Stefano GB, Zhu W, Cadet P, Salamon E, Mantione KJ. Music alters constitutivelv expressed opiate and cytokine processes in listeners. *Med Sci Monit*. 2004; **10**: MSI8-27.
- Taylor-Piliae RE, Chair SY. The use of nursing interventions utilizing music therapy. or sensory information on Chinese patients' anxiety prior to cardiac catheterization. *Eur J Cardiovasc Nurs*. 2002; **1**:203-11.
- Thorgaard B, Henriksen BB, Pedersbaek G, Thomsen 1. Specially selected music the cardiac laboratory- an important tool for improvement of the wellbeing of patients. *Eur J Cardiovasc Nurs*. 2004; **3**:21-6. [pMID: 15053885.]
- Tracy MF, Lindquist R: Watanuki S, Sendelbach S, Kreitzer MJ, Bennan B, *et al.* Nurse attitudes towards the use of complementary and alternative therapies in cru cial care. *Heart Lung*. 2003; **32**:197-209.
- Tusek DL, Cwynar R, Cosgrove DM. Effect of guided imagery on length of stay, pain and anxiety in cardiac surgery patients. *J Cardiovasc Manag*. 1999 March-April; 22-28.
- Umemura M, Honda K. Influence of music on heart rate variability and comfort a consideration through comparison of music and noise. *J. Human Ergo*!. 1998**;** **2**: 30-8.
- Voss JA, Good M, Yates B, Baun MM, Thompson A, Hertzog M. Sedative music reduces anxiety and pain during chair rest after open-heart surgery. *Pain* 2004; **112**:197-203.
- White JM. Effects of relaxing music on cardiac autonomic balance and anxiety after acute myocardial infarction. *AmJ Crit Care*. 1999; **8**:220-7.
- Wong HIC, Lopez-Nahas V; Molassiotis A. Effects of music therapy on anxiety in ventilator-dependent patients. *Heart Lung*. 2001; **30**:376-87.

Role of Chelation Therapy (Biochemical Angioplasty) in Coronary Heart Disease

Coronary heart disease (CHD) is the most common form of heart disease, which is the leading cause of death among American men and women. Each year nearly 380,000 Americans die from CHD. In CHD the coronary arteries, the vessels that provide oxygen-rich blood to the tissues of the heart, become blocked by deposits of a waxy substance called plaque. As plaque builds, the arteries become narrower and less oxygen and nutrients are transported to the heart. CHD can lead to serious problems, such as angina (pain caused by not enough oxygen-carrying blood reaching the heart) and heart attack.

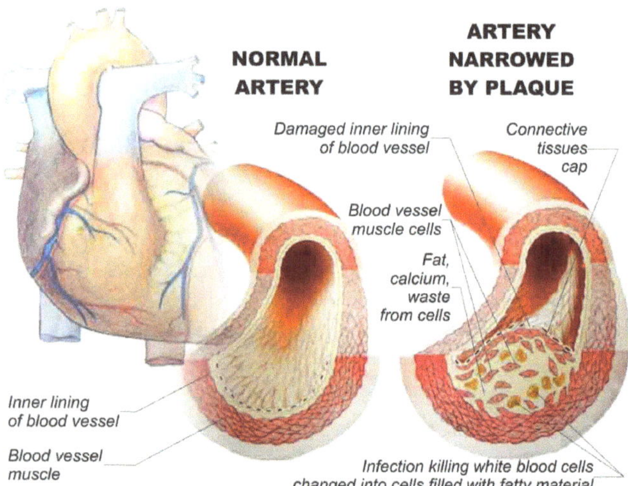

Fig. 28.1: *Showing different mechanisms of obstructed coronary artery*

A heart attack occurs if the flow of oxygen-rich blood to a section of heart muscle is cut off. If blood flow is not restored quickly, the affected section of heart muscle begins to die. Without quick treatment, a heart attack can lead to serious health problems or death.

Factors that can increase the risk of developing CHD include:

- High blood pressure
- High blood cholesterol levels
- Smoking
- Overweight or obesity
- Physical inactivity
- Diabetes
- Insulin resistance
- Metabolic syndrome
- Unhealthy diet
- Family history of CHD
- Older age.

Symptoms of CHD can include chest pain, shortness of breath, lightheadedness, cold sweats, or nausea, but not everyone with CHD has symptoms.

How is CHD diagnosed and treated ?

Diagnosis of CHD is based on personal medical and family histories, risk factors for CHD, a physical exam, and the results from tests and procedures. Doctors who suspect CHD may recommend one or more tests, such as those that check levels of fats, cholesterol, and sugar; electrocardiograms (EKG) to check the heart's electrical activity; "stress" tests to record the heartbeat during exercise; nuclear scanning to check for damaged areas of the heart; and angiography to see if there are blockages or narrowings in the blood vessels that feed the heart. Treatment of CHD includes lifestyle changes—stopping smoking for patients who smoke, following a heart-healthy diet, and engaging in a prescribed exercise program. Medications may also be prescribed, such as aspirin to prevent heart attacks, medications that decrease the workload on the heart, or medicines that reduce blood cholesterol levels or blood pressure. If these efforts are not effective, a patient may need to have the narrowed or blocked arteries re-opened through a procedure called percutaneous coronary intervention (PCI) or bypassed through surgery. PCI involves threading a thin tube into an artery and expanding a balloon-like apparatus as a way to increase the size of the artery so more blood can flow. Bypass surgery is used to treat severe blockages by using veins or arteries from other areas of the body to divert blood flow around the blocked coronary arteries.

Chelation with EDTA for Heart Disease

What is EDTA chelation therapy?

Bio-Chemical Angioplasty also known, as Chelation Therapy is a treatment for coronary artery disease. After a long research and lots of experiments Saaol heart center started to treat patients with BCA and a lifestyle program in 50+ hospitals of Saaol all over India.

Chelation is a chemical process in which a substance is used to bind molecules, such as metals or minerals, and hold them tightly so that they can be removed from the body. In 1900 it was used to remove excess lead from the body for people who has lead poisoning. American organisations came forward to use EDTA Chelation Therapy as a treatment for Coronary artery Disease.

In 1988, a retrospective study of 2870 patients treated with EDTA chelation found that 77% of patients with ischemic heart disease showed "marked" improvement and 91% of patients with peripheral heart disease also showed "marked" improvement. A 1993 retrospective study of 470 patients who underwent EDTA chelation noted that 80% had objective evidence of improvements of their symptoms.

Chelation is a chemical process in which a substance is used to bind molecules, such as metals or minerals, and hold them tightly so that they can be removed from a system, such as the body. In medicine, chelation has been scientifically proven to rid the body of excess or toxic metals. For example, a person who has lead poisoning may be given chelation therapy in order to bind and remove lead from the body before it can cause damage.

In the case of EDTA chelation therapy, the substance that binds and removes metals and minerals is the salts of EDTA (ethylene diamine tetra-acetic acid), a synthetic, or man-made, amino acid that is delivered intravenously. EDTA was first used in the 1950s for the treatment of heavy metal poisoning. Calcium disodium EDTA chelation removes heavy metals and minerals from the blood, such as lead, iron, copper, and calcium, and is approved by the FDA for use in treating lead poisoning and toxicity from other heavy metals.

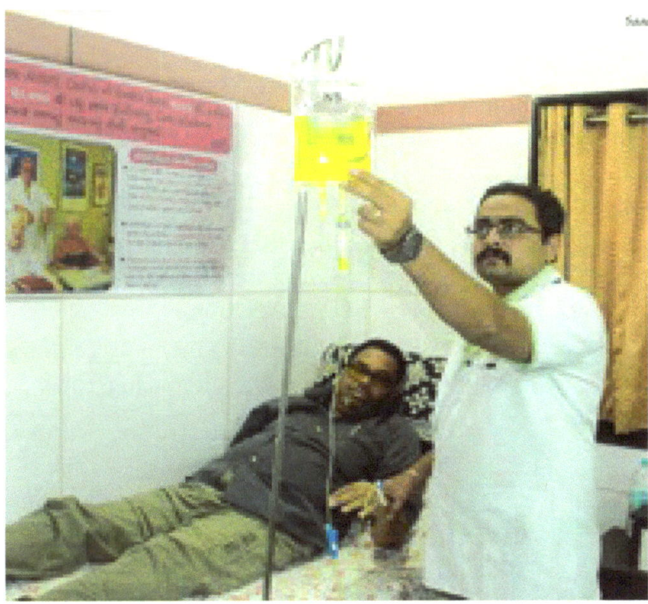

Fig. 28.2: *Showing technique of Chelation with EDTA*

Rather than testing calcium disodium EDTA, TACT used another salt, disodium EDTA, under an FDA license as an Investigational New Drug (IND). Although disodium EDTA it is not approved by the FDA to treat CHD, some physicians and alternative medicine practitioners have recommended its use in chelation as a way to treat CHD.

What are the possible side effects of EDTA chelation therapy?

The most common side effect is a burning sensation at the site where EDTA is delivered into a vein. Rare side effects can include fever, headache, nausea, and vomiting. Even more rare are serious and potentially fatal side effects that can include heart failure, a sudden drop in blood pressure, abnormally low calcium levels in the blood (hypocalcemia), permanent kidney damage, and bone marrow depression (meaning that blood cell counts fall). Hypocalcemia and death may occur, particularly if disodium EDTA is infused too rapidly. Reversible injury to the kidneys, although infrequent, has been reported with EDTA chelation therapy. Other serious side effects can occur if EDTA is not administered by a trained health professional.

How commonly is EDTA chelation therapy used?

The 2007 National Health Interview Survey, conducted by the Centers for Disease Control and Prevention, found that 111,000 adults 18 years of age and older used chelation therapy as a form of complementary medicine in the previous 12 months.

Q: How do you see the future of EDTA/chelation therapy ?

EDTA chelation will become more and more important when its beneficial effects are realised, especially in our modern environment with mercury, lead, manganese, chromium and cobalt overload.

It is very important to realise that "modern medical science" has no means of removing toxic metals from the human body other than by EDTA chelation.

Quacks recommend all sorts of cleansing therapies (colon cleanses etc.), but these are useless and often dangerous.

TACT Study by NIH Reports

TACT study by NIH Reports to American Heart Association About Bio-Chemical Angioplasty TACT (Trial to Assess Chelation Therapy) Study by NIH of EDTA Chelation Therapy Proves Highly Significant Benefits in cardiovascular disease . "Up to 50% prevention of recurrent heart attacks and 43 percent reduction in death rate from all causes." "The patients with diabetes, which made up approximately one third of 1,708 participants, demonstrated a 41 percent overall reduction in the risk of any cardiovascular event. This included a 40 percent reduction in the risk of death from heart disease, reduced risk of nonfatal stroke, or nonfatal heart attack; a 52 percent reduction in recurrent heart attacks; and a 43 percent reduction in death from any cause."

Therapy (TACT). This randomized, placebo-controlled study of 1,708 patients showed that intravenous disodium EDTA chelation therapy decreased subsequent cardiac events with statistical significance, when compared to a control group of similar patients who received placebo. Cardiologists from prestigious medical schools joined a total of 134 medical centers across the U.S. and Canada who participated in this study, at a cost of $30 million. Statistical analysis showed benefits to be highly significant. Cardiac events that were reduced included fewer deaths, fewer heart attacks, and fewer strokes, less need for cardiovascular surgery, and fewer hospitalizations for heart problems. Chelation therapy shown to be safe, without any serious side effects. Patients experienced increasing benefits during the time that they were studied-up to five years thus far. Forty 3-hour intravenous infusions of disodium EDTA were administered during 30 weekly sessions, followed by 10 more treatments once per month. All patients in the study had previously suffered with a well documented heart attack. Results showed effectiveness at reducing their overall death rate, with fewer heart and vascular events. Diabetic patients appeared to do particularly well. The investigators concluded that intravenous EDTA chelation therapy can safely provides important benefits for heart disease patients, who were already on more traditional therapies before receiving chelation. These findings were unexpected by cardiologists, who have long disparaged EDTA chelation therapy. Additional research will be sought to confirmation these findings. Studies to explore the mechanism of action are also needed.

Chelation with Ozone (chelox) for Heart Disease

In an aging population vascular disorders well exemplified by the chronic limb ischemia, chronic heart failure, cerebral ischemia and age-related macular degeneration represent a serious medical and socio-economical problem. While there is always a not easily identifiable first pathogenic noxa, all of these diseases are characterized by ischemia, chronic inflammation and tissue degeneration. Orthodox medicine has provided several optimal drugs targeting various pathological situations but, even with their concomitant applications, it is not possible to reduce the chronic oxidative stress. Here it is proposed to associate the approach of ozonated autohemotherapy as a modifier of the biological response capable to block the pathological progress.

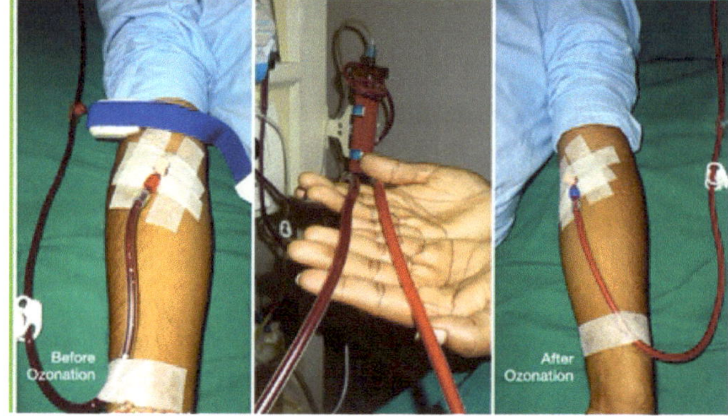

Fig. 28.3: *Showing technique of chelation with Ozone*

Ozone therapy, with its effects on the circulation, is the most effective therapy I have found for heart disease due to blocked arteries. While many patients know of chelation therapy, I have found ozone, and especially the combination of ozone with chelation, to be far superior.

Chelation and ozone treatment (chelox or chezone) for cardiovascular diseases one of the most rewarding conditions to treat

Naturopathic medicine excels at treating many different conditions, because the premise of a holistic approach is to make sure each and every cell is getting the good molecules it needs, and getting rid of the toxic molecules it doesn't. Such an approach makes sense for many patients because it supports health, allowing the body to heal and to respond more appropriately to natural medications.

Of course, the cells derive all of their most basic nutritional needs, including oxygen, from transport of blood in the blood vessels. A large part, but not all, of the cell's metabolic and environmental toxins are also carried away from the cell by the blood.

So when a patient presents with one of the most common forms of cardiovascular disease,coronary artery disease, I immediately see a patient who very likely has tissue that is hungry for oxygen and nutrients. Chezone treatment combines both chelation and ozone to treat this effectively and quickly. Chelox is a generic term for the combination of chelation and an oxidative treatment, where chezone is taught by Frank Shallenberger MD and refers to chelation with ozone therapy. Chezone is a popular and effective treatment for many illnesses, but not frequently offered by other doctors. Here in Vancouver I often get chezone patients from the Seattle area.

Ozone therapy improves oxygen delivery and circulation by:

1. decreasing the viscosity and thickness of the blood, so that it can navigate the small capillaries better, and is easier to pump
2. improves the ability of red blood cells to unload oxygen to the tissues. This persists long after the course of treatments is completed
3. decreases inappropriate inflammation in the blood, allowing for the formation of nitric oxide to help the arteries dilate, further improving blood flow

Chelation therapy improves circulation by:

1. removing heavy metals such as lead, which impair the formation of nitric oxide. Nitric oxide is produced by the lining of the blood vessels as a signal to help arteries relax and dilate, improving circulation
2. delivering high doses of nutrients such as magnesium, acting as a natural calcium channel blocker to keep arteries dilated and relaxed

I will usually put a patient who has coronary artery disease on a naturopathic program that involves both of these treatments. Often, I will combine the two treatments on the same day such that I administer an ozone treatment and follow this immediately with an EDTA chelation treatment (chelox therapy, or chezone). Usually a treatment program would involve up to 20-30 treatments over the course of a few months, but the patient will usually feel a noticeable difference in their symptoms after 3-4 ozone treatments (it can take a while longer if EDTA chelation is done alone).

The ozone procedure generally takes 30 minutes to complete. Once the ozone therapy is complete, an EDTA chelation bag is immediately hung up, taking 45-90 minutes to infuse in.

What to expect?

I was recently asked if there were any testimonials that patients had submitted regarding naturopathic treatment with chelation and ozone for coronary artery disease. I gave my usual response, which is that other patients generally will share their stories if they are seated beside you while getting treatment, but testimonials don't go far in any form of medicine because each patient is different. Then I typically go into how we should be looking at data instead of testimonials, and generally I will give the following infomation which looks into treatments almost identical to my naturopathic programs for coronary artery and heart disease (it is quite repetitive so you may want to skip past the summaries after reading a few):

J Card Surg reported that rat hearts had less damage from reperfusion of blood if the heart was treated with ozone. Reperfusion injury is important in patients who receive a surgical intervention that rapidly restores blood flow. Such injury is thought to be caused by an inability of the heart muscle to adapt to free-radical stress : ozone therapy is known to increase the ability of cells to respond to free radical stress.

Free Radic Biol Med journal reported on 22 patients who had 15 treatments of ozone by the procedure above. They had all had heart attacks within the previous year, and all had evidence of decreased intracellular antioxidant proteins such as glutathione peroxidase. After the treatment course, total cholesterol and LDL cholesterol (bad cholesterol) decreased significantly. More importantly, the antioxidant capability of the blood as measured by glutathione peroxidase increased.

81 patients were studied in Russia, all of whom had detectable blockages in their arteries. After a series of ozone treatments, the blood was less likely to clot, had decreased platelet activity, and had increased levels of enzymes and proteins that dissolved clots.

An Italian study of 72 patients who had blockages in the arteries feeding their legs, looked at different ways of administering ozone versus a control (no treatment group). They found that the ozone treatment groups, but not the control group, had significant improvements in walking speed and difference, and patients could increase walking speed to 2.5 km/hr. The authors believed the positive changes were do to changes in the microcirculation, as in the ability of the blood to unload oxygen.

Another Italian study looked at 15 patients who had blockages in the arteries feeding the legs that were so severe that revascularization surgery (eg bypass) was not an option. They found that ozone therapy was able to decrease the number of patients requiring amputation by 50%.

A Russian study of 85 patients who had progressive angina (chest pain due to lack of blood flow to the heart) and irregular heartbeats showed ultraviolet blood irradiation (similar to ozone therapy, which I also do) increased blood flow to the heart and was associated with favorable clinical improvements.

Another Russian study looked at the use of ultraviolet blood irradiation in cardiac rehab setting. They found the treatment to decrease cholesterol, decrease blood glucose, increase exercise tolerance, and improve the clotting parameters of the blood. Pretty well-rounded results.

A German study of 70 male patients who had severe progressive angina, 2/3rds of which had previously had a heart attack, and many of which who required more than 10 doses of nitroglycerin per day, found that UV blood irradiationimproved the majority of patients. This is after a 2 week trial of intensive drug therapy. They also found that markers of inflammation and infection were markedly cleared after the UV therapy.

There is also plenty of information on chelation therapy and heart disease in patients, and I have summarized some of the literature here in another newsletter.

To answer the question of what to expect for a patient, we can simply say that the condition of the patient improves, usually after a few treatments, although the full course can take a few months. Since we are doing a therapy that improves oxygen delivery, and removes metabolic poisons, the ability of all the cells and tissues to generate energy is restored. The net effect is therefore a decrease in angina symptoms, improvement in blood flow, and more energy.

While it may be that revascularization therapy with bypass surgery or angioplasty gives almost immediate results, such therapy only treats one lesion and does not treat the entire circulation. It's like having a houseful of rusting, corroding pipes, and then waiting for one joint in the plumbing to leak or to get corroded through, instead of slowly, deliberately, effectively treating the entire plumbing system.

This naturopathic approach to coronary artery and heart disease can be summarized in the following:The above series of reactions is how each cell generates energy from calories in our food and the oxygen we breathe.

Ozone stimulates the cycle to run faster, and increases the bottom reaction (oxidative phosphorylation), and improves oxygen delivery.

Chelation therapy removes the metal toxins (in red) that poison and slow down the cycle. The chelation IV bag also provides the nutrients (in green) that feed the cycle.

This is why the combination of ozone therapy and EDTA chelation therapy as a naturopathic program for coronary artery and heart disease is so rewarding. The combination of therapies improves the most fundamental problem in such a disease, which is energy generation. And it does so by providing the nutrients for this to happen, and removing the toxins that block it.

Is chelox / chezone therapy the only thing I have to do?

Of course, chelox / chezone therapy is only part of a comprehensive naturopathic program. During the initial consultation and exam, other important factors in health are addressed, such as dietary and lifestyle factors, particularly graduated exercise. In many cases though, chelox therapy (combination of EDTA chelation and ozone therapy), is the mainstay of the program until symptoms and the condition are improved significantly. Risk factor reduction in terms of lowering cholesterol (within reason), lowering blood pressure, finding the cause of inflammation, still need to be addressed as they are important as well.

What is the frequency of treatments?

Usually, once we have our lab reports back, treatments are given twice a week. Many times out of town patients will require more frequent treatment for practicality reasons, and in these cases chelation is given 3-5 times a week, and ozone therapy 5-7 times a week.

How is the patient monitored?

When I administer the treatment, after the needle is in the vein, I will pull blood every few treatments to ensure that the body is handling the stimulation and detoxification well. Particularly, I make sure the kidneys are handling the detoxification well. Often times, a urine test is done to confirm that the chelation therapy is in fact removing large amounts of metal toxins. This urine test also allows me to give an estimation of the length of treatment.

Bibliography and Acknowledgement

- Bocci V, Paulesu L. Studies on the biological effects of ozone 1. Induction of interferon gamma on human leucocytes. *Haematologica* 1990; **75**(6):510-515.
- Bocci V. Autohaemotherapy after treatment of blood with ozone. A reappraisal. *J Int Med Res* 1994; **22**(3):131-144.
- Carpendale MT, Freeberg J, Griffiss JM. Does ozone alleviate AIDS diarrhea? *J Clin Gastroenterol* 1993; **17**(2):142-145.
- Carpendale MT, Freeberg JK. Ozone inactivates HIV at noncytotoxic concentrations. *Antiviral Res* 1991; **16**(3):281-292.
- Escolar E, Lamas GA, Mark DB, *et al.* The effect of an EDTA-based chelation regimen on patients with diabetes mellitus and prior myocardial infarction in the Trial to Assess Chelation Therapy (TACT). Circulation: *Cardiovascular Quality and Outcomes*. 2014; **7**(1):15–24.
- Fabris G, Tommasini G, Petralia B, *et al.* [Intraforaminal oxygen-ozone therapy]. Rivista di Neuroradiologia 2001; **14**(1):61-66.
- Frankum B, Katelaris CH. Ozone therapy in AIDS--truly innocuous? *Med J Aust* 1993; **159**(7):493.
- Gabriel C, Blauhut B, Greul R, Schneeweis B, Roggendorf M. Transmission of hepatitis C by ozone enrichment of autologous blood. *Lancet* 1996; **347**(9000):541.
- Garber GE, Cameron DW, Hawley-Foss N, Greenway D, Shannon ME. The use of ozone-treated blood in the therapy of HIV infection and immune disease: a pilot study of safety and efficacy. *AIDS* 1991; **5**(8):981-984.
- Lamas GA, Boineau R, Goertz C, *et al.* EDTA chelation therapy alone and in combination with oral high-dose multivitamins and minerals for coronary disease: the factorial group results of the Trial to Assess Chelation Therapy. *American Heart Journal*. 2014; **168**(1):37–44.e5.
- Lamas GA, Boineau R, Goertz C, *et al.* Oral high-dose multivitamins and minerals after myocardial infarction: a randomized trial. *Annals of Internal Medicine*. 2013; **159**(12):797–805.
- *Lamas GA, Goertz C, Boineau R, et al*. Design of the trial to assess chelation therapy (TACT).Am *Heart J*. 2012; **163**(1):7–12.
- Lamas GA, Goertz C, Boineau R, *et al.* Effect of disodium EDTA chelation regimen on cardiovascular events in patients with previous myocardial infarction: the TACT randomized trial. *JAMA*. 2013; **309**(12):1241–1250.
- Marchetti D, La Monaca G. An unexpected death during oxygen-ozone therapy. *Am J Forensic Med Pathol* 2000; **21**(2):144-147.
- Martínez-Sánchez G, Al-Dalain SM, Menéndez S, Re L, *et al.* Therapeutic efficacy of ozone in patients with diabetic foot. *Eur J Pharmacol*. 2005 Oct 31; 523(1-3):151-61.
- Ozmen V, Thomas WO, Healy JT, *et al.* Irrigation of the abdominal cavity in the treatment of experimentally induced microbial peritonitis: efficacy of ozonated saline. Am Surg 1993; **59**(5):297-303.
- Pawlak-Osi?ska K, Ka?mierczak H, Ka?mierczak W, Szpoper M. Ozone therapy and pressure-pulse therapy in Ménière's disease. *Int Tinnitus J*. 2004; **10**(1):54-7.
- Rickard GD, Richardson R, Johnson T, *et al.* Ozone therapy for the treatment of dental caries. Cochrane Database Syst Rev. 2004; (3):CD004153.
- Sweet F, Kao MS, Lee SC, *et al.* Ozone selectively inhibits growth of human cancer cells. Science. 1980 Aug 22;209(4459):931-3.
- Verrazzo G, Coppola L, Luongo C, *et al.* Hyperbaric oxygen, oxygen-ozone therapy, and rheologic parameters of blood in patients with peripheral occlusive arterial disease. *Undersea Hyperb Med* 1995; **22**(1):17-22.

Ayurvedic Detoxification In The Management of Bodly Diseases & Prevention of Heart Ailments With Modern Digital Detox

Ayurveda recommends internal cleansing at every change of seasons. Detox is considered especially beneficial in the spring, because that is the time all of nature is rejuvenating itself.

The principle of rule of balance:- Whatever treatment is recommend in Maharishi Ayurveda, whether it's for purification or for treating an imbalance, we always follow the rule of balance first. This is a principle that is made clear by Charaka, one of the great ayurvedic healers of ancient times. The principle is that the physician should never create a new imbalance in order to repair or fix an imbalance. Whatever herbs we use, whatever purification methods we employ, we should never risk disturbing the doshas (mind/body operating principles) further. Nor do we create an imbalance in the quality and quantity of the dhatus(body tissues) or the quality, quantity and flow of the malas (body wastes). It is also essential that any detox program support the health of the shrotas, the large and small channels that provide the path for toxins to leave the body, so that embedded impurities, once loosened by the purification program, can be flushed out of the body completely and quickly.

The perfect treatment doesn't balance one part of the body at the risk of imbalancing another part. This is the perfection of Maharishi Ayurveda. In following this principle, the detoxification methods of Maharishi Ayurveda flush out the toxins gently without disturbing the body's own natural functioning.

Maharishi Ayurveda recommends two kinds of detoxification programs:

1. Self-detox (including diet, herbal preparations, and daily routine)
2. Detoxification program supervised by an expert trained in Maharishi Ayurveda.

While everyone can benefit from a supervised program such as Maharishi Panchakarma, not everyone should embark on a self-detox program. Which program you choose depends on the nature of your imbalances and the type of toxins lodged in your body.

Different types of toxins that we have to deal with and where they originate

There are three different types of toxins that can impact the physiology:

- Ama
- Amavisha
- Garvisha

Ama is the most common type of toxin, and is the waste product of incomplete digestion. Sticky, white and foul-smelling, it forms in the digestive tract when the food you eat is not digested properly. Ama is usually caused by eating foods unsuitable for your body type or the season; by eating too much or too little; by eating before the previous meal is digested; by going to sleep on a full stomach; or by eating foods that are left over, processed, old or fermented. If ama continues to be produced over a long period of time, it can leave the digestive tract, travel to a weak area elsewhere in the body and settle there. Usually it blocks the shrotas (microcirculatory channels) and disrupts the flow of nutrients to the area as well as the body's natural waste removal systems.

Usually ama develops when agni, the digestive fire, is either weak or irregular. By enhancing agni through dietary changes or by taking ayurvedic herbal supplements, the digestive system itself can burn off simple ama and clear it from the body.

Amavisha is a more reactive form of ama that forms when ama settles in one part of the body for a long time and mixes with the subdoshas, the dhatus or the malas there. This more toxic, reactive type of ama is more dangerous than the simple ama and must be dealt with differently during detoxification.

Garvisha is the third type of toxin, and unlike the other two, garvisha comes from outside the body. Included are environmental toxins such as chemicals, preservatives, poisons, air and water pollution, genetically engineered foods, synthetics and chemicals in clothing, synthetic drugs, chemicals in household cleansers, and heavy metals such as lead, arsenic and asbestos. Garvisha also includes toxins from spoiled foods.

Role of shrotas play in removing these toxins from the body

In detoxification the shrotas play a major role, because the toxins have to leave the body through the large and small channels of the body. So it's very important to maintain the proper health of the shrotas during all the stages of detox while preparing for detox, during the purification process and afterwards.

To understand how the shrotas need to be protected during detoxification, it's important to note that there are three kinds of abnormalities or damage that can happen to the shrotas. The first is blockage of the shrotas with simple ama. This type of toxin is easy to remove through simple purification and detoxification processes. For this person, self-detoxification works quite well, because simple ama can be dissolved through diet, herbal formulas and at-home procedures.

The second type of abnormality involves the more toxic and reactive amavisha. In this situation, the shrotas or channels themselves become hardened and dried with toxins. If your shrotas were pipes, the amavisha would be rust, not only blocking the pipes but actually corroding them as well.

The rust in this analogy is a toxic mixture of ama, amavisha and Shleshaka Kapha, which is the subdosha of Kapha concerned with maintaining proper fluid balance and lubrication of the body. When these three mix together, it causes an excess of moisture, an imbalance that in turn causes Vyana Vata (the subdosha of Vata concerned with circulation) to accelerate its drying effect, causing this toxic sludge to dry onto the channel walls. The channels become dry, inflexible, and narrow. There can also be blockage at the same time. This is the ayurvedic genesis of problems such as atherosclerosis.

Removing this more reactive type of toxin is a more complex problem. Maharishi Ayurveda detoxification procedures take care to first smooth and lubricate the toxins before detoxification. If the detox program doesn't first loosen the toxins, the shrotas could actually rupture when toxins are forced out of the body. At this stage, self-detoxification may still be recommended, but only if there is only a small amount of amavisha.

The third type of damage to the shrotas is the most severe. This results when amavisha becomes even more reactive, or the combination of Shleshaka Kapha, Vyana Vata, amavisha and ama becomes more reactive, or when these toxins are also joined by garvisha, environmental toxins. In this situation the shrotas actually rupture and become seriously damaged. This is the stage in which serious diseases of the shrotas manifest, such as ulcerative colitis, MS, and other autoimmune diseases. At this stage, self-detoxification is never recommended. Instead, it's very important that an individual consult an expert trained in Maharishi Ayurveda, who will supervise a clinical purification treatment such as Maharishi Panchakarma.

The main methods of detoxification used in Maharishi Ayurveda

Maharishi Ayurveda uses the body's own natural detoxification systems. This includes the bowel, kidneys, urine, skin, sweat glands and liver. The detoxification methods are never harsh or forceful, but simply support and enhance the body's own ability to release toxins.

Secondly, in Maharishi Ayurveda, each detox program cleanses all of the body's natural purification systems at once in a coordinated way. If the detox program were to focus on just one system, such as the colon and bowel, that would create an imbalance.

Third, because the Maharishi Ayurveda detoxification program is balanced, natural and effective, it creates a situation in which the body's detoxification system becomes stronger and stronger as time goes on, and thus the body can detoxify itself effectively after the detox treatment is over. For instance, the detox program may include drinking some herbal water steeped with detox herbs, such as Indian sarsaparilla, coriander seed, Manjistha or fennel. These spices have the effect of lubricating and cleansing the channels and supporting the bowel, urinary system, liver and skin. By clearing away the toxins, these herbs increase the alertness, wakefulness and intelligence of the kidneys, liver and other organs and channels. If the person is also following a more intelligent diet and following the ayurvedic routine, all of these therapies together support all of the detoxification systems in the body so they become more and more powerful, more and more efficient and effective. This holistic approach results in the natural balance of the body's detoxification systems, so that all of the detoxification organs become more alert, intelligent and capable of detoxifying the body on a day-to-day basis.

This is in contrast to fragmented detox treatments, in which one single organ such as the liver is flushed of toxins. The liver may become more intelligent by the clearing away of the toxins, but the problem is that toxins and sludge have not been cleansed from the other channels and purification systems of the body in a coordinated manner. Thus toxins are going to accumulate quickly in the liver again, causing the person to feel the need to repeat the process soon afterwards. This type of fragmented treatment doesn't strengthen the body's natural overall ability to detoxify itself. Of course, I don't want to give the impression that a person who uses a Maharishi Ayurveda detoxification program will never need to detoxify again! Everyone today is exposed to influences that create toxins beyond what the body can naturally handle, such as chemicals and preservatives in foods, synthetic drugs and emotional and mental stress. Seasonal changes also create ama. In winter the shrotas shrink, for instance, making it harder for the body to release toxins. During the transition between seasons, the agni (digestive fire) fluctuates, and that can cause some amount of ama to accumulate even if you are very careful about your diet and routine. For this reason, Maharishi Ayurveda recommends that you either self-detox or do Maharishi Panchakarma during each change of seasons, and particularly in the spring. In the spring the body is naturally detoxifying as the impurities flow out of the body, so it is the ideal time to support this detoxification with an herbal program.

Steps for detoxification in Maharishi Ayurveda:- Every ayurvedic detoxification program has three steps:

1. Preparation,
2. Cleansing
3. Post-cleansing therapies.

1.Preparation

Preparation is the most important part of the ayurvedic detox program. To prepare the body for detoxification, it's important to first balance the agni, or digestive fire. If someone has high or sharp agni, they need to take herbs or eat foods to reduce their agni. If the person has low agni, they need to take agni-enhancing herbs, or drink agni-enhancing herbal water. A third situation is irregular agni, meaning sometimes it's high and sometimes it's low, generally associated with a Vata imbalance. For this situation, we need to balance the agni first so it becomes more even.

- Preparation also takes into account the imbalances of the person. If you have more Kapha and are overweight, you will need a Kapha-pacifying diet and herbal water with more warming herbs. If you have a Pitta imbalance, you will need a Pitta-pacifying diet and herbal water with some attention to clearing the channels. For a thin person with Vata aggravation, a lubricating and nurturing diet and herbal water are needed. Lubricating and nurturing foods and herbs help pacify Vata and normalize an irregular agni.
- This careful preparation is unique to Maharishi Ayurveda. The general prevalent understanding is that before detox the only thing you need to do is increase the agni, and many detox programs advise one and all to heighten their agni, regardless of the differences in their constitutions and current imbalances. But you can see that, given the different imbalances and levels of agni, that is not a healthy or even a safe idea.
- For instance, if someone has a sharp digestive fire (tikshnagni), it's extremely important to pacify agni first, because otherwise the detoxification process could create further problems. If the agni is very high, amavisha, or the reactive type of toxic mixture that we called "rust" in the earlier analogy may be present. If you inflame agni in this situation, then during detox the shrotas could be ruptured by amavisha, causing complications and further imbalances.
- A person with Vata vitiation or a very thin person also needs special preparation for detox. Sometimes people who are very thin ask if they are free of toxins. I tell them that they do carry toxins, only their shrotas have become dry due to Vata aggravation, causing the toxins to dry and stick to the shrota walls. So they do need detoxification, but they must prepare properly. If this person starts on a straight detox program that forcefully squeezes out the toxins, that would be inviting danger.
- The Charaka Samhita even contains a verse about this exact situation. It explains that for an underweight person, the malas (body wastes) provide a type of strength, a type of support. So for that person it's necessary to first lubricate, nourish and nurture the body, before embarking on any detox program. This will give the person more stamina and reserves of dhatus (body tissues), so they can tolerate the detoxification

process without inviting risk of serious fatigue, mental irritation or skin eruptions.

2. Cleansing treatment

During the cleansing treatment, which is the second step of detoxification, the person's imbalances at that particular time are also taken into account.

- The health of the person's shrotas, the level of agni (sharp, weak, imbalanced, or balanced), the type of toxins present in the physiology, the balance or imbalance of the doshas – all of these factors need to be considered in determining the type of detox program the person should do – whether self-detoxification is recommended or an administered program such as Maharishi Panchakarma would be better.
- For all types of toxins, the first and foremost treatment is to improve elimination. Herbal Cleanse and Organic Digest Toneare gentle yet effective herbal supplements for cleansing the bowel. Herbal Cleanse contains rare forms of senna leaf and turpeth root (Indian jalap) along with other herbs to aid natural elimination, enhance cellular purification and improve assimilation of nutrients.
- Certain herbs are famous in ayurveda for their detoxifying effect, such as Indian sarsaparilla (hemidesmus indicus) and manjistha (Indian madder). These are contained in Elim-Tox and Elim-Tox-O, which are highly effective in flushing out toxins from the liver, blood, sweat glands and elimination system. Other herbs included in these formulas are Indian tinospora, rose petals and king of bitters (andrographis) to help balance and purify the liver. Indian sarsaparilla, red sandalwood and Neem leaf strengthen purification of toxins through the sweat glands and the skin. Other herb groups support elimination through the urinary tract, and still others support elimination of toxins through the stool and urine by lubricating the digestive tract. You can see that just this one product (either Elim-Tox or Elim-Tox-O) purifies all of the major elimination organs and systems in the body.
- Elim-Tox is faster acting, and is ideal if you have only simple ama. If you have a Pitta imbalance, or have some amount of amavisha, take Elim-Tox-O instead. It is slower-acting than Elim-Tox, but is safer for Pitta-based people because it first pacifies the reactivity of Pitta and amavisha before flushing out the toxins.
- Finally, Organic Genitrac helps flush out ama from the genitourinary tract. It targets the genitourinary channels to help eliminate toxins through the urine.
- So you can see that by using these three products together – Herbal Cleanse (or Organic Digest Tone), Elim-Tox (or Elim-Tox-O) and Organic Genitrac – you will be cleansing all of the body is detoxification organs and the shrotas simultaneously to provide a holistic and balanced effect.

3. Post-detoxification Management

The third step, or post-detoxification, is important because this is the optimum time to take rasayanas, the ayurvedic elixirs that rejuvenate the body and stop aging, such as Maharishi Amrit Kalash. With the toxins cleared out of the organs and channels of the body, the body is more awake and alert and can utilize the benefits of the rasayana more than ever before.

Which type of detox program is needed.

you can get an idea where your toxins are located, and whether you can purify them easily with the

- Self-Detox Program
- Expert trained in Maharishi Ayurveda

One simple rule is that a person who has a Kapha imbalance or body type with simple ama, with no symptoms of stiffness, no irritation, no symptoms of amavisha and garvisha, is the ideal candidate to do self-detoxification. People who have ama and only small amounts of amavisha can also do self-detox safely.

Recommendations for self-detoxification at home

The first thing to do is to prepare for detoxification by following these recommendations for diet, spices, and daily routine. Spring is the best time to detoxify, so you can start right away.

Preparation for Self-Detox (Fifteen Days)

I. Follow the Detox Diet

The cusp between winter and spring is the ideal time to do an at-home internal cleansing program, to allow your body to release the toxins that may have built up over the long cold winter.

A complete ayurvedic cleansing program includes 15 days of preparation and 45 days of actual cleansing. Ayurvedic healers recommend paying special attention to your diet during these two phases to avoid overtaxing your digestion and to enable purification to occur easily and completely.

Maharishi Ayurveda does not recommend fasting or entirely liquid diets such as juices, because that may cause your agni (digestive fire) to become imbalanced.

Here are some suggestions from The Council of Maharishi Ayurveda Physicians for diet management during detox:

Avoid ama-producing foods

Ama is the product of incomplete digestion it represents sticky toxic matter that can clog the channels of your body that carry nutrients to the cells and waste out of the body. Since cleansing is done to clear ama out of the body, you'll want to stay away from foods that build more ama in the body. From the ayurvedic perspective, leftovers, and "dead" foods such as processed, packaged, canned and frozen foods all create ama because they are very hard for your body to digest.

Non-organic foods:- genetically-modified foods; foods grown with chemicals, pesticides and chemical fertilizers; and foods with chemical additives also introduce toxins into your body and are confusing for the natural "intelligence" of your digestive system, and should therefore be avoided.

Avoid heavy dairy products such as aged hard cheese or yogurt, foods that are deep-fried or oily, raw foods of any kind, heavy desserts, and foods that contain refined sugar and honey, as these are harder to digest and create ama. Avoid yeasted breads, dry breads such as crackers, and fermented foods.

Eat ama-reducing foods

Favor vegetarian foods that are light, warm, cooked and easily digestible. Freshly-made flatbreads, freshly-made light soups and dhals, organic vegetables cooked with spices, and freshly-made grains such as quinoa are ideal. Mung dhal pacifies all three doshas and is nutritious, yet easy to digest.

Certain fruits, vegetables and spices are especially helpful during cleansing, so you'll want to eat a serving or two every day during the preparation and cleansing phases:

Fruits: Eat cooked prunes and figs at breakfast along with a stewed apple or pear. In general, most sweet juicy fruits are excellent cleansers.

Vegetables: Eat lots of cooked leafy greens. Chop the greens and cook them with Detox Spice Mix for best results. Brussels sprouts and cabbage are also helpful.

Grains: Light yet nutritious whole grains such as quinoa, barley, amaranth and small helpings of rice are recommended. Kanji, made by boiling rice with lots of water, is an excellent hot beverage and helpful for flushing toxins out of the body through the urine.

Spices: Ginger, turmeric, coriander, fennel and fenugree khelp open up the channels of the body and support the flushing of toxins via the skin, urinary tract, colon and liver. Add spices to soups and dhals as they cook, or sauté the spices in a little ghee and add to dishes when the cooking process is completed.

Lassi: made by combining fresh yogurt with water and digestion-boosting spices, is an excellent lunchtime beverage.

Choose foods according to your body type or imbalances

Ayurvedic healers recommend tailoring your diet year-round to your constitution and your imbalances. This is particularly true during cleansing to help regulate your digestive fire (agni). For detailed information on diets and foods for pacifying each of the three doshas, visit Vata, Pitta, or Kapha.

Drink plenty of hot water through the day

Warm water helps flush toxins out of the body through the urine. To derive healing benefits from the water you drink, add detoxifying spices to the water. Here is a recipe for Detoxifying Tea from The Council of Maharishi Ayurveda Physicians : After the 45 days of cleansing are over, take a few days to gradually introduce heavier foods and ease back into your regular diet. This is also the perfect time to start taking Rasayanas (ayurvedic formulations for overall health and vitality) like Amrit, Organic Digest Tone, or Vital Man or Vital Lady. Now that the channels of your body are clear, your body will make maximum use of the overall healing benefits of these tonics.

II. Follow the Detox Routine

1. Get enough rest:- You may need more sleep while detoxifying. It's also important to go to bed early (before 10 p.m.) and get up early (before 6 a.m.), as both staying up late and sleeping late in the morning can flood the shrotas with toxins. Practice the Transcendental Meditation® program regularly.
2. Exercise each day.
    - Gentle exercise such as yoga asanas and walking can support detoxification by improving digestion and elimination and moving toxins out of the body. Walking for twenty minutes or half an hour is ideal, because it allows you to breathe deeply, purify the respiratory system and supply the cells with cleansing prana. Walking in the early morning especially helps move toxins out of the body.
    - Yoga asanas are designed to purify and enliven

different organs of the body, and they also enhance digestion and elimination, as does all exercise. Pranayama breathing exercises are also excellent for cleansing the respiratory system and other organs. During the preparation for detox and the actual self-detox program, it's best to avoid strenuous exercise.

3. Massage daily:- One of the most important purification procedures in Maharishi Ayurveda is warm oil massage (abhyanga), and you can do it every day on your own. Abhyanga loosens impurities from the shrotas and tissues, allowing them to flow into the digestive tract, where they can be easily eliminated through the bowel. While you're detoxifying, take a little extra time with your morning massage, and you'll magnify the results many times. Use warm massage oil with herbs added, such as Youthful Skin Massage Oil, as the herbs are chosen to penetrate the surface of the skin and reach the deeper layers and tissues, purifying and nourishing the shrotas of the skin. By gently massaging the whole body, you're also gently purifying other organs as well. Increasing circulation also helps purify the blood. Always follow your abhyanga with a warm (not hot) bath. If you don't have time for a bath, a shower can substitute.

III. Follow Ama-Reducing Eating Habits

All through the year, and especially while detoxifying, it's important to follow the ayurvedic eating guidelines for reducing ama. These include:

1. Do not fast or skip meals during any part of the self-detoxification program.
2. Eat at the same time every day so your agni can "fire up" for the meal.
3. Eat your main meal at noon and lighter meals at breakfast and dinner.
4. Eat while sitting down in a settled atmosphere; pay attention to the food when you eat (no TV, no phones, no reading).
5. Engage in pleasant conversation with friends or family (no business meetings or emotional discussions).
6. Eat only when the previous meal has been digested (no grazing or untimely snacking this really disrupts digestion). Eat only when you are hungry again.
7. Sit quietly for a minute at the beginning of the meal (saying grace before meals is one way to do this), and wait for a couple of minutes after eating before leaving the table. This gives your digestion a settled start.
8. Leave a little space in your stomach at the end of the meal to give your digestion room to function. Maharishi Ayurveda recommends that you regularly eat to only ¾ of your capacity. This last guideline is especially important when you're on a detoxification program. You don't want to overeat when your body is detoxifying.

Self-Detox Program (45 days)

Throughout the Self-Detox Program of 45 days, continue to follow the ama-reducing diet, daily routine and eating habits mentioned in the section Preparing for Detox.

- Take two to five tablets of Organic Digest Tone before going to bed each night to cleanse the bowel, or two to four capsules of Herbal Cleanse.
- Take two tablets of Elim-Tox morning and evening to cleanse the liver, the blood, the sweat glands and the elimination system. Take Elim-Tox-O instead if you have any symptoms of amavisha or if you have a Pitta imbalance.
- Take two tablets of Organic Genitrac morning and evening. This will purify the urinary tract and assist the removal of toxins. (Note - If you take Amrit, cut your dosage in half when on the cleansing program. Also, it is best not to combine Elim-Tox with Bio-Immune or Radiant Skin, because these formulations have overlapping actions and benefits.)

Post-Detox Program

- After spending 15 days preparing for detox and 45 days actually doing the self-detox program, you should feel much lighter, more blissful, and more energetic. You may even have shed some unwanted pounds. Give yourself time to gradually transition into your normal routine and eating habits. Take time to gradually add heavier foods to your diet, and be sure to get enough rest for a few days after detox is over. Follow your normal ayurvedic routine and recommended diet for your body type.
- Take rasayanas such as Maharishi Amrit Kalash and Vital Lady or Vital Man. Now that your shrotas are clear, the rasayanas are most effective in reaching the cells and deeply nourishing and rejuvenating your entire physiology.

Special Recommendations for Cleansing the Body's Main Organs of Purification.

If you feel your impurities are located in either the bowel, the urinary tract or the skin, you can follow these special recommendations while preparing to detox and during the actual self-detox program. You can also follow these recommendations whenever you feel toxins building up in that particular area.

1. Detoxifying the Bowel

Constipation or irregular bowel movements causes the malas (body waste such as fecal matter) to be reabsorbed by the body. This creates toxins in the rasa dhatu (nutritive fluid), the rakta dhatu (blood), and from there the other dhatus. Regular bowel movements provide the primary day-to-day detoxification channel.

If the stool is very dry or slow, try adding more ghee to the diet and drink Herbal Water for Constipation (see recipe below). Add spices to your food, using the Herbal Spice Mixture for Slow Bowel Movement (see below). This will also support digestion and liver function. Eat foods with more soft fibers such as oatmeal, tender leafy greens, summer squashes, and cooked or soaked prunes and figs. Avoid a Vata-aggravating diet or drying diet, and avoid drying foods such as crackers, dried cereal, raw foods and any foods that are drying for the bowel. Take Herbal Cleanse, Organic Digest Tone or Psyllium seed husks (take one teaspoon soaked in one cup of warm water before bed) to scrub out the bowel.

- Slow Bowel Movement Herbal Water
- Slow Bowel Movement Herbal Spice Mix

2. Detoxifying the Urine

The kidneys and urinary tract form an essential purification system in the body. If you do not have a diagnosed problem with the prostate, kidneys, or water retention, but even so you feel that you are retaining water and that the flow of urine is not quite normal, you can detoxify the urine and kidneys using Urinary Tract Cleansing Herbal Water. You can also add some white daikon radish to your vegetables, as this helps purify the urine and normalize its flow, so you're not retaining any toxins. It does this without irritating or adding pressure to the urinary tract. The kidneys and urinary tract can also be cleaned by spacially prepared urinary tract cleansing herbal water

3. Detoxifying the Skin

If you harbor toxins under the skin or in the fat or blood tissue, this will manifest as excessive oiliness, breakouts or extreme photosensitivity. For this situation, drink Skin Detox Herbal Water every day. Also use the Skin Detox Spice Mix on your vegetables and grains. This can be done with the following;-

- Skin Detox Herbal Water
- Skin Detox Spice Mix

In can if person have all three problems;- If you have all three problems,

- Choose any one type of herbal water to start with which ever problem you feel is most predominant should be takled first.
- **Also, taking Elim-Tox-O helps all three:** it purifies the skin, the bowel and the urinary tract.
- Organic Premium Amla Berry with lunch and dinner,
- Organic Genitrac and the Skin Detox Spice Mix are additional recommendations.
- Eating cooked leafy greens is an excellent dietary addition for all three types of detoxification.

Measures in purifying the liver: The liver is an essential organ for screening toxins. It is the liver's job to scan and identify toxins in the nutritive fluid and store them so they donot enter the blood. The liver is responsible for the purity of the blood and for keeping ama from mixing with it. However, if the liver becomes overloaded with too many chemicals, preservatives or additives from foods or other toxins, it will no longer be able to screen the toxins. By purifying and strengthening the liver, this important function of protecting the blood from toxins can be restored.

In case if you have a sluggish liver, it's best to check with an ayurvedic expert. It's better to take the physician's advice for this important organ. All of the programs we have already mentioned, especially

1. Using the spice turmeric in food, will help strengthen and purify the liver.
2. Elim-Tox-O and Elim-Tox also help protect and strengthen the liver.
3. choose one formula that's right for you.

Detox prevention program. Measures to Prevent toxic accumulation in the body

Prevention is the key to health, so the best plan is to prevent toxic build-up.

- Follow the diet and daily routine for your imbalances;
- Exercise every day to improve your digestion and elimination;
- Do a daily abhyanga to flush out toxins through the skin;
- Drink the herbal water suitable for your imbalances;
- Meditate every day to remove stress. Daily practice of the Transcendental Meditation technique is highly beneficial in dissolving mental and emotional ama, and thus is a necessary part of any detox prevention program. Mental and

emotional stress have a physiological counterpart : the hormones and biochemicals that flood your body whenever you feel anxious, fearful, or angry. Research on the Transcendental Meditation technique shows that it reduces cortisol levels and other measures of anxiety in the body. Other research shows that it lowers blood pressure and reduces negative emotions such as fear, aggression, and anger. Even diseases caused by amavisha, such as heart disease, hypertension and stroke, are found to significantly improve with the practice of the Transcendental Meditation technique, as reported in the American Heart Disease journals Stroke and Hypertension.

- Finally, the ayurvedic seasonal routines and dietary guidelines are key parts of any prevention program. By following simple seasonal guidelines, you can help mitigate the toxins that accumulate due to seasonal changes.

Digital addiction disorder and Detox therapy

Internet addiction disorder (IAD), also known as problematic Internet use or pathological Internet use, refers to excessive Internet use that interferes with daily life. Addiction, defined by Webster Dictionary as a «compulsive need for and use of a habit-forming substance characterized by tolerance and by well-defined physiological symptoms upon withdrawal», was traditionally used to depict a person›s dependence on the substance. More recently, the concept has been applied to behavioral dependence including internet use. The problem of Internet addiction evolves together with the development and spread of the Internet. As adolescents (12–17 years) and emerging adults (18–29 years) access the Internet more than any other age groups and undertake a higher risk of overuse of the Internet, the problem of Internet addiction disorder is most relevant to young people.

Excessive use of the Internet has been found by various studies to disrupt individuals' time use and have a series of health consequences. But the existence of Internet addiction as a mental disorder is not yet well recognized. The current version of Diagnostic and Statistical Manual of Mental Disorders (DSM-V) noted that Internet gaming disorder (one type of IAD) is a condition that requires more research in order to be considered as a full disorder in 2013

What is Digital detox.

It refers to a period of time during which a person refrains from using electronic connecting devices such as smartphones and computers. It is regarded as an opportunity to reduce stress, focus more on social interaction and connection with nature in the physical world. Claimed benefits include increased mindfulness, lowered anxiety, and an overall better appreciation of one's environment.

Smartphones, laptops and tablets, combined with the increasing wireless Internet accessibility, enable technology users to constantly be connected to the digital world. Constant online connectivity may have a negative impact on the users' experience with electronic connecting devices and result in a wish to temporarily refrain from communication technology usage.

In one study in Mind, 95% of those interviewed said their mood improved after putting down their phones to spend time outside, changing from depressed, stressed, and anxious to more calm and balanced.

The motivations behind digital detoxing vary. In some cases the motivation is negative emotional responses to the technology usage, such as dissatisfaction or disappointment of the technology device and its functions. In other cases, users see the technology as a distracting factor that consumes time and energy, and want to take back control over their everyday lives. Some people have moral, ethical or political reasons to refrain from technology usage, such as fear of violation of their privacy. Furthermore, a concern of developing addictive behavior in terms of tech addiction or Internet addiction disorder is one of the motivations for disconnecting for a period of time.

Constant engagement with digital connecting devices at the workplace is claimed to lead to increased stress levels and reduce productivity Certain characteristics of the technology make it more difficult to distinguish work from leisure. Moreover, being continually connected increases the amount of interruptions at work. Allowing employees to disconnect for a part of the day in order to truly focus on their work without disturbance from colleagues is claimed to be beneficial to the productivity and work environment.

The connecting devices' multitasking character has a serious impact on the learning ability. Multitasking implies operating on a surface level, which only involves the short-time memory Using multiple connecting devices as learning platforms is therefore not beneficial. A reduction of information choices enables the brain to focus more on the quality of the information rather than the hastiness of it.

Terminology

Digital addict

It is used to refer to a person who compulsively uses digital technology, which would manifest as another form of addiction if that technology was not as easily accessible to them. Colloquially, it can be used to describe a person whose interaction with technology is verging on excessive, threatening to absorb their attention above all else and consequently having a negative impact on the well-being of the user. The primary theory is digital technology users develop digital addiction by their habitual use and reward from computer applications. This reward triggers the reward center in the brain that releases more dopamine, opiates, and neurochemicals, which overtime can produce a stimulation tolerance or need to increase stimulation to achieve a "high" and prevent withdrawal. Used as a conversational phrase, digital addict describes an increasingly common dependence on devices in the digital age.

The notion of "Internet Addictive Disorder" was initially conjured up by Dr. Ivan K. Goldberg in 1995 as a joke to parody the complexity and rigidity of American Psychiatric Association's (APA) «Diagnostic and Statistical Manual of Mental Disorders (DSM)." In his first narration, Internet addictive disorder was described as having the symptoms of "important social or occupational activities that are given up or reduced because of Internet use," "fantasies or dreams about the Internet," and "voluntary or involuntary typing movements of the fingers." The definition of Internet addiction disorder has troubled researchers ever since its inception. In general, no standardized definition has been provided despite that the phenomenon has received extensive public and scholar recognition. Below are some of the commonly used definitions. In 1998, Dr. Jonathan J. Kandell defined Internet addiction as "a psychological dependence on the Internet, regardless of the type of activity once logged on."

English psychologist Mark D. Griffiths (1998) conceived Internet addiction as a subtype of broader technology addiction, and also a subtype of behavioral addictions

Dr. Keith W. Beard (2005) articulates that "an individual is addicted when an individual's psychological state, which includes both mental and emotional states, as well as their scholastic, occupational and social interactions, is impaired by the overuse of [Internet]"

Diagnosis of Internet addiction

DSM-based instruments

Most of the criteria utilized by research are adaptations of listed mental disorders (e.g., pathological gambling) in the Diagnostic and Statistical Manual of Mental Disorders (DSM)handbook. Dr. Ivan K. Goldberg, who first broached the concept of Internet addiction, adopted a few criteria for IAD on the basis of DSM-IV, including "hoping to increase time on the network" and "dreaming about the network. By adapting the DSM-IV criteria for pathological gambling, Dr. Kimberly S. Young (1998) proposed one of the first integrated sets of criteria, Diagnostic Questionnaire (YDQ), to detect Internet addiction. A person who fulfills any five of the eight adapted criteria would be regarded as Internet addicted:

- Preoccupation with the Internet
- A need for increased time spent online to achieve the same amount of satisfaction;
- Repeated efforts to curtail Internet use;
- Irritability, depression, or mood lability when Internet use is limited
- Staying online longer than anticipated
- Putting a job or relationship in jeopardy to use the Internet
- Lying to others about how much time is spent online
- Using the Internet as a means of regulating mood.

While Young's YDQ assessment for IA has the advantage of simplicity and ease of use, Keith W. Beard and Eve M. Wolf (2001) further asserted that all of the first five (in the order above) and at least one of the final three criteria (in the order above) be met to delineate Internet addiction in order for a more appropriate and objective assessment

Young further extended her 8-question YDQ assessment to the now most widely used Internet Addiction Test (IAT), which consists of 20 items with each on a 5-point Likert scale. Questions included on the IAT expand upon Young's earlier 8-question assessment in greater detail and include questions such as "Do you become defensive or secretive when anyone asks you what you do online?" and "Do you find yourself anticipating when you go online again?". A complete list of questions can be found in Dr. Kimberly S. Young's 1998 book Caught in the Net : How to Recognize the Signs of Internet Addiction and A Winning Strategy for Recovery and Drs. Laura Widyanto and Mary McMurran's 2004 article titled The Psychometric Properties of the Internet Addiction Test. The Test score ranges from 20 to 100 and a higher value indicates a more problematic use of the Internet:

- 20–39 = average Internet users,
- 40–69 = potentially problematic Internet users
- 70–100 = problematic Internet users.

Over time, a considerable number of screening instruments have been developed to diagnose Internet addiction, including the Internet Addiction Test (IAT) the Internet-Related Addictive Behavior Inventory (IRABI) the

Chinese Internet Addiction Inventory (CIAI) the Korean Internet Addiction Self-Assessment Scale (KS Scale), the Compulsive Internet Use Scale (CIUS),] the Generalized Problematic Internet Use Scale (GPIUS) the Internet Consequences Scale (ICONS),[36] and the Problematic Internet Use Scale (PIUS). Among others, the Internet Addiction Test (IAT) by Young (1998) exhibits good internal reliability and validity and has been used and validated worldwide as a screening instrument.

Although the various screening methods are developed from diverse contexts, four dimensions manifest themselves across all instruments:

- **Excessive use:** compulsive Internet use and excessive online time-use;
- **Withdrawal symptoms:** withdrawal symptoms including feelings such as depression and anger, given restricted Internet use;
- **Tolerance:** the need for better equipment, increased internet use, and more applications/ software;
- **Negative repercussions:** Internet use caused negative consequences in various aspects, including problematic performance in social, academic, or work domains.

More recently, researchers Mark D. Griffiths (2000) and Dr. Jason C. Northrup and colleagues (2015) claim that Internet per se is simply the medium and that the people are in effect addicted to processes facilitated by the Internet. Based on Young›s Internet Addiction Test (IAT) Northrup and associates further decompose the internet addiction measure into four addictive processes : Online video game playing, online social networking, online sexual activity, and web surfing. The Internet Process Addiction Test (IPAT)] is created to measure the processes to which individuals are addicted.

Screening methods that heavily rely on DSM criteria have been accused of lacking consensus by some studies, finding that screening results generated from prior measures rooted in DSM criteria are inconsistent with each other. As a consequence of studies being conducted in divergent contexts, studies constantly modify scales for their own purposes, thereby imposing a further challenge to the standardization in assessing Internet addiction disorder

Single-question instruments

Some scholars and practitioners also attempt to define Internet addiction by a single question, typically the time-use of the Internet. The extent to which Internet use can cause negative health consequences is, however, not clear from such a measure. The latter of which is critical to whether IAD should be defined as a mental disorder.

Classification

As many scholars have pointed out, the Internet serves merely as a medium through which tasks of divergent nature can be accomplished. Treating disparate addictive behaviors under the same umbrella term is highly problematic.

Dr. Kimberly S. Young (1999) asserts that Internet addiction is a broad term which can be decomposed into several subtypes of behavior and impulse control problems, namely,

- **Cybersexual addiction:** compulsive use of adult websites for cybersex and cyberporn;
- **Main article:** Internet sex addiction.
- **Cyber-relationship addiction:** Over-involve ment in online relationships;
- **Net compulsions:** Obsessive online gambling, shopping or day-trading;
- **Information overload:** Compulsive web surfing or database searches;
- **Computer addiction:** Obsessive computer game playing.

Treatment: therapies

From smartphones to sat navs, our lives are full of screens. We wake up to them, we come home to them, and we carry them around in our pockets all day. So perhaps it›s unsurprising that experts are warning that this constant exposure could be damaging our health.

“Technology may be incredibly useful and educational and it undoubtedly allows us much creativity, connectivity and enjoyment,” says Charlotte Walsh, partner at Digital Detox. “But if it begins to distract you from doing what you should be doing - like your job or your education - or it negatively affects your relationships, or costs you more money than you can afford, then it starts to become dangerous. If it is negatively impacting your life you need to evaluate what you do online, when and with whom.»

In numbers | Internet addiction

The average person checks their phone 200 times a day - that’s once every six and a half minutes 73% of Brits say they’d struggle to go a day without checking their phone or computer

One in four people spend more time online than they do asleep 70% of 16-24-year-olds say they prefer texting to talking The average teenager sends 3,400 electronic messages a month from their bed

But how easy is it to start and, more importantly, stick to a much-needed digital detox? "To avoid becoming a slave to your smartphone, you do need a level of self-discipline - and, occasionally, a complete break," explains Walsh.

How to make your digital detox a success

1. Make a gadget list

"Before you commit to a detox, try making two lists," advises Dr Sally-Ann Law, a psychologist and personal life coach. "Firstly, list all of your gadgets. This will show you how dependent you are on technology. Secondly, make a list of all the things that you enjoy doing in life, but aren't doing presently." "This will help you realise that, if you cut down your technology use, you'll gain back hours of time to do things that you find considerably more meaningful than constantly checking Facebook. Some estimates show that we spend the equivalent of three weeks every year on social media and checking emails - time we could be at home or on holiday."

2. Give yourself an allowance

"If you establish a maximum daily time allowance for your devices then you will be more likely to stick to your detox," suggests Dr Richard Graham, a Technology Addiction Specialist at Nightingale Hospital. If you establish a maximum daily time allowance for your devices, then you will be more likely to stick to your detoxDr Richard Graham "By restricting the time you spend using technology, you can focus on the 'real world' much more, and will be encouraged to enjoy social interactions in person rather than through a screen."

3. Don't set unachievable targets

Although an allowance is important, London-based life coach Carole Ann Rice believes that digital detoxes are something one needs to ease into. "In order to completely sever your dependency, it would be a good idea to first simply set small limits for each day.

Be this during exercise time, your lunch break, or when out shopping, if you slowly eliminate technology from various parts of your day, your detox will be easier to stick at. Habitual rituals help us achieve our targets, but only if they are achievable themselves."

4. Commit to changing one habit at a time

"Choose one technology habit to change at a time," advises Dr Law. "Maybe this would be banning all devices from the dining table, or from the bedroom, or only checking emails every two hours." Choose one technology habit to change at a time, and make sure that you stick to it for at least a week no matter what, and then move onto tackling another. Dr Sally Ann Law But whatever it is, make sure that you stick to it for at least a week no matter what - and then move onto tackling another habit." Keep going like this, eliminating your dependencies incrementally, until you feel more in control," says Dr Law.

5. Ensure you get enough sleep

"Try storing devices in a different room to your bedroom overnight," suggests Dr Graham. "This will stop yourself using them straight before sleep, and first thing in the morning - which is important as sleep issues can sometimes coexist with technology addiction."

Make sure you turn all screens off at least two hours before bed - that means no phone, no laptop, no iPad. "Your bedroom is for sleeping - so don't turn it into a cinema, a shopping centre, a bank or a casino."

6. Make an effort to give others your attention

"You should make the effort to give people your undivided attention," says Rice. "Focus on how rude people will think you are if you're constantly checking your phone or texting away - and this will make your more likely to give them 100 per cent of your attention." If you're still struggling, take away temptation. "Try timing your emails so they only download to your smartphone every two or three hours. This will mean that your time and energy isn't dissipated by constant distractions, and you can then deal with your day's emails and notifications in a concentrated period of allotted time per day."

7. Find a detox buddy

"Things are always easier when you team up with someone," says Dr Law, "So why not pair up with a 'detox buddy'? With this support, you can discuss your progress, encourage each other to keep going and spend time together face-to-face rather than messaging through a screen. A detox buddy will keep you honest."

8. Leave your gadgets at home

"We are ever-curious about what others are up to then we compare and despair," says Rice. "So try leaving your gadgets at home, or just going out without your headphones once in a while. You may find that you miss very little, and will have more time to do more with your life than spending it watching other people's worlds through a screen. Carole Ann Rice "Rather than thinking life without your iPod is boring, get used to listening to birdsong when out on a run. "You may find that you miss very little, and will have more time to do more with your life than spending it watching other people's worlds through a screen."

9. Tell everyone what you're doing

"The more people you tell about your detox, the more people will be watching you - and the less you will want to fail," Dr Graham explains. "Setting an example to friends or family is a great way to motivate yourself. Try leaving phones on silent or switched off during meal times - something which is particularly important for children and young people who learn behaviour from their parents."

Current interventions and strategies used as treatments for Internet addiction stem from those practiced in substance abuse disorder. In the absence of "methodologically adequate research", treatment programs are not well corroborated. Psychosocial treatment is the approach most often applied. In practice, rehab centers usually devise a combination of multiple therapies

Psychosocial Treatment

Cognitive-Behavioral Therapy

The cognitive-behavioral therapy with Internet addicts (CBT-IA) is developed in analogy to therapies for impulse control disorder . Several key aspects are embedded in this therapy:

- Learning time management strategies;
- Recognizing the benefits and potential harms of the Internet;
- Increasing self-awareness and awareness of others and one's surroundings;
- Identifying "triggers" of Internet "binge behavior," such as particular Internet applications, emotional states, maladaptive cognitions, and life events;
- Learning to manage emotions and control impulses related to accessing the Internet, such as muscles or breathing relaxation training;
- Improving interpersonal communication and interaction skills;
- Improving coping styles
- Cultivating interests in alternative activities.

Three phases are implemented in the CBT-IA therapy:

- **Behavior modification to control Internet use:** Examine both computer behavior and non-computer behavior and manage Internet addicts' time online and offline;
- **Cognitive restructuring to challenge and modify cognitive distortions:** Identify, challenge, and modify the rationalizations that justify excessive Internet use;
- **Harm reduction therapy to address co-morbid issues:** Address any co-morbid factors associated with Internet addiction, sustain recovery, and prevent relapse.
- Symptom management of CBT-IA treatment has been found to sustain 6 months post-treatment.
- Restore Recoverytm is a training program that aims to standardize the CBT-IA application and assist practitioners› practice in assessing and treating Internet addiction disorder.

Motivational Interviewing

- The motivational interviewing approach is developed based on therapies for alcohol abusers. This therapy is a directive, patient-centered counseling style for eliciting behavior change through helping patients explore and resolve ambivalence with a respectful therapeutic manner. It does not, however, provide patients with solutions or problem solving until patients› decision to change behaviors.
- Several key elements are embedded in this therapy.

Asking open-ended questions;

- Giving affirmations
- Reflective listening.
- Other psychosocial treatment therapies include reality therapy, Naikan cognitive psychotherapy, group therapy, family therapy, and multimodal psychotherapy

Transcutaneous Electrical Nerve Stimulation

Scholars have also evaluated the effect of 2/100-Hz transcutaneous electrical nerve stimulation (TENS) on Internet addicts. Two Chinese studies found that 2/100- Hz TENS, which adjusts the release of central neurotransmitter, can effectively reduce the online time of adolescent Internet addicts and mitigate IA syndrome.

Pharmacologic Therapy

Given that multiple psychiatric disorders frequently coexist with Internet addiction disorder, pharmacological therapies are used to address the shared mechanism. Several studies have been carried out in this respect. One study also suggests that desires exhibited in online gaming addiction (IGD) might have the same neurobiological mechanism as that of substance dependence. Although some evidence has emerged, the general efficacy of pharmacologic therapy in treating IA is yet to be established.

Digital Detox Week

In 1994, the week was first championed by TV-Free America, and promoted by Adbusters magazine and other organizations. TV-Free America then became Center for SCREEN-TIME Awareness. CSTA was an organization that encouraged all people to use electronic screen media responsibly and then have more time for a healthy life and more community participation. It was a grassroots alliance of many different organizations, with participation in over 70 nations around the world. Screen Free week happens in Canada.

CCFC changed the name of TV-Turnoff to Screen-Free Week in 2010, since entertainment media (and advertising) are increasingly delivered through a variety of screens (computers, hand-held devices, etc.), and not just traditional television commercials. In 2008 Adbusters changed the name of TV Turnoff Week to Digital Detox Week to reflect the growing predominance of computers and other digital devices.

Screen-Free Week (formerly TV Turnoff Week and Digital Detox Week) is an annual event where children, families, schools and communities are encouraged to turn off screens and "turn on life". Instead of relying on television programming for entertainment, participants read, daydream, explore, enjoy nature, and spend time with family and friends. Over 300 million people have taken part in the turnoff, with millions participating each year.

In 2010, Campaign for a Commercial-Free Childhood (CCFC) became the home of Screen-Free Week at the request of the Board of the Center for SCREEN-TIME Awareness (CSTA), which ran the initiative since 1994 (first as TV-Free America). CCFC launched a new website and developed a new Organizer›s Kit, fact sheets, and other materials for Screen-Free Week 2011 and beyond. The Screen-Free Week Organizer›s Kit is available as a free download

International Network Into Problematic Internet Usage

European Union under its Horizon 2020 umbrella has just launched a new United Kingdom-led four year European Cooperation in Science and Technology (COST) Action Programme (CA 16207), to advance networked interdisciplinary research into problematic internet usage across Europe and beyond. The first steps will be to reach consensus on the reliable definition of the problem, devise age-appropriate assessment instruments to measure its severity, plan studies to clarify its clinical course and impact on health and quality of life as well as to clarify the underpinning brain-based mechanisms to support the development of screening biomarkers to identify those who are vulnerable before the problematic use becomes too entrenched and ultimately to identify targets to guide the development of new and effective interventions. The Action welcomes research-active scientists working in the field. Actions website Net&Me is due to be launched by the end of Feb 2018.

Bibliography and Acknowledgement

- Digital detox: definition of digital detox in Oxford dictionary (British & World English). Oxforddictionaries.com. Retrieved 2014-07-20.
- DSM-5. www.psychiatry.org. Retrieved 2018-02-19.
- Gaming disorder. World Health Organization. Retrieved 2018-03-02.
- How Does Nature Impact Our Wellbeing? | Taking Charge of Your Health & Wellbeing. Taking Charge of Your Health & Wellbeing. Retrieved 2017-06-08.
- How To Do A Digital Detox. Forbes. 2014-06-13. Retrieved 2014-07-20.
- PsycNET. psycnet.apa.org. Retrieved 2018-02-21.
- "Turning Off the TV" article at The Washington Post. April 24, 2006. Accessed December 23, 2008.
- Internet Addiction: Metasynthesis of 1996–2006 Quantitative Research. CyberPsychology & Behavior. 12 (2): 203–207
- Anderson, E. L.; Steen, E.; Stavropoulos, V. (2017). "Internet use and Problematic Internet Use: A systematic review of longitudinal research trends in adolescence and emergent adulthood". *International Journal of Adolescence and Youth.* **22** (4): 430–454.
- Ayyagari, R., Grover, V., & Purvis, R. 2011. Technostress: Technological antecedents and implications. *MIS Quarterly*, **35**(4), 831-858.
- Bakken, Inger Johanne; Wenzel, Hanne Gro; Götestam, K. Gunnar; Johansson, Agneta; Øren, Anita (2009-04-01). "Internet addiction among Norwegian adults: A stratified probability sample study". *Scandinavian Journal of Psychology*. **50** (2): 121–127.
- Beard, Keith W. (2005-02-01). "Internet Addiction: A Review of Current Assessment Techniques and Potential Assessment Questions". *CyberPsychology & Behavior*. **8** (1): 7–14.
- Beard, Keith W.; Wolf, Eve M. (2001-06-01). "Modification in the Proposed Diagnostic Criteria for Internet Addiction". *CyberPsychology & Behavior.* **4** (3): 377–383.
- Black, D. W.; Belsare, G.; Schlosser, S. (December 1999). "Clinical features, psychiatric comorbidity, and health-related quality of life in persons reporting compulsive computer use behavior". *The Journal of Clinical Psychiatry*. **60** (12): 839–844.
- Block, Jerald J. (2008-03-01). "Issues for DSM-V: Internet Addiction". *American Journal of Psychiatry.* **165** (3): 306–307.
- Brabazon, T. (2012). Time for a digital detox? From information obesity to digital dieting. Fast Capitalism, 9.1.
- Brand, Matthias (2017). Internet Addiction. Studies in Neuroscience, Psychology and Behavioral Economics. Springer, Cham. pp. 19–34.
- Brenner, V. (1997). "Psychology of computer use: XLVII. Parameters of Internet use, abuse and addiction: the first 90

days of the Internet Usage Survey". *Psychological reports*. **80** (3): 879–882.

- Byun, Sookeun; Ruffini, Celestino; Mills, Juline E.; Douglas, Alecia C.; Niang, Mamadou; Stepchenkova, Svetlana; Lee, Seul Ki; Loutfi, Jihad; Lee, Jung-Kook (2008-12)
- Campanella, M.; Mucci, F.; Baroni, S.; Nardi, L.; Marazziti, D. 2015. "Prevalence of Internet Addiction: A Pilot Study in a Group of Italian Students" (PDF). *Clinical Neuropsychiatry*. **4:** 90–93.
- Caplan, Scott E. (2010). "Theory and measurement of generalized problematic Internet use: A two-step approach". *Computers in Human Behavior*. **26** (5): 1089–1097.
- Chang, Man Kit; Law, Sally Pui Man (2008). "Factor structure for Young's Internet Addiction Test: A confirmatory study". *Computers in Human Behavior*. **24** (6): 2597–2619.
- Chao-Cheng; Chen, Jen-Yeu (2001-10-01). "Internet Addiction Disorder Among Clients of a Virtual Clinic". *Psychiatric Services*. **52** (10): 1397 1397.
- Cheng, Cecilia; Li, Angel Yee-lam (2014-12-01). "Internet Addiction Prevalence and Quality of (Real) Life: A Meta-Analysis of 31 Nations Across Seven World Regions". Cyberpsychology, Behavior, and Social Networking. **17** (12): 755–760.
- Cheryl Pawlowski (2000). Glued to the tube: the threat of television addiction to today's society. Naperville, Ill: Sourcebooks. ISBN 1-57071-459-2.
- Chou, Chien; Condron, Linda; Belland, John C. (2005-12-01). "A Review of the Research on Internet Addiction". Educational Psychology Review. **17** (4): 363–388.
- Chou, Chien; Hsiao, Ming-Chun (2000). "Internet addiction, usage, gratification, and pleasure experience: the Taiwan college students' case". *Computers & Education*. **35** (1): 65–80
- Clark, Deborah J.; Frith, Karen H. (September 2005). "The Development and Initial Testing of the Internet Consequences Scales (ICONS)". CIN: Computers, Informatics, Nursing. **23** (5): 285.
- Demetrovics, Zsolt; Szeredi, Beatrix; Rózsa, Sándor (2008-05-01). "The three-factor model of Internet addiction: The development of the Problematic Internet Use Questionnaire". *Behavior Research Methods*. **40** (2): 563–574.
- Durkee, Tony; Kaess, Michael; Carli, Vladimir; Parzer, Peter; Wasserman, Camilla; Floderus, Birgitta; Apter, Alan; Balazs, Judit; Barzilay, Shira (2012-12-01). "Prevalence of pathological internet use among adolescents in Europe: demographic and social factors". *Addiction*. **107** (12): 2210–2222.
- Ellen Currey-Wilson (2007). The Big Turnoff: Confessions of a TV-Addicted Mom Trying to Raise a TV-Free Kid. Chapel Hill, NC: Algonquin Books. ISBN 1-56512-539-8.
- Floros, Georgios; Siomos, Konstantinos; Stogiannidou, Ariadni; Giouzepas, Ioannis; Garyfallos, Georgios (2014). "Comorbidity of psychiatric disorders with Internet addiction in a clinical sample: The effect of personality, defense style and psychopathology". *Addictive Behaviors*. **39** (12): 1839–1845..
- Gómez, Patricia; Rial, Antonio; Braña, Teresa; Golpe, Sandra; Varela, Jesús (2017-02-24). "Screening of Problematic Internet Use Among Spanish Adolescents: Prevalence and Related Variables". *Cyberpsychology, Behavior, and Social Networking*. **20** (4): 259–267.
- Griffiths, M. (2000). "Internet addiction-time to be taken seriously?". Addiction research. **8** (5): 413–418.
- Hawi, Nazir S. (2012). "Internet addiction among adolescents in Lebanon". *Computers in Human Behavior*. **28** (3): 1044–1053.
- Heo, Jongho; Oh, Juhwan; Subramanian, S. V.; Kim, Yoon; Kawachi, Ichiro (2014-02-05). "Addictive Internet Use among Korean Adolescents: A National Survey". PLOS ONE. **9**(2): e87819.
- Holden, Constance (2001-11-02). "'Behavioral' Addictions: Do They Exist?". Science. 294 (5544): 980–982.
- Huang, Zheng; Wang, Mo; Qian, Mingyi; Zhong, Jie; Tao, Ran (2007-12-01). "Chinese Internet Addiction Inventory: Developing a Measure of Problematic Internet Use for Chinese College Students". *CyberPsychology & Behavior*. **10** (6): 805–812.
- Jean Lotus; Burke, David (1998). Get a Life!. Bloomsbury Publishing PLC. ISBN 0-7475-3689-9.
- Kandell, Jonathan J. (1998-01-01). "Internet Addiction on Campus: The Vulnerability of College Students". *Cyber Psychology & Behavior*. **1** (1): 11–17.
- Kawabe, Kentaro; Horiuchi, Fumie; Ochi, Marina; Oka, Yasunori; Ueno, Shu-ichi (2016-09-01). "Internet addiction: Prevalence and relation with mental states in adolescents". *Psychiatry and Clinical Neurosciences*. **70** (9): 405–412.
- Kershaw, Sarah (2005-12-01). "Hooked on the Web: Help Is on the Way". The New York Times. ISSN 0362-4331. Retrieved 2018-02-28.
- Ko, Chih-Hung; Yen, Ju-Yu; Chen, Cheng-Sheng; Chen, Cheng-Chung; Yen, Cheng-Fang (February 2008). "Psychiatric Comorbidity of Internet Addiction in College Students: An Interview Study". CNS Spectrums. **13** (2): 147–153.
- Kohli, Sahaj (2014-07-16). "Here's One Big Sign It's Time To Reevaluate Your Relationship With Your Phone". Huffingtonpost.com. Retrieved 2014-07-20.
- Kuss, D.; Lopez-Fernandez, O. (2016). "Internet-use related addiction: The state of the art of clinical research". *European Psychiatry*. **33**: S303.
- Lopez-Fernandez, Olatz (2015-09-01). "How Has Internet Addiction Research Evolved Since the Advent of Internet Gaming Disorder? An Overview of Cyberaddictions from a Psychological Perspective". *Current Addiction Reports*. **2** (3): 263–271.
- Marie McClendon (2001). Alternatives to TV Handbook. Whole Human Beans Co. ISBN 0-9712524-0-8.
- Meerkerk, G.-J.; Van Den Eijnden, R. J. J. M.; Vermulst, A. A.; Garretsen, H. F. L. (2008-12-10). "The Compulsive Internet Use Scale (CIUS): Some Psychometric Properties". CyberPsychology & Behavior. **12** (1): 1–6.
- Morrison, S., & Gomez, R. (2014). Pushback: The Growth of Expressions of Resistance to Constant Online Connectivity. In iConference 2014 Proceedings (p. 1-15).

- Niemz, Katie; Griffiths, Mark; Banyard, Phil (2005-12-01). "Prevalence of Pathological Internet Use among University Students and Correlations with Self-Esteem, the General Health Questionnaire (GHQ), and Disinhibition". CyberPsychology & Behavior. **8** (6): 562–570.
- Northrup, Jason C.; Lapierre, Coady; Kirk, Jeffrey; Rae, Cosette (2015-07-28). "The Internet Process Addiction Test: Screening for Addictions to Processes Facilitated by the Internet". Behavioral Sciences. **5** (3): 341–352.
- Postman, Neil (1994). The Disappearance of Childhood. London: Vintage. ISBN 0-679-75166-1.
- Postman, Neil (1985). Amusing Ourselves to Death: Public Discourse in the Age of Show Business. USA: Penguin. ISBN 1-670-80454-1.
- S., Young, Kimberly (1998). Caught in the net : how to recognize the signs of Internet addiction--and a winning strategy for recovery. New York:. OCLC 38130573. Wiley. ISBN 9780471191599
- Shapira, Nathan A.; Goldsmith, Toby D.; Keck, Paul E.; Khosla, Uday M.; McElroy, Susan L. (2000). "Psychiatric features of individuals with problematic internet use". Journal of Affective Disorders. **57** (1–3): 267–272.
- Shek, Daniel T.L.; Yu, Lu (2016). "Adolescent Internet Addiction in Hong Kong: Prevalence, Change, and Correlates". *Journal of Pediatric and Adolescent Gynecology*. **29** (1): S22–S30.
- Smith, J. L. (2013, December 28). Switch off – it's time for your digital detox. The Telegraph.
- Soule, L. C.; Shell, L. W.; Kleen, B. A. (2003). "Exploring Internet addiction: Demographic characteristics and stereotypes of heavy Internet users". *Journal of Computer Information* Systems. **44** (1): 64–73.
- Stone, Richard (2009-06-26). "China Reins in Wilder Impulses in Treatment of 'Internet Addiction'". *Science*. 324 (5935): 1630–1631.
- Wallis, David (1997-01-06). "Just Click No". The New Yorker. ISSN 0028-792X. Retrieved 2018-02-21.
- Weinstein, Aviv; Lejoyeux, Michel (2010). "Internet Addiction or Excessive Internet Use" (PDF). *The American Journal* . of Drug and Alcohol Abuse. 36: 277–283.
- Widyanto, Laura; Griffiths, Mark D.; Brunsden, Vivienne (2010-11-10). "A Psychometric Comparison of the Internet Addiction Test, the Internet-Related Problem Scale, and Self-Diagnosis". *Cyberpsychology, Behavior, and Social Networking*. **14** (3): 141–149.
- Widyanto, Laura; McMurran, Mary (2004). "The Psychometric Properties of the Internet Addiction Test". *CyberPsychology & Behavior*. **7** (4): 443–450.
- Widyanto, Laura; McMurran, Mary (2004-08-01). "The Psychometric Properties of the Internet Addiction Test". *CyberPsychology & Behavior.* **7** (4): 443–450.
- Winn, Marie (2002). The plug-in drug: television, computers, and family life. New York: Penguin Books. ISBN 0-14-200108-2.
- Wölfling, K.; Bühler, M.; Leménager, T.; Mörsen, C.; Mann, K. (2009-09-01). "Glücksspiel- und Internetsucht". Der Nervenarzt (in German). **80** (9): 1030–1039.
- Wu, Xiao-Shuang; Zhang, Zhi-Hua; Zhao, Feng; Wang, Wen-Jing; Li, Yi-Feng; Bi, Linda; Qian, Zhen-Zhong; Lu, Shan-Shan; Feng, Fang (2016). "Prevalence of Internet addiction and its association with social support and other related factors among adolescents in China". *Journal of Adolescence*. **52**: 103–111.
- Yang, Shu Ching; Tung, Chieh-Ju .2007. "Comparison of Internet addicts and non-addicts in Taiwanese high school". Computers in Human Behavior. **23** (1): 79–96.
- Yellowlees, Peter M.; Marks, Shayna (2007). "Problematic Internet use or Internet addiction?". Computers in Human Behavior. **23** (3): 1447–1453.
- Young, Kimberly (2017). Internet Addiction. Studies in Neuroscience, Psychology and Behavioral Economics. Springer, Cham. pp. 3–18.
- Young, Kimberly S. (1998-01-01). "Internet Addiction: The Emergence of a New Clinical Disorder". *Cyber Psychology & Behavior*. **1** (3): 237–244.
- Young, Kimberly S. (1999-10-01). "The Research and Controversy Surrounding Internet Addiction". *Cyber Psychology & Behavior*. **2** (5): 381–383.

Telomere Length In Slowing Ageing Process With Herbal Medicines In Cardiovascular Diseases.

The length of telomeres, which are located at the ends of chromosomes, reflects the lifespan of a cell. Telomere length decreases with each cell division and this process is necessary for appropriate DNA replication in eukaryotes. The regular shortening of telomere length will eventually lead to exposure of the genome and trigger the expression of proteins involved in apoptosis. These events make up the phenomenon called cellular senescence. Cellular senescence is associated with the onset and development of certain diseases. In this context, it is interesting to explore telomere "dynamics" in ischaemic and non-ischaemic cardiovascular diseases, and to determine whether these structures could be potential pharmacological targets(destroyed to treat a tumour or restored in the case of heart failure to preserve the integrity of myocardial cells).Several epidemiologic surveys have reported an association of short telomere length (TL) with CVD and cardiovascular mortality For instance, the Cardiovascular Health Study reported that each shortened kilobase pair of TL corresponded to a threefold increased risk of MI and stroke]. A recent systematic review and meta-analysis reported a constant positive association of decreased leukocyte TL (LTL) with cardiometabolic outcomes, where one standard deviation (SD) decrease in LTL was significantly associated with a 21%, 24%, and 37% increased risk of stroke, MI, and type 2 diabetes mellitus, respectively In this review, we discuss and review the current knowledge of the role of telomeres in CVDs.

Telomeres and Telomerase

In humans, telomeres consist of hundreds to thousands of repetitive sequences of TTAGGG at chromosomal ends for maintaining genomic integrity. Because the DNA replication is asymmetric along double strands, a sequence at the 3′-hydroxyl end would lose 30–200 nucleotides with each DNA replication and cell division. Telomeres provide a repetitive noncoding sequence at the 3′ end to prevent the loss of critical genetically encoded information during replication. Moreover, telomeres are coated with a complex of six capping proteins (telomere repeat-binding factor 1 (TRF1), telomere repeat-binding factor 2 (TRF2), repressor activator protein 1 (Rap1), TRF1 and TRF2 interacting nuclear protein 2 (TIN2), Tripeptidyl-peptidase 1 (TPP1), and protection of telomere 1 (POT1)), also known as shelterin proteins, which are packed into a compact T-loop structure to prevent the DNA repair machinery from mistaking telomeres for double-stranded DNA breaks. Therefore, TL have been proposed as a mitotic clock that measures how many times a cell has divided.

The human telomerase is responsible for maintaining and elongating TL and consists of the telomerase RNA component (TERC) and telomerase reverse transcriptase (TERT), the catalytic component. The TERT uses the TERC as a template to synthesize new telomeric DNA repeats at a single-stranded overhang to maintain TL. Some cells such as germ cells, stem cells, hematopoietic progenitor cells, activated lymphocytes, and most cancer cells have a high level of telomerase activity to overcome telomere shortening and maintain limitless cell division. However, somatic cells generally have a low or undetectable level of telomerase activity with limited longevity. The TL and integrity are regulated through the interplay between the telomerase and shelterin proteins. Telomerase activity decreases with age but increases markedly in response to injury. In the mammalian heart, telomerase expression is low but functionally significant. A substantial increase in telomerase expression was detected in cardiomyocytes, endothelial cells and fibroblasts of cryoinjured adult mice hearts, which implies that telomerase plays a role in regulating tissue repair and regenerative.

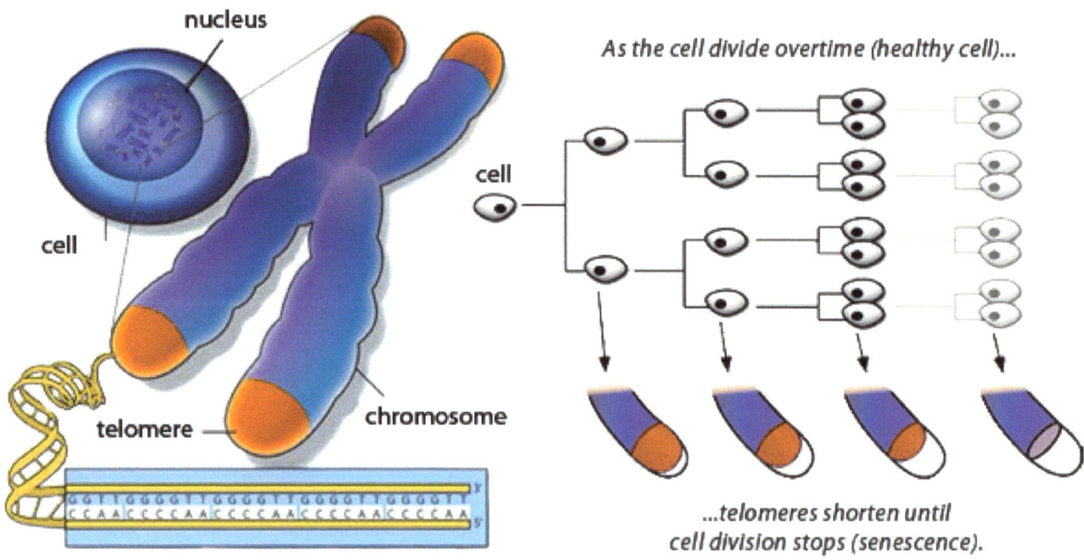

Fig. 30.1:*showing normal characteristics of telomere on chromosome (left) and their physiological progressive shortening until cell division stops (right)*

When a telomere is shortened to a critical length, the cell enters cellular senescence, which initiates a series of changes in the gene expression of replicative cell-cycle inhibitors and inhibits proliferation and then finally into apoptosis as known as replicative senescence. By contrast, stress-induced premature senescence (SIPS) is triggered by external stimuli, including oxidizing agents and radiation, leads to the premature activation of the cellular senescence process not associated with telomere shortening. The senescent cells alter their morphology and secretary phenotype in autocrine and paracrine patterns. This active altered secretion pattern has been termed as the senescence-associated secretory phenotype (SASP). They secrete IL-6 and IL-8, intercellular adhesion molecule 1 (ICAM-1), metalloproteases, monocyte attractants, plasminogen activator inhibitor 1, and vascular endothelial growth factor. Senescent cells contribute to inflammation and promote apoptosis, tissue remodeling, and repair through their SASP. Hence, chronic inflammation initiates a vicious cycle that enhances telomere dysfunction and the accumulation of senescent cells. Cell senescence aggravates chronic inflammation and accelerates aging and the development of aging-associated diseases

Telomere biology

Location and function of telomeres

Telomeres are composed of nucleotides and are located at the end of chromosomes in eukaryotic cells. They cap the termination of the double strands of DNA and thus preserve the integrity and stability of the genome during replication. Telomeres are made up of a repetitive sequence of six nitrogenous bases rich in guanine (TTAGGG). This sequence is repeated over several thousand base pairs at the 3′ end of DNA (4 to 15 kilobases in humans). In most human somatic cells, the length of the telomeres decreases by 20 to 200 base pairs with each cell division. This loss of genetic material corresponds to the phenomenon called "the end replication problem". If this shortening of telomeres is not repaired, it eventually leads to cessation of the cell cycle and cell death by apoptosis. The synthesis of telomere DNA requires the activity of specialized enzyme complexes : telomerases. These complexes are made up of various proteins (TRAF1, TRAF2, Ku86, TIN2, etc.). Their function is to lengthen telomeres by the synthesis of two supplementary TTAGGG sequences at their ends. Typically, telomerase activity is diminished or even absent in most adult somatic cells, the exception being cells with a strong potential for division, like active lymphocytesand certain types of stem cells .

Regulation of telomere length

The maintenance of telomere length depends on several factors, including the composition in associated proteins, the level of oxidative stress and the level of telomerase activation as well as telomere length itself . This is why telomere length varies considerably from one species to another and from one individual to another. Moreover, it seems that telomere length may be affected by certain genetic factors, notably linked to chromosome X : this was shown in a study by Nawrot et al. in 2004 involving a cohort of families.

Telomerase activity, however, seems to be one of the key elements in the maintenance of telomere integrity. Indeed, cells with short telomeres and an absence of telomerase activity become senescent and go into apoptosis more quickly than do cells with telomeres that are long enough not to require telomerase activity to survive. Inversely, some cells are deficient in TERC, TERT and other proteins necessary for telomerase function. This is illustrated by the transfection of primary B and T lymphocytes from patients with dyskeratosis congenita with exogenous TERC, which restored telomerase activity and increased telomere length.

Moreover, the role of the Rad54, which is involved in DNA repair, in the regulation of telomere length was brought to light recently. Indeed, Rad54-deficient mice presented severe telomere shortening, and this in the absence of any modification in telomerase activity . These findings tend to show that Rad54 protein is involved in a mechanism that maintains the integrity of telomeres independently of telomerases. The regulation of telomere length also depends on the level of methylation of certain histones, namely histones H3 and H4, associated with subtelomeric regions. The methylation of these histones decreases access to telomere sequences and thus diminishes telomerase activity. Therefore, proteins that play a role in the regulation of these methylations have an impact on telomere length. For example, proteins of the retinoblastoma family increase the methylation of subtelomeric regions and thus diminish telomere length]. In contrast, retinoblastoma protein 2, which depresses the activity of DNA methytransferase, responsible for the methylation of subtelomeric regions, plays a role in increasing telomere length .

The existence of telomeric RNA (called TERRA or TelRNA), which is transcribed by RNA polymerase II, has been shown recently. These telomeric RNA transcriptionsmay have a negative impact on telomere length . Finally, one of the major mechanisms of telomere shortening is the activity of exonucleases 5′-3′. Indeed, the role of these exonucleases is to degrade the RNA primer used in the replication of the DNA necessary for DNA polymerase activity. This deterioration creates lesions in which the DNA is in the single strand form within the replication loop. The presence of single-strand DNA prevents the formation of Okazaki fragmentsand thus elongates the DNA, but can lead to an increase in : damage to DNA; the risk of fusion of chromosome extremities and the activation of p53-dependent responses to DNA damage . The maintenance of telomere length within eukaryotic cells is thus a complex phenomenon that involves a wide range of factors. Several mechanisms acting in a synergistic fashion thus appear to stabilize telomere length. The different mechanisms mentioned above involved in the regulation of telomere length

Oxidative stress

One of the principal mechanisms involved in telomere shortening is represented by the level of free radical oxidative stress. Oxidative damage to telomeric DNA appears as the formation of an adduct of guanine, 8-oxodG, which is involved in the initiation of disturbances in the maintenance of telomere length. Moreover, ROS, and especially the hydroxyl radical, induce breaks in DNA and deteriorate DNA base repair . Unlike the rest of the genome, telomeres seem to be unable to repair breaks in single-strand DNA. Because of this, telomeres are particularly sensitive to the accumulation of the guanine oxide adduct. This sensitivity to oxidation in telomeres was revealed by Oikawa et al. in two studies. The first, in 1999, concerned the exposure of DNA from calf thymus to hydrogen peroxide associated with copper (II). The results showed the presence of DNA lesions especially at the level of the 5′-GGG-3′ triplet. The second study, in 2001 showed that the exposure of fibroblasts to ultraviolet A also induced damage, highlighted by the presence of 8-oxodG localized at telomeres. Moreover, the presence of non-matched bases within the telomeric sequence interferes with the DNA replication mechanisms necessary for the maintenance of structure integrity. Oxidative stress may thus induce premature shortening of telomeres independently of age. Telomeres are unable to repair oxidized DNA, which therefore accentuates the damage caused by ROS. Petersen et al. showed that lesions caused by hydrogen peroxide were repaired slowly and incompletely at the level of the telomeres, which is not the case at the level of the mini-satellites. One of the hypotheses put forward is that TRF2 binding at the level of the telomere could prevent DNA repair enzymes from reaching the site. Moreover, TRF2 interacts with polymerase β and thus has a potential negative effect on the repair of DNA damage. TRF2 also inhibits ataxia telangiectasia muted kinase phosphorylation, which is involved in the initiation process of DNA repair . One important point, which must always be underlined, is the in vivo concomitance between increased production of ROS and the development of an inflammatory process. In this context, the proinflammatory cytokines produced can cause telomere shortening directly. In this field, several studies have shown that telomeraseactivity correlated inversely with levels of tumour necrosis factor alpha. The latest, via the activation of two transcription factors (nuclear factor-kappa B and activator protein 1), is responsible for an increase in the expression of proinflammatory genes . In this context, the studies of Beyne-Rauzy et al. showed that the reduction in telomere length induced by exposure of cells to tumour necrosis factor alpha brought about a negative regulation in the level of expression of human

Activating Your Longevity Genes: The Sirtuins

For centuries, nearly every culture has searched for a way to slow and even reverse the aging process. Greek writers pursued the Fountain of Youth as far back as the fifth century BCE. India still recognizes the ancient science of longevity called Ayurveda, which is believed to add years to your life by nourishing and detoxing the body. My favorite success story of all, however, is that of a Chinese herbalist named Li Ching-Yuen, who, according to some records, was born in 1736 and died 256 years later. Cut to the twenty-first century, and we're just as focused on discovering the mechanisms that prevent and reverse aging as our global ancestors were. In fact, one of the most studied proteins in the past ten years that's been found to aid the aging process is called sirtuin, or silent information regulator. Sirtuins control the rate at which we age, and the length of our lifespan, meaning that on many levels they are our bodies anti-aging regulators. They've been dubbed "longevity genes," One of the most studied sirtuins is called SIRT1. Among other sources, it's found in garlic, Panax ginseng, and Polygonum multiflorum, an anti-aging herbal supplementgrown in China that research has shown demonstrates anti-aging properties that activate a variety of biological processes in the body. There has been some controversy recently regarding possible liver damage resulting from the internal use of Polygonum multiflorum. These three anti-aging herbs were an integral part of Master Li's regimen, switching on his SIRT1 when he used them! Even if he lived half the years that sources claim, it's still an impressive number and one that supports the longevity-enhancing properties of herbs, in a time long before science showed us how.

Cardiomyocytes

An experimental study reported that telomerase knockout mice (TERC /) have progressively shortened telomeres in the later generation along with attenuation in myocyte proliferation and an increase in apoptosis. In addition, these mice exhibit ventricular dilation, thinning of the wall, and cardiac dysfunction, mimicking the end-stage dilated cardiomyopathy in humans. By contrary, forced expression of TERT in the cardiac muscle of mice promotes cell proliferation, hypertrophy, and survival

Furthermore, enhanced telomerase activity in insulin-likegrowth factor-1 transgenic mice has been shown to delay cellular aging and promote cell growth, thus preventing ventricular dysfunction. In humans, endomyocardial biopsies from patients with HF reveal shortened telomeres, increased cellular senescence, and cell death. Telomere dysfunction and increased susceptibility to apoptosis in cardiac myocytes is thought to be underlying mechanism of HF. The hypothesis has tested in cultured human cardiomyocytes, which defective expression of TRF2, a telomere end-capping protein, triggered telomere erosion, activation of the DNA damage checkpoint kinase, Chk2 and apoptosis.

Several studies have indicated that the heart undergoes the regeneration of some cardiac myocytes throughout life However, the proliferative and regenerative potential of cardiac progenitor cells partially depend on the integrity of telomeres and activity of telomerase. Stem cells in young cardiac myocytes have active telomerase and stable TL, whereas stem cells in the aging heart exhibit telomere attrition and express cell senescence markers. Hence, the decrease in the cardiac myocyte regeneration potential and accumulation of old dying cells finally lead to cardiac pumping failure. These findings indicate that telomere biology play an important role in regulation of regenerative capacity in myocardium and involved in the pathophysiology of HF.

Endothelial Progenitor Cells

The repair mechanisms for vascular atherosclerosis are dependent on endothelial progenitor cells (EPCs), which originate from hematopoietic stem cells (HSCs) in the bone marrow. The shortening of the TL of HSCs caused by inflammation or oxidative stress limits the number and function of EPCs and impairs the replicative potential in the injured part of the vasculature. However, EPCs with human TERT transduction have enhanced mitogenic and migratory activity in cell cultures and improved neovascularization in murine model of hindlimb ischemia. These findings demonstrate that EPCs with enhanced telomerase activity could be a novel therapeutic strategy for patients with severe ischemia heart disease and post infarct cardiomyopathy. Furthermore, we observed mutations in circadian gene Per 2 caused vascular senescence and impaired impairs ischemia-induced revascularization through the alteration of EPC function, which may explained the clinical observation of the link of alteration of the circadian and cardiovascular diseases.

Implications for Cardiovascular Diseases

Measurement of Telomere Length

Peripheral leukocyte DNA has been most commonly used in epidemiological studies to measure TL because a blood sample can be easily obtained. A consistent synchrony exists between LTL and somatic cells, including vascular cells, within people. The two methods most commonly used in clinical studies are Southern blotting and quantitative polymerase chain reaction (qPCR). Southern blotting has an advantage of measuring the absolute LTL, including the proportion of very short telomeres. Cells with very short TL are closely associated with cellular senescence, regardless of mean TL, because only one critically short telomere can force a cell to enter senescence.

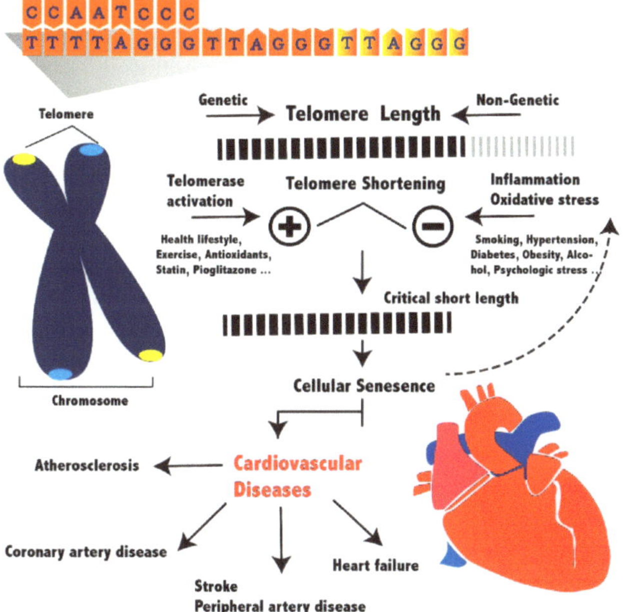

Fig.30.2: *Schematic overview of telomere length and cardiovascular diseases. Individual variations of telomere length are affected by genetic and non-genetic factors. Critically short telomeres lead to cellular senescence and dysfunction, which contribute to atherogenesis and reduce repair and regenerative capacity in cardiovascular system. Disease promoting factors, such as smoking and hypertension, accelerate telomere shortening through inflammation or increased oxidant stress. However, disease protective factors, such as exercise and statin use, can activate telomerase activity and maintain telomere length.*

However, Southern blotting requires numerous DNA samples (2–3 μg per assay) and is time-consuming and expensive. Thus, qPCR is used in most epidemiological studies. The fundamental difference in laboratory methods among individual studies might contribute to controversial results. Recently, a study compared these laboratory methods performed in two independent laboratories to measure the same samples. Both the q-PCR and Southern blotting provided highly reproducible and correlated results.

Genetic Factors

TL is largely inherited and is modulated by several intrinsic and environmental factors throughout life. Rare mutations in genes that maintain and regulate TL have been identified in monogenic catastrophic diseases with premature tissue degeneration and organ dysfunction, such as dyskeratosis congenita, idiopathic pulmonary fibrosis, and aplastic anemia. Extensive inter-individual variations in LTL in the general population may attributed to single-nucleotide polymorphisms (SNPs), which have been identified in genomewide association studies (GWASs). In a meta-analysis of 37,684 people, seven loci were identified to be associated with mean LTL. Five of these loci on genes are involved in telomere biology, including chromosomes 3q26.2 (TERC), −5p15.33 (TERT), 4q32.2 (nuclear assembly factor 1), 10q24.33 (oligonucleotide/oligosaccharide-binding fold containing 1), 18, and 20q13.3 (regulator of telomere elongation helicase 1). In another meta-analysis of 9190 people, two novel genomic regions that were identified to be associated with LTL variation are near a conserved telomere maintenance complex component 1 (CTC1) on chromosome17p13.1 and zinc finger protein 676 on 19p12\.

Cardiovascular Risk Factors

The amount of telomere lost during each cell division varies among people. Previous evidence indicated that increased oxidative stress and chronic inflammation are associated with a higher telomere loss and accelerated telomere shortening. Several common risk factors for CVD such as smoking, diabetes mellitus, hypercholesterolemia, hypertension, obesity, physical inactivity, alcohol consumption and psychosocial problems have been associated with short TL. However, the mechanism underlying the association of telomere shortening with these risk factors remains hypothetical. Most studies have reported that telomere shortening is associated with these risk factors through increased tissue inflammation and oxidative stress For example, animal studies demonstrated that hyperglycemia attenuates nitric oxide production in endothelial cells, promotes inflammation and oxidative stress, and accelerates LTL shortening and vascular atherosclerotic processes. In additional, we found disrupted circadian rhythm results in loss of rhythmic telomerase activities with shortened TL and premature aging in mice. Similar observations also showed in the emergency physicians working in rotating shifts.

However, some dietary and lifestyle factors such as marine omega-3 fatty acid, antioxidants, vitamin intake, physical activity and healthy lifestyle were reported to decrease rates of LTL shortening. These factors might contribute to reduced reactive oxygen species, inhibit inflammation, increase endothelial nitric oxide synthase (eNOS) activity, and increased telomerase activity. In an experimental study, voluntary wheel running in mice for three weeks upregulated the activity of telomerase, increased the expression of TRF2, and reduced the expression of vascular apoptosis regulators. However, these exercise-induced changes were absent in both $TERT^{-/-}$ and endothelial nitric oxide synthase $(eNOS)^{-/-}$ mice, indicating the beneficial effects are medicated by TERT and eNOS. A human study also reported that comprehensive lifestyle changes significantly increased telomerase activity and consequently telomere maintenance capacity in human immune system cells.

Consequently, telomere shortening is a reflection of cellular aging and a marker of the health status of the aging population . Absolute TL at birth is determined by genetic materials from both parents. During aging, the mean TL declines with cell replication and turnover. The process of telomere shortening is accelerated by exposure to disease-promoting factors such as smoking, obesity, and psychosocial stress. Furthermore, telomerase activation has been considered a possible target for reversing the telomere shortening.

Coronary Artery Diseases

Several studies in diverse populations have reported an association of shorter telomeres in circulating leukocytes with CAD . The precise mechanisms connecting short telomeres and CAD are yet to be established. Current evidence from epidemiologic and experimental studies supports the role of telomeres in CAD development. First, cardiovascular risk factors such as smoking, hypertension, insulin resistance, and hyperlipidemia, are associated with short LTL. Second, the progression of atherosclerotic plaques in vasculature have been shown to be associated with short TL and cell senescence in vascular cells such as endothelial and vascular smooth muscle cells. Furthermore, short mean LTL represents a greater degree of telomere attrition and senescence in immune cells. Low grade systemic inflammation, which is thought to be mediated by immunosenescence, has been shown to be associated with numerous age-related conditions, including atherosclerosis and cardiovascular diseases.

However, many studies are cross-sectional design and because most cardiovascular risk factors also affect LTL, the causal or consequential relationship between shorter TL and CAD remains controversial. Recently, some prospective longitudinal studies may support the hypothesis that telomere shortening causes CAD, rather than telomere shortening is a consequence of CAD. In a large prospective WOSCOPS study , compared with people in the highest tertiles of LTL, those in the lowest tertiles of LTL had a 44% increased risk of coronary artery events in a mean follow-up period of 5.5 years after adjustment for risk factors for CAD. In addition, a recent meta-analysis of prospective studies reported that the estimated relative risk of the shortest versus the longest third of LTL was 1.4 (95% confidence interval : 1.15–1.70). LTL was measured in these prospective trials before the diagnosis of a CVD, thus avoiding the concern of the confounding of reverse causality. Furthermore, reports about the association of genetic variants affecting TL with the risk of CAD also provide evidence for the causal association. The genotypes are randomly determined during conception and thus their associations could be not susceptible to bias and confounding. A meta-analysis of 14 GWASs including up to 22,233 patients with CAD and 64,762 controls revealed that seven SNPs have been identified for the variation in mean LTL. For example, a mean TL decrease of 117 base pairs per TERC telomere-shortening allele accounts for approximately 10% drop in functional telomere reserves in a typical middle-aged adult, and thus increases susceptibility to telomere dysfunction and replicative senescence. The effect of inter-individual variations in LTL is also illustrated in this meta-analysis, which found that the allele associated with shorter LTL increases the risk of CAD; one SD decrease in LTL was estimated to increase the CAD risk by 21%.

LTL in patients with CAD has prognostic value. A prospective cohort study of 780 patients conducted for a follow-up period of 4.4 years reported an association of decreased LTL with all-cause mortality, with an adjusted hazard ratio of 1.8 in the lowest TL quartile compared with the highest TL quartile. Moreover, LTL has been observed to be shorter in patients with premature acute MI (aged <50 years) than in healthy, age-matched controls. According analysis in previous studies, patients with MI have TL that is equivalent to that in controls older than 8–12 years. This might partially explain some young patients with MI without traditional cardiovascular risk factors. Biological aging can reflect the effects of cumulative oxidative stress and inflammatory burden on the aging vasculature. Compared with chronological aging, biological aging may provide superior risk stratification for CVDs. Accurate risk assessment is essential to provide appropriate therapeutic interventions and to further reduce the occurrence of morbid cardiovascular events. New network analysis systems, including genetic traits, imaging characters, and biological risk factors, should be developed for determining the risk of atherosclerosis. We think LTL could be a sensitive score in the risk prediction system, and additional clinical trials are required to validate the observation and hypothesis.

In the coronary intervention field, researchers observed shorter LTL and increased proinflammatory activity in high-risk unstable plaque (calcified thin-capped fibroatheroma) on virtual histology intravascular ultrasound in patients with acute coronary syndrome also. Furthermore, delayed re-endothelialization after drug-eluting stent (DES) implantation with uncovered stent struts can increase the risk of stent thrombosis. A small clinical trial reported an inverse association of LTL with the percentage of uncovered stent struts, as assessed through optical coherence tomography. Shorter LTL may indicate functional exhaustion and impaired proliferative capacity of EPCs, which are responsible for re-endothelialization after a vascular injury. Additional large-scale prospective studies should be conducted to investigate the clinical application of LTL as a predictive marker for stent thrombosis and target vessel outcomes after DES implantation.

Heart Failure

In a clinical study of 803 patients, LTL was decreased by approximately 40% in patients with HF, and TL in the patients with HF was related to the disease severity. A study investigating the association of a lower left ventricular ejection fraction with decreased TL reported an association of one SD decrease in TL with a 5% lower ejection fraction. Moreover, LTL was significantly associated with cardiovascular outcomes in patients with ischemic HF.

HF with a normal ejection fraction was not well recognized until the two previous decades. Approximately half of patients hospitalized for HF have a normal ejection fraction, and outcomes in these patients are equivalent to those in patients with a lower ejection fraction. Aging leads to an increase in the deposition of extracellular matrix components, principally collagen, with an increase in the ratio of type I to type III collagen and a decrease in the elastin content, contributing to impaired ventricular relaxation. Furthermore, blunted beta-adrenergic responsiveness, excitation–contraction coupling, and altered calcium-handling proteins contribute to diastolic dysfunction. Studies have reported that the left ventricular relaxation function deteriorates with normal aging and is positively associated with LTL. Older people with shorter LTL have a significantly lower E/A ratio.

Association with Other CVDs

- Sudden cardiac death (SCD)
- Idiopathic pulmonary arterial hypertension
- In patients with degenerative aortic valve stenosis,

Therapeutic Consideration

From the implications of current understanding of telomere biology, potential therapeutic interventions such as the maintenance of TL and modulation of telomerase activity to reverse telomere attrition and cellular senescence, is emerging as a novel strategy for treating atherosclerosis and CVD. Experimental studies have reported that the manipulation of telomerase activity and TL enhances or reverses senescence and aging-associated phenotypes. For example, telomerase activation therapy after MI successfully prevented ischemic HF in mice. However, studies of targeting telomerase therapy in humans are still scarce. A small chemical compound TA-65, extracted from Astragalus membranaceus, is the first described telomere activator. One human study demonstrated dietary supplementation of TA-65 increasing several indicators of health in cardiovascular system and metabolism. Further longitudinal study is mandatory to investigate the anti-aging effects and potential long-term adverse effects.

Several studies demonstrated the effects of TL maintenance and senescence prevention in certain drugs, which have been used for decades exert clinically beneficial on CVD. For example, statins, 3-hydroxy-3-methylglutaryl-coenzyme A reductase inhibitors, exert various pleiotropic effects to prevent the development of atherosclerotic plaque. They mitigate the genomic damage through potentiation of the DNA repair capacity and upregulation of glutathione synthesis to fight oxidative stress. Furthermore, they can enhance telomerase activity and protect telomere through upregulating TRF2 in endothelial cells and EPCs. A more specific analysis of human T-lymphocytes showed that atorvastatin in pharmacologically relevant doses led to a transient increase in telomerase activity in T-cells. This effect, which could be blocked by inhibitors of Akt and Phosphatidylinositol-4,5-Bisphosphate 3 (PI3)-Kinase, was more pronounced in the CD4-positive ($CD4^+$) than in the CD8-positive ($CD8^+$) T-cell subset

Angiotensin II has been reported to induce oxidative DNA damage and accelerate cellular senescence in cultured human VSMCs. Therefore, angiotensin-converting enzyme inhibitor or angiotensin II inhibitor can be used to reduce oxidative stress and subsequent DNA damage and senescence. Additionally, pioglitazone, a peroxisome proliferator-activated receptor agonist, can increase the activity of telomerase and expression of TRF-2 as well as reduce the expression of the senescence markers p16, cell-cycle checkpoint kinase 2, and p53.

Anti-Aging Implications of Astragalus Membranaceus (Huangqi): A Well-Known Chinese Tonic

Astragalus membranaceus (Huangqi):- as one of the most important Qi tonifying adaptogenic herbs in Trational Chinese Medicine, has a long history of medicinal use. Astragalus membranaceus was originally described in the Shennong›s Classic of Materia Medica, the earliest complete Pharmacopoeia of China written from the Warring States Period to Han Dynasty [11,12]. It is valued for its ability to strengthen the primary energy of the body which we know as the immune system, as well as the metabolic, respiratory and eliminative functions. This fact is being increasingly substantiated by pharmacological studies showing that it can increase telomerase activity, and has antioxidant, anti-inflammatory, immune-regulatory, anticancer, hypolipidemic, antihyperglycemic, hepatoprotective, expectorant, and diuretic effects Specifically, constituents of the dried roots of Astragalus spp. Radix Astragali provide significant protection against heart, brain, kidney, intestine, liver and lung injury in various models of oxidative stress-related disease.

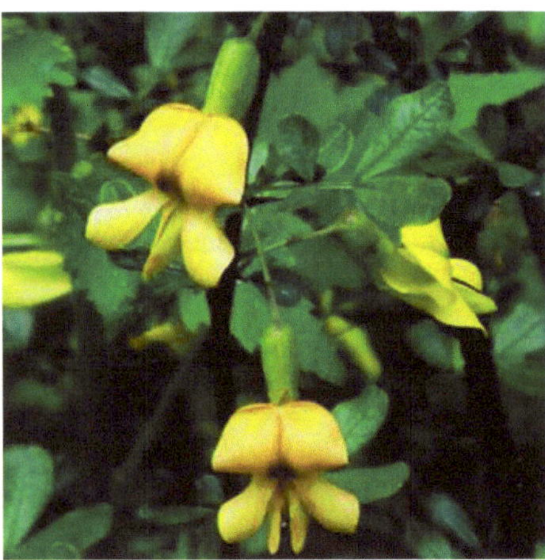

Fig. 30.3: *Astragalus (Astragalus Membranaceus) - Start Astragalus seeds and grow this herbaceous perennial plant that is native to the northern and eastern parts of China as well as Mongolia and Korea. It is is the pea family and produces smą pea-ike yeow flowers. Astragaus has a long history, many centuries in fact, as a medicinal herb in Chinese medicine. Research in modern day is aso finding hepu benefits rom t he A stragaus h erb p ant. The Astragalus herb is also known as Milk Vetch or Chinese Milk Vetch.*

In order to clarify the potential application of Astragalus membranaceus in anti-aging, we summarize the effect and mechanism of its extracts and effective component monomer against aging and age-related disease. This information could help clinicians and scientists develop novel target-specific and effective therapeutic agents that are deprived of major systemic side effects, so as to establish a better treatment regimen in the battle against aging.

5 Reasons To Add Astragalus To Your Anti-Aging Supplement Plan

Scientists now believe that checking the length of your telomeres is the best way to determine healthy aging and gain clues about how long you might live. For my patients, I test biological age versus chronological age—how old you are by the calendar, versus how old you are by measuring telomere length through a blood test.

Can We Lengthen Telomeres?

Life Length laboratory was founded in Madrid, Spain by María Blasco, Ph.D., one of the world's foremost researchers on the function of telomeres in aging. This is the best test found to determine the median telomere length.

Though the role of telomeres in aging is still not completely understood, scientists believe that cells with the shortest telomeres trigger a process that causes a dramatic change in how normal cells function. Cells with the shortest telomeres die prematurely. Telomere shortening is prevented by the activation of telomerase, an enzyme vital for tissue regeneration. Long telomeres reflect high telomerase activity, and are considered a good predictor of greater tissue regeneration and longevity. What can we do about shortened telomeres? Will longer telomeres actually make people younger? A handful of chemical and natural compounds hold promise as telomere extenders. Researchers have screened thousands of natural compounds and chemicals for their effects on telomeres. One of the more interesting compounds comes from the traditional Chinese herbal medicine Huang Qi : astragalus (*Astragalus membranaceus*).

In Traditional Chinese Medicine (TCM), astragalus is considered a Qi tonic, a natural substance that increases energy in the body. You can buy the dried herb is any Chinese herb store and also on the Internet. It's not the whole plant, or even the TCM prepared forms that fascinates researches, but special compounds found in astragalus extracts. These active compounds are classified as isoflavones, saponins, and polysaccharides, and all three have therapeutic properties. It's the saponins that have attracted the most attention for their effects on telomeres, however.

Astragalus Lengthens Telomeres

Astragaloside IV (AG-IV), an astragalus saponin, has shown benefits in reversing cell damage. It also helps promote tissue healing, improves immune response against viral infections in HIV-patients, inhibits the spread of lung and colon cancer, promotes nerve regeneration, and manages inflammation. It also activates telomerase. Cycloastragenol (CGA), a derivative of AG-IV with even more activating potential on telomerase, is as close as we know to a telomere activator. Research suggests that CGA may have wide use in the treatment of degenerative diseases, as well as for aging. The commercial telomere activator called TA-65, a natural product derived from CGA, has shown benefits on bone and cardiovascular health. In a 2014 French study, TA-65 lengthened flight feathers on birds. TA-65 activates telomerase and increases T-cells that are important immune cells that fight against infection and cancer.

Strategies for Protecting Telomeres

Diet and Supplementation: one way that our body maintains healthy DNA is through the process of methylation. In simple terms, methylation is a process by which certain chemicals called 'methyl groups' are added to various constituents of proteins, DNA, and other molecules. These chemical groups are used to keep them in good 'working' condition by preventing telomeres from getting too short; this prevents genetic mutations to DNA.

1. Researchers reporting in The Journal of Nutrition found that high blood levels of folate (800 mcg each day), plus vitamin B12 (500 to 1000 mcg daily) along with all of the B vitamins are linked to longer telomeres.
2. In addition, proteins from nuts and seeds can be potent methyl group donors. For maximum benefit, raw nuts are better than roasted because heat damages the volatile oils and other nutrients in nuts.
3. Vitamin C has been shown to slow the shortening of telomeres at doses between 1 – 3 grams daily.
4. Research on the minerals zinc (25-50 mg per day) and magnesium (400-800 mg per day) show that they are vital to DNA replication during cell division. A lack of these nutrients can lead to DNA damage and telomere shortening.
5. Mixed tocotrienols (a full spectrum form of Vitamin E) at a dose of 400 to 800 IU per day can actually restore the length of telomeres and prevent their loss by helping produce the enzyme telomerase.

Green tea: a 2010 study of elderly Chinese subjects found that increased green tea intake may be associated with a potential increase in lifespan through regulating telomere length. In this report, published in the *British Journal of Nutrition*, a total of 976 men and 1,030 women aged 65 and older were initially assessed in 2006. In addition to questions regarding lifestyle habits and diet, the blood of these research volunteers was tested for telomere length.

Following measurements of the average difference in telomere length between those who consumed the highest amount of green tea and those who consumed the lowest, the researchers determined a potential lifespan difference of five years between these two groups. The results of this study mainly favoured the telomeres of men, with less significant results being found in the female tea drinkers.

Chinese herbs: after screening over 250,000 different compounds in an attempt to find a way to boost telomerase production, scientists discovered a chemical in a Chinese herb that seems to fit the bill. Named TA65, this plant compound has preliminary research that is very promising, but with a price tag of $600 per bottle only those with deep pockets are able to purchase the capsules, while others are holding out for more research. The good news is that the herb that TA65 was isolated from is a common longevity tonic.

Astragalus membranaceus is a herb that the ancient Chinese used to boost resistance to illness.

Astragalus membranaceus, commonly called Huang Qi in Mandarin, is an age old herb that the ancient Chinese used to put a spring in their step and boost resistance to illness. This is the herb that TA65 was isolated from, and every year something new comes out about the power of this plant. With its sweet taste and relatively mild overall flavour, it blends easily into soups and teas. Though the level of TA65 in a preventive daily dose of 10 grams of Astragalus is likely pretty small, it still works well in the prevention of a list of diseases. If combined with the previously mentioned diet/supplements, regular tea consumption, and meditation, Astragalus could go a long way to boost your lifespan and resistance to disease.

Meditation: the positive mental shifts that happen during a meditation session have been associated with greater production of telomerase. A study called the Shamatha Project measured telomerase levels as the end of a three-month intensive meditation retreat. Telomerase activity was about a third higher in the meditation group in comparison to a control group of individuals who did not meditate. The meditation group also found many beneficial psychological effects from meditation including a better sense of control, mindfulness, and a stronger understanding of long-term goals and values. Members also experienced a decrease in negative emotions and neurotic behaviour. The Shamatha Project is one of the most detailed studies to have ever been done on meditation.

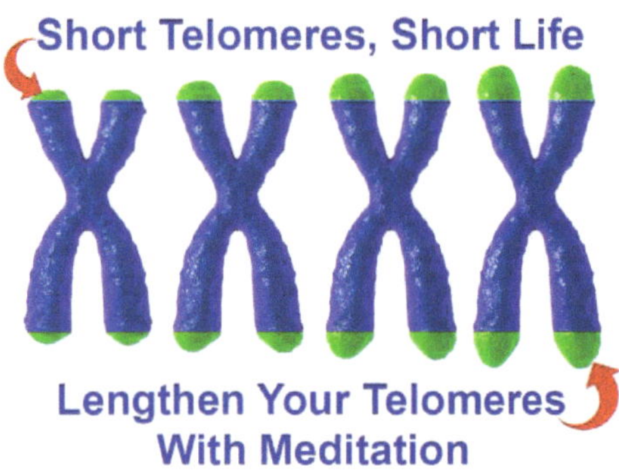

Fig. 30.4: *Illustration showing positive effect of Meditation in lengthening the telomere*

Historically, some of the herbal medicines that lead to slow aging

The Shen Nong Ben Cao Jing is perhaps the most esteemed fundamental text of herbal medicine in China, and is one of the 10 premodern classics of medicine selected by the People's Republic of China for concentrated research of prehistoric medical information. Shen Nong was one of the three fundamental patriarchs of the modern Chinese civilization architecture, with Huang Di and Fu Xi, both of whom are also well known with their association to Traditional Chinese Medicine and what became Daoism. The Shen Nong Ben Cao Jing, or Shen Nong's Fundamental Herbal Classic Text, often called the Divine Farmer's Material Medica Classic, or the Divine Farmer's Almanac, for some reason, lists the slowing of aging, or promotion of longevity, as one of the key qualities of a number of classic herbs. While modern research is still pursuing this efficacy in the chemistry of these herbs, and some of them may not seem particularly dramatic in their so-called "anti-aging" effects, we might consider them as part of a more complex holistic regimen. Most of these herbs are in the general category of Kidney and Adrenal tonics, showing that astute knowledge of these ancient Daoist physicians, recognizing that the kidney and adrenal system deteriorates with aging.

In modern times, the focus of research into herbal medicine to promote healthy aging, or longevity, called Yang Sheng in Daoist history, has been more focused on adaptogenic and yang tonic herbs such as Rhodiola rosea, Siberian ginseng, Ganoderma lucidum (LIng zhi or Reishi mushroom) and Panax Ginseng, with much research proving the benefits of chemicals in these herbs to achieve a variety of goals in healthy aging. Ayurvedic herbs such as Withania somniflora (Ashwaghanda) and Bocopa monieri have also been much studies and proven to benefit healthy aging. A more comprehensive and holistic approach has been found to be most effective, though, and this is reflected in the use of herbal formulas in Chinese Herbal Medicine, with an array of chemicals and effects acting synergistically. Intelligent formulas to promote healthy aging address neuroprotective concerns, hormonal balance, adaptation to stress of all types, cardiovascular health, and improved immune function with better control of inflammatory cytokines. A number of gentle but effective herbs have a long history of inclusion in this comprehensive strategy, as do a number of nutrient medicines discovered in modern research.

Since the prescriptions for these herbs in the Shen Nong Manual called for prolonged taking of the herb, formulas may be devised, obtained from a professional TCM herbalist, and prepared with a classic double-boil extraction method. In this preparation, the herbs would be placed in a one pint jar filled with water, with a tight lid, that is then placed into another pan of water that also has a tight lid. The water in the outer pan is brought to a near boil, and then kept at a very low temperature, or flame, for a few hours, bringing the water in the jar to a near boil, but not with the high heat that would break down the herbal chemistry dramatically. The complete herbal chemistry is water extracted this way. Many older patients in China still use this method for longevity herbal formulas, and sip the water in the pint jar daily. The patient and the physician could choose from the classically prescribed herbs below to find an individualized formula for prolonged taking. Some of these herbs are bitter, and honey may be added to the water to improve taste, although the taste of the herbal medicine is not the point, but rather the effects.

Modern research has recommended such herbs as Rhodiola rosea (Hong jin tian), Astragalus (Huang qi), Ginseng, and Cornelian cherry (Shan zhu yu) as well, to slow cellular aging, and these types of tonic herbs may be added to enhance effects. The following are translated excerpts from the esteemed early Chinese herbal classic named after the patriarch Shen Nong:

Chrysanthemum morifolii, or Ju hua, is a flower that is bitter and balanced, and is used mainly to treat the pathologies of the head, such as dizziness, headache, eye pain, and swelling. The classic text states that prolonged taking of Ju hua may aid circulation, make the body light, slow aging and prolong life. This genus of chrysanthemum grows in rivers and swamps.

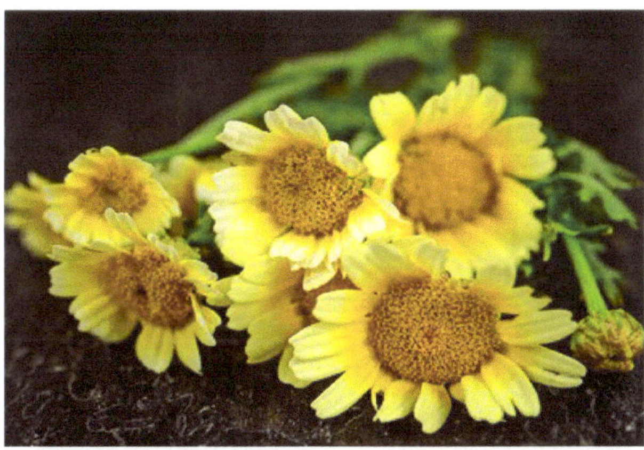

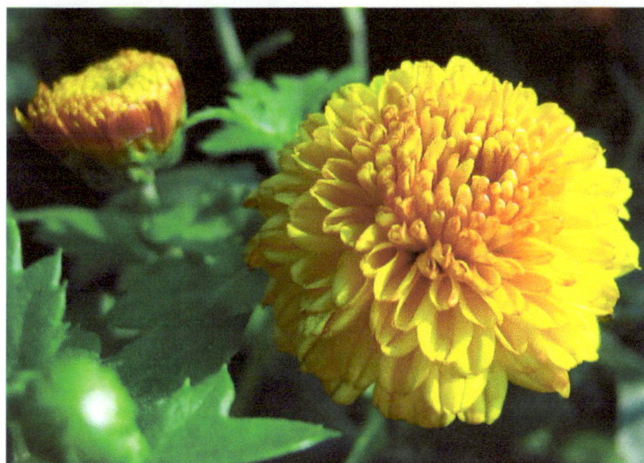

Fig. 30.5: *showing Chrysanthemum green leaves(top) The briant yeowowers are aso tasty! A beautiu Orienta heirloom, very colorful.(bottom)*

Achyranthis bidentatae, or Niu xi, is a root that is bitter and balanced, mainly treating rheumatic disorders and chronic pain of the knees and legs with stiffness. The classic text states that prolonged taking may make the body light and slow aging. The genus of Achyrathis grows in rivers and valleys, and is also called Bai bei, or hundredfold.

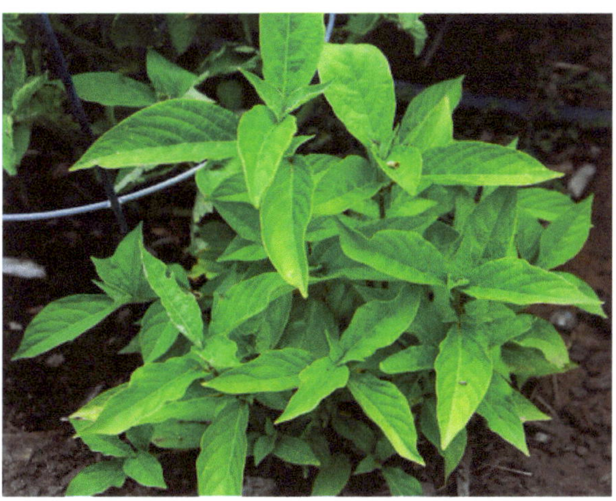

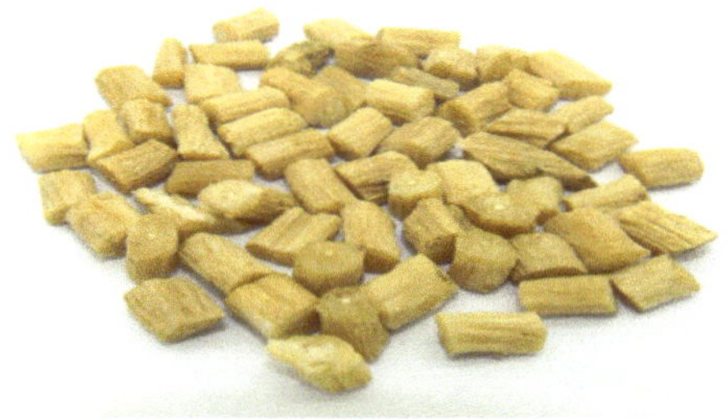

Fig. 30.6: *showing leaves of Achyranthis bidentatae, or Niu xi,plant (top) and dried roots(bottom)*

Angelicae pubescentis, or Du huo, is a root that is bitter and balanced, and is used mainly to relieve pain and stiffness, but also problems with the central nervous system, and in females fibroids and other conglomerations. Prolonged taking may make the body light and slow aging. This genus grows in rivers and valleys.

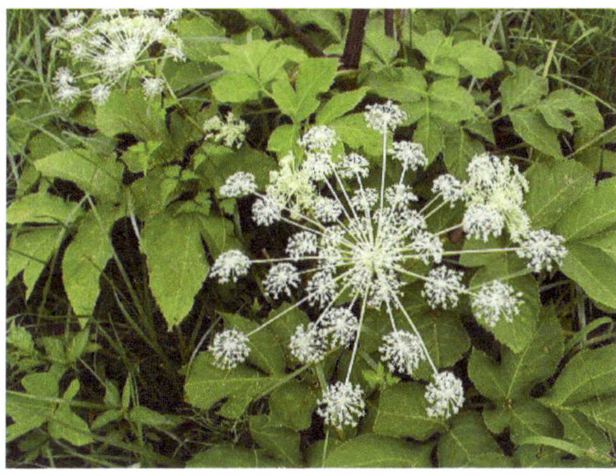

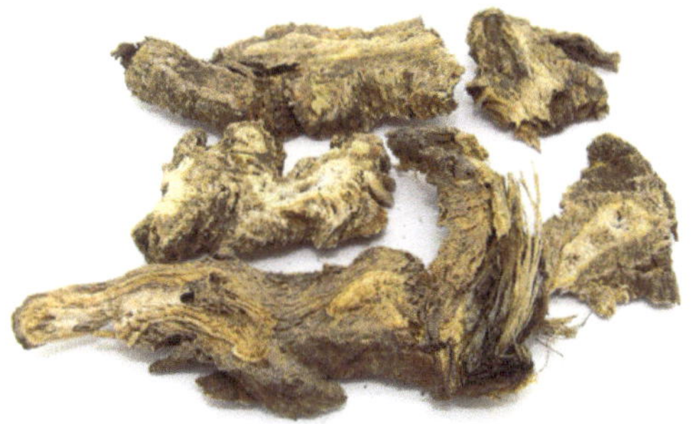

Fig. 30.7: *showing leaves and flowers (top) and dried form (bottm) of Angelicae pubescentis, or Du huo herb*

Cimicifugae, or Sheng ma (Black cohosh is an analogue), is sweet and balanced, and mainly treats toxins, especially parasitic toxins. Prolonged taking may prevent premature death from chronic disease, make the body light, and lengthen life. This genus grows in mountains and valleys.

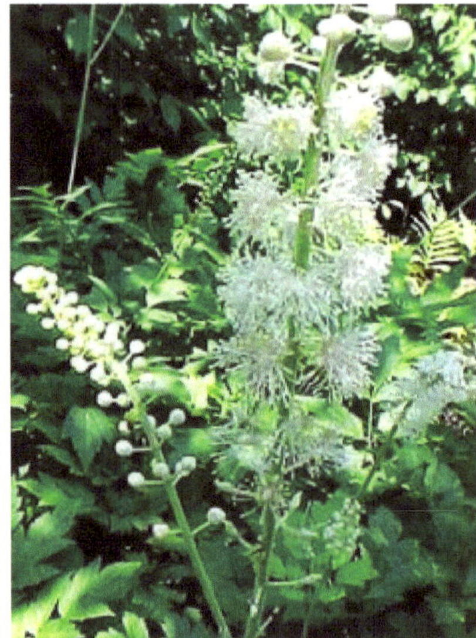

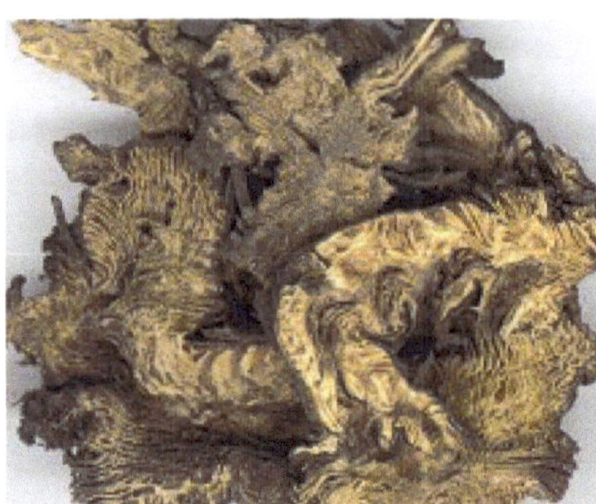

Fig.30.8:*showing leaves and flowers (top) and dried form (bottom) of Cimicifugae, or Sheng ma (Black cohosh) herb*

Artemisia keiskeanae, or An lu zi, is the seed of a genus of artemesia, and mainly was used to treat blood stasis in the main organs, swelling and edema of the abdomen, and rheumatic illness. Prolonged taking may make the body light, prolong life, and prevent senility (dementia). This genus grows in rivers and valleys.

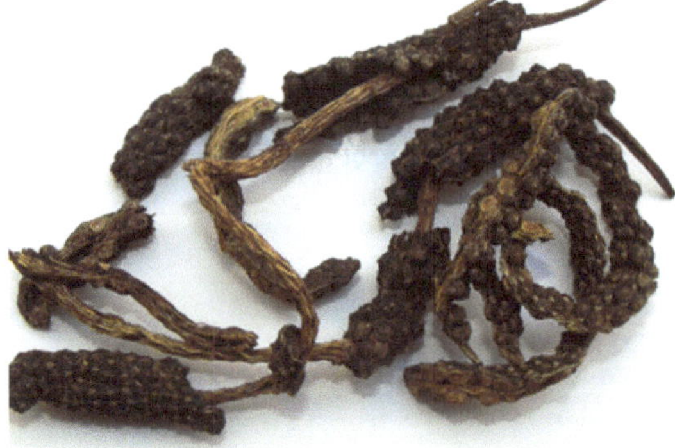

Fig. 30.9: *showing seeds of Artemisia keiskeanae, or An lu zi plant*

Artemisia argyi, or Bai hao, or Ai ye, is a leafy herb that is sweet and balanced, and mainly treats antigens in the main yin organs, supplements deficiency, promotes hair growth and restoration of hair color, and treats anxious depression with constant hunger but reduced appetite. Prolong taking may sharpen the vision and hearing, and prevent senility.

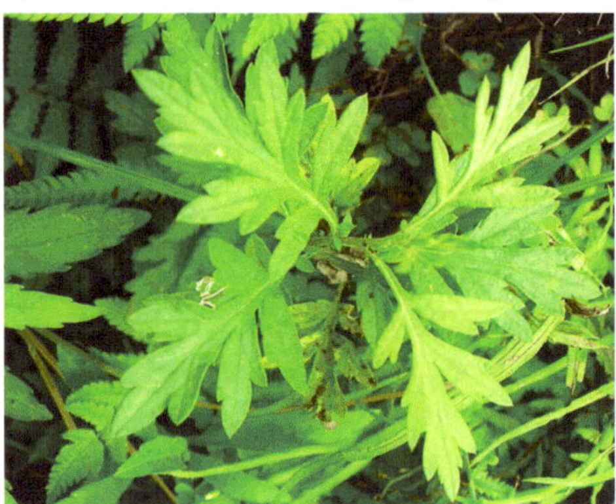

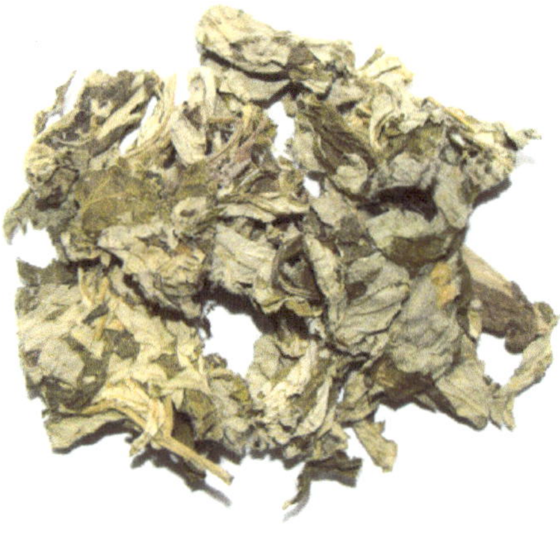

Fig. 30.10: *showing leavesof plant (top) and dried leaves form (bottom) of Artemisia argyi, or Bai hao, or Ai ye herb*

Plantaginis, or Che qian zi, is the seed of the plantago, and is sweet and cold, mainly used to treat urinary difficulties and swelling. Prolonged taking may make the body light and slow aging. This genus grows in plains and swamps.

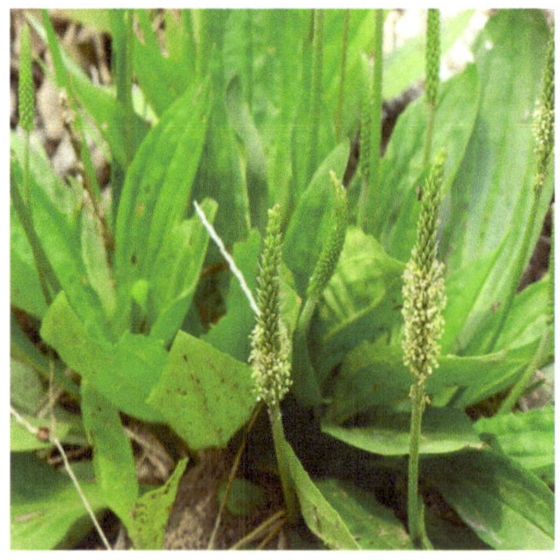

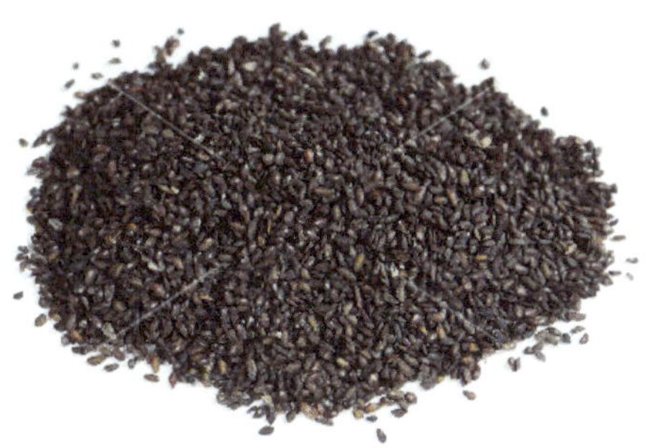

Fig. 30.11:*showing leaves and flowers of plant (top) and dried seeds of (bottom) Plantaginis, or Che qian zi, herb*

Cuscutae chinensis seed, or Tu si zi, is acrid and balanced, and is mainly used to supplement insufficiency, boost the qi and physical strength, and regain lost weight. Prolonged taking may improve the vision, make the body light, and prolong life. This genus grows in mountains and valleys.

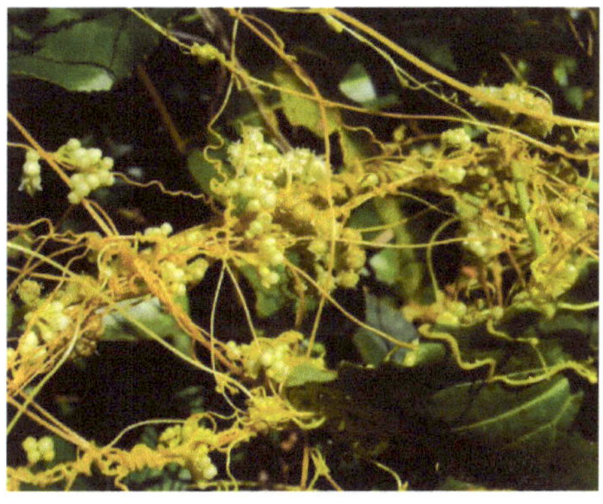

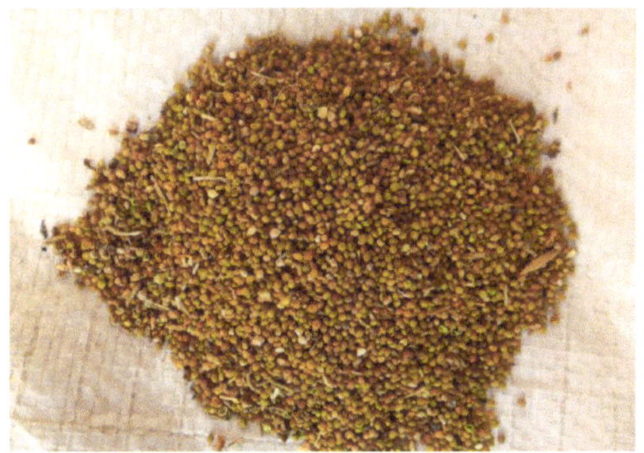

Fig. 30.12: *showing leaves and seeds of plant (top) and dried seeds of (bottom) Cuscutae chinensis seed, or Tu si zi, herb*

Junci baltici, or Shi long chu (also known as Dipsacus, or Cao xu duan), is a bitter and cooling herb that treats chronic parasitic disease, urinary difficulties, and rheumatic pain. Prolonged taking may make the body light, sharpen the vision and hearing, and prolong life. (Dipsaci are thistles).

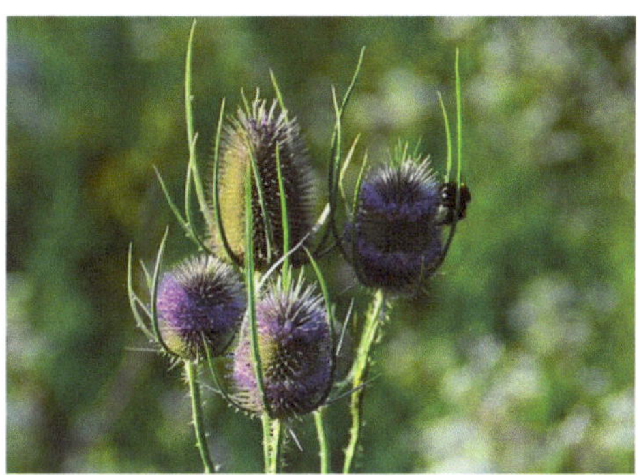

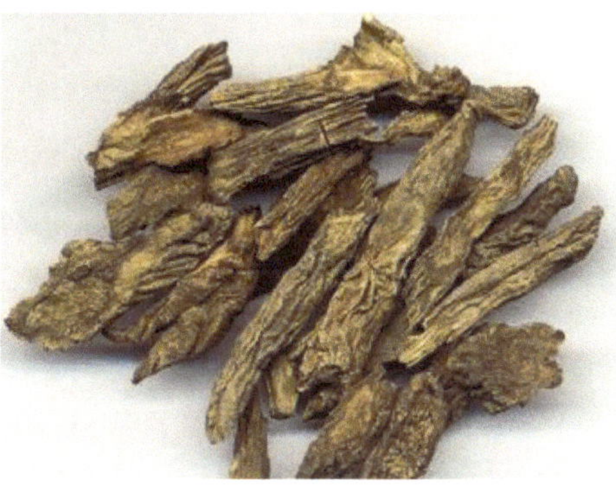

Fig. 30.13: *showing leaves and seeds of plant (top) and dried form of (bottom) Junci baltici, or Shi long chu (also known as Dipsacus, or Cao xu duan), herb*

Vacarriae segetalis seed, or Wang bu liu xing, is bitter and balanced, and mainly treats wounds, bleeding, and pain. Prolonged taking may make the body light, slow aging, and increase longevity. This genus grows in mountains and valleys.

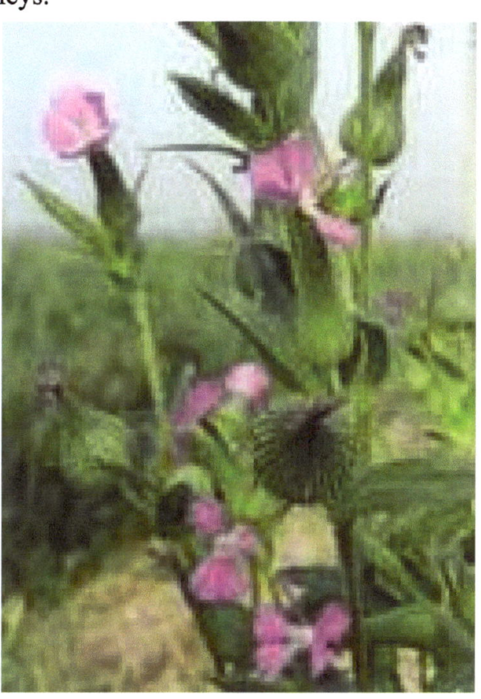

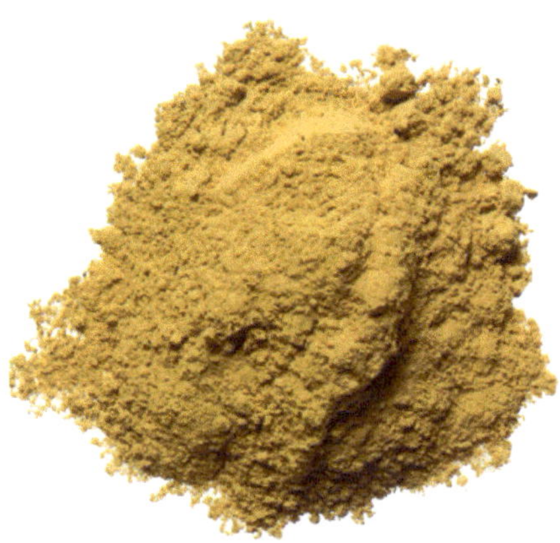

Fig. 30.14:*showing leaves and flowers of plant (top) and dried powder form (bottom) of Vacarriae segetalis seed, or Wang bu liu xing herb*

Eupatorii chinensis, or Lan cao (may be analogous to boneset), is acrid and balanced, and mainly is used to treat chronic parasitic diseases and difficult urination. Prolonged taking may make the body light, slow aging, and better communicate with spirit light. Its other name is Shui xiang, or Water fragrance, and is grows in pools and swamps.

Sesame seed sprouts, Sesami indici, or Qing xiang, is sweet and cold, and mainly treats antigens in the yin organs and arthritic pains, strengthening the tendons, ligaments and joints. Prolonged taking may sharpen the hearing and vision, prevent senility, and increase longevity. Sprouting the black sesame seed may be most beneficial.

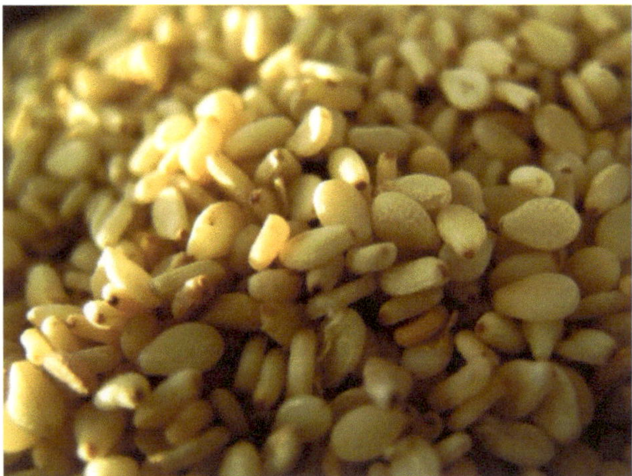

Fig. 30.15:*showing Sesame seed sprouts, Sesami indici, or Qing xiang*

Artemisia capillaris, or Yin chen hao, is a bitter herb that mainly treats joundice and liver disease. Prolonged taking may make the body light, boost the qi, and slow aging.

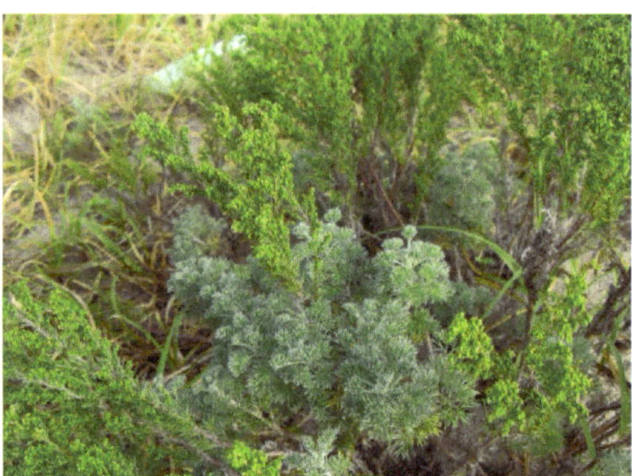

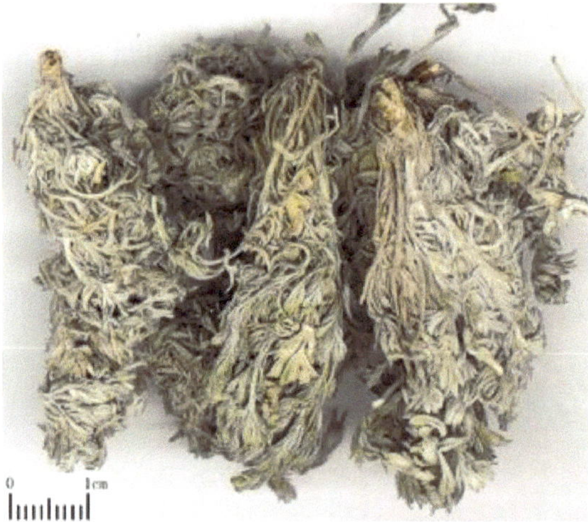

Fig. 30.16: *showing Artemisia capillaris, or Yin chen hao, plant (top) and dried leaves (bottom)*

Abutilonis seu malvae, or Gu huo (also Dong kui zi), is a seed that is sweet and warming, and mainly treats chronic pain and swelling. Prolonged taking may make the body light, increase life span, and slow aging. This genus grows in rivers and swamps.

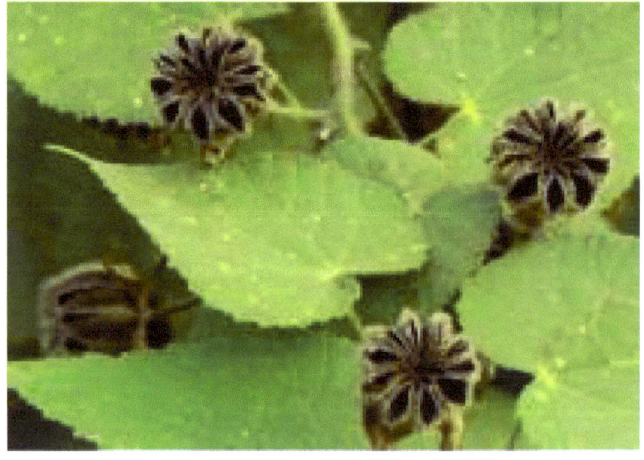

Fig. 30.17: *showing Dong kui zi),plant*

Magnoliae liliflorae, or Xin yi hua, is a flower that is acrid and warming, and is used mainly to treat inflammatory conditions, dizziness and headache, and black patches on the face. Prolonged taking may make the body light, brighten the vision, increase longevity, and slow aging.

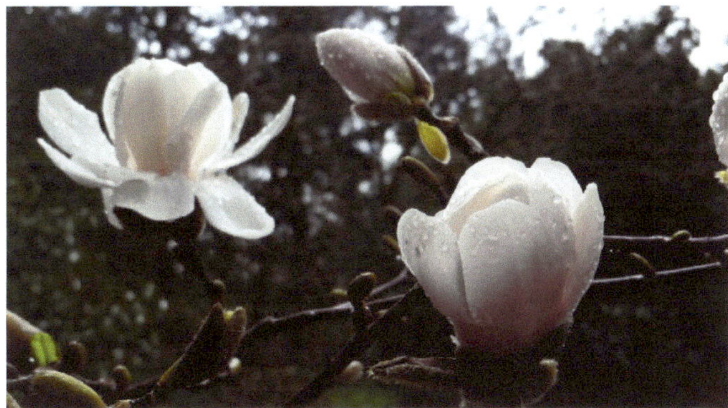

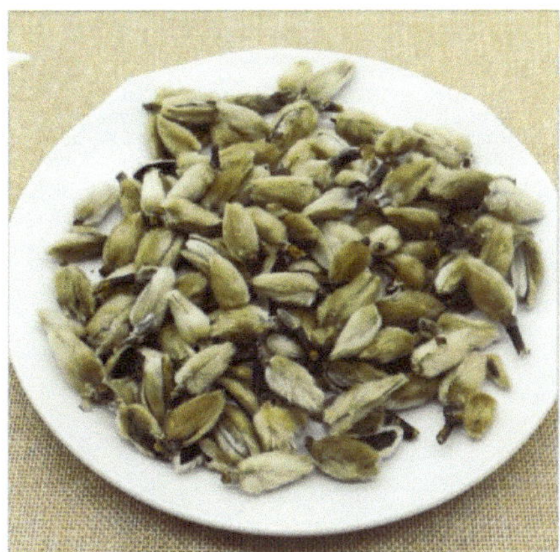

Fig. 30.18: *showing Magnoliae liliflorae, or Xin yi hua,, plant with flowers (top) and dried form (bottom)*

Lycium chinensis, or Gou qi zi (wolfberry), is a small red fruit that is bitter and cooling, and is used mainly to treat deep internal heat, diabetes, and general infirmity. Prolonged taking may benefit the tendons and joint tissues, make the body light, and slow aging. The root of this plant may be the beneficial part in this recommendation, which would indicate the Chinese herb Di gu pi. Numerous studies have shown Lycium fruit has chemicals that are cardioprotective, immunomodulatory, neuroprotective, and exhibit anticancer benefits. Studies of Di gu pi have shown inhibitory activity against pathogenic bacteria and fungi.

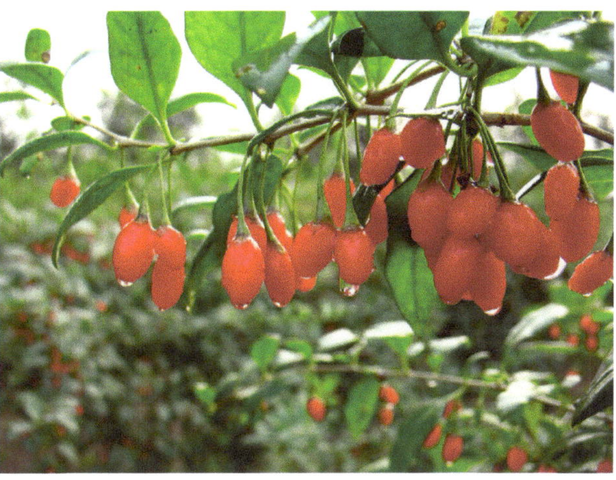

Fig. 30.19: *showing Lycium chinensis, or Gou qi zi (wolfberry),plant ,red fruit and leaves*

Zanthoxylum peperiti pericarp, or Qin jiao, is acrid and warm, and maintly treats arthritic complaints, chronic toxins and antigens, and benefits the growth of hair, teeth and brightens the vision. Prolonged taking may make the body light, render a good facial complexion, slow aging, and prolong life. This genus grows in rivers and valleys.

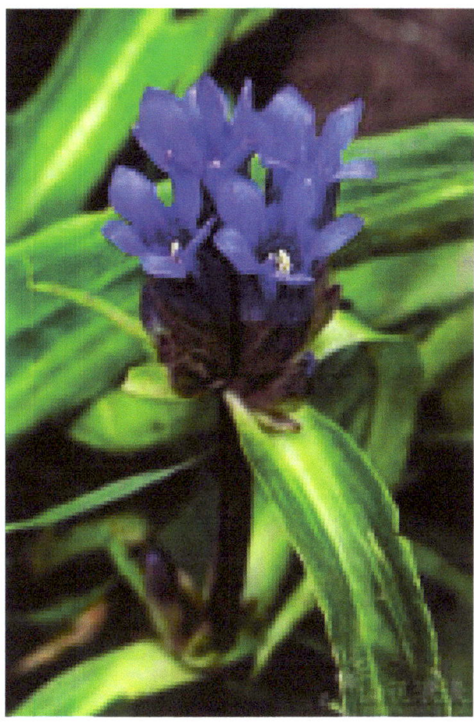

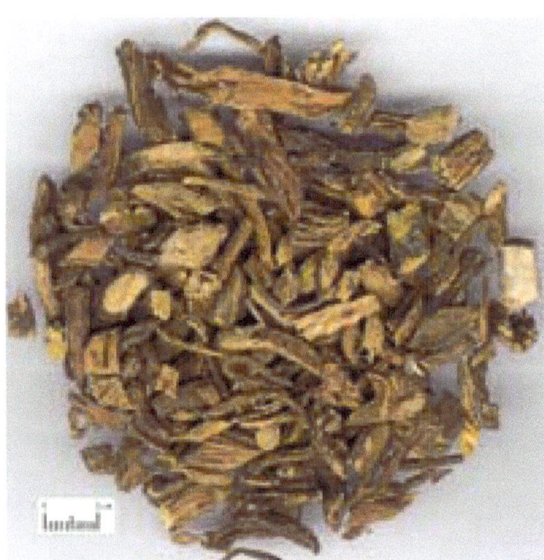

Fig. 30.20:*showing Zanthoxylum peperiti pericarp, or Qin jiao plant with flowers (top) and dried form (bottom)*

Zanthoxylum bungeani pericarp, or Shu jiao, is acrid and warm, and mainly treats chronic disease of the lung, and rheumatic disease. Prolonged taking may keep the hair from turning white, make the body light, and increase the life span.This genus grows in rivers and valleys.

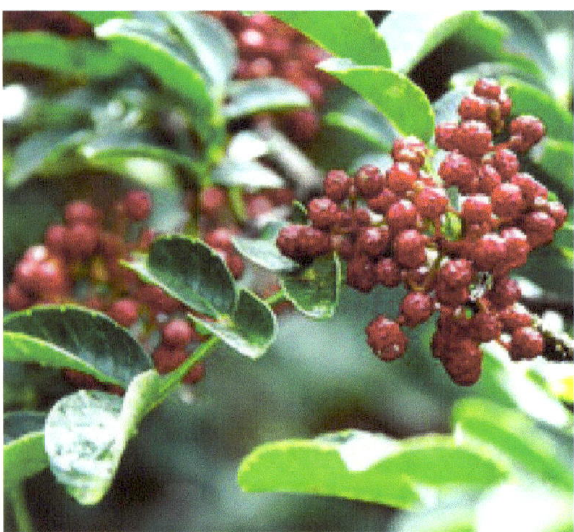

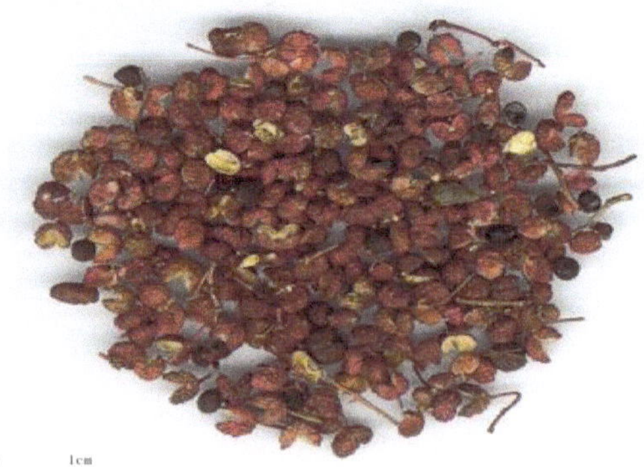

Fig. 30.21: *showing Zanthoxylum bungeani pericarp, or Shu jiao plant with seeds (top) and dried form (bottom)*

Sclerotium polypori umbellati, or Zhu ling, is sweet and balanced, and mainly treats malaria, other chronic parasitic disease, and inhibited urination. Prolonged taking may make the body light, and slow aging.

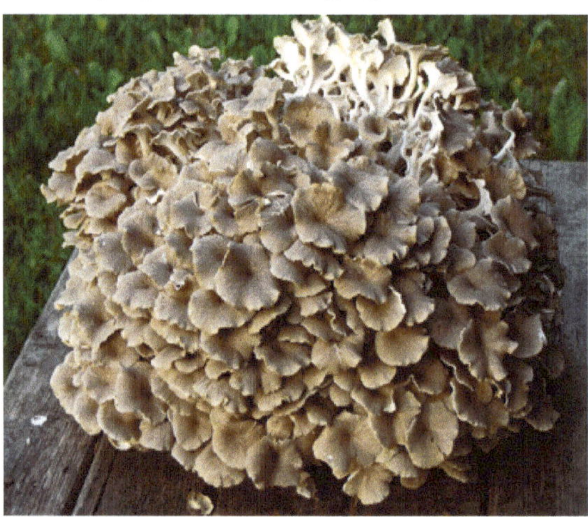

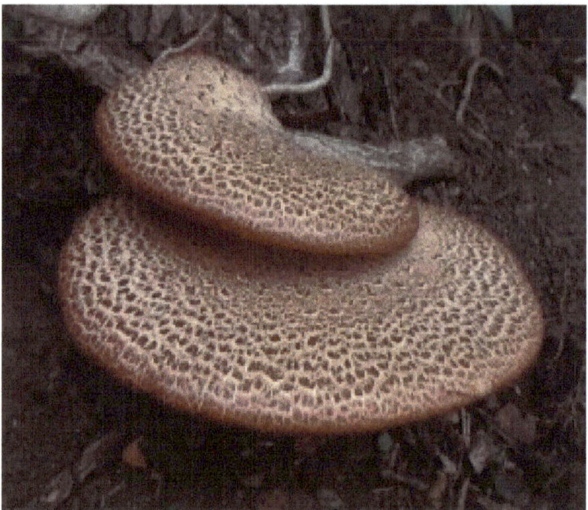

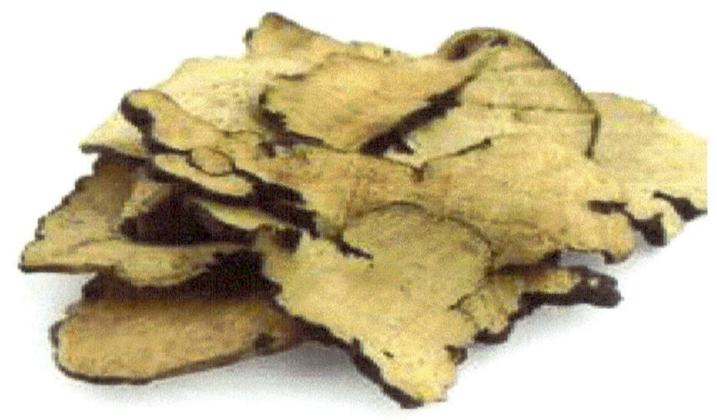

Fig. 30.22: *showing Sclerotium polypori umbellati, or Zhu ling,plant with leafs (top & middle) and dried form (bottom)*

Panax ginseng, or Asian ginseng

The other Chinese herb I love for SIR1 activation and all around anti-aging supplementation is called Panax ginseng, or Asian ginseng, and known in Chinese as ren shen, man root. It is one of the royal herbs in Chinese herbalism. Once considered so valuable that wars were fought over the right to the areas it grew in, ginseng does deserve its reputation. Among its many anti-aging properties, ginseng is a highly effective activator of SIRT1 in every cell of your body. In fact, this extraordinary root stimulates cellular function, and at the same time increases all hormones, particularly the sex hormones, which are so vital to looking young.

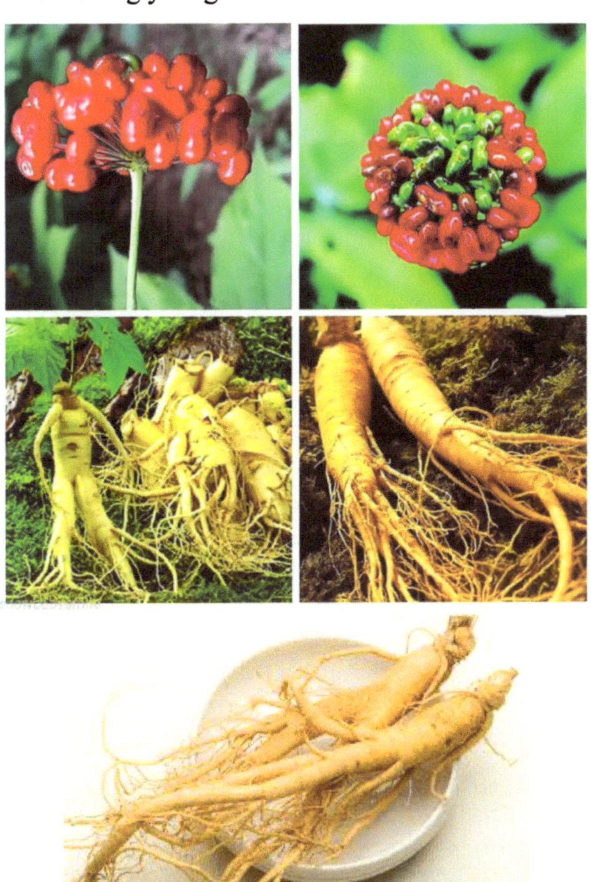

Fig. 30.23: *showing all forms of Panax ginseng, or Asian ginseng (top) and dry mature herb (bottom)*

Resveratrol

Resveratrol is a sirtuin-activating, anti-aging compound that's found in red wine and may provide an explanation to what's known as the "French paradox" that is, the finding that the French, who eat a diet full of saturated fat, have surprisingly low levels of heart disease. Resveratrol, one of the most potent sirtuin activators discovered so far, is found in red wine. In March 2013, Harvard researchers found that resveratrol is capable of slowing aging. This has important implications for human longevity as Resveratrol is readily available as an anti-aging supplement.

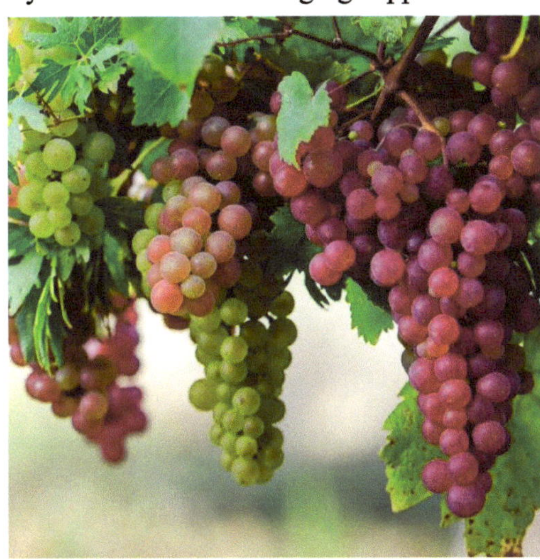

Fig. 30.24:*showing mature red grapes which is a source of Resveratrol*

Resveratrol, or trans-3, 5, 4'-trihydroxystilbene, is an anti-aging antioxidant found in the skin of many fruits, including blueberries, peanuts, and, when eaten with the thin, papery red skin, even rhubarb. It is particularly found in the red grape, and in the red wine made from these grapes. Levels of resveratrol in red wine vary according to grape type and country of origin. The highest levels are found in wines from cooler countries, with the highest being from Bordeaux, and lower levels found in red wines from California. The pinot noir grape produces the highest levels of resveratrol, but cabernet sauvignon from the cooler regions and Italian sangiovese are also very high in this anti-aging compound.

Resveratrol supplementation from foods or otherwise activates the sirtuin anti-aging pathway. This pathway is a chain of biochemical reactions, which, when activated, actually slows down aging. This stimulation is complex and appears to require resveratrol in its natural state, with many cofactors intact—as it's found in plants. It is far less active in its chemically purified form. What's more, every one of your cells contains an energy-producing factory called a mitochondrion (plural, mitochondria), and optimal mitochondrial function is essential to long life, energy, and a youthful appearance—and sure enough, resveratrol stimulates the sirtuin that affects aging mitochondria.

Ashwagandha

Ashwagandha (Withania somnifera) has become one of the most popular Ayurvedic herbs in the Western world. And it is no wonder, with all the benefits this beloved root has to offer! Ashwagandha has been used in Ayurveda for thousands of years as a rasayana (rejuvenative) and it is renowned as an adaptogenic herb, which means it is used to help the body resist physiological and psychological stress by adapting to the needs of the body. Take our free Ayurvedic Profile™ quiz to see if ashwagandha is one of the herbs recommended for you.

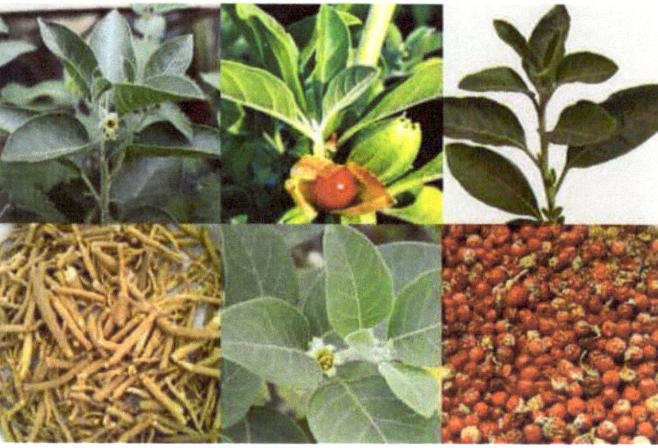

Fig. 30.25: *showing all forms of Ashwagandha plant*

Health Benefits of Ashwagandha

Ashwagandha is used to tone, support, and revitalize bodily functions. It has been revered over time for its dual capacity to energize and calm at the same time. Stress can cause fatigue, often manifesting as "hyper" signs like agitation and difficulty sleeping. By providing a nourishing, yet energizing effect, ashwagandha can support a healthy nervous system. With the use of ashwagandha, stress doesn't impact the nervous system with such intensity, and the "hyper" signs of stress and agitation will naturally resolve over time. In this way, ashwagandha has a rejuvenating and calming influence on the nervous system and, consequentially, on the entire being. This quality of ashwagandha makes it a prime supplement to use in the toning and rejuvenation process. In addition to its dual energizing/calming effect, ashwagandha offers a number of benefits:

- Supports a healthy immune system
- Calms mental processes
- Fosters healthy sleep patterns
- Benefits a healthy reproductive system in both males and females
- Supports sustained energy levels, strength, and vitality, including with physical activity*
- Supports a healthy back and joints
- Promotes thyroid health
- Promotes healthy functioning of the adrenals and therefore prolongs the life

Summary

Telomere shortening and dysfunction play a crucial role in the pathogenesis of aging associated CVDs. Critically short telomeres can lead to cellular senescence and apoptosis, which contribute to the development of atherosclerosis and predispose people to plaque instability. Both genetic and environmental factors have been associated with individual variations in TL. Cardiovascular risk factors such as smoking, diabetes mellitus, hypertension, obesity, sedentary lifestyle, and stress have been considered to increase oxidative stress or inflammation, consequently accelerating TL shortening. However, healthy lifestyle and physical activity are protective factors and maintain TL. In clinical practice, shorter LTL reflects the burden of oxidative stress and inflammation, and might be an effective biomarker for risk stratification for atherosclerosis and CVDs. The association of LTL with CAD has been reported in several prospective epidemiological studies, although conclusive evidence of causal relationship is still lacing. However, for subclinical atherosclerosis, ischemic stroke, and PAD, available data are controversial. The role of telomeres in disease pathogenesis should be explored according to some crucial clinical implications of pilot studies, such as coronary artery stenting, SCD, idiopathic pulmonary hypertension, and degenerative aortic stenosis. Furthermore, targeting telomerase or additional telomere-associated proteins may provide a novel therapeutic strategy for neovascularization in patients with ischemic heart diseases and for restoring replicative capacity in those with HF. Additional basic and well-designed clinical studies are required to validate these observations and further expand our knowledge the complexities of telomere dynamics in humans.

Bibliography and Acknowledgement

- Akasheva D.U., Plokhova E.V., Tkacheva O.N., Strazhesko I.D., Kruglikova A.S., Pykhtina V.S., Dudinskaya E.N., Skvortsov D.A., Egshatyan L.V., Brailova N.V., *et al.* Age-related changes of left ventricular diastolic function, NT-proBNP level and their association with leukocyte telomere length. Kardiologiia. 2015;55:59–65.
- *Ann N Y Acad Sci*, **1019** (2004), pp. 278-284
- *Ann N Y Acad Sci*, **908** (2000), pp. 99-110
- Armstrong E.J., Xing L., Zhang J., Zheng Y., Shunk K.A., Yeh R.W., Farzaneh-Far R., Yu B., Jang I.K. Association between leukocyte telomere length and drug-eluting stent strut coverage by optical coherence tomography. *J. Am. Coll. Cardiol.* 2012;**59**:2218–2219.
- Aurigemma G.P. Diastolic heart failure—A common and lethal condition by any name. *N. Engl. J. Med.* 2006;355:308–310. doi: 10.1056/NEJMe068128.

- Aviv A., Hunt S.C., Lin J., Cao X., Kimura M., Blackburn E. Impartial comparative analysis of measurement of leukocyte telomere length/DNA content by Southern blots and qPCR. Nucleic *Acids Res*. 2011
- B. van Steensel, A. Smogorzewska, T. de Lange TRF2 protects human telomeres from end-to-end fusions Cell, 92 (1998), pp. 401-413 [16]
- Banerjee B., Peiris D.N., Koo S.H., Chui P., Lee E.J.D., Hande M.P. Genomic imbalances in key ion channel genes and telomere shortening in sudden cardiac death victims. *Cytogenet. Genome Res*. 2008;122:350–355.
- Bär C., Bernardes de Jesus B., Serrano R., Tejera A., Ayuso E., Jimenez V., Formentini I., Bobadilla M., Mizrahi J., de Martino A., *et al*. Telomerase expression confers cardioprotection in the adult mouse heart after acute myocardial infarction. *Nat. Commun*. 2014
- Baragetti A., Palmen J., Garlaschelli K., Grigore L., Pellegatta F., Tragni E., Catapano A.L., Humphries S.E., Norata G.D., Talmud P.J. Telomere shortening over 6 years is associated with increased subclinical carotid vascular damage and worse cardiovascular prognosis in the general population. *J. Intern. Med*. 2015;277:478–487.
- Barasch E., Gottdiener J.S., Aurigemma G., Kitzman D.W., Han J., Kop W.J., Tracy R.P. The relationship between serum markers of collagen turnover and cardiovascular outcome in the elderly: The Cardiovascular Health Study. Circ. *Heart Fail*. 2011; **4**:733–739.
- Behjati M., Hashemi M., Salehi M., Kelishadi R. Can leukocyte telomere length (LTL) be considered as an index in application of neural network in the atherosclerosis risk stratification? *Int. J. Cardiol*. 2010;144:136–137.
- Bekaert S., de Meyer T., Rietzschel E.R., de Buyzere M.L., de Bacquer D., Langlois M., Segers P., Cooman L., van Damme P., Cassiman P., *et al*. Telomere length and cardiovascular risk factors in a middle-aged population free of overt cardiovascular disease. *Aging Cell*. 2007;6:639–647.
- Benetos A., Gardner J.P., Zureik M., Labat C., Xiaobin L., Adamopoulos C., Temmar M., Bean K.E., Thomas F., Aviv A. Short telomeres are associated with increased carotid atherosclerosis in hypertensive subjects. *Hypertension*. 2004;43:182–185. doi: 10.1161/01. HYP.0000113081.42868. f4. [PubMed][Cross Ref]
- Benetos A., Okuda K., Lajemi M., Kimura M., Thomas F., Skurnick J., Labat C., Bean K., Aviv A. Telomere length as an indicator of biological aging: The gender effect and relation with pulse pressure and pulse wave velocity. *Hypertension*. 2001;**37**:381–385.
- Bennaceur K., Atwill M., Al Zhrany N., Hoffmann J., Keavney B., Breault D., Richardson G., von Zglinicki T., Saretzki G., Spyridopoulos I. Atorvastatin induces T cell proliferation by a telomerase reverse transcriptase (TERT) mediated mechanism. *Atherosclerosis*. 2014; 236:312–320.
- Bernardes de Jesus B., Vera E., Schneeberger K., Tejera A.M., Ayuso E., Bosch F., Blasco M.A. Telomerase gene therapy in adult and old mice delays aging and increases longevity without increasing cancer. *EMBO Mol. Med*. 2012;4:691–704.
- Blackburn E.H. Switching and signaling at the telomere. *Cell*. 2001; **106**:661–673.
- Blackburn E.H., Epel E.S., Lin J. Human telomere biology: A contributory and interactive factor in aging, disease risks, and protection. *Science*. 2015; 350:1193–1198.
- Blasco M. Telomere length, stem cells and aging. Nat. Chem. Biol. 2007; **3**:640–649.
- Boccardi V., Paolisso G. Telomerase activation: A potential key modulator for human healthspan and longevity. *Ageing Res. Rev*. 2014;15:1–5.
- Borlaug B.A., Paulus W.J. Heart failure with preserved ejection fraction: Pathophysiology, diagnosis, and treatment. *Eur. Heart J*. 2011;32:670–679.
- Breitschopf K., Zeiher A.M., Dimmeler S. Pro-atherogenic factors induce telomerase inactivation in endothelial cells through an Akt-dependent mechanism. *FEBS Lett*. 2001; **493**:21–25.
- Brouilette S., Singh R.K., Thompson J.R., Goodall A.H., Samani N.J. White cell telomere length and risk of premature myocardial infarction. Arterioscler. Thromb. *Vasc. Biol*. 2003; **23**:842–846.
- Brouilette S.W., Moore J.S., McMahon A.D., Thompson J.R., Ford I., Shepherd J., Packard C.J., Samani N.J. Telomere length, risk of coronary heart disease, and statin treatment in the West of Scotland Primary Prevention Study: A nested case-control study. *Lancet*. 2007;369:107–114.
- Brouilette S.W., Whittaker A., Stevens S.E., van der Harst P., Goodall A.H., Samani N.J. Telomere length is shorter in healthy offspring of subjects with coronary artery disease: Support for the telomere hypothesis. *Heart*. 2008; **94:**422–425.
- Burnett-Hartman A.N., Fitzpatrick A.L., Kronmal R.A., Psaty B.M., Jenny N.S., Bis J.C., Tracy R.P., Kimura M., Aviv A. Telomere-associated polymorphisms correlate with cardiovascular disease mortality in Caucasian women: The Cardiovascular Health Study. Mech. *Ageing Dev*. 2012; 133:275–281.
- Butler M.G., Tilburt J., Devries A., Muralidhar B., Aue G., Hedges L., Atkinson J., Schwartz H. Comparison of chromosome telomere integrity in multiple tissues from subjects at different ages. Cancer Genet. *Cytogenet*. 1998; **105**:138–144.
- C.M. Azzalin, P. Reichenbach, L. Khoriauli, *et al*. Telomeric repeat containing RNA and RNA surveillance factors at mammalian chromosome ends Science, 318 .2007. 798-801
- Calvert P.A., Liew T.V., Gorenne I., Clarke M., Costopoulos C., Obaid D.R., O'Sullivan M., Shapiro L.M., McNab D.C., Densem C.G., *et al*. Leukocyte telomere length is associated with high-risk plaques on virtual histology intravascular ultrasound and increased proinflammatory activity. Arterioscler. Thromb. *Vasc. Biol*. 2011; **31:**2157–2164.
- Campisi J. Cellular senescence: Putting the paradoxes in perspective. Curr. Opin. *Genet. Dev*. 2011; 21:107–112.
- Carty C.L., Kooperberg C., Liu J., Herndon M., Assimes T., Hou L., Kroenke C.H., LaCroix A.Z., Kimura M., Aviv A., *et al*. Leukocyte Telomere Length and Risks of Incident Coronary

Heart Disease and Mortality in a Racially Diverse Population of Postmenopausal Women. Arterioscler. Thromb. *Vasc. Biol.* 2015; **35:**2225–2231.

- Chang E., Harley C.B. Telomere length and replicative aging in human vascular tissues. *Proc. Natl. Acad. Sci.* USA. 1995; **92**:11190–11194.
- Chen C.H., Nakayama M., Nevo E., Fetics B.J., Maughan W.L., Kass D.A. Coupled systolic-ventricular and vascular stiffening with age: Implications for pressure regulation and cardiac reserve in the elderly. *J. Am. Coll. Cardiol.* 1998; **32**:1221–1227.
- Chen S., Lin J., Matsuguchi T., Blackburn E., Yeh F., Best L.G., Devereux R.B., Lee E.T., Howard B.V., Roman M.J., Zhao J. Short leukocyte telomere length predicts incidence and progression of carotid atherosclerosis in American Indians: The strong heart family study. Aging. 2014; **6**:414–427.
- Chen W.D., Wen M.S., Shie S.S., Lo Y.L., Wo H.T., Wang C.C., Hsieh I.C., Lee T.H., Wang C.Y. The circadian rhythm controls telomeres and telomerase activity. *Biochem. Biophys. Res. Commun.* 2014;451:408–414.
- Cherkas L.F., Aviv A., Valdes A.M., Hunkin J.L., Gardner J.P., Surdulescu G.L., Kimura M., Spector T.D. The effects of social status on biological aging as measured by white-blood-cell telomere length. *Aging Cell.* 2006;5:361–365.
- Cherkas L.F., Hunkin J.L., Kato B.S., Richards J.B., Gardner J.P., Surdulescu G.L., Kimura M., Lu X., Spector T.D., Aviv A. The association between physical activity in leisure time and leukocyte telomere length. *Arch. Intern. Med.* 2008;168:154–158.
- Chimenti C., Kajstura J., Torella D., Urbanek K., Heleniak H., Colussi C., Di Meglio F., Nadal-Ginard B., Frustaci A., Leri A., et al. Senescence and death of primitive cells and myocytes lead to premature cardiac aging and heart failure. *Circ. Res.* 2003; **93**:604–613.
- Codd V., Nelson C.P., Albrecht E., Mangino M., Deelen J., Buxton J.L., Hottenga J.J., Fischer K., Esko T., Surakka I., et al. Identification of seven loci affecting mean telomere length and their association with disease. *Nat. Genet.* 2013;**45**:422–427.
- Collerton J., Martin-Ruiz C., Kenny A., Barrass K., von Zglinicki T., Kirkwood T., Keavney B. Telomere length is associated with left ventricular function in the oldest old: The Newcastle 85+ study. *Eur. Heart J.* 2007; **28**:172–176.
- Comporti M., Signorini C., Leoncini S., Gardi C., Ciccoli L., Giardini A., Vecchio D., Arezzini B. Ethanol-induced oxidative stress: Basic knowledge. *Genes Nutr.* 2010; **5**:101–109.
- Condorelli G., Jotti G.S., Pagiatakis C. Fibroblast senescence as a therapeutic target of myocardial fibrosis. *J. Am. Coll. Cardiol.* 2016; **67:**2029–2031.
- D'Mello M.J.J., Ross S.A., Briel M., Anand S.S., Gerstein H., Paré G. Association between shortened leukocyte telomere length and cardiometabolic outcomes: Systematic review and meta-analysis. Circ. Cardiovasc. Genet. 2015;**8**:82–90.
- De Lange T. Shelterin: The protein complex that shapes and safeguards human telomeres.Genes Dev. 2005;19:2100–2110. doi: 10.1101/gad.1346005.
- Dock J.N., Effros R.B. Role of CD8 T cell replicative senescence in human aging and in HIV-mediated immunosenescence. *Aging Dis*. 2011;**2**:382–397.
- E.H. Blackburn Switching and signaling at the telomere Cell, 106. 2011; 661-673
- Effros R.B., Dagarag M., Spaulding C., Man J. The role of CD8+ T-cell replicative senescence in human aging. *Immunol. Rev*. 2005; 205:147–157.
- Ellehoj H., Bendix L., Osler M. Leucocyte Telomere length and risk of cardiovascular disease in a cohort of 1,397 danish men and women. *Cardiology*. 2016;**133**:173–177.
- Epel E.S., Merkin S.S., Cawthon R., Blackburn E.H., Adler N.E., Pletcher M.J., Seeman T.E. The rate of leukocyte telomere shortening predicts mortality from cardiovascular disease in elderly men. *Aging.* 2009;**1**:81–88.
- Erusalimsky J.D., Kurz D.J. Cellular senescence in vivo: Its relevance in ageing and cardiovascular disease. *Exp. Gerontol.* 2005;**40**:634–642.
- Fadini G.P., Agostini C., Sartore S., Avogaro A. Endothelial progenitor cells in the natural history of atherosclerosis. *Atherosclerosis*. 2007;**194:**46–54.
- Farzaneh-Far R., Lin J., Epel E.S., Harris W.S., Blackburn E.H., Whooley M.A. Association of marine omega-3 fatty acid levels with telomeric aging in patients with coronary heart disease. *JAMA*. 2010;303:250–257.
- Fitzpatrick A.L., Kronmal R.A., Gardner J.P., Psaty B.M., Jenny N.S., Tracy R.P., Walston J., Kimura M., Aviv A. Leukocyte telomere length and cardiovascular disease in the cardiovascular health study. *Am. J. Epidemiol.* 2007; **165**:14–21.
- Franceschi C., Bonafè M., Valensin S., Olivieri F., de Luca M., Ottaviani E., de Benedictis G. Inflamm-aging: An evolutionary perspective on immunosenescence. *Ann. N. Y. Acad. Sci.* 2000;908:244–254.
- González-Suárez E., Geserick C., Flores J.M., Blasco M.A. Antagonistic effects of telomerase on cancer and aging in K5-mTert transgenic mice. Oncogene. 2005;24:2256–2270.
- Gorenne I., Kavurma M., Scott S., Bennett M. Vascular smooth muscle cell senescence in atherosclerosis. *Cardiovasc. Res.* 2006;**72**:9–17.
- Graakjaer J., Pascoe L., Der-Sarkissian H., Thomas G., Kolvraa S., Christensen K., Londoño-Vallejo J.A. The relative lengths of individual telomeres are defined in the zygote and strictly maintained during life. *Aging Cell.* 2004;**3**:97–102.
- Haendeler J., Hoffmann J., Diehl J.F., Vasa M., Spyridopoulos I., Zeiher A.M., Dimmeler S. Antioxidants inhibit nuclear export of telomerase reverse transcriptase and delay replicative senescence of endothelial cells. *Circ. Res.* 2004;**94**:768–775.
- Harley C.B., Liu W., Flom P.L., Raffaele J.M. A natural product telomerase activator as part of a health maintenance program: Metabolic and cardiovascular response. *Rejuvenation Res.* 2013;**16**:386–395.

- Haver V.G., Mateo Leach I., Kjekshus J., Fox J.C., Wedel H., Wikstrand J., de Boer R.A., van Gilst W.H., McMurray J.J.V., van Veldhuisen D.J., *et al.* Telomere length and outcomes in ischaemic heart failure: Data from the COntrolled ROsuvastatin multinational Trial in Heart Failure (CORONA) *Eur. J. Heart Fail.* 2015;**17**:313–319.
- Haycock P.C., Heydon E.E., Kaptoge S., Butterworth A.S., Thompson A., Willeit P. Leucocyte telomere length and risk of cardiovascular disease: Systematic review and meta-analysis. *BMJ.* 2014
- Hemann M.T., Strong M.A., Hao L.Y., Greider C.W. The shortest telomere, not average telomere length, is critical for cell viability and chromosome stability. Cell. 2001;107:67–77.
- Herbert K.E., Mistry Y., Hastings R., Poolman T., Niklason L., Williams B. Angiotensin II-mediated oxidative DNA damage accelerates cellular senescence in cultured human vascular smooth muscle cells via telomere-dependent and independent pathways. *Circ. Res.* 2008;102:201–208.
- Hoffmann J., Haendeler J., Aicher A., Rössig L., Vasa M., Zeiher A.M., Dimmeler S. Aging Enhances the Sensitivity of Endothelial Cells Toward Apoptotic Stimuli Important Role of Nitric Oxide. *Circ. Res.* 2001;89:709–715.
- Hoffmann J., Shmeleva E.V., Boag S.E., Fiser K., Bagnall A., Murali S., Dimmick I., Pircher H., Martin-Ruiz C., Egred M., et al. Myocardial ischemia and reperfusion leads to transient CD8 immune deficiency and accelerated immunosenescence in CMV-seropositive patients. *Circ. Res.* 2015;116:87–98.
- Huda N., Tanaka H., Herbert B.S., Reed T., Gilley D. Shared environmental factors associated with telomere length maintenance in elderly male twins. *Aging Cell.* 2007; **6**:709–713.
- Huzen J., Peeters W., de Boer R.A., Moll F.L., Wong L.S.M., Codd V., de Kleijn D.P.V., de Smet B.J.G.L., van Veldhuisen D.J., Samani N.J., et al. Circulating leukocyte and carotid atherosclerotic plaque telomere length: Interrelation, association with plaque characteristics, and restenosis after endarterectomy. Arterioscler. Thromb. *Vasc. Biol.* 2011; **31**:1219–1225.
- Izikki M., Hoang E., Draskovic I., Mercier O., Lecerf F., Lamrani L., Liu W.Y., Guignabert C., Fadel E., Dorfmuller P., *et al.* Telomere maintenance is a critical determinant in the physiopathology of pulmonary hypertension. *J. Am. Coll. Cardiol.* 2015; **66**:1942–1943.
- J. Karlseder, D. Broccoli, Y. Dai, *et al.* p53- and ATM-dependent apoptosis induced by telomeres lacking TRF2 Science, 283 (1999), pp. 1321-1325
- J.M. Houben, H.J. Moonen, F.J. van Schooten, *et al.* Telomere length assessment: biomarker of chronic oxidative stress? Free *Radic Biol Med*, **44** (2008), pp. 235-246
- Jaco, P. Munoz, F. Goytisolo, *et al.* Role of mammalian Rad54 in telomere length maintenance Mol Cell Biol, **23** (2003), pp. 5572-5580
- Jaskelioff M., Muller F.L., Paik J.H., Thomas E., Jiang S., Adams A.C., Sahin E., Kost-Alimova M., Protopopov A., Cadiñanos J., *et al.* Telomerase reactivation reverses tissue degeneration in aged telomerase-deficient mice. *Nature.* 2011;469:102–106.
- Jurk D., Wilson C., Passos J.F., Oakley F., Correia-Melo C., Greaves L., Saretzki G., Fox C., Lawless C., Anderson R., *et al.* Chronic inflammation induces telomere dysfunction and accelerates ageing in mice. *Nat. Commun.* 2014
- K. CollinsMammalian telomeres and telomerase *Curr Opin Cell Biol*, 12 (2000), pp. 378-383
- K. Liu, M.M. Schoonmaker, B.L. Levine, *et al.* Constitutive and regulated expression of telomerase reverse transcriptase (hTERT) in human lymphocytes *Proc Natl Acad Sci U S A*, 96 (1999), pp. 5147-5152
- Kajstura J., Rota M., Cappetta D., Ogórek B., Arranto C., Bai Y., Ferreira-Martins J., Signore S., Sanada F., Matsuda A., *et al.* Cardiomyogenesis in the aging and failing human heart. *Circulation.* 2012;**126**:1869–1881.
- Karlseder J., Smogorzewska A., de Lange T. Senescence induced by altered telomere state, not telomere loss. Science. 2002; 295:2446–2449.
- Kissel C.K., Lehmann R., Assmus B., Aicher A., Honold J., Fischer-Rasokat U., Heeschen C., Spyridopoulos I., Dimmeler S., Zeiher A.M. Selective functional exhaustion of hematopoietic progenitor cells in the bone marrow of patients with postinfarction heart failure. *J. Am. Coll. Cardiol.* 2007; **49**:2341–2349.
- Kurz D.J., Hong Y., Trivier E., Huang H.L., Decary S., Zang G.H., Lüscher T.F., Erusalimsky J.D. Fibroblast growth factor-2, but not vascular endothelial growth factor, upregulates telomerase activity in human endothelial cells. Arterioscler. Thromb. *Vasc. Biol.* 2003; **23**:748–754.
- Leri A., Franco S., Zacheo A., Barlucchi L., Chimenti S., Limana F., Nadal-Ginard B., Kajstura J., Anversa P., Blasco M.A. Ablation of telomerase and telomere loss leads to cardiac dilatation and heart failure associated with p53 upregulation. EMBO J. 2003; **22**:131–139.
- M. Kirwan, R. Beswick, T. Vulliamy, *et al.* Exogenous TERC alone can enhance proliferative potential, telomerase activity and telomere length in lymphocytes from dyskeratosis congenita patients *Br J Haematol*, **144** (2009), pp. 771-781
- M. Okano, S. Xie, E. LiCloning and characterization of a family of novel mammalian DNA (cytosine-5) methyltransferases *Nat Genet*, **19** (1998), pp. 219-220
- M.A. BlascoThe epigenetic regulation of mammalian telomeres *Nat Rev Genet*, **8** (2007), pp. 299-309
- M.D. Edo, V. AndresAging, telomeres, and atherosclerosis *Cardiovasc Res,* **66** (2005), pp. 213-221
- Mangino M., Hwang S.J., Spector T.D., Hunt S.C., Kimura M., Fitzpatrick A.L., Christiansen L., Petersen I., Elbers C.C., Harris T., *et al.* Genome-wide meta-analysis points to CTC1 and ZNF676 as genes regulating telomere homeostasis in humans. Hum. *Mol. Genet.* 2012;21:5385–5394.
- Matsumoto Y., Adams V., Walther C., Kleinecke C., Brugger P., Linke A., Walther T., Mohr F.W., Schuler G. Reduced number and function of endothelial progenitor cells in patients with

aortic valve stenosis: A novel concept for valvular endothelial cell repair. *Eur. Heart J.* 2009; **30**:346–355.

- Matthews C., Gorenne I., Scott S., Figg N., Kirkpatrick P., Ritchie A., Goddard M., Bennett M. Vascular smooth muscle cells undergo telomere-based senescence in human atherosclerosis: Effects of telomerase and oxidative stress. *Circ. Res*. 2006; **99**:156–164.
- Minamino T., Kourembanas S. Mechanisms of telomerase induction during vascular smooth muscle cell proliferation. *Circ. Res.* 2001; **89**:237–243.
- Minamino T., Miyauchi H., Yoshida T., Ishida Y., Yoshida H., Komuro I. Endothelial cell senescence in human atherosclerosis: Role of telomere in endothelial dysfunction. *Circulation.* 2002;105:1541–1544.
- Moyzis R.K., Buckingham J.M., Cram L.S., Dani M., Deaven L.L., Jones M.D., Meyne J., Ratliff R.L., Wu J.R. A highly conserved repetitive DNA sequence, (TTAGGG)n, present at the telomeres of human chromosomes. *Proc. Natl. Acad. Sci. USA*. 1988;85:6622–6626.
- Mozaffarian D., Benjamin E.J., Go A.S., Arnett D.K., Blaha M.J., Cushman M., De Ferranti S., Després J., Fullerton H.J., Howard V.J., *et al.* Heart disease and stroke statistics-2015 update: A report from the American Heart Association. *Circulation*. 2015;131:E29–E322.
- Müezzinler A., Zaineddin A.K., Brenner H. Body mass index and leukocyte telomere length in adults: A systematic review and meta-analysis. *Obes. Rev*. 2014;15:192–201.
- Murasawa S., Llevadot J., Silver M., Isner J.M., Losordo D.W., Asahara T. Constitutive human telomerase reverse transcriptase expression enhances regenerative properties of endothelial progenitor cells. Circulation. 2002;106:1133–1139.
- Nat Struct Mol Biol, 15 (2008), p. 998
- O'Donnell C.J., Demissie S., Kimura M., Levy D., Gardner J.P., White C., D'Agostino R.B., Wolf P.A., Polak J., Cupples L.A., et al. Leukocyte telomere length and carotid artery intimai medial thickness R the framingham heart study. Arterioscler. *Thromb. Vasc. Biol.* 2008;28:1165–1171.
- Oh H., Taffet G.E., Youker K.A., Entman M.L., Overbeek P.A., Michael L.H., Schneider M.D. Telomerase reverse transcriptase promotes cardiac muscle cell proliferation, hypertrophy, and survival. *Proc. Natl. Acad. Sci. USA.* 2001;98:10308–10313. doi: 10.1073/pnas.191169098.
- Oh H., Wang S.C., Prahash A., Sano M., Moravec C.S., Taffet G.E., Michael L.H., Youker K.A., Entman M.L., Schneider M.D. Telomere attrition and Chk2 activation in human heart failure. *Proc. Natl. Acad. Sci. USA*. 2003;100:5378–53783.
- Okuda K., Khan M.Y., Skurnick J., Kimura M., Aviv H., Aviv A. Telomere attrition of the human abdominal aorta: Relationships with age and atherosclerosis Atherosclerosis. 2000;152:391–398.
- Ornish D., Lin J., Daubenmier J., Weidner G., Epel E., Kemp C., Magbanua M.J.M., Marlin R., Yglecias L., Carroll P.R., Blackburn E.H. Increased telomerase activity and comprehensive lifestyle changes: A pilot study. *Lancet. Oncol.* 2008; **9:**1048–1057.
- Ostan R., Bucci L., Capri M., Salvioli S., Scurti M., Pini E., Monti D., Franceschi C. Immunosenescence and immunogenetics of human longevity. *Neuroimmunomodulation.* 2008;**15**:224–240.
- P. Fotiadou, O. Henegariu, J.B. SweasyDNA polymerase beta interacts with TRF2 and induces telomere dysfunction in a murine mammary cell line *Cancer Res*, 64 (2004), pp. 3830-3857
- Panayiotou A.G., Nicolaides A.N., Griffin M., Tyllis T., Georgiou N., Bond D., Martin R.M., Hoppensteadt D., Fareed J., Humphries S.E. Leukocyte telomere length is associated with measures of subclinical atherosclerosis. *Atherosclerosis*. 2010;211:176–181.
- Pernice F., Floccari F., Caccamo C., Belghity N., Mantuano S., Pacilè M.E., Romeo A., Nostro L., Barillà A., Crascì E., et al. Chromosomal damage and atherosclerosis. A protective effect from simvastatin. *Eur. J. Pharmacol*. 2006;532:223–229.
- Poch E., Carbonell P., Franco S., Díez-Juan A., Blasco M.A., Andrés V. Short telomeres protect from diet-induced atherosclerosis in apolipoprotein E-null mice. FASEB J. 2004;18:418–420.
- Poss K.D., Wilson L.G., Keating M.T. Heart regeneration in zebrafish. Science. 2002;298:2188–2190. doi: 10.1126/science.1077857.
- R. Benetti, S. Gonzalo, I. Jaco, *et al.* A mammalian microRNA cluster controls DNA methylation and telomere recombination via Rbl2-dependent regulation of DNA methyltransferases
- Raschenberger J., Kollerits B., Hammerer-Lercher A., Rantner B., Stadler M., Haun M., Klein-Weigel P., Fraedrich G., Kronenberg F. The association of relative telomere length with symptomatic peripheral arterial disease: Results from the CAVASIC study. Atherosclerosis. 2013;229:469–474.
- Richardson G.D., Breault D., Horrocks G., Cormack S., Hole N., Owens W.A. Telomerase expression in the mammalian heart. FASEB J. 2012;26:4832–4840.
- Rojas A., Romay S., González D., Herrera B., Delgado R., Otero K. Regulation of endothelial nitric oxide synthase expression by albumin-derived advanced glycosylation end products. Circ. Res. 2000;86:E50–E54.
- Rosenzweig A. Medicine. *Cardiac regeneration. Science.* 2012;338:1549–1550
- S. Kawanishi, S. OikawaMechanism of telomere shortening by oxidative stress
- S. Oikawa, S. KawanishiSite-specific DNA damage at GGG sequence by oxidative stress may accelerate telomere shortening *FEBS Lett,* 453 (1999), pp. 365-368
- S. Oikawa, S. Tada-Oikawa, S. KawanishiSite-specific DNA damage at the GGG sequence by UVA involves acceleration of telomere shortening Biochemistry, 40 (2001), pp. 4763-4768
- S. Petersen, G. Saretzki, T. von Zglinicki Preferential accumulation of single-stranded regions in telomeres of human fibroblasts *Exp Cell Res*, 239 (1998), pp. 152-160
- S. Schoeftner, M.A. BlascoA 'higher order' of telomere regulation: telomere heterochromatin and telomeric RNAs *EMBO J*, 28 (2009), pp. 2323-2336

- Samani N.J., Boultby R., Butler R., Thompson J.R., Goodall A.H. Telomere shortening in atherosclerosis. *Lancet.* 2001;358:472–473.
- Samani N.J., van der Harst P. Biological ageing and cardiovascular disease. *Heart.* 2008; **94**:537–539.
- Samper E., Flores J.M., Blasco M.A. Restoration of telomerase activity rescues chromosomal instability and premature aging in TERC? mice with short telomeres. *EMBO Rep.* 2001;2:800–807. doi: 10.1093/embo-reports/kve174.
- Sampson M.J., Winterbone M.S., Hughes J.C., Dozio N., Hughes D.A. Monocyte telomere shortening and oxidative DNA damage in type 2 diabetes. *Diabetes Care.* 2006;**29**:283–289.
- Sano H., Nagai R., Matsumoto K., Horiuchi S. Receptors for proteins modified by advanced glycation endproducts (AGE)—Their functional role in atherosclerosis. Mech. Ageing Dev. 1999;107:333–346.
- Satoh M., Ishikawa Y., Takahashi Y., Itoh T., Minami Y., Nakamura M. Association between oxidative DNA damage and telomere shortening in circulating endothelial progenitor cells obtained from metabolic syndrome patients with coronary artery disease. *Atherosclerosis.* 2008;198:347–353.
- Savva G.M., Pachnio A., Kaul B., Morgan K., Huppert F.A., Brayne C., Moss P.A.H. Cytomegalovirus infection is associated with increased mortality in the older population. *Aging Cell.* 2013;12:381–387.
- Schmidt A.M., Hori O., Brett J., Yan S.D., Wautier J.L., Stern D. Cellular receptors for advanced glycation end products. Implications for induction of oxidant stress and cellular dysfunction in the pathogenesis of vascular lesions. Arterioscler. Thromb. 1994;14:1521–1528.
- Schupp N., Schmid U., Heidland A., Stopper H. Rosuvastatin protects against oxidative stress and DNA damage in vitro via upregulation of glutathione synthesis. *Atherosclerosis.* 2008;199:278–287.
- Shmeleva E.V., Boag S.E., Murali S., Bennaceur K., Das R., Egred M., Purcell I., Edwards R., Todryk S., Spyridopoulos I. Differences in immune responses between CMV-seronegative and -seropositive patients with myocardial ischemia and reperfusion. Immun. Inflamm. Dis. 2015;3:56–70.
- Slagboom P.E., Droog S., Boomsma D.I. Genetic determination of telomere size in humans: A twin study of three age groups. *Am. J. Hum. Genet.* 1994;55:876–882.
- Spyridopoulos I., Haendeler J., Urbich C., Brummendorf T.H., Oh H., Schneider M.D., Zeiher A.M., Dimmeler S. Statins enhance migratory capacity by upregulation of the telomere repeat-binding factor TRF2 in endothelial progenitor cells. *Circulation.* 2004;110:3136–3142.
- Spyridopoulos I., Hoffmann J., Aicher A., Brümmendorf T.H., Doerr H.W., Zeiher A.M., Dimmeler S. Accelerated telomere shortening in leukocyte subpopulations of patients with coronary heart disease: Role of cytomegalovirus seropositivity. *Circulation.* 2009;120:1364–1372.
- Strandberg T.E., Saijonmaa O., Tilvis R.S., Pitk 1 K.H., Strandberg A.Y., Miettinen T.A., Fyhrquist F. Association of telomere length in older men with mortality and midlife body mass index and smoking. J. Gerontol. A. Biol. Sci. Med. Sci. 2011;66:815–820.
- Strandberg T.E., Strandberg A.Y., Saijonmaa O., Tilvis R.S., Pitk 1 K.H., Fyhrquist F. Association between alcohol consumption in healthy midlife and telomere length in older men. The Helsinki Businessmen Study. Eur. J. Epidemiol. 2012;27:815–822.
- T. Richter, G. Saretzki, G. Nelson, et al. TRF2 overexpression diminishes repair of telomeric single-strand breaks and accelerates telomere shortening in human fibroblasts United Nations World Population Ageing 1950–2050. [(accessed on 1 May 2016)].
- T. von ZglinickiOxidative stress shortens telomeres Trends Biochem Sci, 27 (2002), pp. 339-344
- T. von ZglinickiRole of oxidative stress in telomere length regulation and replicative senescence
- T.S. Nawrot, J.A. Staessen, J.P. Gardner, et al. Telomere length and possible link to X chromosome Lancet, 363 (2004), pp.507-510
- Torella D., Rota M., Nurzynska D., Musso E., Monsen A., Shiraishi I., Zias E., Walsh K., Rosenzweig A., Sussman M.A., et al. Cardiac stem cell and myocyte aging, heart failure, and insulin-like growth factor-1 overexpression. Circ. Res. 2004;94:514–524.
- Valdes A.M., Andrew T., Gardner J.P., Kimura M., Oelsner E., Cherkas L.F., Aviv A., Spector T.D. Obesity, cigarette smoking, and telomere length in women. Lancet. 2005;366:662 664.
- Van der Harst P., van der Steege G., de Boer R.A., Voors A., Hall A.S., Mulder M.J., van Gilst W.H., van Veldhuisen D.J. Telomere length of circulating leukocytes is decreased in patients with chronic heart failure. J. Am. Coll. Cardiol. 2007;49:1459–1464.
- Vasa M., Breitschopf K., Zeiher A.M., Dimmeler S. Nitric oxide activates telomerase and delays endothelial cell senescence. Circ. Res. 2000;87:540–542.
- Von Zglinicki T. Oxidative stress shortens telomeres. Trends Biochem. Sci. 2002;27:339–344.
- Wang C.Y., Wen M.S., Wang H.W., Hsieh I.C., Li Y., Liu P.Y., Lin F.C., Liao J.K. Increased vascular senescence and impaired endothelial progenitor cell function mediated by mutation of circadian gene Per2. Circulation. 2008;118:2166–2173.
- Weng N.P. Regulation of telomerase expression in human lymphocytes. Springer Semin. Immunopathol. 2002;24:23–33. doi: 10.1007/s00281-001-0093-4.
- Werner C., F rster T., Widmann T., P ss J., Roggia C., Hanhoun M., Scharhag J., B chner N., Meyer T., Kindermann W., et al. Physical exercise prevents cellular senescence in circulating leukocytes and in the vessel wall. Circulation. 2009;120:2438–2447.
- Zou Y., Sfeir A., Gryaznov S.M., Shay J.W., Wright W.E. Does a sentinel or a subset of short telomeres determine replicative senescence? Mol. Biol. Cell. 2004;15:3709–3718.

Stem Cell and GeneTherapies Are As Alternative Treatments In Cardiovascular Diseases

Section 1. Stem Cell Transplantation

Despite the development of improved therapies and the significant advances in the understanding of the basis of disease pathogenesis, millions of people all over the World are living with life-threatening cardiovascular diseases. Recent breakthroughs suggest exciting directions that are likely to produce more effective therapies for the treatment of cardiovascular disease. One such area, cell transplantation (grafting of healthy cells into the diseased heart), holds enormous potential as an approach to cardiovascular pathophysiology. Once thought to be a scientific long shot, cell transplantation is becoming recognized as a viable strategy to strengthen weak hearts and limit infarct growth. The technology could also be used for the long-term delivery of beneficial recombinant proteins to the heart, which is a strategy to complement molecular biology advances and provide an alternative strategy for gene therapy. In an attempt to reduce the invasiveness of cell transfer, catheter-based techniques have been rapidly developed They basically rely on three routes:

- Endoventricular
- Intracoronary
- Transvenous,

The guidance of cell delivery being achieved with electromagnetic mapping, coronary angiography, and endovascular ultrasounds, respectively. In our experience, the latter technique has been found particularly user-friendly and we are currently testing its potential benefits in a sheep model of myocardial infarction. However, although these percutaneous approaches have been expeditiously applied in patients, they have actually undergone limited preclinical testing.

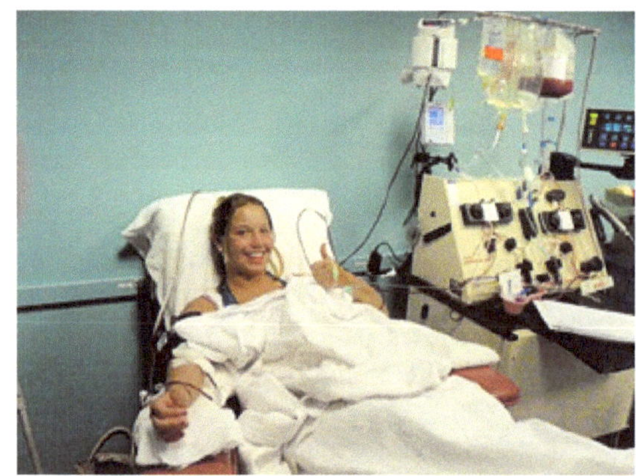

Fig. 31.1: *Transplantation (transfer of SC) is a safe, and usually painless procedure. It should be conducted in a sterile environment by a professional medical personnel. Usually, an ambulatory procedure. Within a day the patient usually returns to normal life. Ongoing monitoring of the patient is usually carried out on an 'out-patient' basis.*

Thus, the extent of intramyocardial cell trapping following endoventricular injections has not been fully investigated, nor is the ability of intracoronarily injected bone marrow cells to gain access to myocardial tissue, even if their transendothelial migration is thought to be enhanced by high-pressure infusion and angioplasty balloon inflation to prevent backflow. Indeed, viability of cells following passage through the catheters has usually been assessed but their functionality (i.e., ability of skeletal myoblasts and bone-marrow cells to differentiate into myotubes and cardiac/vascular cells, respectively), which is an equally important end point, as well as their long-term survival have often been underlooked. For example, in a recent study follow-up of myoblasts injected through an endoventricular catheter was limited to 10 days. Likewise, there are also limited data regarding the functional efficacy of these techniques and only found one experimental study in which the effects of transen docardially injected bone marrow cells were extensively investigated. Clearly, there is still much work to be done in this area, particularly for comparing the results of percutaneous cell delivery with that of the surgical approach, which remains the benchmark against which alternate modes of cell transplantation should be tested. This remark does not only apply to percutaneous approaches but also to biografts made of bioresorbable cell-seeded scaffolds, which could represent an effective means of repairing wall defects in adult and pediatric open-heart operations.

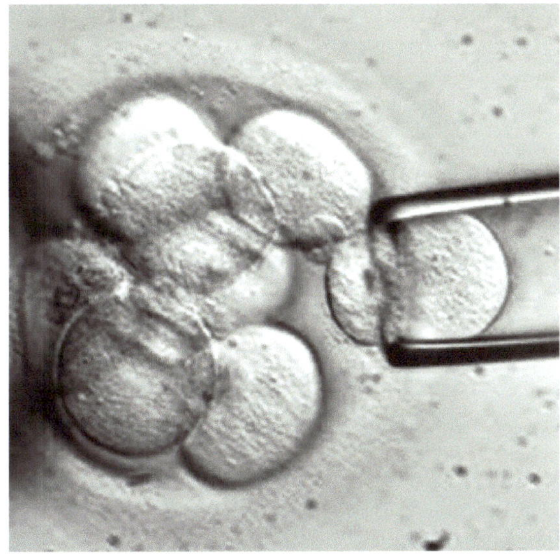

Fig. 31.2: *Histopahthological photograph showing hematopoietic stem cell ready for transplantation.*

The Problem of Cell Death

Regardless of the route of delivery, cell death remains a major problem of cell transplantation common to all cell lineages. Thus, up to 90% of transplanted cardiomyocytes have been shown to die within the first 24 hours. The mechanisms of this high death rate are multiple and include particularly physical strain during injections, ischemia due to the poor vascularity of the target scar, and apoptosis. As it is uncertain whether multiplication of surviving cells can catch up to this initially high attrition rate, the development of cell survival-enhancing strategies appears critical for optimizing the functional benefits of the procedure. Two of them are of potentially great clinical relevance. The first consists of enhancing angiogenesis to limit the ischemic component of cell death, an approach based on the observation that the survival of cardiomyocytes grafted into highly vascularized granulation tissue is two-fold greater than that observed after grafting into acutely necrotic myocardium. In practice, increased angiogenesis can be achieved by pretransplantation transfection of cells with genes encoding vascular growth factors, direct co injection of these factors or concomitant revascularization of cell-transplanted segments (an approach which appears sound but only be confirmed when efficacy is demonstrated by ongoing randomized trials committed to avoiding bypass surgery in these segments to avoid confounding factors in the interpretation of outcome measures). The second strategy aimed at increasing the survival rate of transplanted cells relies on limitation of apoptosis, which can be successfully achieved by heat shocking cells just prior to their implantation. Finally, it is also likely that even though an immune response is unlikely to occur in the case of autologous transplantation, the inflammatory state created by needle punctures can contribute to cell damage. This mechanism is expected to be still greater if it superimposes upon the inflammation that occurs during the early phase of infarction. Conversely, late injections may equally reduce the effectiveness of the procedure if they are performed once the remodeling process has been completed. These observations suggest that there is probably an optimal time window for cell transplantation following myocardial infarction and that bracketing this time frame is another means of optimizing the benefits of the procedure.

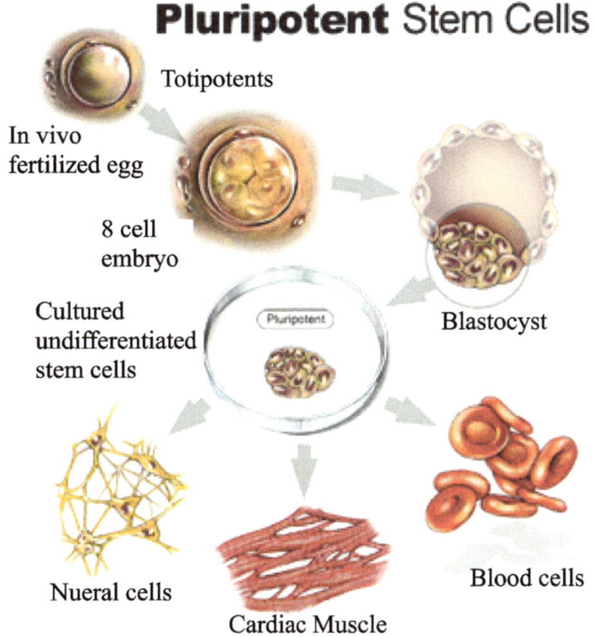

Fig. 31.3: *Diagrammatic representation of morphology of a pluripotent stem cell .*

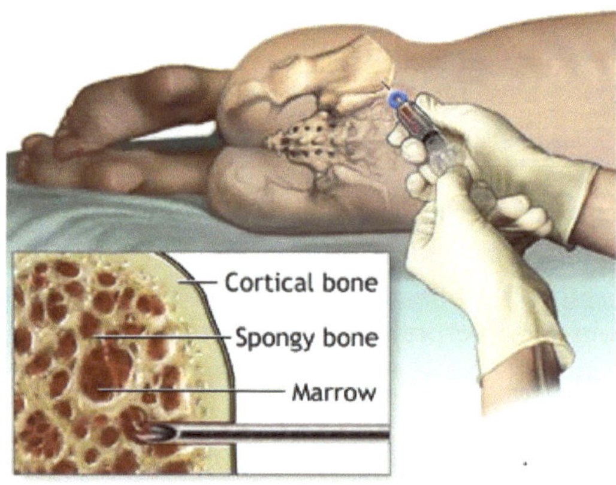

Fig. 31.4:*Technique of bone marrow aspiration. A small amount of bone marrow is removed during a bone marrow aspiration. The procedure is quick but uncomfortable, and is generally well-tolerated by both children and adults. The marrow can be studied to determine the cause of anemia, the presence of leukemia or other malignancies, or the presence of some "storage diseases," in which abnormal metabolic products are stored in certain bone marrow cells.*

Bone Marrow-Derived Cells

The number of clinical studies of bone-marrow cell transplantation is growing tremendously, with some of them being reported in peer-reviewed journals while others are limited to isolated and anectodal cases agressively announced through Internet-mediatedpress releases. So far, surgical approaches have entailed intramyocardial implantation of bone marrow mononuclear cells or CD 133 + progenitors at the time of concomitant coronary artery bypass grafting whereas catheter-based approaches have consisted of intracoronary injections of mononuclear cells coupled with balloon angioplasty and stenting in patients with acute myocardial infarction or endoventricular stand alone injections in ischemic patients targeted for increased angiogenesis. Overall, these phase I studies should be credited for documenting the feasibility of the procedure, the apparent lack of adverse events, and the similarity of results with both blood-derived and bone marrow-derived cells.

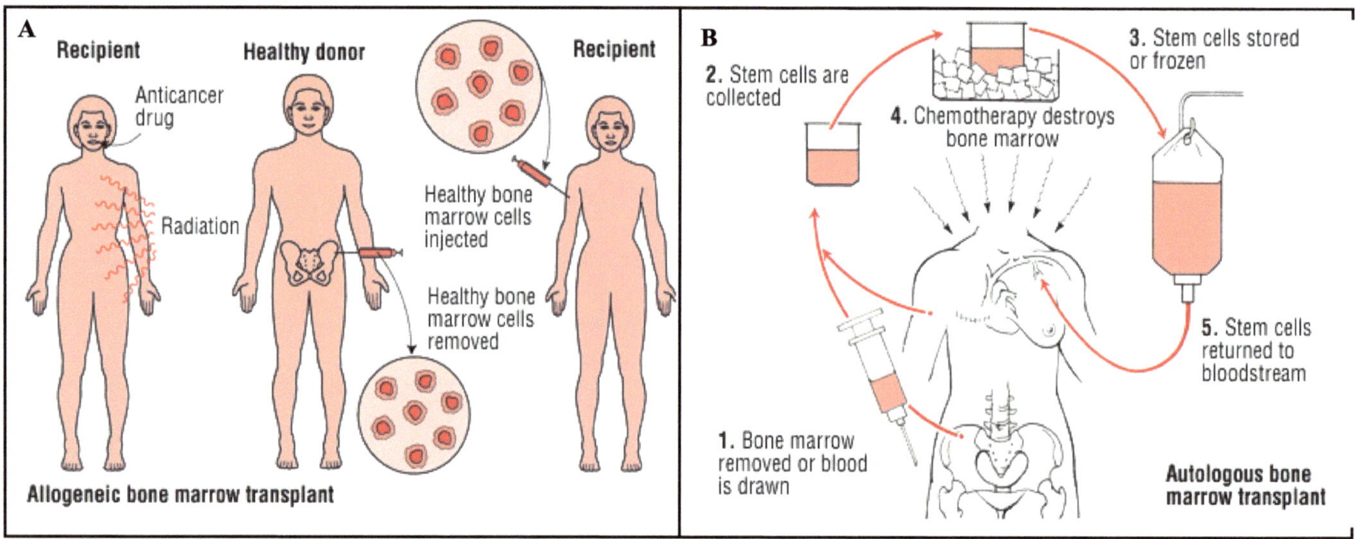

Fig 31.5: *Illustrations (A) Showing allogeneic bone marrow transplant (B)Showing autologous bone marrow transplant*

The claims for efficacy, based on improved perfusion and function, are more questionable in the absence of control randomized groups of patients, particularly if one keeps in mind the powerful placebo effect seen in end-stage ischemic heart disease-a remark equally relevant to the previously mentioned trials of skeletal myoblast transplantation. Hopefully, a forthcoming phase II trial involving intracoronary injections of bone marrow (fresh or briefly cultivated) or placebo solution in patients withacute myocardial infarction should allow more objective assessment of the expected benefits of this modality of cell therapy. preparation, stem cells can be transplanted by cardiologists. Via a special balloon catheter, stem cells are injected into the coronary artery supplying the infarcted zone. There, they ideally develop to new heart muscle cells and regenerate heart muscle functionality by reducing the area of the infarcted zone

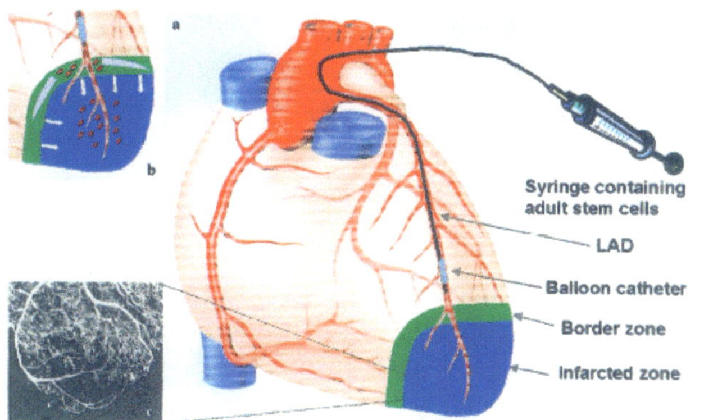

Fig. 31.6 *Cardiac Stem Cell Therapy After a patient has obtained standard cardiac therapy (e.g. balloon dilatation of occluded coronary arteries, stent implantation), harvesting and transplantation of stem cells is carried out in the following way : During the days after the infarct, the patient obtains medication causing stem cells to be flushed out into the bloodstream.Blood tests are made and examined every day. If they indicate that the peak of stem cells in the blood is reached (after about 4-6 days), stem cells will be harvested.Stem cells are "filtered out" from the patient's blood by special dialysis equipment and then prepared by molecular biologists of the Blood Center. After approximately 5 hours of filtering and*

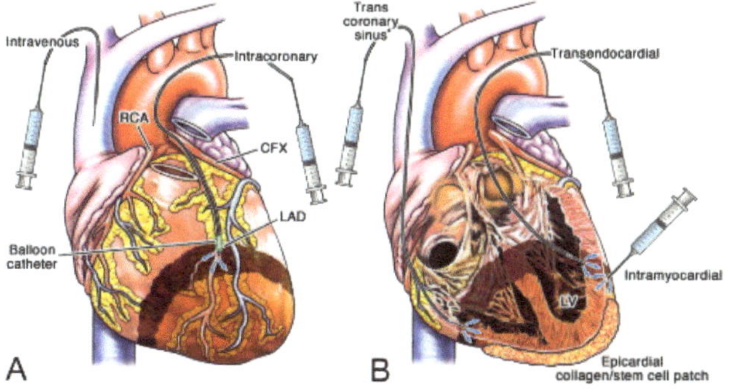

Fig.31.7: *Various Transplantation Methods in Heart Disease (A) Intracoronary and (B) intramyocardial transplantation methods in heart disease. Depicted are clinically used methods for vascular and myocardial cell delivery in cardiac intervention and cardiac surgery. CFX = circumflex artery; LAD = left anterior descending artery; LV = left ventricle; RCA = right coronary artery*

The recent observation that the majority of endothelialprogenitor cells are derived from the monocyte/macrophage pathway also makes it clinically relevant to. know whether injection of these cells, alone or as part of the mononuclear cell mix, carries a specific risk related to the recognized role of macrophages in atherosclerotic plaque instability and rupture. Cellular transplantation appears as a promising means of 'rejuvenating" infarcted myocardium through the engraftment of cells that may positively affect heart function by various mechanisms involving elastic, contractile, and paracrine effects. Although still scarce, laboratory investigations also suggest that the regenerating capacity of the transplanted cells could also be relevant to nonischemic cardiomyopathies, thereby contributing to expanding the potential for cell replacement therapy. As mentioned in this review, several basic issues remain to be addressed to better characterize the optimal cell type, define the most effective mode and timing of cell delivery, optimize graft survival and understand the mechanism(s) of action of the donor cells. In parallel, the initial encouraging efficacy data collected in a still limited number of patients need to be validated by large prospective randomized trials complying with the stringent methodologic rules commonly applied to drug trials. Only such an approach will conclusively establishwhether the hopes currently raised by cellular transplantation are met, to what extent the cell-related regeneration process affects patient function and clinical outcome and, consequently, the place this novel strategy may occupy within the armamentarium of techniques designed to treat heart failure.

Three important clinical studies have been published. One entailed surgical implantation of skeletal myoblasts and reported improved functional outcomes without adverse events but

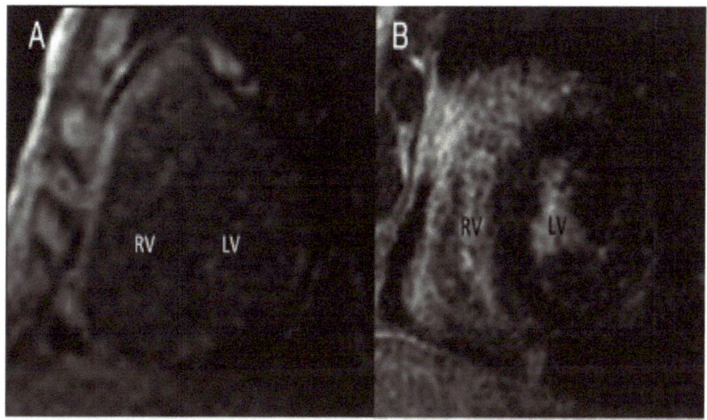

Fig. 31.8: *A, Baseline midventricular short axis magnetic resonance imaging (MRI) obtained 10 minutes after administration of intravenous gadolinium shows diffusely abnormal nulling of the myocardium with a characteristic dark blood pool, consistent with cardiac amyloidosis. B, Three years after stem cell transplant, postgadolinium midventricular short axis MRI image shows normal nulling of the myocardium with faint patchy areas of residual delayed enhancement. RV indicates right ventricle; LV, left ventricle.*

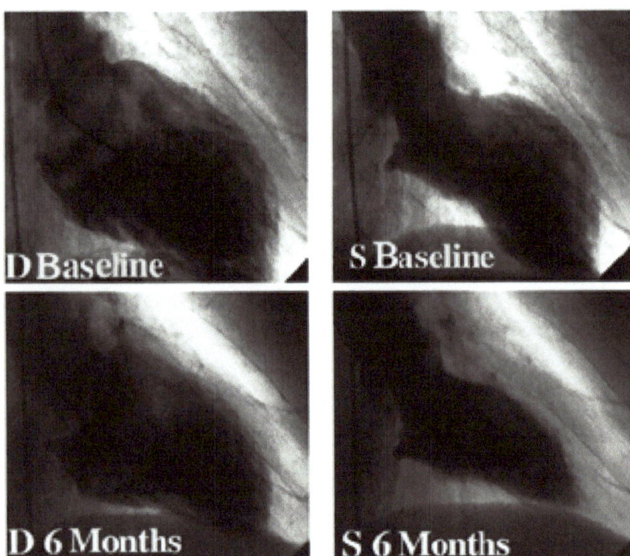

Fig.31.9: *Ventriculography at baseline (akinesia in anterior region) and after 6 months (with clear improvement in contractility of anterior region) for patient D indicates diastole; S, systole*

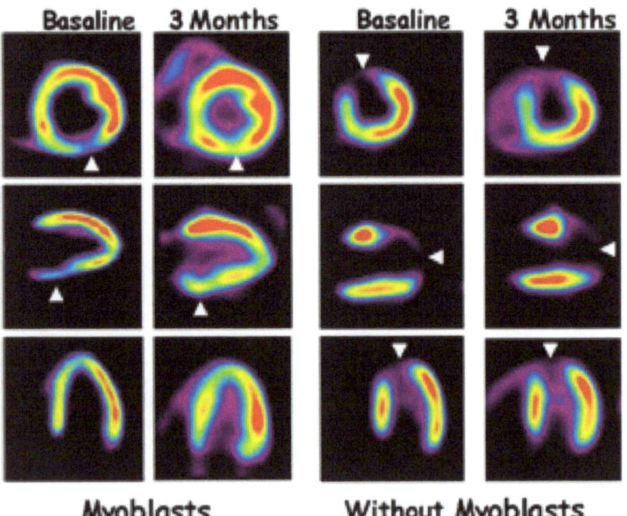

Fig.31.10: *F-18-fluorodeoxyglucose (FDG) positron emission tomography (PET) imaging. The left-hand panel corresponds to the PET image in a post-myocardial infarction patient. The arrowheads point to a deficit of FDG uptake that would indicate an image of necrosis. At 3 months after revascularization surgery and autologous myoblasts implantation, a highly significant improvement in FDG uptake can be seen which would indicate greater viability. The right-hand panel corresponds to a patient who underwent revascularization surgery without cell transplantation and in whom improved tissue viability cannot be seen.*

interpretation of the data is confounded by the fact that the cell-transplanted segments were also concomitantly revascularized. Two other studies have looked at the effects of bone marrow derived mononuclear or mesenchymal stem cells injected directly into the coronary arteries shortly after myocardial infarction. The strength of these two trials is that they have been randomized although only the latter included a placebo-controlled group. Both have reported improvement in function and perfusion, thereby supporting the concept that these cell types may be beneficial in acutely infarcted patients undergoing concomitant revascularization of the culprit vessel. Their conclusions, however, still require validation by additional, larger-scale placebo-controlled, double-blind randomized trials.

Section 11 Gene Therapy for Cardiovascular Disease

The field of cardiovascular gene transfer has developed rapidly during the past 5 years. Important advances have been made in vector development, in vivo gene delivery, and definition of potential therapeutic targets. Despite substantial progress, a number of technical issues need to be addressed before gene therapy is applied safely and broadly to cardiovascular diseases. In this review, major advances in cardiovascular gene transfer are summarized. In addition, technical issues required for translation of preclinical studies of gene transfer into clinical protocols are discussed.

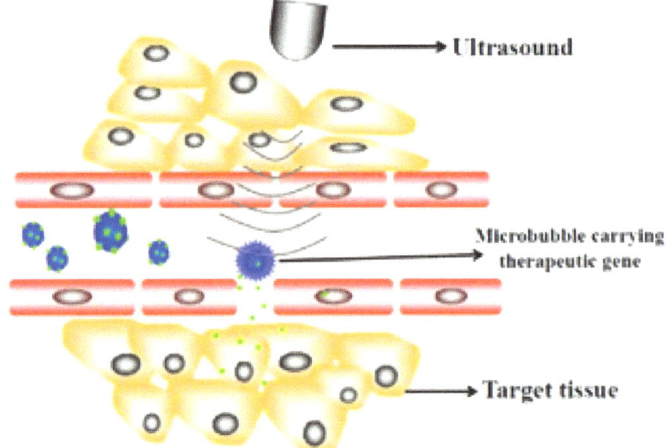

Fig. 31.11: *Schematic diagram of gene therapy mediated by UTMD. Microbubbles carrying therapeutic gene are destroyed at the site of the target tissue, resulting in sonoporation and delivery of the drug directly to the target cell. The process of sonoporation induced by US application leads to transiently holes in cell membrane and capillary, which facilitates the uptake of therapeutic gene.*

Advances in recombinant DNA technology, including gene transfer, have stimulated hope that this technology can be used to improve the practice of cardiovascular medicine. Applications of this technology that affect the clinical management of patients include the development of new therapeutic products, engineered by the overexpression of genes, such as recombinant tissue-type plasminogen activator. Recombinant DNA technology has also provided techniques that have been used to create animal models of cardiovascular diseases. These models permit definition of the role of specific gene products in the pathogenesis of cardiovascular diseases. Characterization of its molecular basis has led to a more precise definition of diseases and the potential for relevant clinical treatments. The development of molecular genetic interventions to treat cardiovascular diseases depends on technical advances in the development of methods of gene delivery; achievement of long-term, highly efficient, and targeted expression to relevant cells of the cardiovascular system; and design of vectors that are safe for long-term human administration

Methods of Gene Delivery

The transduction and expression of genes in appropriate cell types represent important steps in the development of gene therapy. Therefore, investigations have focused on the development of methods to deliver and express genes in vascular cells and cardiac myocytes. Viral vectors (retroviruses and adenoviruses), viral conjugate vectors (adenovirus-augmented receptor-mediated vectors and hemagglutinating virus of Japan [HVJ] liposomes), and nonviral vectors (cationic liposomes, polymers, and injection of plasmid DNA) have been used. To optimize gene delivery to target cells, characteristics of the cell must be considered, such as proliferative capacity and location within the target tissue. Vascular cells (endothelial and smooth muscle cells) and cardiac myocytes differ particularly in proliferation features, and therefore different strategies have been used to transduce these cells.

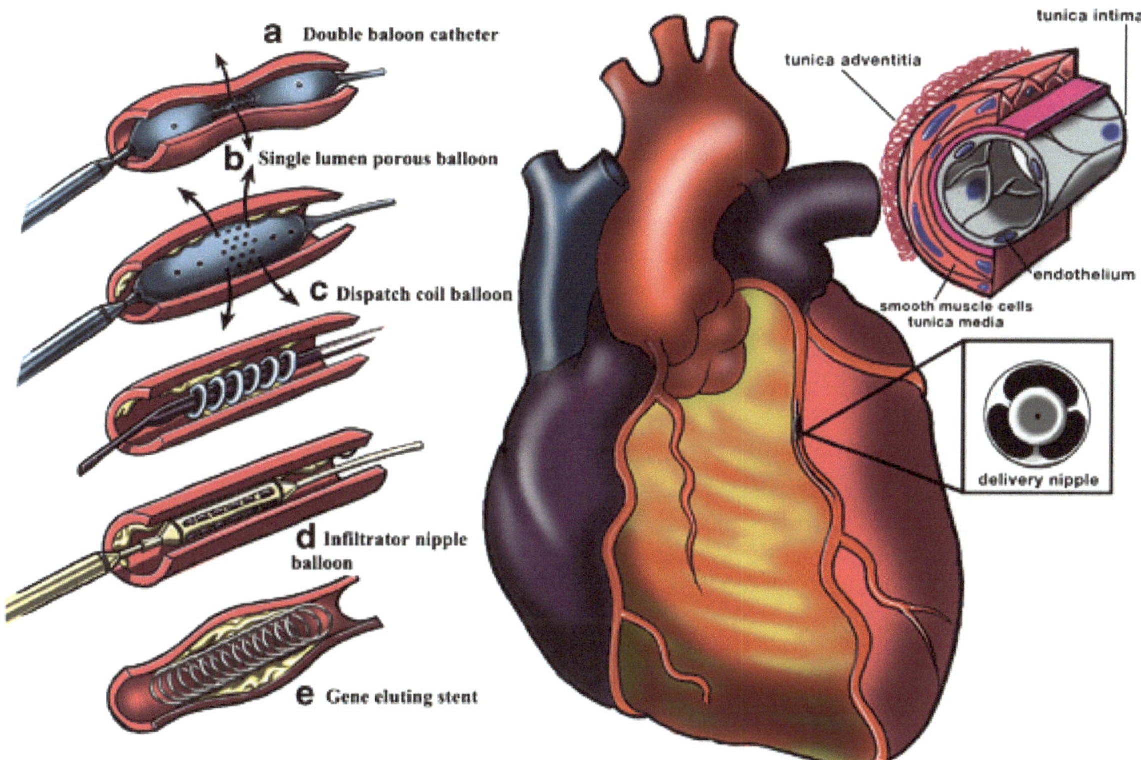

Fig. 31.12: *showing different catheters and stent for transvascular intracoronary wall gene delivery.*

Vascular Cells

Retroviral Vectors

Because vascular cells are accessible through the blood stream, percutaneous, site-specific gene delivery was developed for local arterial segments. Retroviral vectors were initially used in in vivo vascular gene transfer studies. Interest in retrovirus-mediated gene transfer was based on the use of these vectors in gene transfer to other organ systems, including bone marrow stem cells,liver,and the skin, where in some target cells, these vectors transduce a large proportion of target cells. In the case of retroviral vectors, the viral vector stably integrates into chromosomal DNA of the target cell, resulting in potentially stable gene expression, although integration into chromosomal DNA could potentially result in insertional mutagenesis.These vectors are most appropriate for ex vivo gene transfer for cardiovascular disease,which involves removal of the relevant target cells, i.e, endothelial cells or hepatocytes from the host, transfection of the cells in vitro, and subsequent reintroduction of the modified cells into the animal or patient. It is unknown whether stable high-level gene expression in vivo will be achieved with retrovirally transduced cells.

Several features of retroviral gene transfer may limit its application to cardiovascular medicine, particularly with respect to direct in vivo gene therapy. Replication of target cells is necessary for proviral integration. Recent studies suggest that viral integration may depend on mitosis, not just DNA synthesis. Successful retrovirus-mediated gene transfer to vascular cells may require induction of proliferation in target endothelial or smooth muscle cells, at least for short periods of time. In uninjured arteries, endothelial and smooth muscle cell proliferation occurs slowly, and therefore retroviral integration would occur at a low frequency. After vascular injury or stimulation, such as with a balloon catheter, injured vascular cells may be transduced at higher rates. Previous studies have suggested that retroviral transduction of vascular cells can be used successfully in vivo. Limitations of this gene delivery vector include its low frequency of gene transfer and the relative lability of retroviral particles compared with other viruses. Retroviral particles are rapidly inactivated in vivo in primates, presumably by the presence of complement in serum.Because of the instability of retroviral particles and the inability of retroviruses to integrate in nonreplicating cells, retroviral vectors may have limited use for direct gene transfer in vivo, although there may be a role for these vectors for ex vivo gene transfer to vascular stents or prosthetic grafts.

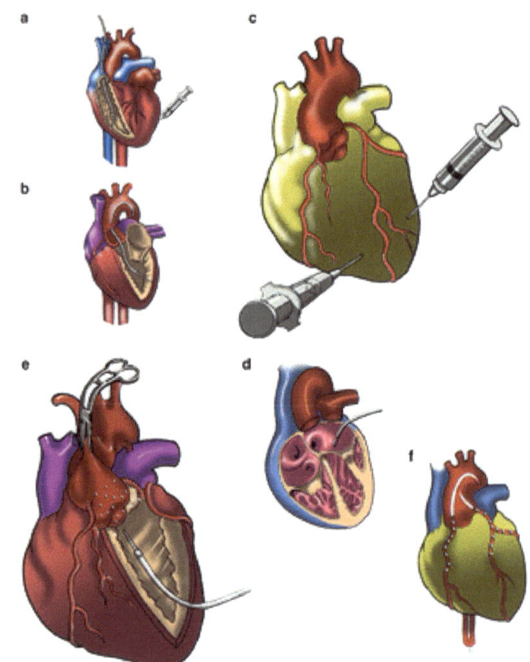

Fig.31.13: *Direct and transvascular techniques of gene delivery. (a) Intramyocardial injection via the intracavitary catheter in right ventricle. (b) Intramyocardial injection via the intracavitary catheter in left ventricle. (c) Intramyocardial injection via the syringe. (d) Transvascular intracavitary delivery. (e) Transvascular nonselective intracoronary delivery with aortic cross-clamping. (f) Transvascular selective antegrade intracoronary delivery.*

Table 31.1: *Key features of gene therapy and viral vectors.*

Viral vectors	Integration	Long-term gene expression	Immune response	Comments
Adenovirus	–	–	+	Broad tropism, easy to produce high titre stocks, widely characterised in vivo
Adeno-associated virus (AAV)	+	+	–	Limited cloning capacity, nonpathogenic, integrate randomly in the absence of the *rep* gene
Lentivirus	+	+	–	Retrovirus-derived, pseudotyping with heterologous coat proteins improves biosafety
Retrovirus	+	+	–	Only infects dividing cells

Adenoviral Vectors

To improve the frequency of direct gene transfer into arteries, recent investigations have focused on adenoviral vectors. The adenovirus genome is composed of linear, double-stranded DNA of approximately 36 kb in length. The gene products are organized into early (E1-E4) and late (L1-L5) regions, based on expression before or after initiation of DNA replication. Expression of viral genes depends on cellular transcription factors and expression of the adenoviral E1 region, which encodes a transactivator of viral gene expression. The E3 region encodes viral proteins that regulate immuno surveillance in vivo. Adenoviruses have a lytic life cycle, characterized by attachment to an adenoviral glycoprotein receptor on mammalian cells and cell entry by receptor-mediated endocytosis. Adenoviruses escape degradation in lysosomes due to adenoviral capsid proteins, and viral DNA is transported to the nucleus. In the nucleus, adenoviral genome persists in an unintegrated form. During the lytic infection, viral genome replicates to several thousand copies per cell.

Adenovirus serotypes 2 (Ad-2) and 5 (Ad-5) have been developed as viral vectors for gene transfer the *E1A* and *E1B* genes from the viral genome. Vectors are produced by homologous recombination in 293 cells or any cell line that contains an integrated copy of the adenoviral *E1* gene. A foreign cDNA with eukaryotic regulatory sequences is introduced into a bacterial plasmid containing a region of the left adenoviral genome that is deleted of the *E1* gene. This plasmid is cotransfected into 293 cells with an incomplete adenoviral genome. Homologous recombination between the two DNAs generates a recombinant genome in which the *E1* gene is replaced by the foreign DNA. Viral stock is propagated in 293 cells to high titer, approximately 10 to 10 particles per milliliter.

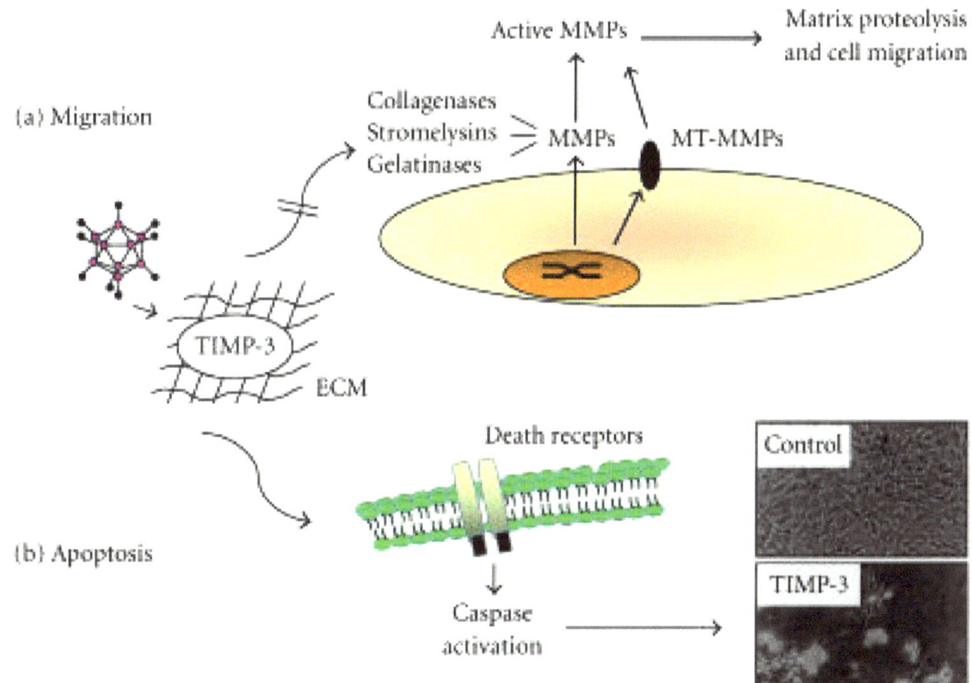

Fig. 31.14: *Gene therapy by overexpression of TIMP-3. Following Ad-mediated gene delivery to vascular smooth muscle cells, TIMP-3 is secreted and is found located with the extracellular matrix (ECM). From here, TIMP-3 is available to exert two distinctly different phenotypes through its metalloproteinase inhibitory effects. (a) Matrix metalloproteinases (MMPs, including collagenases, stromelysins, gelatinases, and membrane-type metalloproteinases [MT-MMPs]) are upregulated following vascular injury. TIMPs, through their native MMP inhibitory activity, are able to bind to and retard pro-MMP-to-active enzyme conversion and combined with the ability to block active MMP activity, matrix proteolysis and hence cell migration is inhibited [45]. (b) TIMP-3, uniquely amongst the TIMP family, is also able to promote smooth muscle cell death through death receptor-induced caspase activation and induction of apoptosis [46]. Micrographs courtesy of Mark Bond, Bristol Heart Institute, UK.*

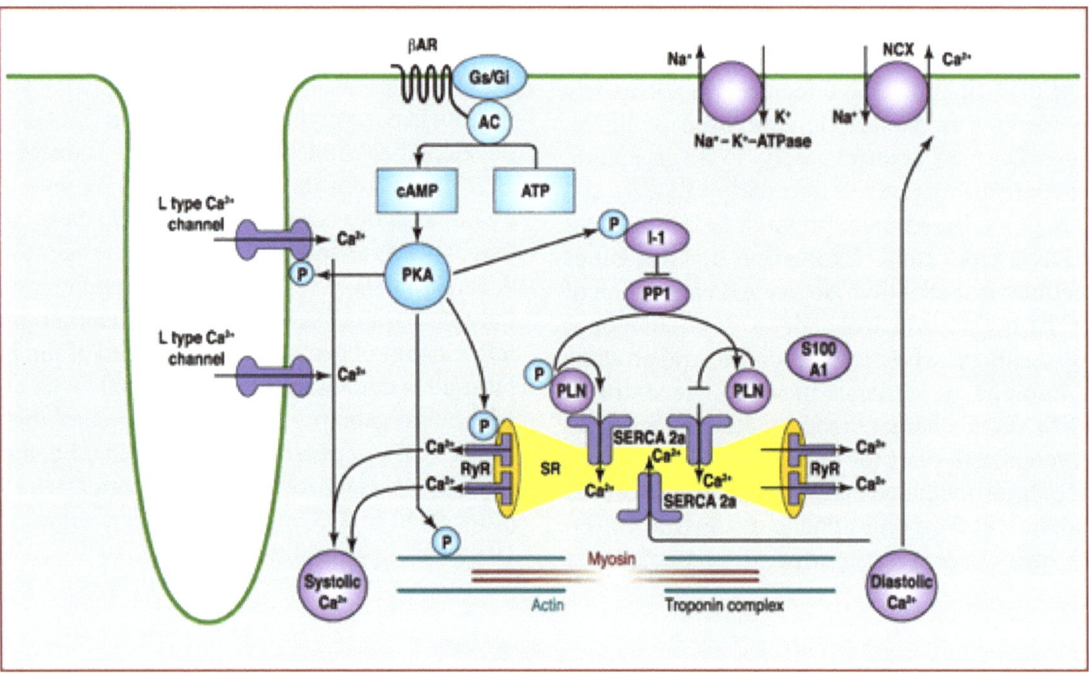

Fig.31.15:*Excitation-contraction signaling in cardiomyocytes with emphasis on targets for gene therapy. Interplay between calcium handling (purple) and ?-adrenergic (blue) systems is illustrated. AC : adenylyl cyclase; ATP : adenosine triphosphate; ?-AR : beta adrenergic receptor; I-1 : (protein phosphatase) inhibitor-1; cAMP : cyclic adenosine monophosphate; Gs : stimulatory G protein; Gi : inhibitory G protein; NCX : sarcolemnal sodium/calcium exchanger; PKA : protein kinase A; PLN : phospholamban; PP : protein phosphatase; RyR : ryanodine receptor; SERCA : sarcoplasmic/endoplasmic reticulum calcium ATPase; SR : sarcoplasmic reticulum*

Adenoviruses effectively infect mammalian cells, including nondividing cells in vitro and in vivo. Physiological levels of recombinant proteins have been secreted into the circulation after adenoviral infection of skeletal muscle.The virus particle is relatively stable and amenable to purification and concentration at a high titer. Integration of adenoviral DNA sequences into chromosomal DNA of the target cell occurs at a low frequency, and adenoviral DNA is maintained in an extrachromosomal form. Extrachromosomal replication of the vector reduces the likelihood of mutation by random integration and dysregulation of cellular genes.

Despite these advantages, there are limitations to current, or “first-generation,” adenoviral vectors. In most models, gene expression is transient after adenoviral infection, generally less than 3 weeks, and inflammation is observed in organs expressing the transgene. Gene expression in vascular cells is transient as well, usually persisting for only several weeks. Although transient gene expression may be well suited to vascular therapies requiring expression of a gene product over a short period of time, development of an immune response to adenoviral proteins is a major limitation to the use of these vectors. Recent studies in genetically defined strains of mice have demonstrated that viral proteins, expressed from the E1-deleted adenoviral genome, are presented as foreign antigens and lead to the generation of cytolytic T lymphocytes that destroy adenovirus-infected cells.Insertion of a temperature-sensitive mutation within the E2A region of E1-deleted adenoviral vectors results in lack of expression of late viral gene products at nonpermissive temperatures, resulting in prolonged gene expression (e”70 days) and blunted cytolytic T-cell infiltration in mouse liver. In arterial gene transfer studies using first-generation adenoviral vectors, mononuclear cell infiltrates have been occasionally observed in the adventitia of peripheral26 and pulmonary arteries of pigs, but medial and intimal inflammation, necrosis, and aneurysm formation have not been observed. Further studies are required to examine the use of first-generation adenoviral vectors for vascular gene transfer studies. It is likely that further modifications in these vectors, including deletions in the E2 and E4 regions and modifications in the E3 region, will diminish host immune responses.

Adenovirus-Augmented, Receptor-Mediated Gene Delivery

Viral vector conjugate systems may have application in vascular gene therapy and include adenovirus-augmented, receptor-mediated gene delivery. This vector uses inactivated adenovirus complexed to a receptor ligand to facilitate entry of DNA to a cell.This vector consists of two components. DNA condenses with polylysine, which in turn is bound to inactivated virus.The virus is coupled to a ligand such as transferrin. The transferrin ligand binds to a transferrin receptor in a cell, and the transferrin viral polylysine DNA complex enters the cell by receptor-mediated endocytosis. The inactivated adenovirus functions to disrupt lysosomes in the host cell, reducing DNA degradation and releasing DNA into the cytoplasm. The use of these vectors for vascular gene transfer is being investigated.

Cationic Liposomes

Most nonviral methods of gene transfer rely on normal mechanisms used by cells for the uptake and cellular transport of macromolecules. These methods rely on receptor-mediated endocytotic pathways or fusion of cell membranes. One example is cationic liposomes, which are positively charged artificial lipid vesicles that incorporate negatively charged DNA and deliver nucleic acid to cells through fusion with cell membranes or receptor-mediated endocytosis. Plasmid DNA is released in the cytoplasm and transported to the nucleus where it is maintained in an unintegrated form. Cationic liposomes interact spontaneously and rapidly with polyanions, such as DNA and mRNA, to form liposome complexes. Cationic liposome reagents used in vascular gene transfer studies include DOTMA/DOPE (Lipofectin), DC-cholesterol, DOSPA/DOPE (Lipofectamine), and DMRIE/DOPE. Expression of recombinant genes in vivo after liposomal transfection has been reported in rats, rabbits, dogs, and pigs . Cationic liposomes produce more efficient gene delivery compared with neutrally charged or anionic liposomes,but current formulations, including DOSPA/DOPE, are less efficient than adenoviral vectors. Further modifications in plasmids and chemical formulations of liposomes appear to have promise in improving transfection efficiency. Cationic liposomes have a favorable safety profile for in vivo administration. Liposome vectors contain no viral sequences, and there are no cDNA size constraints in vector construction. In addition, this vector is straightforward to prepare for clinical use. Cell division is not required for liposome transfection, although the efficiency appears to be increased in proliferating cells.

HVJ Liposome Conjugates

Recent studies suggest that complexing inactivated HVJ with liposomes improves transfection efficiencies of vascular smooth muscle cells in in vitro and in vivo models of vascular injury, including the injured rat carotid artery. These vectors have also been successfully used for hepatic and renal in vivo gene transfer. It is likely that further modifications to vectors used for vascular gene transfer will include components of viral and nonviral vectors that optimize delivery, improve gene expression, and minimize toxic side effects.

Polymers

Additional strategies for the local delivery of therapeutic agents include impregnating oligonucleotides into polymer gels and applying the polymer to the external surfaces of arteries.Although pharmacokinetics of oligonucleotide delivery and retention have not been precisely defined, the data suggest that there is sufficient retention of oligonucleotide to inhibit c-*myb* and PCNA RNA expression within 24 hours after balloon injury and inhibit intimal thickening after 2 weeks. Plasmid DNA and adenoviral vectors have been applied directly to polyethylene balloons coated with a hydrogel polymer. Although there is some loss of plasmid DNA from the balloon during transit through the circulation, DNA is distributed transmurally after inflation of the balloon. Modifications in polymers to provide slow release of therapeutic agents hold promise for site-specific delivery of oligonucleotides and vectors to arterial segments.

Myocyte Gene Transfer

Dissection of molecular mechanisms governing myocardial differentiation has been performed in neonatal cardiac myocytes in culture, in part because these cells are relatively amenable to gene transfer with plasmid-based transfections. Recombinant gene expression in adult myocardium in vivo requires an expression vector with high-level activity in adult cardiac myocytes and a method for introducing this vector into myocardial cells.

Because cardiac myocytes are terminally differentiated cells, they require a vector that is not dependent on cell replication for delivery and expression. The analysis of foreign genes within intact adult myocardium has been performed by direct injection of plasmid DNA. Although direct injection of genes is a simple procedure and permits examination of the behavior of genes in vivo, this technique is limited by transfection of a small number of cells within several millimeters around the injection site. Expression of recombinant genes is temporally limited as well, with expression peaking within several weeks and declining rapidly thereafter. Episomal persistence of the introduced DNA and the postmitotic state of adult cardiac myocytes, which prevent integration of genes into chromosomes, limit stability of the transgene.

Table 31.2: *Gene therapy strategies for the treatment of cardiovascular diseases.*

Disease	Therapeutic approach	Target
Atherosclerosis	Antiatherogenic	LCAT, apoAI, apoE mRNA
Vein graft failure, ischaemia, thrombosis	Diffusable/secreted gene products	VEGF, FGF, eNOS, antithrombotic agents, SOD, heme oxygenase
Vein graft failure	Inhibitors of smooth muscle cell migration/proliferation	p53, TIMPs, Rb, p21
Thrombosis	Prevention of thrombus formation	TFPI, tPA
Restenosis	Suicide genes	Tk
Hypertension	Antisense oligonucleotides	Angiotensinogen, AT_1 receptor, ACE
Vein graft failure	Decoys	Soluble VCAM, E2F
Hypertension	Reduction in blood pressure	Kallikrein, ANP, eNOS, endothelin

Some limitations of in vivo plasmid DNA injection have been addressed by adenoviral vectors. Adenoviruses effectively infect nonreplicating mammalian cells, including skeletal and cardiac myotubes. These viruses are grown and purified in high titer. These properties result in highly efficient gene transfer into adult cardiac myocytes in vitroand in vivo. Quantitative comparisons of chloramphenicol acetyl transferase (CAT) activity resulting from injection of a CAT plasmid or an adenoviral vector encoding CAT revealed that the amount of CAT activity resulting from adenovirus infection was 10 to 100 fold higher compared with plasmid DNA. Similar findings were observed comparing adenoviral vectors and plasmids encoding *lacZ*. Although adenoviral vectors produce efficient gene transfer into the myocardium, expression is transient, peaking at 1 to 2 weeks. Acute inflammatory responses have been observed in hearts injected with adenovirus,although inflammation along the injection path has also been noted after injection of plasmid DNA. Further investigations will identify factors that account for the transient nature of gene expression and will characterize potential proinflammatory effects of this vector

Animal Models of Gene Transfer

Vascular Gene Transfer

In the past 5 years, there has been great interest in expressing recombinant DNA and other nucleic acids in blood vessels in vivo. The goals of these studies have been to define gene function and to develop new therapeutic strategies for vascular diseases. The feasibility of direct gene transfer to arteries in vivo was demonstrated using viral (retrovirus) and nonviral (liposomes) vectors in several animal species, including pigs, rabbits, and dogs. These studies reported a low efficiency of gene transfer, generally 1% or less of vascular cells in vivo. More recent studies have suggested that the efficiency of gene transfer into arteries can be improved with adenoviral vectors; increased expression of reporter genes has been reported in sheep, rat, rabbit, and pig vessels. Endothelial cells of normal arteries and endothelial and smooth muscle cells in injured arteries have been transduced at efficiencies approximately 10 to 100 fold higher than reported for retroviral and liposome vectors. A major limitation to adenoviral gene transfer in the vasculature has been transient expression; in most studies, expression of reporter gene has been observed for 7 to 14 days and is diminished or lost by 28 days. Lack of persistence of gene expression may result from cytolytic responses directed against infected cells. Transient gene expression, however, may be desirable for vascular diseases, like restenosis after angioplasty, which are characterized by cellular proliferation peaking in the first several weeks after arterial injury. Several observations concerning the delivery of recombinant genes and patterns of gene expression can be drawn from these studies. Infusion of vector into normal arteries with an intact endothelium results in transfection of intimal cells (primarily endothelial cells). Injury to the vessel and/or application of pressure to the vector infusate results in delivery of DNA transmurally and gene expression in the media.Several catheters have been used in gene transfer studies, including double-balloon catheters, porous balloon catheters, and hydrogel catheters, and the patterns of gene expression within an artery may differ depending on the design of the catheter, animal species, and type of artery transduced. Direct gene transfer has been used to create somatic transgene models to define gene function in arteries. In this system, genes can be expressed within arterial segments, and their biological function can be investigated. This approach has proved useful for investigation of genes whose direct in vivo effects have been difficult to analyze. For example, transfection of a recombinant angiotensin-converting enzyme gene into rat arteries using HVJ liposomes promotes angiotensin II–mediated vascular hypertrophy. After transfer of a recombinant endothelial cell–type nitric oxide (NO) synthase (ec-NOS) gene into balloon-injured rat carotid arteries, NO production was associated with a reduction in intimal thickening.Gene transfer approaches have also proved useful in the analysis of atrial natriuretic peptide, type 2 angiotensin II receptor, and VCAM-1.

Growth factors and cytokines stimulate vascular cell proliferation and vessel formation in vivo. Although the genes encoding many factors have been cloned and their mechanism of action defined in vitro, definition of their role in vivo has been more difficult to analyze. Several recombinant growth factor genes, including platelet-derived growth factor–B (PDGF-B), a secreted form of acidic fibroblast growth factor (FGF-1), and an active form of transforming growth factor–²1 (TGF-²1) have been expressed by direct gene transfer in porcine arteries, and the function of these gene products has been analyzed. Expression of a PDGF-B gene in porcine arteries stimulated intimal hyperplasia characterized by smooth muscle cell proliferation. Synthesis and secretion of FGF-1 were associated with expansion of the intima as well as intimal angiogenesis. Arteries transfected with a TGF-²1 gene demonstrated increased procollagen synthesis in the intima and media as early as 4 days after gene transfer compared with control arteries transfected with a reporter gene. Although these recombinant genes stimulate vascular cell proliferation in vivo, they exert otherwise distinct effects on smooth muscle cell proliferation, angiogenesis, and extracellular matrix formation. These studies suggest that intimal thickening may represent a common response to gene expression of multiple growth factors, which in turn exert different effects on vessel repair.

Another approach to investigating the pathogenesis of vascular cell proliferation in vivo is to examine gene products that inhibit cell proliferation. Local delivery of an antiproliferative agent during the peak of smooth muscle cell proliferation or extracellular matrix synthesis after balloon injury might limit expansion of the intima. Several approaches have been explored in this setting, including recombinant chimeric toxins, antisense oligonucleotide strategies,and gene transfer.

One approach to the selective elimination of dividing cells is to express a herpes virus thymidine kinase (HSV-tk) gene in smooth muscle cells after balloon injury. Thymidine kinase, when expressed in transduced cells, converts ganciclovir, a nucleoside analogue, into an active toxic form, and subsequent incorporation of phosphorylated ganciclovir into cellular DNA induces chain termination in dividing cells, causing cell death. A bystander effect, demonstrated in smooth muscle and endothelial cells, confers susceptibility to ganciclovir in neighboring dividing cells, leading to inhibition of cell growth in nontransduced neighboring cells as well. Adenoviral vectors encoding a HSV-tk gene or no cDNA insert were introduced into porcine arteries immediately after balloon injury, and a course of ganciclovir or saline was initiated. Three weeks after balloon injury and adenoviral infection, a significant reduction in intima-to-media area ratios (54% to 59%) was observed. A reduction in intimal BrdC (5-bromo-deoxycytosine) incorporation of 40% was observed in HSV-tk ganciclovir-treated animals compared with HSV-tk saline-treated animals 7 days after gene transfer, indicating that inhibition of smooth muscle cell proliferation contributed to this effect. A significant reduction in intima-to-media area ratios in the HSV-tk ganciclovir-treated animals was observed 6 weeks after treatment, suggesting that the decrease in intimal hyperplasia was stable. In addition, no major systemic toxicities were observed associated with adenoviral infection and ganciclovir treatment. These data suggest that expression of an enzyme that catalyzes the formation of a cytotoxic drug locally within an artery may limit smooth muscle cell proliferation after balloon injury.

In balloon-injured rat carotid arteries, introduction of adenoviral vectors encoding HSV-tk immediately after balloon injury or 7 days later and treatment with ganciclovir also result in significant reductions in intima-to-media area ratios. Reendothelialization was present in rat and porcine arteries infected with HSV-tk adenoviral vectors and treated with ganciclovir, and significant toxicities were not observed in treated arteries or systemic organs. Additional approaches to limiting smooth muscle cell proliferation after vascular injury include targeting of nuclear cell cycle regulatory pathways, including the retinoblastoma gene product (Rb). Studies in injured rat carotid and porcine femoral artery models suggest that expression of a nonphosphorylatable, constitutively active form of Rb after adenoviral infection limits intimal smooth muscle proliferation for at least 3 weeks after vascular injury.

Myocardial Gene Transfer

Recent exciting developments hold promise for transduction of adult myocytes in vivo. Initial studies demonstrated the feasibility of expression of reporter genes in rat and canine myocardium by direct injection of plasmid DNA, but these studies were limited by low efficiencies that hindered investigations of gene expression in myocytes. The observation that adenoviruses infect nondividing cells has heightened interest in these vectors for gene transfer to adult myocardium. Indeed, recent studies have demonstrated higher levels of gene expression in rat myocardium after direct injection of adenovirus vectors compared with injection of plasmid DNA alone. Adult myocardium in vivo has also been transduced by intravascular administration of adenoviral vectors encoding reporter genes Gene expression was observed in both the coronary vasculature and the adjacent myocardium. Levels of gene expression in the myocardium were 10 to 50 fold higher compared with direct DNA plasmid injection. Although adenoviral vectors provide efficient gene transfer, gene expression in the

Table 31.3: *Gene Therapy Targets for Heart Failure*

Molecular Target	Stage in Development	Findings	Model Assessed
Sarcoendoplasmic Reticulum calcium-ATPase 2a (SERCA2a)	Clinical trials, phase 2	Decreased HF symptoms, increased functional status, and reversal of negative LV remodeling	Human
Stromal-derived factor-1 (SDF-1)	Clinical trials, phase 1/2	Safe and improved 6-minute walk test, quality of life, and NYHA class	Human
Adenylyl cyclase 6 (ADCY6)	Preclinical	Increased LV function, increased cAMP levels, reversal of dysfunctional β-AR signaling, and increased survival Improved LV contractility	Mice Pig
βARKct-carboxy terminal peptide from GRK2	Preclinical	Heart failure rescue Improved β-AR signaling and contractile dysfunction	Rabbit Human cardiomyocytes
S100A1	Preclinical	Increased reuptake SR Ca2+, lowered Ca2+ leak, enhanced cardiac function, and reversed LV remodeling	Rat cardiomyocytes
Parvalbumin (PVALB)	Preclinical	Increased rate of Ca2+ removal and improved relaxation rate	Rat

HF indicates heart failure; LV, left ventricle; NYHA, New York Heart Association; βARKct, *β-adrenergic receptor kinase; β-AR, β-adrenergic; SR, sarcoplasmic reticulum.*

myocardium is transient. In most studies, reporter gene expression peaked at 1 week, diminished at 2 weeks, and was present at low levels after 1 month in adult myocytes. The mechanisms for loss of gene expression, including immune responses, are not completely understood.

Gene transfer to the myocardium has proven to be a useful tool in understanding cardiac gene regulation in vivo. For example, transcriptional elements regulating basal and thyroid hormone–responsive cardiac ±-myosin heavy chain (±-MHC) gene expression in adult rat hearts in vivo have been studied; Sequences upstream of the rat ±-MHC gene linked to a luciferase reporter were injected into adult rat hearts, and thyroid hormone responsiveness was evaluated. The thyroid hormone responsive element was necessary, but not sufficient, to confer positive and negative regulation of thyroid hormone. Direct injection of constructs into the myocardium is a model system for investigating DNA elements and regulatory pathways that control gene expression and growth in the heart.

An additional promising area is the direct injection of adenoviral vectors into skeletal muscle for production of secreted proteins. Myoblasts, transduced by retroviral vectors expressing human growth hormone, injected into skeletal muscle produced physiological levels of human growth hormone in the serum. Recent studies suggest that physiological levels of recombinant erythropoietin are secreted into the circulation after intramuscular injection of adenovirus into skeletal muscle of neonatal mice or adult SCID mice.Neonatal and adult SCID mice injected once with 10 to 10 plaque-forming units demonstrated significant dose-dependent elevations in serum human erythropoietin levels and increased hematocrit levels that were stable over the 4-month time course of the experiments, and no evidence of a localized inflammatory response or systemic infection was present. Intramuscular injection of adenoviral vectors may be useful for the treatment of inherited disorders of deficient serum proteins.

Clinical Benefits of Gene Therapy for Cardiovascular Disease

Gene transfer enables the overexpression of candidate therapeutic genes either locally or systemically. Cardiovascular disease targets under investigation include therapeutic angiogenesis in ischaemic myocardium and limb muscles, treatment of hypertension, vascular bypass graft occlusion, and prevention of postangioplasty restenosis. Cardiovascular diseases are diverse and as such have unique traits requiring precise tailoring of gene therapy strategies to a particular disease. Those features which may vary include mode of delivery, type of vector, length of gene expression, and target tissue. Unlike other inherited genetic defects which may require more long-term gene transfer, transient, nonintegrative gene expression has been shown to be sufficient to promote neovascularization in the case of angiogenesis. This may also apply to antiproliferative strategies for the prevention of neointima formation postangioplasty, for the prevention of in-stent restenosis, or for gene therapy of coronary artery bypass graft failure. However, complex diseases with substantial polygenic influences such as essential hypertension will require sustained gene overexpression.

Cardiovascular Disease Targets For Gene Therapy

Many diseases affecting the cardiovascular system are amenable to gene therapy protocols. Indeed, success has been achieved experimentally. Here, we briefly review the therapeutic strategies relating to the treatment of ischaemia, late vein graft failure, atherosclerosis, thrombosis, and hypertension.

Ischaemia

Peripheral ischaemic diseases are commonly associated with the lower extremities and can be characterized by an impaired blood supply resulting from narrowed or blocked arteries, which subsequently starve tissues of the necessary nutrients and oxygen. Similarly, inadequate blood flow to the heart gives rise to myocardial ischaemia. This may occur if coronary flow is reduced by the presence of an atherosclerotic plaque, a blood clot or an artery spasm. Surgical bypassing and percutaneous revascularization have alleviated many of the symptoms but is not suitable for all patients due to the extension of arterial occlusion and microcirculation impairment. Amputation and heart transplants are the only forms of treatment for ischaemia and therefore gene therapy provides an alternative solution The two main therapeutic genes under investigation are the angiogenic growth factors (VEGF) and fibroblast growth factor (FGF). Research has focused on delivering these agents to the site of ischaemia. VEGF is a heparin binding glycoprotein, which is a principal angiogenic factor for endothelial cells. The delivery of VEGF to target cells lends itself to gene transfer since it is naturally secreted from cells and therefore can achieve its biological effect with a limited number of transfected cells). Gowdak *et al.* demonstrated that intramuscular injection of AdVEGF121 resulted in significant lengthening of arterioles and capillaries of nonischaemic limbs in the rat and rabbit. Furthermore, tissue perfusion in animals receiving gene delivery two weeks prior to experimental induction of skeletal muscle ischaemia by removal of the femoral artery was preserved. Clinically, Ad-mediated transfer of VEGF has been demonstrated to improve the endothelial function and to lower the extremity flow reserve in patients with peripheral arterial disease. In this case, AdVEGF121 was delivered intramuscularly and endothelial function determined 30 days postinjection .

In a phase-I clinical trial involving a group of 21 patients given $AdVEGF_{121}$ by direct myocardial injection into the ischaemic region, no adverse effects were detected locally or systemically. Furthermore, angiography suggested an improvement in the area where the vector had been delivered and patients described alleviation in angina symptoms. More recently, the AGENT trial has addressed the safety and anti-ischaemic effects of administering Ad-FGF4 in patients suffering from angina. Single intracoronary infusion of Ad-FGF4 was shown to result in improved exercise times assessed using the exercise treadmill test compared to the placebo group and no adverse side effects. A single intramuscular injection of AAV-VEGF has been shown in the rat ischaemic hindlimb model to produce an increase in capillary growth, a significant increase in mean blood flow of the ischaemic limb, and a higher average skin temperature An intracardiac injection of $AAV\text{-}VEGF_{165}$ has also been shown to induce angiogenesis in the ischaemic myocardium without any evidence of angioma formation.

Although VEGF has positive effects on the promotion of angiogenesis, there are pertinent safety considerations. It has been shown that VEGF may enhance atherosclerotic plaque development through an increase in focal macrophage levels. Macrophages then induce those growth factors and cytokines, which mediate intimal hyperplasia and contribute to plaque instability through enhancing levels of matrix metalloproteinases (MMPs) and other hydrolytic enzymes. Other potential risks of therapeutic angiogenesis include the production of nonfunctional, leaky vessels, and stimulation of angiogenesis in tumours. Animal studies in mice highlight the need for regulated expression of VEGF as persistent unregulated VEGF expression following intraventricular injection resulted in the formation of intramural vascular tumours at the site of myoblast implantation. The development of tissue-specific vectors and promoters may help to minimise the risks from these adverse reactions.

Protection from reperfusion injury

Reperfusion of ischaemic myocardium resulting from dissolution of the blockage by clinical intervention, may in turn further injure the damaged tissue as a result of reperfusion injury. Reperfusion leads to oxidative stress in the tissue and hence may itself require intervention. Hypoxic regulatable elements and overexpression of agents, which scavenge free radicals or reduce oxidative stress, have been targeted using gene therapy protocols. To produce long-term myocardial protection Melo *et al.* used

AAV to deliver the cytoprotective heme oxygenase gene by intramyocardial injection into rat hearts. They found that eight weeks after administration of the AAV-hHO-1 when acute coronary artery ligation was performed the treated rats had a dramatic reduction in myocardial infarction size. Phillips *et al.* also devised a cardioprotective strategy using a "vigilant vector" AAV construct. This involves a heart specific promoter, MLC2v, which only expresses mRNA in the heart. The vector also includes a hypoxia regulatory element (HRE) which can act as an "on" switch so that production of the transgene antisense AT1R only occurs when ischaemia is detected. This would result in long-term protection of cardiac function during bouts of ischaemia [39]. In an acute model of oxidative stress, the effects of expression of superoxide dismutase (SOD) from adenoviral vectors was investigated [40]. High doses of Ad-SOD3 (3 × 1010 pfu) resulted in a 3-fold elevation of serum SOD activity and was protective against hepatic ischaemia-reperfusion injury.

Late vein graft failure

As one of the most commonly performed surgical procedure at some 400,000 cases worldwide each year, coronary artery bypass grafts (CABG) are effective at relieving symptoms of angina and prolong life for those patients with multiple vessel disease. Vein grafts are inserted into the arterial circulation and undergo a sequence of adaptive physiological changes. Early thrombotic occlusion occurs in 10% of grafts with patency rates of 50% over 10 years due to the onset of intimal thickening and atheromas. Early thrombosis occurs in the first few weeks after grafting, particularly at the distal anastomosis due to vessel wall injury. Drug treatments include aspirin and other antiplatelet agents, which reduce but do not eliminate early occlusions but are often associated with hemorrhagic side effects. Late vein graft failure is characterized by progressive medial thickening and neointima formation. Therefore, vein graft failure limits the clinical success of coronary bypass grafting in terms of symptoms and mortality. Remodelling of the vascular wall by MMPs promotes SMC migration and proliferation, ultimately leading to neointima formation and a narrowing of the vessel lumen. The main therapeutic targets in the context of late vein graft failure are those affecting SMC migration and proliferation. Vein graft lends itself ideally to gene therapy, as there is a clinical therapeutic window whereby surgically prepared vein can be genetically modified prior to grafting. Many candidate therapeutic target genes have been studied experimentally with the aim to prevent the formation of neointimal lesions associated with late vein graft failure. SMC proliferation and migration and matrix degradation are integral to lesion formation and hence, among those classes of gene investigated are antiproliferative, proapoptotic, antiinflammatory, or antimigratory agents.

The Prevent clinical trial aimed to assess the efficacy of intraoperative gene therapy in patients receiving bypass vein grafts. By blockading the cell transcription factor E2F with decoy oligodeoxynucleoties at the time of grafting, they were able to significantly reduce the incidence of post-operative occlusion. E2F upregulates up to a dozen cell cycle genes and its inhibition inhibits target cell cycle gene expression and DNA synthesis. The success of this trial in reducing bypass graft failure in a high risk cohort underlines the important role that gene therapy could play in the prevention of vein graft failure.

MMPs have been shown to be an integral part of neointima formation, and overexpression of the naturally occurring tissue inhibitors of MMPs (TIMPs) is a possible approach. Ad-mediated transfer of TIMPs has been demonstrated in a number of models of vein graft failure. In a mouse model, local delivery of Ad-TIMP-2 was found to reduce vein graft diameter . In contrast, using the pig saphenous vein-carotid artery interposition graft model, George *et al.* demonstrated that while Ad-mediated TIMP-2 delivery was ineffective at reducing vein graft neointima formation, TIMP-3 had a profound inhibitory effect on lesion formation. This was attributed, in part, to its proapoptotic effect in the medial and neointimal layers. Encouragingly, the results from the porcine model were translated into a human ex vivomodel of vein graft failure with an 84% reduction in neointima formation following local delivery of Ad-TIMP-3 . Similarly, TIMP-1 was also shown to have an inhibitory effect on lesion formation in this model.

Endothelial nitric oxide synthase (eNOS) is important to vascular homeostasis and plays a vasoprotective role by inhibiting platelet and leukocyte adhesion, inhibiting SMC proliferation and migration, and in turn promoting endothelial survival. Local eNOS delivery would, in theory, arrest the proliferative response to vascular injury. Nitric oxide (NO) bioactivity is substantially reduced postbypass graft surgery whilst levels of NO scavenging superoxide are increased. It is therefore likely that the loss of NO may contribute to vascular remodelling events in the vein graft . West *et al.* showed that Ad-nNOS gene transfer in a rabbit vein graft model favourably affected vein graft remodelling by inhibiting the early inflammatory changes and reducing late intimal hyperplasia. They observed an increase in NOS activity, a reduction in adhesion molecule expression and inflammatory cell infiltration, and a reduction in basal superoxide generation.

Targeting SMC proliferation has also been shown to be effective using gene therapy protocols. In a rabbit model of vein grafting, Ad-mediated expression of a constitutively active form of the retinoblastoma gene product (AdΔRb) reduced neointima formation four weeks after surgery by 22% In the human saphenous vein model of vein graft, targeting SMC by overexpression of wild-type p53 both induced apoptosis and inhibited SMC migration resulting in a reduction in lesion formation. Likewise, overexpression of C-type natriuretic peptide, which inhibits SMC growth by Ad resulted in accelerated graft re-endothelialisation and reduced thrombosis and neointima formation. Kibbe *et al.* inhibited intimal hyperplasia in porcine vein grafts by incubation with Ad-iNOS for 30 minutes prior to surgery. This effect was sustained up to 21 days postgrafting. While these strategies all show short-term effects, long-term studies are fundamentally important owing to the long-term nature of bypass graft failure.

Thrombosis

Defects in the vessel wall, namely, endothelial cell dysfunction can result in a reduction of antithrombotic activity leading to clot formation. The two main groups of anti-thrombotic genes are those with antiplatelet or anticoagulant activity. Prostacylin (PGI2), nitric oxide (NO) and thrombin inhibitors all act through the inhibition of platelet adhesion and aggregation, in conjunction with the prevention of vascular SMC proliferation and vasoconstriction. The anti-thrombotic treatment, tissue plasminogen activator (tPA), which has anticoagulant properties and is used to lyse existing clots, may be a useful therapeutic gene for antithrombotic therapy (Table 1). The short half-life of tPA could be overcome with sustained overexpression from a gene therapy vector. Other anticoagulant gene products include hirudin, thrombomodulin, antistasin and, tissue factor pathway inhibitor (TFPI). Hirudin is perhaps the most potent inhibitor of thrombin, the enzyme responsible for fibrinogen cleavage, platelet activation, and SMC proliferation. The advantage of local expression of antithrombotic therapeutic genes is that not only is thrombolysis promoted at specific sites in the artery, but also the side effects of the conventional anticoagulant are avoided. Clinical conditions amenable to antithrombotic gene therapy include CABG, percutaneous transluminal coronary angioplasty, peripheral artery angioplasty, and intravascular stenting. Intravascular clot formation is a major cause of acute myocardial infarction and contributes to the majority of sudden deaths in patients with coronary artery disease. Successful thrombolysis for acute thrombosis is dependent on prompt treatment and delays in vector administration and expression of antithrombotic factors suggests that antithrombotic gene therapy is more likely to play a role in the prevention of reocclusion and chronic arterial narrowing. Cyclo-oxygenase-1 (COX-1), the rate limiting enzyme in the synthesis of PGI2, was overexpressed by local delivery of Ad to porcine carotid arteries immediately postangioplasty. This was shown to increase the levels of PGI2 and, in turn, inhibit thrombosis in injured vessels. By manipulating the coagulation cascade integral in thrombus formation, a number of positive gene therapy studies have been reported. In a rabbit stasis/injury model of arterial thrombosis, local overexpression of thrombomodulin using Ad was assessed. In addition to reducing thrombosis, the vector did not induce inflammatory damage at the site of delivery [56]. Work by the same group targeting tissue-type plasminogen activator (tPA) also demonstrated effective prevention of thrombus formation. Local gene transfer of TFPI into rabbit carotid arteries using an Ad vector prior to experimental thrombosis induction completely inhibited the formation of thrombi without affecting systemic coagulation status. Similar data were described in the porcine carotid artery model following local delivery of Ad-TFPI.

Atherosclerosis

Due to the complexity and interplay of genetic and environmental factors in the development of atherosclerosis, it is unlikely that localized gene therapy will be a useful approach in the primary prevention of the disease. Inefficient intravascular gene transfer efficiency through atherosclerotic lesions and lipid-rich atheromas has been attributed to the very low numbers of transfectable cells and the high connective tissue content. An extensive list of therapeutic genes exists for the treatment of atherosclerosis including LDL- or VLDL-receptor gene transfer to overcome LDL-receptor efficiency, a major inherited genetic defect and a determinant of atherosclerosis. Patients with defective enzymes vital for lipoprotein metabolism such as lipoprotein and hepatic lipases would benefit from gene transfer of DNA producing the correct enzymes. A reduction in the level of atherogenic apolipoprotein (apo) B100 is possible after gene transfer of the apoB mRNA editing enzyme, whilst lipoprotein A could be lowered with synthesis inhibiting ribozymes. Apolipoprotein AI (apoAI) and lecithin-cholesterol acyltransferase (LCAT) are important factors in the removal of excess cholesterol and the subsequent reduction in the incidence of atherosclerotic lesions. Through in vitro bicistronic expression of these two genes from AAV plasmid vectors, it was shown that increased synthesis of apoAI and LCAT could play a role in reducing atherosclerotic risk.

The apoE−/− transgenic mouse is a well-established experimental model for atherosclerosis as it develops severe hypercholesterolaemia and atherosclerotic lesions similar to humans. Harris *et al.* (2002) found that they could detect apoE mRNA in the muscle from a single intramuscular injection into the apoE−/− mouse, but could not detect circulating recombinant apoE in the plasma [62]. However circulating antibodies were detected against the human apoE. The most significant finding of this study was three months after administration of the AAV-apoE they found a significant reduction (approximately 30%) in atherosclerotic plague density in the aortas of treated animals compared to the controls. These results suggest that only low levels of apoE are required to produce protection against atherosclerosis.

Attenuation of lesion development has been demonstrated using Ad-mediated overexpression of heme oxygenase-1 TIMP-1 platelet-activating factor acetylhydrolase (PAF-AH)—the enzyme responsible for the inactivation of PAF and apoE itself, administered intravenously [66]. Of particular significance, Kim *et al.* recently described the lifetime correction of hypercholesterolaemia in apoE−/−mice following a single intravenous injection of a helper-dependent Ad vector. Follow-up of 2.5 years old mice demonstrated 100% coverage of the aorta with atherosclerotic plaques in control mice with almost no lesion development in treated animals.

Hypertension

Systemic hypertension is a common multifactorial disorder primarily manifesting itself as chronic high blood pressure and is a major risk factor for atherosclerosis, peripheral vascular disease stroke, and many other complications associated with structural damage to the cardiovascular system. Drugs for controlling high blood pressure are effective over a 24-hour period, are nonspecific and cause side effects. It is well established that the hyperactive renin-angiotensin system (RAS) is a key factor in primary hypertension and gene therapy strategies have concentrated on those genes in the RAS controlling regulation of blood pressure.

Due to its multifactorial nature, gene therapy for hypertension has yet to be demonstrated clinically. Many gene therapy interventions have, however, been employed successfully in the laboratory. Targeting elements involved in the oxidative stress pathways, Alexander et al. and Fennell et al. have demonstrated an improvement of endothelial function in the SHRSP with local delivery ofAd-Enos or Ad-extracellular SOD. Angiotensin II- induced hypertension and accompanying endothelial dysfunction were studied by Nakane et al. Gene transfer of Ad-eNOS but not SOD (copper/zinc or extracellular SOD) was shown to restore endothelial function ex vivo in aortic rings from treated rabbits. Ad-eNOS delivery into the rostral ventrolateral medulla of SHRSP and WKY rats resulted in a significant reduction in blood pressure in both rats. A continuous supply of tissue kallikrein by a single intramuscular injection of Ad produced a significant delay of elevated blood pressure for five weeks in the SHR. An increase in vasodilator proteins such as kallikrein, eNOS, and atrial natriuretic peptide (ANP) in animal models has correlated with a reduction in blood pressure.

Antisense targeting angiotensinogen and the angiotensin type-1 (AT1) receptor attempted to decrease those genes responsible for vasoconstriction. AAV-plasmids have been used to deliver antisense AT1-R to SHR rats They showed that a single intracardiac injection was sufficient to reduce blood pressure by 30 mm Hg when compared to the controls over a five-week period The effect of AAV-AGT-AS on the development of hypertension in SHR rats has also been examined. The rats were injected with AAV-AGT-AS five days after birth as the development of hypertension in SHR rats commences between the eighth and tenth week after birth. A significant slowing of the development of hypertension for six months was observed but there was no complete inhibition of the rise in blood pressure

Biologic Pacemaker - Role of Gene and Cell Therapy in Cardiac Arrhythmias

Gene therapy could create "biological pacemaker":- Researchers say they've found a way to transform ordinary pig heart muscle cells into a "biological pacemaker," a feat that might one day lead to the replacement of electronic pacemakers in humans. "Rather than having to undergo implantation with a metallic device that needs to be replaced regularly and can fail or become infected, patients may someday be able to undergo a single gene injection and be cured of slow heart rhythm forever," said senior study author Dr. Eugenio Cingolani, director of the Cedars-Sinai Heart Institute's Cardiogenetics-Familial Arrhythmia Clinic, in Los Angeles.

Using gene therapy, the researchers altered a peppercorn-sized area in the heart muscle of pigs to create a new "sino-atrial node" the bundle of neurons that normally serves as the heart's natural pacemaker.

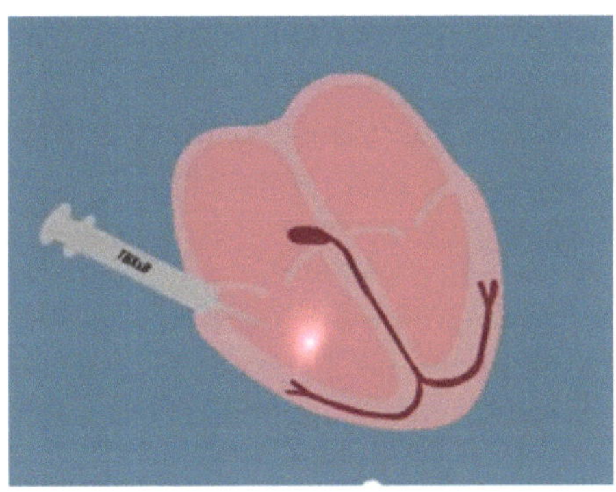

Fig 31.15: *Showing Gene therapy is a procedure where genes (or segments of DNA) are inserted into a cell and the cell then takes up the gene and incorporates it into its own genome*

The technique kept alive a handful of pigs suffering from complete heart block, a condition in which the heart beats very slowly or not at all due to problems in the heart's electrical system.

The biological pacemaker also appeared to function as well as an original sino-atrial node and better than typical electronic pacemakers, said study co-author Dr. Eduardo Marban, director of the Cedars-Sinai Heart Institute, in Los Angeles. "When we exercise, our hearts go faster. When we rest, our hearts slow down," Marban said. "The pigs with the biological pacemaker faithfully reproduced these responses, which were absent in 'control' pigs that had been treated only with an electronic pacemaker."

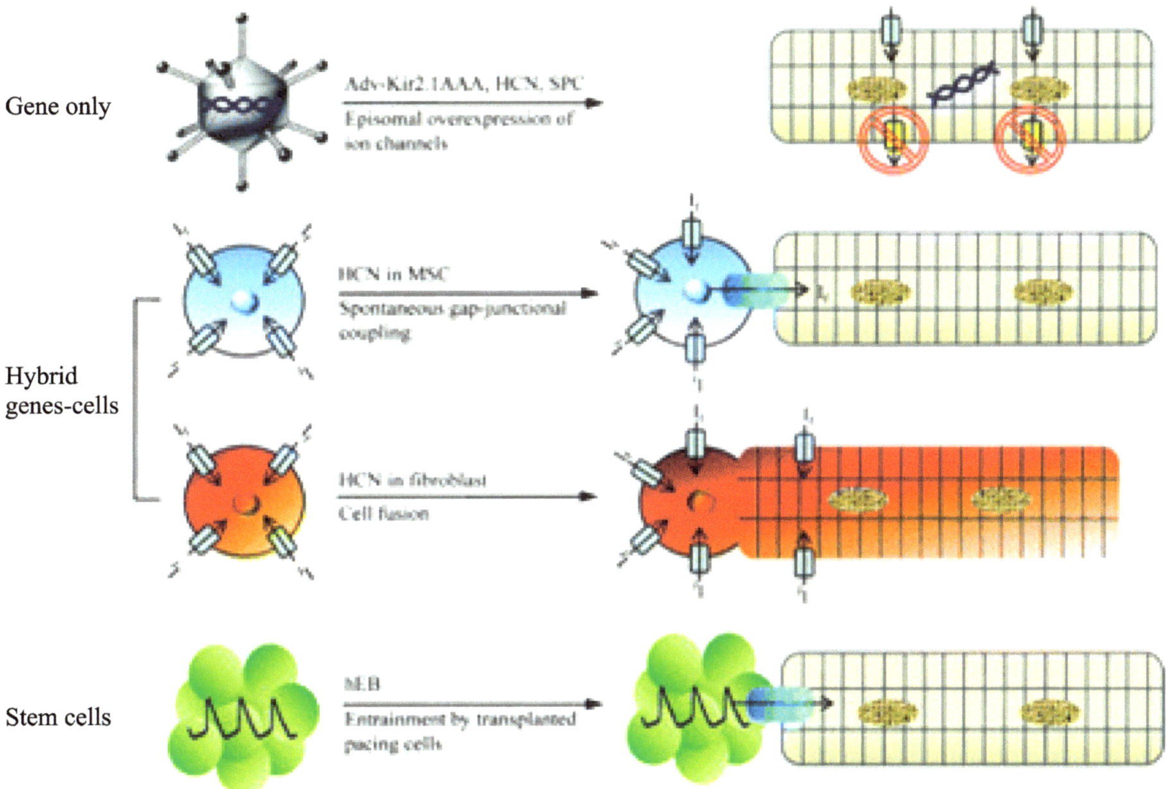

Fig. 31.16: *A summary of different approaches to creating a biological pacemaker. First approach (top row) is a strict gene therapy in which Kir2.1AAA, HCN, or synthetic pacemaker channel genes are overexpressed in myocytes via adenoviral delivery. Kir2.1 dominant negative proteins suppress repolarizing, outward currents whereas pacemaker channels directly contribute to diastolic membrane potential depolarization. Delivering If by MSCs requires gap-junctional coupling between myocytes and MSCs (second row). In the cell fusion approach (third row), If and the pacemaker activity arise from the HCN channels expressed on the cell membrane of the heterokaryon, without the need for gap-junctional coupling. Spontaneously beating human EBs and cardiospheres transduce their pacemaker activity to cardiomyocytes via electrotonic cell–cell coupling (fourth row).*

About 300,000 electronic pacemakers are placed in humans in the United States each year, at an annual cost of $8 billion, Marban said. They work by sending electrical pulses to the heart if it is beating too slowly or if it misses a beat. The key to the new procedure is a gene called TBX18, which converts ordinary heart cells into specialized sino-atrial node cells, Marban said. The heart's sino-atrial node initiates the heart beat like a metronome, using electric impulses to time the contractions that send blood flowing through people's arteries and veins, the scientists explained. People with abnormal heart rhythms suffer from a defective sino-atrial node.

Researchers injected the gene into a very small area of the pumping chambers of pigs' hearts. The gene transformed the heart cells into a new pacemaker.

"In essence, we create a new sino-atrial node in a part of the heart that ordinarily spreads the impulse, but does not originate it," Marban said. "The newly created node then takes over as the functional pacemaker bypassing the need for implanted electronics and hardware."

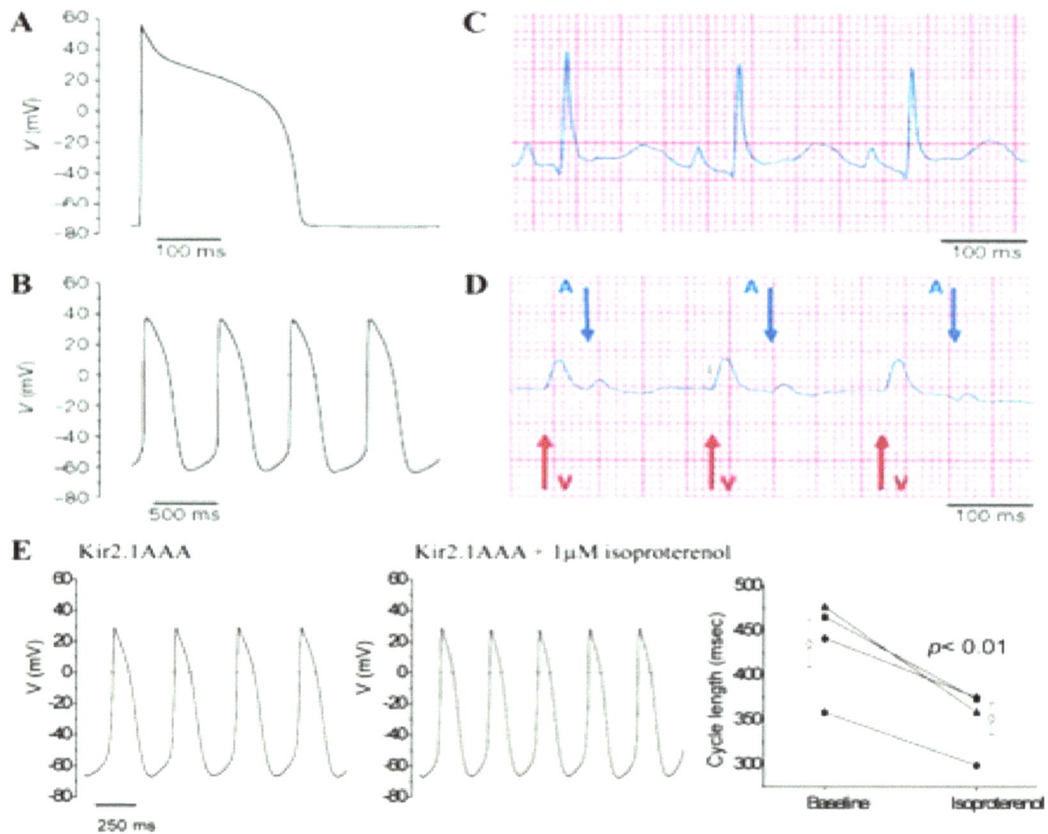

Fig. 31.17: *Suppression of Kir2.1 channels unmasks latent pacemaker activity in ventricular cells. A, APs evoked by depolarizing external stimuli in control ventricular myocytes. B, Spontaneous APs in Kir2.1AAA-transduced myocytes with depressed IK1. C, Baseline electrocardiograms in normal sinus rhythm. D, Ventricular rhythms 72 hours after gene transfer of Kir2.1AAA. P waves (A and arrow) and wide QRS complexes (V and arrow) march through to their own rhythm. A through D are reproduced from Miake et al. with permission.37 E, Guinea pig ventricular myocytes in which Kir2.1AAA was overexpressed (left) and exposed acutely to 1 umol/L isoproterenol (with courtsy from J. Miake, H. B. Nuss, and E.M.)*

Pigs were used in the research because their hearts are very similar in size and shape to those of humans, said lead study author Dr. Yu-Feng Hu, a fellow at the Cedars-Sinai Heart Institute.

Within two days of receiving the gene injection, pigs had significantly stronger heartbeats than pigs that did not receive the gene. The effect persisted for the duration of the 14-day study. Toward the end of the two weeks, the treated pigs' heart rates began to falter somewhat, but remained stronger than that of the pigs who did not receive the gene injection.

The research team hopes to advance to human trials within three years, Cingolani said. However, results from animal trials often can't be duplicated in humans.

If the approach does work in humans, one expert said biological pacemakers could have several uses. They could be used as a "bridge" to help patients whose electronic pacemaker has to be removed or replaced, said Dr. David Friedman, chief of heart failure services at North Shore-LIJ's Franklin Hospital in Valley Stream, N.Y. "Many people with electronic pacemakers that help maintain normal heart rhythm experience short periods when their pacemaker is compromised due to infection or other problems that render it non-functional," Friedman explained. "This gene therapy may someday fill that gap, expanding the arsenal of currently experimental gene and stem cell therapies that symbolize the 'holy grail' of treatments for a wide array of heart conditions."

Cingolani said the therapy could also be used to treat fetuses with congenital heart block, who cannot receive a traditional pacemaker because they are still in the womb. This condition affects one out of every 20,000 fetuses. In mammalian heart, the sino-atrial (SA) node is the pacemaker region, which contains a family of ionic currents that contributes to the pacemaker potential. Using SA nodal cells, experiments have shown that dysrhythmias are easily elicited under conditions involving calcium overload that occur during ischemia and cardiac failure. Clinically these SA nodal dysfunctions cause bradyarrhythmias in general and are associated with syncope but rarely with death. To initiate pacemaker function an inward current (If) carried by sodium through a family of channels that are hyperpolarization-activated and cyclic nucleotide-gated (HCN channels)

Recent advances in molecular and cellular biology, specifically in the areas of stem cell biology and tissue engineering have initiated the development of a new field in molecular biology, regenerative medicine, seeks to develop new biological solutions, using the mobilization of endogenous stem cells or delivery of exogenous cells to replace or modify the function of diseased, absent, or malfunctioning tissue. As far as adult cardiomyocytes have limited regenerative capacity it represents an attractive candidate for these emerging technologies. Therefore, dysfunction of the specialized electrical conduction system may result in inefficient rhythm initiation or impulse conduction leading to significant bradycardia that may require the implantation of a permanent electronic pacemaker. Replacement of the dysfunctional myocardium by implantation of external heart muscle cells is emerging as a novel paradigm for restoration of the myocardial electromechanical properties, but has been significantly limited by the paucity of cell sources for human heart cells and by the relatively limited evidence for functional integration between grafted and host cells. Human embryonic stem cell lines may provide a possible solution for the cell sourcing problem.

Although electronic pacing is an excellent therapy, still have disadvantage like the need for monitoring and replacement, indwelling catheter-electrodes in the heart, possibility of infection, and lack of autonomic responsiveness, geometric limitations with respect to pediatric patients make it warrant a search for better alternatives The biological pacemaker, a tissue that spontaneously or via engineering confers pacemaker properties to regions of the heart, is an exciting alternative. Several approaches have been taken in attempting to produce biological pacemakers. These can be considered in 3 headings:

1. The use of viral vectors to deliver genes to regions of the heart such that a pacemaker potential resulting in spontaneous impulse initiation evolves in the region of gene administration.
2. The use of embryonic stem cells grown along a cardiac lineage and manifesting the electrophysiologic properties of sinus node cells
3. The use of mesenchymal stem cells as platforms to carry pacemaker genes to the heart, relying on gap junctional coupling such that the stem cell and a coupled myocyte form a single functional unit to generate pacemaker function

Why biological pacemakers needed

Although electronic pacemakers reduced mortality associated with complete heart block and morbidity of sinoatrial node dysfunction, still they have disadvantages:

1. The imposed limitations on the exercise tolerance and cardiac rate-response to emotion. Despite the use of paradigms to improve heart rate response during increased physical activity, there is no substitute currently available for the autonomic modulation of heart rate.
2. In pediatrics, patient age and size, the mass of the power pack, and the size and length of the electrode catheter are important considerations. The hardware must be tailored to the growth of the patient.
3. The placement site of the stimulating electrode in the ventricle and the resultant activation pathway may have beneficial or deleterious effects on electrophysiologic or contractile function.
4. The long-but-limited life battery expectancy, requiring testing and replacement at periodic intervals.
5. Infection may require removal and/or replacement of

the pacemaker.

6. Various devices including neural stimulators metal detectors and magnetic resonance imaging equipment have been reported to interfere at times with electronic pacemaker function.
7. So a biological alternative that might last for the life of the patient, respond to physiologic demands for different heart rates at different times, and activate the heart via a pathway tailored to the anatomy of disease in any individual is an exciting possibility.

An ideal biological pacemaker should;

1. Create relatively acepted physiologic rhythm for the life of the individual.
2. Needs no battery or electrode, and no replacement.
3. Effectively compete in direct comparison with electronic pacemakers.
4. Have no inflammatory or infectious potential.
5. Not carcinogenic.
6. Adapt to changes in physical activity and/or emotion with appropriate rapid changes in heart rate.
7. Propagate through an optimal pathway of activation to maximize efficiency of contraction and cardiac output.
8. Not arrythmogenic.
9. Potentially curative.

Strategies for building a biological pacemaker:- Three strategies reported till now to create biological pacemaker activity:

1. Up-regulation of adrenergic neurohumoral actions on heart rate
2. Reduction of repolarizing current
3. Increasing inward current during diastole

All three strategies had their foundations in 21th century pharmacology and physiology. In studies of autonomic modulation, increased heart rate via beta-adrenergic catecholamines or sympathetic stimulation through an increase in pacemaker current in the sinus node and in accessory pacemakers, whereas increasing vagal tone or stimulating muscarinic receptors decreased heart rate (Di Francesco *et al.* 1986, Campbell *et al.* 1989). In studies of ionic determinants of pacemaker activity, augmentation of hyperpolarizing, outward currents decreased pacemaker rate (Di Francesco *et al.* 1995), suggesting that the opposite intervention, i.e. decreasing hyperpolarizing, outward currents, would increase rate (Miake *et al.* 2002). Pharmacological experiments demonstrated that suppressing inward current carried by the T-type or L-type Ca channel slows pacemaker rate. (Lasker *et al.* 1997, Robinson, Di Francesco 2001). What are needed are the tools to apply this knowledge to the molecular and genetic determinants of the pacemaker potential.

The necessary information was provided in part via the identification and cloning of the gene products that determine the beta adrenergic receptors, the inward rectifier current, and the pacemaker current. Also of central importance was the development of tools for; 1- gene therapy, wherein genes encoding the molecular subunits of interest are inserted via plasmids or viral vectors into cells of the myocardium; 2- cell therapy via the use of embryonic stem cells, whose differentiation is directed into myocardial precursors manifesting pacemaker activity, or mesenchymal stem cells used as platforms to implant channels into cardiac myocytes. A critical factor is the development of models in which to test pacemaker constructs. In vitro models of cells in culture are a standard for testing a variety of gene therapies it has been found that infecting neonatal rat ventricular myocytes with replication-deficient adenoviral constructs incorporating the gene of interest (with or without coexpression of GFP) provides a cost-effective and reproducible assay Using a variation on this model for testing the ability of stem cells to transmit the electrical signal of interest .It has been considered that a 100 times or more overexpression of current and a statistically significant effect on beating rate as standards that discriminate efficacy, More research is required to establish uniform guidelines permitting reliable correlation of in vitro and in vivo effectiveness. As an intact animal screen, the use of guinea pig (Miake *et al.* 2002), swine (Edelberg *et al.* 2001), and dog (Qu *et al.* 2003, Plotnikov *et al.* 2004, Potapova *et al.* 2004) has been reported. The use of dog is based on its cardiac size, tractability as a chronic model, and similar electrophysiologic properties to those of man.

Cell therapy for the treatment of cardiac arrhythmias:- An alternative approach to overcome the shortcomings of gene therapy may be the use of genetically modified cell grafts that can be initially transfected ex vivo with excellent long-term efficiency and then transplanted to the in vivo heart.

This will require the following:

1. Establish the proper cell sources for transplantation.
2. Assessment of the phenotypic structural and functional properties of the cell grafts, in vitro.
3. Establish transplantation strategies to deliver the cells to the desired locations.
4. Achieve the desired in vivo effect by assuring the survival of the cell grafts, their integration and interactions with host tissue, and their proper function.

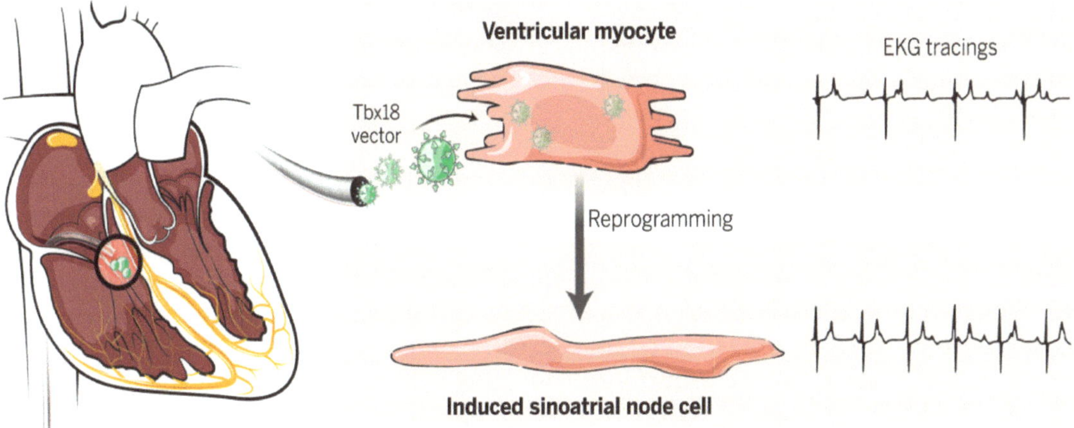

Fig. 31.18: *Tbx18 adenovirus reprograms heart muscle cells into sinoatrial node cells. Reprogrammed cells then generate electrical impulses to restore normal heart rate. Image from Science, 345 (6194): 268-269.*

Cell therapy can be applied for the treatment of cardiac arrhythmias at three different levels:

1. Replace absent or malfunctioning cells of the conduction system.
2. Modify the myocardial electrophysiological substrate by using cell grafts genetically engineered to express specific ionic channels, which can couple and modify the electrophysiological properties of host tissue through electrotonic interactions.
3. Modify the myocardial environment by local secretion of specific recombinant proteins.

A major limitation for the development of such cell replacement strategies is the paucity of cell sources for human cardiomyocytes. The use of the recently described human embryonic stem cell lines may be solution to this cell-sourcing problem (Gepstein 2002). These unique cell lines have the capability to be propagated in vitro in the undifferentiated state in large quantities and to be coaxed to differentiate to a plurality of cell lineages, including cardiomyocytes (Kehat *et al.* 2001a). This differentiating system is not limited to the generation of isolated cardiac cells, but rather a functional cardiac syncytium is generated with a stable pacemaker activity and electrical propagation (Kehat *et al.* 2002). that can also respond to adrenergic and cholinergic stimuli. The ability to generate, ex vivo, different subtypes of human cardiomyocytes (with pacemaking-, atrial-, ventricular-, or Purkinje-like phenotypes) (Mummery *et al.* 2003) that could lend themselves to genetic manipulation may be of great value for future cell therapy strategies aiming to regenerate or to modify the conduction system. The ability of the grafted cells (pacemaker cells or conductive tissue) to integrate structurally and functionally with host tissue is a sole requirement. The human ES cell derived cardiomyocytes were able to integrate ex vivo both structurally and functionally with preexisting cardiac tissue and to generate a single functional syn cytium (Kehat *et al.* 2001 b). Whereas it is not surprising that cardiomyocyte cell grafts can form intercellular connections with host cells (Isner 2002). Recent studies have demonstrated that other cell types such as fibroblasts (Rook *et al.* 1992, Fast *et al.* 1996, Gaudesius *et al.* 2003) are also capable of forming gap junctions with host cardiomyocytes and that specific electrotonic interactions can be generated between these cells. The feasibility of using genetically engineered fibroblasts, transfected to express the voltage-gated potassium channel Kv1.3, to modify the electrophysiological properties of cardiomyocyte cultures have been examined, in a study, using a high-resolution multi-electrode array mapping technique to assess the electrophysiological and structural properties of primary neonatal rat ventricular cultures. The transfected fibroblasts were demonstrated to significantly alter the electrophysiological properties of the cardiomyocyte cultures. These changes were manifested by a significant reduction in the local extracellular signal amplitude and by the appearance of multiple local conduction blocks (Feld *et al.* 2002). The location of all conduction blocks correlated with the spatial distribution of the transfected fibroblasts as assessed by vital staining and all of the electrophysiological changes were reversed following the application of a specific Kv1.3 blocker.

Genetically engineered cell grafts, transfected to express potassium channels, can couple with host cardiomyocytes and alter the local myocardial electrophysiological properties by reducing cardiac automaticity and prolonging refractoriness. Investigators studied the ex vivo, in vivo, and computer simulation studies to determine the ability of transfected fibroblasts to express the voltage-sensitive potassium channel Kv1.3 to modify the local myocardial excitable properties. Co-culturing of the transfected fibroblasts with neonatal rat ventricular myocyte cultures resulted in a significant reduction (68%) in the spontaneous beating frequency of the cultures compared with baseline values and co-cultures seeded with naive fibroblasts. In vivo grafting of the transfected fibroblasts in the rat ventricular myocardium significantly prolonged the local effective refractory period from an initial value of 84 +/-8 ms (cycle length, 200 ms) to 154+/-13 ms (P<0.01). Marga toxin partially reversed this effect (effective refractory period, 117 +/-8 ms; P <0.01). In contrast, effective refractory period did not change in nontransplanted sites (86+/-7 ms) and was only mildly increased in the animals injected with wild-type fibroblasts (73+/-5 to 88+/-4 ms; P<0.05). Similar effective refractory period prolongation also was found during slower pacing drives (cycle length, 350 to 500 ms) after transplantation of the potassium channels expressing fibroblasts (Kv1.3 and Kir2.1) in pigs. (Yankelson *et al.* 2008).

The possible utilization of cell grafts (fibroblasts, different stem cell derivatives, or other cell sources) that can be genetically manipulated ex vivo to display specific electrophysiological characteristics and then grafted to the in vivo heart may possess a number of theoretical advantages over direct gene therapy. These advantages may be related to a better efficiency and control of the transfection process ex vivo, the ability to screen the phenotypic properties of the cells before transplantation, and the possible achievement of long-term effect because cardiac cell grafts were demonstrated to survive for prolonged periods following transplantation (Muller-Ehmsen *et al.* 2002). Yet, determining the optimal way for the delivery of the cells, controlling their survival following transplantation, assuring appropriate integration of the cells with host tissue, and developing means to control the required electrophysiological effect are all important obstacles for the future use of this approach as a therapeutic strategy.

Ischemic heart disease represents one of the most important conditions predisposing to arrhythmias. A variety of preclinical and clinical studies have demonstrated the potential utility of gene therapy in the management of chronic ischemic patients through the local secretion of angiogenic growth factors such as vascular endothelium growth factor (VEGF) and fibroblast growth factor (Isner 2002). Cell therapy strategies may similarly play a dual role in promoting angiogenesis. First, cells transfected ex vivo may be used for sustained local release of recombinant proteins with angiogenic properties following in vivo grafting. Second, transplantation of specific cell types such as endothelial progenitor cells may contribute directly to the neovascularization process. The improved understanding of the molecular pathways involved in the development of heart failure allow definition of several molecular targets for gene therapy to improve systolic and diastolic properties of failing myocytes. To focus on modulating calcium homeostasis, manipulating the beta-adrenergic receptor signaling pathways, and improving cardiomyocyte resistance to apoptosis need to be looked for in future strategies. Similarly, cellular cardiomyoplasty and tissue engineering approaches to regenerate functional myocardium also represent a novel approach for the treatment of heart failure

Future prospective in biological pacing system

Improvement in the understanding of the mechanisms underlying many of cardiac arrhythmias and the development of molecular and cellular tools suggest a future role for gene and cell therapies for treatment of different cardiac arrhythmia. Bridging the gap between the proof-of-concept and the clinical application will require important methodological developments as well as extensive animal experiments. Newer refinements in vector development and design are needed to have better transduction in cardiovascular tissue. Cell specific regulatory elements and promoters to selectively target the cardiac tissue is a potential area of interest (Beck *et al.* 2004). Bacterial gene delivery as an alternative to viral vectors has been proposed (Palffy *et al.* 2006). Hybrid vectors, gutted vectors and new generation non viral vectors may hold the key to future. Evidence from both viral and stem cell approaches state that proof of concept is there. Trials can be designed that permit us to test biological versus electronic pacemakers in relative safety in patients who are protected from failure of the biological unit. Tandem pacing is the proposed way to proceed clinically (patients with chronic atrial fibrillation and complete heart block); i.e. implant both a biological pacemaker and an electronic demand pacemaker in the same individual, this has been tested in dogs in complete heart block an adenoviral HCN2 construct (into the left bundle-branch system) were delivered and an electronic demand unit, the electrode of which was placed in the right ventricular endocardial apex (Bucchi *et al.* 2006). The biological pacemaker fired 70%of the time and was catecholamine responsive. Moreover, when the biological unit slowed, the electronic unit took over; similarly, the electronic unit sensed the biological unit well and discontinued its function when the biological function emerged, the memory function of the electronic unit can track the function of the biological unit, providing a record for the cardiologist. Given the imperfections that still reside with electronics, the possibility of a system with no wires, no hardware, and a software that is of the body's own ion channels and autonomic nervous system offers something more appealing, if it can be made to function at the level needed and for the time required. As mentioned above, rate responsiveness is here, and improved and leadless systems have arrived as well. Therefore, there are two competitive approaches evolving. Which will dominate, traditional electronics upgraded to achieve still newer levels of success or biologics, is unknown, and the future will answer.

Bibliography and Acknowledgement

- Barr E, Carroll J, Kalynych AM, Tripathy SK, Kozarsky K, Wilson JM, Leiden JM. Efficient catheter-mediated gene transfer into the heart using replication-defective adenovirus. *Gene Ther.* 1994; **1**:51-58.
- Cornetta K, Moen RC, Culver K, Morgan RA, McLachlin JR, Sturm S, Selegue J. Amphotropic murine leukemia retrovirus is not an acute pathogen for primates. *Hum Gene Ther.* 1990; **1**:15-30.
- Nabel EG, Plautz G, Boyce FM, Stanley JC, Nabel GJ. Recombinant gene expression in vivo within endothelial cells of the arterial wall. *Science.*1989;244:1342-1344.
- 10Hu CH, Wu GF, Wang XO *et al.* Transplanted human umbilical cord blood mononuclear cells improve left ventricular function through angiogenesis in myocardial infarction. *Chin Med J* (Engl). 2006; **119**(18):1499-506.
- Berkner KL. Expression of heterologous sequences in adenoviral vectors. *Curr Top Microbiol Immunol.* 1992; **58**:39-66.
- Bonanno G, Mariotti A, Procoli A, *et al.* Human cord blood CD133+ cells immunoselected by a clinical-grade apparatus differentiate in vitro into endothelial- and cardiomyocyte-like cells. Transfusion. 2007; **47**(2):280-
- Chen SL, Fang WW, Ye F, Liu YH, Qian J, Shan SJ, Zhang JJ, Chunhua RZ, Liao LM, Lin S, Sun JP. Effect on left ventricular function of intracoronary transplantation of autologous bone marrow mesenchymal stem cell in patients with acute myocardial infarction. *Am J Cardiol* 2004; 94:92-95.
- Cheng F, Zou P, Handong Y. Induced differentiation of human cord blood mesenchymal stem/progenitor cells into cardiomyocyte-like cells in vitro. *J Huazong Univ Sci and Tech.* 2003; 23(2):154-157.
- Cone RD, Mulligan RC. High-efficiency gene transfer into mammalian cells: Generation of helper-free recombinant retrovirus with broad mammalian host range. *Proc Natl Acad Sci U S A.* 1984;81:6349-6353.
- Engelhardt JF, Simon RH, Yang Y, Zepeda M, Weber-Pendleton S, Doranz B, Grossman M, Wilson JM. Adenovirus-mediated transfer of the CFTR gene to lung of nonhuman primates: biological efficacy study. *Hum Gene Ther.*1993;4:759-769.
- Engelhardt JF, Ye X, Doranz B, Wilson JM. Ablation of E2A in recombinant adenoviruses improves transgene persistence and decreases inflammatory response in mouse liver. *Proc Natl Acad Sci U S* A. 1994;91:6196-6200.
- Flugelman MY, Jaklitsch MT, Newman KD, Casscells W, Bratthauer GL, Dichek DA. Low-level in vivo genetransfer into the arterial wall through a perforated balloon catheter. *Circulation.* 1992;3:1110-1117.
- Garver RI Jr, Chytil A, Courtney M, Crystal RG. Clonal gene therapy: transplanted mouse fibroblast clones express human ±1- antitrypsin gene in vivo. Science. 1987;237:762-764.
- Gerard RD, Herz J. Adenovirus-mediated low density lipoprotein receptor gene transfer accelerates cholesterol clearance in normal mice. *Proc Natl Acad Sci U S A.* 1993;90:2812-2816.
- Graham FL, Prevec L. Adenovirus-based expression vectors and recombinant vaccines. In: Ellis RW, ed. Vaccines: New Approaches to Immunological Problems. Boston, Mass: Butterworth-Heinemann; 1992:363-390.
- Grossman M, Raper SE, Kozarsky K, Stein EA, Engelhardt JF, Muller D, Lupien PJ, Wilson JM. Successful ex vivo gene therapy directed to liver in a patient with familial hypercholesterolaemia. *Nat Genet.* 1994;6:335-341.
- Guzman RJ, Lemarchand P, Crystal RG, Epstein SE, Finkel T. Efficient and selective adenovirus-mediated gene transfer into vascular neointima.*Circulation*. 1993;88:2838-2848.
- Henning RJ, Abu-Ali H, Balis JU, Morgan MB, Willing AE, Sanberg PR. Human umbilical cord blood mononuclear cells for the treatment of acute myocardial infarction. Cell Transplant. 2004;13(7-8):729-39.
- Herreros J, Prosper F, Perez A, Gavira JJ, Garcia-Velloso MJ, Barba J, Sanchez PL, Canizo C, Rabago G, Marti-Climent JM, Hernandez M, Lopez-Holgado N, Gonzalez-Santos JM, Martin-Luengo C, Alegria E. Autologous intramyocardial injection of cultured skeletal mus cle-derived stem cells in patients with non-acute myocardial infarction. *Eur Heart J* 2003; 24:2012-2020.
- J, Guetta E, Feinberg MS et al. Human umbilical cord blood-derived CD133+ cells enhance function and repair of the infarcted myocardium. *Stem Cells.* 2006;24(3):772-80.
- Lee SW, Trapnell BC, Rade JJ, Virmani R, Dichek DA. In vivo adenoviral vector-mediated gene transfer into balloon-injured rat carotid arteries. *Circ Res.* 1993;73:797-807.
- Lemarchand P, Jones M, Yamada I, Crystal RG. In vivo gene transfer and expression in normal uninjured blood vessels using replication-deficient recombinant adenovirus vectors. *Circ Res.* 1993;72:1132-1138.
- Yang Y, Nunes FA, Berencsi K, Furth EE, Gonczol E, Wilson JM. Cellular immunity to viral antigens limits E1-deleted adenoviruses for gene therapy. Proc Natl Acad Sci U S A. 1994;91:4407-4411.
- Zabner J, Petersen DM, Puga AP, Graham SM, Couture LA, Keyes LD, et al. Safety and efficacy of repetitive adenovirus-mediated transfer of CFTR cDNA to airway epithelia of primates and cotton rats. Nat Genet. 1994;6:75-83.

Integrating Spirituality Into Patient Care: An Essential Element of Modern Health Care System

The World Health Organization (WHO) defined human health in a broader sense in its 1948 constitution as «a state of complete physical, mental and social well-being and not merely the absence of disease or infirmity But recently recognizing the role of spirituality in health wellness. This definition has been revised to ;- "Health is a dynamic state of complete physical, mental, spiritual and social well being and not merely the absence of disease or infirmity."

Spirituality and health is a growing field of healthcare. It grew out of courses in spirituality and health developed for medical students in the United States. Research in this area over the last 30 years has also formed an evidence base for spirituality and health. Studies have demonstrated an association between spiritual beliefs and values and a variety of healthcare outcomes. More recent research has also shown a strong desire on the part of patients to have their spirituality addressed as part of their care. Studies also show that spiritual care has an impact on patient decision making, particularly in end-of-life care. The Association of American Medical Colleges developed a broad definition of spirituality as well as learning objectives and guidelines for teaching. Standards in organizations such as the American College of Physicians support physicians treating the whole person, that is, the body, mind, and spirit. In 2009, National Competencies in Spirituality and Health education were developed in the United States with schools currently working on curriculum projects based on these competencies. Models are being developed for all members of the healthcare team to address patient distress, in cooperation with chaplains as spiritual care experts. The goals are to develop a biopsychosocial and spiritual assessment and treatment as part of compassionate whole-person care of all patients.

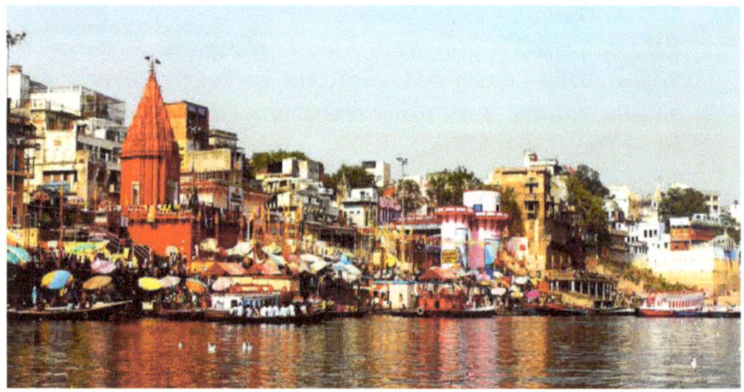

Fig. 32.1: *Photograph of Dashashwamedh Ghat on the banks of river Ganga in Varanasi city (UP). Antient faith is that one who prays at Lord Shiva temple after taking bath in holy Ganga ,he/she gets salvation and aquaires Mokhasha ie freedom from repeated birth and death*

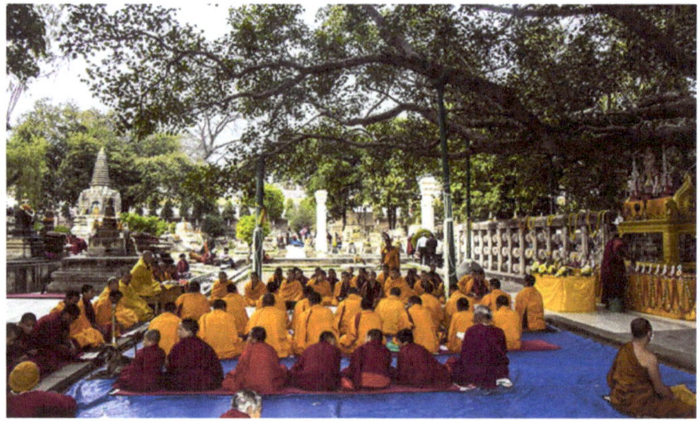

Fig.32.2: *Photograph of Bodh Gaya . Devotees are worshiping Lord Buddha under the Banyian tree where Lord Buddha got enlightenment and delivered his lecture to his disciples about the existence of almighty God.*

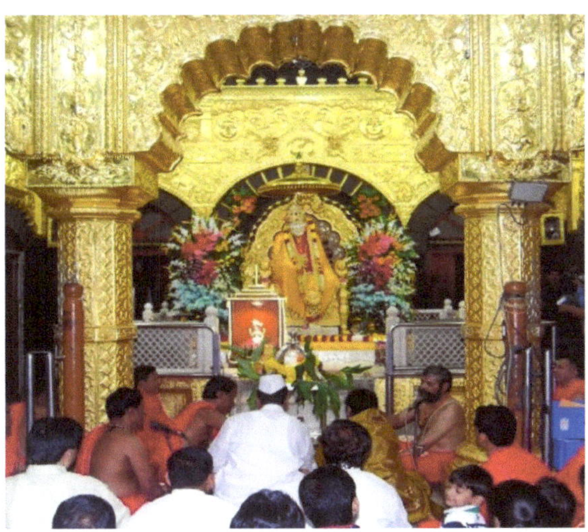

Fig. 32.3: *Photograph of Sai Baba at Shirdi temple, a place of great spiritual faith and wellness*

What is Whole-Person Care?

- Transcends control of a disease process and the relief of symptoms
- Aims at full health, understood as the recovery of an integrated and authentic self
- Maintains focus on the patient as a whole person, regardless of how intractable, expensive, or complicated the patient's problems might appear to be

NCP Guidelines Address 8 Domains of Care.

1. Structure and processes
2. Physical aspects
3. Psychological and psychiatric aspects
4. Social aspects
5. Spiritual, religious, and existential aspects
6. Cultural aspects
7. Imminent death
8. Ethical and legal aspects

Consensus: Design and Definition

40 national leaders representing physicians, nurses, chaplains and clergy, psychologists, social workers, other spiritual care providers, and healthcare administrators

- Develop a consensus - driven definition of spirituality
- Make recommendations to improve spiritual care in palliative care settings
- Identify resources to advance the quality of spiritual care

World Health Organisation has already realized the need of the 4th dimension of health, i.e. the spiritual health to be considered as an important element of health. In the words of Derek Yach (World Health Assembly May, 1998):"From the inception, it was felt that the 4th Dimension of health was missing from its definition. The special group of the WHO Executive Board (1998) proposed that the Preamble of the Constitution should be amended as follows"

"Health is a dynamic state of complete physical, mental, spiritual and social well being and not merely the absence of disease or infirmity. During one of my lectures on "Life style modification and Health" I was asked to describe spiritual health. Although spiritual health means something different to everyone, below is my response hoping that it might offer some insight in addition to an expanded definition of health beyond diet and exercise. Again, this is my own perspective on spiritual health, which is a dynamic and ever evolving field of learning in medical science and hence not to be considered as absolute truth.

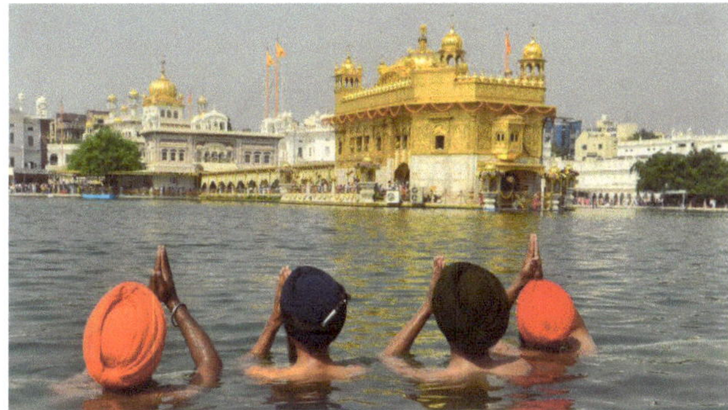

Fig. 32.4: *Another example. Photograph of Golden temple at Amritsar (Pb) ,a place of great religious faith.*

The traditional meaning of spirituality is a process of re-formation which "aims to recover the original shape of man, the image of God". One can define spiritual health as nothing but peacefulness, simplicity, empathy, compassion to name a few. It might really sound to be true and interesting. It does happen with me too, whenever, I am around a spiritually healthy person, I feel peaceful, inspired, relaxed and safe. It is said, a spiritually healthy person is very much in tune with the present moment and doesn't live in the past or in the future, but instead fully accepts the current moment as the only "real" moment in which to experience and enjoy life in totality.

Interestingly, spirituality and health is a growing field of healthcare. It grew out of courses in spirituality and health developed for medical students in the United States. Research in this area over the last 30 years has also formed an evidence base for spirituality and health. Studies have demonstrated an association between spiritual beliefs of patients and values and a variety of healthcare outcomes. More recent research has also shown a strong desire on the part of patients to have their spirituality addressed as part of their medical care.

Empirical evidence is also available to indicate a direct relation between spirituality and positive health outcomes. Positive values, attitudes, belief and strength that one acquires through spiritual practices contribute to health and happiness. Spiritual practices have a positive correlation with survival, low blood pressure, fewer symptoms of anxiety and depression, less severe medical illness, better quality of life etc. As researchers clearly suggest that spiritual practices enhance the level of self-confidence, assertiveness and such other qualities which help accelerate the process of recovery from illness and surgery in general. One such specific studies of heart transplant patients showed that those who participated in spiritual activities besides complying with suggested medical prescriptions registered faster all round improvement.

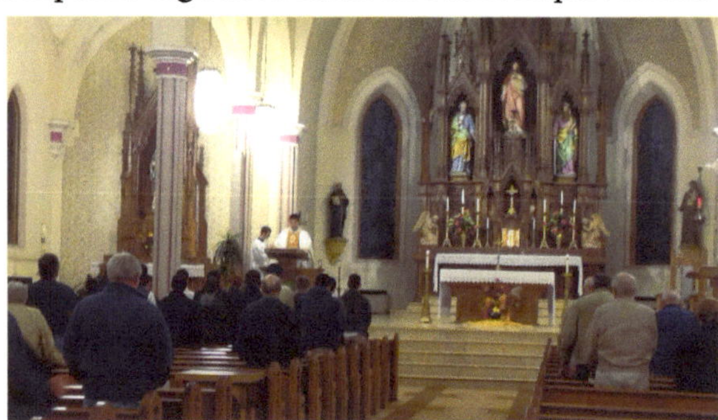

Fig. 32.5: *Photograph of a Church, a place of great religious faith for Christians. They have gathered infront of Lord Jesus praying for forgiveness of their sins and grant them wholesome wellness*

In 1992, 3 medical schools offered courses on spirituality and health in America. In 2001, 75 of the 125 schools offered courses. At The George Washington University School of Medicine, spirituality is interwoven with the rest of the curriculum throughout the 4 years of medical school so that the students learn to integrate it into all of their care. Most of the other schools follow this model of integrating spirituality into on-going parts of the medical school curriculum.

Researchers suggest a positive relation between spiritual practices and positive health outcomes, like greater self-confidence, assertiveness and fewer symptoms of anxiety and depression. Evidence shows that spiritual well-being is positively related with self-ratings of physical health and vitality. Physicians do consider such factors in their medical care practice.

Research indicates a close relationship between love for God or feeling of being loved by some Higher Reality with greater self-esteem, higher levels of self-efficacy, sense of mastery, less depression, less physical disability and greater self-rated health. The John Templeton

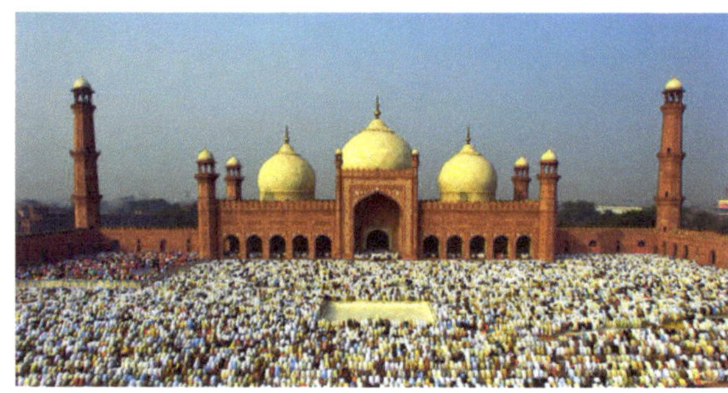

Fig. 32.6: *Photograph of a Meeca masjid ,a place of great religious faith for muslims.Scientists have shown that praying to Mecca five times a day, if done properly, can reduce pain in the lower back.*

Foundation, USA has invested on more than 24 research studies on forgiveness 'Unconditional love is the most powerful stimulant of the immune system – the truth is; love heals'

For the last two decades, modern system of medicine has started realizing the mind–body axis of the disease and health. Empirical evidence is available to indicate a direct relation between religious involvement, spirituality and positive health outcomes. Positive values, attitudes, beliefs and strength that one acquires through spiritual practices contribute to health and happiness. Spiritual practices have a positive correlation with survival, low blood pressure, less remission time from depression, less number of cigarettes smoked per day per week, less severe medical illness, better quality of life and cooperativeness.

In a cross-sectional study on "Spirituality and health: a knowledge, attitude and practice study among doctors of North India", found that 65.65% had a strong or very strong belief in the spiritual dimension of health; 55.22% believed in the preventive role of spirituality; 80% believed in the curative role of spirituality and a similar proportion held the view that spirituality has an important role in day-to-day patient care. The most significant finding was that 93.48% of the doctors believe that a spiritual person deals better with stress

WHO's quest to integrate spiritual health in the development agenda of United Nations and in the core value system of peoples' life can be easily discerned in the words of Stuckelberger "Addressing the scientific link between religion, spirituality and health has too often been a 'forgotten subject' or avoided for irrational, emotional or 'political' reasons. It is time for the scientific community to integrate religious and spiritual factors, which have guided human behavior over centuries, into health and human science

7 Ways to improve Your Spiritual Wellness

The spiritual element of wellness can be the most personal piece of the puzzle when trying to place all seven dimensions of wellness together. Generally, people like to live a life with meaning and purpose. When these goals are met, it puts harmony in one's life, and the others they surround themselves with.

So, what can you do to improve your spiritual wellness? It's best to figure out what techniques work for you. Since spiritual wellness involves one's values, beliefs, and purpose, it can be achieved in several ways—both physically and mentally.

1. Explore your spiritual core:- By exploring your spiritual core, you are simply asking yourself questions about the person you are and your meaning. Ask yourself : Who am I? What is my purpose? What do I value most? These questions will lead you down a road where you will think more in-depth about yourself and allow you to notice things about yourself that will help you achieve fulfillment.

2. Look for deeper meanings:- Looking for deeper meanings in your life and analyzing occurring patterns will help you see that you have control over your destiny. Being aware of this can help you achieve a happy and healthy life.

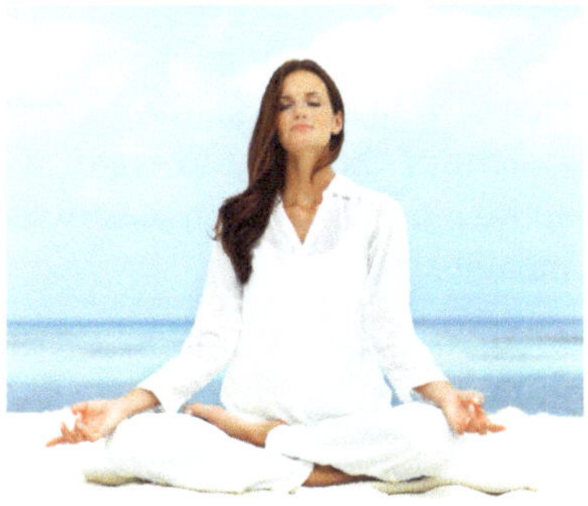

Fig. 32.7: *Photograph of a young lady performing Yoga for her health wellness*

3. Get it out:- Expressing what is on your mind will help you to maintain a focused mind. After a long day or a significant event, you may feel confused and not be able to make sense of your feelings. By writing down your thoughts, you may be able to think clearer and move forward.

4. Try yoga:- Yoga is a physical technique that can help improve your spiritual wellness by reducing emotional and physical strains on your mind and body. Yoga is taught at all different levels and can help lower stress, boost the immune system, and lower blood pressure as well as reduce anxiety, depression, fatigue, and insomnia.

5. Travel:- It's true! Taking time for yourself to travel to a comforting place or somewhere new can do wonders for your mind. When you are at a place where your mind can keep out distractions and help you reflect and rest, you will have a better connection with yourself. This allows you to weed out stressors and set your mind on the right path for overall wellness. Some activities to take part in when on a trip can be exercising, speaking with a counselor or advisor, meditation, or taking a temporary vow of silence.

6. Think positively:- Once you start viewing things in your life in a positive manner, you will find yourself thinking differently and refocusing your mind to a happy, healthy place. When you eliminate negativity and re-frame how you think of certain things and situations, you'll notice yourself being more relaxed.

7. Take time to meditate:- While managing your time and daily tasks can be hard, it is crucial to devote time to connecting with yourself. Whether in the morning when you wake up, during your lunch break, or before you go to sleep, take five to 10 minutes to meditate each day. Fitting mediation and relaxation into your lifestyle will free your mind and foster a stronger relationship with your spiritual wellness.

What is Gayatri Mantra?

Originally written in the Vedas, the mantra is made up of 24 syllables that are meant to have both a psychological and physiological effect on our body. Here are 10 reasons chanting the Gayatri Mantra is good for your health.

ॐ भूर् भुवः स्वः तत् सवितुर् वरेण्यम्।
भर्गो देवस्य धीमहि धीयो यो नः प्रचोदयात्॥

Research on Gayatri Mantra

This Mantra awakens you to the real life. This Mantra is the vital force of life. It is a spring and mine of endless energy. Through this Mantra you know your powers and potential and work for better life. This Mantra ends all pains, miseries and brings happiness in life. It lightens, empowers, enriches and elevates our life. It is a source of tremendous energy. It makes you shine like Sun and Cool like Moon. For the last almost 20 years (since 1998) AIIMS is doing research on the *Gayatri Mantra*. It has been found as the *Magic Mantra* and a *Magic Medicine/ Panacea* for curing and healing all the ills and ailments of body, mind, heart and soul. Not only this it dramatically enhances your brain power and the overall quality of life. It enhances your life longevity too. This mantra rejuvenates and refreshes your cells and genes. This mantra generates new waves in the brain. Now even medical journalism and the science of medicine has stamped its startling impact on life.

This mantra does wonders and miracles in our life, We must daily recite/chant this mantra for better life. It to be treated as an integrated and inseparable part of daily diet. It is diet of life. It infuses in your life new energy. It is diet for maintaining a good physical, mental, emotional, psychological and spiritual health. This mantra has an unique and special significance in our life. This mantra is recited on all the auspicious occasions. It is one of the top mantras in all. This mantra helps you in harnessing your hidden potential.

How Gayatri Mantra is improving the Physical and Mental Health of People?

Gayatri mantra benefits have played an important role in improving the professional and personal lives of the people. In spite of hectic pressure, they remain committed to their goals and remain positive in face of failures. Chanting verses plays a crucial role in the well being of the people. If you are in depression find solace in the Gayatri Prayer and feel happy as well as contented.

Who has not heard of gayatri mantra? Probably every body does however not many are aware about the great benefits it provides. Composed in Sanskrit, the verses appear to be parts of a conventional poem but the effects of reciting them are long lasting and extra ordinary. So, let us find out how they benefit us in our daily lives. Perform Gayatri mantra Jaap in the morning and evening to attain peace of mind. The divine word cleanses the soul of the impurities in the form of bad thoughts. Kids and adult can improve their focus and concentration with the chanting of mantras. Relish the calmness and interact with the subconscious mind as each word seems to come deeply from within the soul.

Calmness of the mind:

Modern life is replete with tension that might impact not only mental but physical health. Chanting mantras bring calmness to the brain switching it off from the hustle and bustle of surroundings. It helps people to meet the challenges of life with renewed confidence. While chanting word OM, the body right from the tongue to skull reverberates ensuring the passage of the air. The body releases relaxing hormones to calm the soothing nerves.

Enhances the concentration:

People realize gayatri mantra benefits in the form of increased concentration and memory power. It plays an important role in activating the three chakras which include eye, throat and crown. They are important parts of the body connecting brain, Penial glands and the eyes. Once the vibrations travel inside the body, they increase the focus and the concentration power of the individual.

Improvement in respiration:

While chanting gayatri manthram, people tend to perform deep breathing. It helps to clear congestion of the wind pipe and also improves the health of the lungs. Increased level of oxygen in blood enhances the stamina of the person during the performance of the physical and mental tasks.

Relaxation:

Mantras are instrumental in facilitating breathing; therefore they improve the functioning of the cardiac muscles. Apart from synchronizing heart beats, they are instrumental in controlling the blood pressure. People who have the habit of regularly reciting mantras rarely get affected with heart related disorders.

Nervous system:

One of the most important effects of the Gayatri mantra Jaap is that it vibrates the inner organs of the body making the nervous system robust. It can stimulate the neurotransmitters to transfer impulses and enhances the alert level of the body. In addition, the verses also improve the immune system of the body to ward of diseases. By using the mantras, the body can easily withstand the physical and mental stress.

Could chanting ancient Sanskrit mantras increase the size of your brain?

Scientists have put forward a theory that memorising ancient mantras could increase the size of brain regions associated with cognitive function. In a study led by neuroscientist and postdoctoral researcher Dr James Hartzell, the brain's massive grey matter density and cortical thickness was found to increase in those who had learnt and routinely recited the Sanskrit texts for the past decade.

For the study, Dr Hartzell, who coined the term, 'The Sanskrit Effect', compared the brains of 21 male participants with those of 21 professional Vedic Sanskrit Pandits who had memorised the Yajurveda Saṃhitā text and trained since childhood to memorise, recite and master the exact pronunciation of the ancient texts. What he and his research team found was massive grey matter density and cortical thickness increases in Pandit brains in language, memory and visual systems.

"The findings provide unique insight into the brain organisation implementing formalized oral knowledge systems," Dr Hartzell told SBS Hindi.

"In the cerebellum – which is the back lower part of the brain which coordinates both your motor and your cognitive functions – we found that 33 percent of the Pandits' cerebellum grey matter was denser or more increased compared to the [other participants], which was remarkable."

"We had never seen any studies that showed such a large increase in the Hippocampus and this is incredibly important for understanding how memory works in the brain." he told SBS Hindi.

"We don't know yet, the answer to the question, whether the difference in the brain could be because of memorizing such a large text or because memorising a text in the Sanskrit language is having an impact.

"One is that the Sanskrit tradition itself says that the sound of the Sanskrit language, the mantras, the meaning and the sound all of this has a very specific effect different from other languages, different than Hindi, English, Tibetan or Pali and so on, so the tradition makes that claim and that's a very well worked out idea in the tradition."

Study of Mahamrityunjaya Mantra Chanting on Severe Traumatic Brain Injured Patient.

At Delhi's Ram Manohar Lohia hospital, Selected comatose patients with serious brain injury have undergone a treatment that is not a usual part of hospital regimens— the chanting of an ancient Vedic mantra that is believed to ward off untimely death. This treatment, condoned by the hospital, is part of a study for which the Indian government has sanctioned research funds.

In 2014, Dr Ashok Kumar, then a resident neuropharmacologist at the All India Institute of Medial Sciences, proposed a pilot study on the "role of intercessory prayer in determining the outcome after severe traumatic brain injury." Intercessory prayers are offered by people on behalf of someone else. The prayer in question is the Mahamrityunjaya chant, a mantra from the Rig Veda, one of the oldest texts of Hinduism. Kumar's study attempted to determine whether the chanting of this mantra on behalf of patients with severe traumatic brain injury, or STBI, would play a role in improving their health outcomes. STBI is caused by external trauma to the head, such as from a fall, a car crash or an otherwise violent movement of the head.

महा मृत्युंजय मन्त्र

ॐ त्र्यम्बकं यजामहे सुगन्धिं पुष्टिवर्धनम्
उर्वारूकमिव बन्धनान् मृत्योर्मुक्षीय मा मृतात्

महा मृत्युंजय मन्त्र का अर्थ

समस्त संसार के पालनहार
तीन नेत्रो वाले शिव की हम अराधना करते है
विश्व मे सुरभि फैलाने वाले भगवान शिव
मृत्यु न कि मोक्ष से हमे मुक्ति दिलाएं

To carry out this study, Kumar applied to the Indian Council of Medical Research, or ICMR, for a research fellowship. The ICMR is the apex body in India for the formulation and promotion of biomedical research and is overseen by the ministry of health and family welfare. In March 2016, the ICMR approved the fellowship, and sanctioned Rs 28,000 per month for the study. The funds were awarded for one year starting October 2016, and then renewed for the next two years.

Kumar had initially proposed that the project be conducted at AIIMS, where he was then employed. However, Kumar said the ethics committee at AIIMS rejected the project as "unscientific." He then proposed the project to the Ram Manohar Lohia hospital. The ethics committee at RML sanctioned the project after six rounds of queries about different aspects of the study, which Kumar had to answer. In a written submission to the RML ethics committee, Kumar said that the study aims to "evaluate whether intercessory prayer has any direct or indirect effect on an unconscious STBI patient and reduces the psychological stress and serum cytokines level and improves the patient outcome." Cytokines are small secreted proteins released by cells that impact the interactions and communications between cells. Traumatic brain injury triggers an immune response which activates a number of cells and cytokines which may contribute to secondary brain damage.

"In the Ramayana, before Lord Rama built the bridge to Lanka, he offered the Mahamrityunjaya mantra," Kumar, presently a senior research fellow at RML's neurosurgery department, told me. "In ancient India, when soldiers got injured in war, this mantra was used to revive them. There are lots of studies among Christians that people with breast cancer and cardiovascular disease who go to church have improved outcomes. Hindu civilisation is more ancient than Christianity and the aim of this project is to prove that there is scientific basis to Hindu belief."

The hypothesis of Kumar's study is that "intercessory prayer generates spiritual vibrations, which are believed to be involved in the development of positive faith, and reduce psychological stress, which might be associated with cytokines reduction and a better STBI outcome." He conducted the study for nearly three years from October 2016 to April 2019 at the RML hospital. It involved 40 patients divided into two groups of twenty. Intercessory prayer was conducted for one group while the other group served as a control group whose treatment continued without any prayers offered on their behalf. The objective was to compare the medical outcomes of both groups. Written permission was taken from the relatives of the patients for whom the prayers were conducted. The project called for the Mahamrityunjaya chant to be recited 1.25 lakh times over a period of seven days per patient. There were two criteria to select patients—the prayers needed to commence within 24 hours of the injury, and the patient needed a score of between 4 and 8 on the Glasgow scale—in other words, a state of severe coma. The Glasgow scale measures the level of consciousness in a person following traumatic brain injury, from severe, which is 8 or less, to mild, which is between 13 and 15. Since the doctors at the RML hospital did not know the intricacies of the chant, Kumar roped in teachers from the Lal Bahadur Shastri Rashtriya Sanskrit Vidyapeetha, a university in Delhi that imparts instruction in traditional Sanskrit. The Vidyapeetha is a public institution under the ministry of human resource development. "Their head of department of medical astrology was very interested and fine-tuned the Mahamrityunjaya chant for our project," Kumar said, referring to the Vidyapeetha. "The name of the patient, date of birth, place of birth and gotra"—a Hindu system of patrilineal kinship—"were included in the chant." A professor from the Vidyapeetha came with Ganga jal—water from the Ganga River—to do shuddhi, or purification, for the selected patient, and then offered the prayer on the patient's behalf at a temple in the Vidyapeetha premesis. Meanwhile, at the RML hospital, Kumar took blood samples before and after the seven-day prayer period.

Bibliography and Acknowledgement

- Bansal R., Maroof K.A., Parashar P., Pant B. Spirituality and health: a knowledge, attitude and practice study among doctors of North India. *Spiritual Health Int*. 2008; **9**:263–269.
- Bernardi L, Sleight P, Bandinelli G, Cencetti S, Fattorini L, Wdowczyc-Szulc J, *et al.* Effect of rosary prayer and yoga mantras on autonomic cardiovascular rhythms: Comparative study. *BMJ*. 2001; **323**:1446–9.
- Bhatta KV. 4th ed. South Canara: Kaitanje Prakashan; 2004. Shri Gayatri Mantra Rahasya.
- Derrickson BS. The spiritual work of the dying: a framework and case studies. *Hosp J*. 1996;**11**:11–30.
- Filbey FM, Russell T, Morris RG, Murray RM, McDonald C. Functional magnetic resonance imaging (fMRI) of attention processes in presumed obligate carriers of schizophrenia: Preliminary findings. *Ann Gen Psychiatry*. 2008;7:18.
- Harshananda S. 3rd ed. Chennai: Ramkrishna Math; 2010. Upanayana, Sandhya Vandana and Gayatri Mantra Japa.
- Kalyani BG, Venkatasubramanian G, Arasappa R, Rao NP, Kalmady SV, Behere RV, *et al.* Neurohemodynamic correlates of 'OM' chanting: A pilot functional magnetic resonance imaging study. *Int J Yoga*. 2011;4:3–6.
- Leighton S. When mortality calls, don't hang up. *Spiritual Life*. 1996; **22**(3):150–157.
- Moberg D. Spiritual well-being of the dying. In: Lesnoff-Caravaglia G, editor. Aging and the Human Condition. New York: Human Science Press; 1982.
- Natu MV, Agarwal AK. Testing of stimulant effects of coffee on the psychomotor performance: An exercise in clinical pharmacology. *Indian J Pharmachol*. 1997; **29**:11–4.
- Shimomura T, Fujiki M, Akiyoshi J, Yoshida T, Tabata M, Kabasawa H, *et al.* Functional brain mapping during recitation of Buddhist scriptures and repetition of the Namu Amida Butsu: A study in experienced Japanese monks. *Turk Neurosurg*. 2008; **18**:134–41.
- Sripad G, Nagendra HR, Bhatta R, Vivekananda S, Samsthana YA, Bhawan E, *et al.* Effect of vedic chanting on memory and sustained attention. *Indian J Tradit Knowl*. 2006;5:177–80.
- Stuckelberger A. 2005. Spirituality, Religion and Health United Nations Geneva Panel Report: "Spirituality, Religion and Social Health" 58th World Health Assembly in Geneva. http://www.rcrescendo.org/11.Siritualitetpastorale/GINEBRA/SPIRITUALITY.pdf Available from: *J Relig Health*. 5 Sep 2013.
- Sushrutha S, Manjunath NK, Bhatta R. Karnataka: 2009. Changes in higher brain functions following recitation of gayatri mantra. M. Sc dissertation Swami Vivekananda Yoga Anushandhan Samsthana, Bangaluru.
- Telles S, Nagarathna R, Nagendra HR. Autonomic changes while mentally repeating two syllables: One meaningful and the other neutral. *Indian J Physiol Pharmacol*. 1998;42:57–63.
- Weiss EM, Siedentopf C, Golaszewski S, Mottaghy FM, Hofer A, Kremser C, *et al.* Brain activation patterns during a selective attention test-a functional MRI study in healthy volunteers and unmedicated patients during an acute episode of schizophrenia. *Psychiatry Res*. 2007;154:31–40.
- Yach D. 2008. Report from the World Health Organization: Closing the Gap in a Generation: Health Equity Through Action on the Social Determinants of Health.http://en.wikipedia.org/wiki/Social_determinants_of_health Available from: Levin J. Wiley, A Division of Bennett, Coleman and Co. Ltd; New Delhi: 2001.

Herbal Medicine In Treatment of Cardiovascular Diseases (Review)

Herbs have been used as medical treatments since the beginning of civilization and some derivatives (eg, aspirin, reserpine, and digitalis) have become mainstays of human pharmacotherapy. For cardiovascular diseases, herbal treatments have been used in patients with congestive heart failure, systolic hypertension, angina pectoris, atherosclerosis, cerebral insufficiency, venous insufficiency, and arrhythmia. However, many herbal remedies used today have not undergone careful scientific assessment, and some have the potential to cause serious toxic effects and major drug-to-drug interactions. With the high prevalence of herbal use in the United States today, clinicians must inquire about such health practices for cardiac disease and be informed about the potential for benefit and harm. Continuing research is necessary to elucidate the pharmacological activities of the many herbal remedies now being used to treat cardiovascular diseases. Since the beginning of human civilization, herbs have been an integral part of society, valued for both their culinary and medicinal properties. Herbal medicine has made many contributions to commercial drug preparations manufactured today including ephedrine from Ephedra sinica (ma-huang), digitoxin from Digitalis purpurea(foxglove), salicin (the source of aspirin) from Salix alba (willow bark), and reserpine from Rauwolfia serpentina (snakeroot), to name just a few. A naturally occurring β-adrenergic blocking agent with partial agonism has been identified in an herbal remedy. The recent discovery of the antineoplastic drug paclitaxel from Taxus brevifolia (pacific yew tree) stresses the role of plants as a continuing resource for modern medicine.

However, with the development of patent medicines in the early part of the 20th century, herbal medicine has been losing ground to new synthetic medicines touted by scientists and physicians to be more effective and reliable. Nevertheless, about 3% of English-speaking adults in the United States still report having used herbal remedies in the preceding year.This figure is probably much higher for non–English-speaking Americans. Despite this heavy use of herbal medicines in the United States, health practitioners often fail to ask about their use when taking clinical histories. It is imperative that physicians become more aware of the wide array of herbal medicines available, as well as learning more about their beneficial and adverse effects.

Table 33.1: *Potential applications for therapy in cardiovascular conditions of some common Herbal Medicines*

Herb	Possible Cardiovascular Indications
Hawthorn (*Crataegus* species)	Heart failure, angina, hyperlipidemia
Garlic (*Allium sativum*)	Hypertension, hyperlipidemia, antithrombotic
Danshen (*Salvia miltiorrhiza*)	Angina, ischemic stroke, hyperlipidemia, antithrombotic
Lingzhi (*Ganoderma lucidum*)	Hyperlipidemia, hypertension, diabetes
Ginkgo (*Ginkgo biloba*)	Cerebral insufficiency, peripheral vascular disease, antithrombotic
Foxglove (*Digitalis* species)	Heart failure, atrial fibrillation
Ginseng (*Panax* species)	Angina, hypertension, diabetes

Part of the problem for both consumers and physicians has been the paucity of scientific data on herbal medicines used in the United States. As a result, those who wish to obtain factual information regarding the therapeutic use or potential harm of herbal remedies would have to obtain it from books and pamphlets, most of which base their information on traditional reputation rather than relying on existing scientific research. One may wonder why the herbal industry never chose to simply prove its products safe and effective. The answer is primarily economical. With the slim chance of patent protection for the many herbs that have been in use for centuries, pharmaceutical companies have not provided financial support for research on the merits of herbal medicine. At the same time, the National Institutes of Health have only been able to offer limited funding for this purpose.

Congestive Heart Failure

A number of herbs contain potent cardioactive glycosides, which have positive inotropic actions on the heart. The drugs digitoxin, derived from either *D purpurea* (foxglove) or *Digitalis lanata*, and digoxin, derived from *D lanata* alone, have been used in the treatment of congestive heart failure for many decades. Cardiac glycosides have a low therapeutic index, and the dose must be adjusted to the needs of each patient. The only way to control dosage is to use standardized powdered digitalis, digitoxin, or digoxin. When 12 different strains of *D lanata* plants were cultured and examined, their total cardenolide yield ranged from 30 to almost 1000 nmol/1 g. As is evident, treating congestive heart failure with nonstandardized herbal drugs would be dangerous and foolhardy.

Some common plant sources of cardiac glycosides include *D purpurea* (foxglove, already mentioned), *Adonis microcarpa* and *Adonis vernalis* (adonis), *Apocynum cannabinum* (black Indian hemp), *Asclepiascurassavica* (redheaded cotton bush), *Asclepias friticosa* (balloon cotton), *Calotropis precera* (king's crown), *Carissa spectabilis* (wintersweet), *Cerebra manghas* (sea mango), *Cheiranthus cheiri* (wallflower), *Convallaria majalis* (lily of the valley, convallaria), *Cryptostegia grandiflora* (rubber vine), *Helleborus niger* (black hellebore), *Helleborus viridus*, *Nerium oleander* (oleander), *Plumeria rubra* (frangipani), *Selenicerus grandiflorus* (cactus grandiflorus), *Strophanthus hispidus* and *Strophanthus kombe* (strophanus), *Thevetia peruviana* (yellow oleander), and *Urginea maritima* (squill) Even the venom glands of the animal *Bufo marinus* (cane toad) contain cardiac glycosides. Recently, the digitalislike steroid in the venom of the *B marinus* toad was identified as a previously described steroid, marinobufagenin. Marinobufagenin demonstrated high digoxinlike immunoreactivity and was antagonized with an antidigoxin antibody.

Accidental poisonings and even suicide attempts with ingestion of cardiac glycosides are abundant in the medical literature. Some herbal remedies (eg, Siberian ginseng) can elevate synthetic digoxin drug levels and cause toxic effects. In the United States, there are about 15,000 intoxications due to accidental or intentional ingestion of poisonous plants annually In 1993, 2388 toxic exposures in the United States were reported to be due to plant glycosides. Of these, the largest percentage were attributed to oleander (ie, 25%). In the case of oleander, all plant tissues, including the seeds, roots, stems, leaves, berries, and blossoms, are considered extremely toxic. In fact, death in humans has been reported following ingestion of as little as 1 oleander leaf. The clinical manifestations of oleander intoxication, as well as other natural glycosides, is virtually identical to digoxin overdose. Morbidity and mortality are mainly related to cardiotoxic adverse effects that usually include life-threatening ventricular tachyarrhythmias, bradycardia, and heart block. The diagnosis should rely on the clinical presentation of unexplained hyperkalemia, and cardiac, neurologic, and gastrointestinal symptoms.

The diagnosis can be further supported by the detection of the substance digoxin in a radioimmunoassay for digoxin. However, the extent of cross-reactivity between the cardiac glycosides from herbal sources and antibodies used in the radioimmunoassays has not been clearly defined. For this reason, digoxin assays may serve to confirm the suspected diagnosis but not to quantify the severity. Once the diagnosis has been established, the use of digoxin-specific Fab antibody fragments may be helpful in the treatment of severe intoxication. Other modalities, such as dialysis, cannot be easily facilitated because, like digoxin, natural glycosides are distributed extensively into peripheral tissues.

Hypertension

The root of *R serpentina* (snakeroot), the natural source of the alkaloid reserpine, has been a Hindu Ayurvedic remedy since ancient times. In 1931, Indian literature first described the use of *R serpentina* root for the treatment of hypertension and psychoses; however, the use of *Rauwolfia* alkaloids in Western medicine did not begin until the mid1940s. Both standardized whole root preparations of *R serpentina* and its reserpine alkaloid are officially monographed in the United States Pharmacopeia A powdered whole root of 200 to 300 mg orally is equivalent to 0.5 mg of reserpine Reserpine was one of the first drugs used on a large scale to treat systemic hypertension. It acts by irreversibly blocking the uptake of biogenic amines (norepinephrine, dopamine, and serotonin) in the storage vesicles of central and peripheral adrenergic neurons, thus leaving the catecholamines to be destroyed by the intraneuronal monoamine oxidase in the cytoplasm. The depletion of catecholamines accounts for reserpine's sympatholytic and antihypertensive actions. Reserpine's effects are long lasting, since recovery of sympathetic function requires synthesis of new storage vesicles, which takes days to weeks. Reserpine lowers blood pressure by decreasing cardiac output, peripheral vascular resistance, heart rate, and renin secretion. With the introduction of other antihypertensive drugs with fewer central nervous system adverse effects, the use of reserpine has diminished.

The daily oral dose of reserpine should be 0.25 mg or less, and as little as 0.05 mg if given with a diuretic. Using the whole root, the usual adult dose is 50 to 200 mg/d administered once daily or in 2 divided doses

Rauwolfia alkaloids are contraindicated for use in patients with previously demonstrated hypersensitivity to these substances, in patients with a history of mental depression (especially with suicidal tendencies), in patients with active peptic ulcer disease or ulcerative colitis, and in patients receiving electroconvulsive therapy. The most common adverse effects are sedation and inability to concentrate and perform complex tasks. Reserpine may cause mental depression, sometimes resulting in suicide, and its use must be discontinued at the first sign of depression. Reserpine's sympatholytic effect and its enhancement of parasympathetic actions account for its well-described adverse effects : nasal congestion, increased gastric secretion, and mild diarrhea.

Stephania tetrandra is an herb sometimes used in traditional Chinese medicine to treat hypertension. Tetrandrine, an alkaloid extract of *S tetrandra*, has been shown to be a calcium ion channel antagonist, paralleling the effects of verapamil. Tetrandrine blocks T and L calcium channels, interferes with the binding of diltiazem and methoxyverapamil at calcium-channel binding sites, and suppresses aldosterone production.

A parenteral dose (15 mg/kg) of tetrandrine in conscious rats decreases mean, systolic, and diastolic blood pressures for more than 30 minutes; however, an intravenous 40-mg/kg dose killed the rats by myocardial depression. In stroke-prone hypertensive rats, an oral dose of 25 or 50 mg/kg produced a gradual and sustained hypotensive effect after 48 hours without affecting plasma renin activity In addition to its cardiovascular actions, tetrandrine has reported antineoplastic, immunosuppressive, and mutagenic effects.

Tetrandrine is 90% protein-bound with an elimination half-life of 88 minutes, according to dog studies; however, rat studies have shown a sustained hypotensive effect for more than 48 hours after a 25- or 50-mg oral dose. Tetrandrine causes liver necrosis in dogs orally administered 40 mg/kg of tetrandrine 3 times weekly for 2 months, reversible swelling of liver cells with a 20-mg/kg dose, and no observable changes with a 10-mg/kg dose. Given the evidence of hepatotoxicity, many more studies are necessary to establish a safe dosage of tetrandrine in humans.

More recently, tetrandrine has been implicated in an outbreak of rapidly progressive renal failure, termed *Chinese herb nephropathy*. Numerous individuals developed the condition after using a combination of several Chinese herbs as part of a dieting regimen. It has been hypothesized that the cause may be attributed to misidentification of *S tetrandra*; nonetheless, questions still remain as to the role of tetrandra in the development of this serious toxic effect.

The root of *Lingusticum wallichii* is used in traditional Chinese medicine as a circulatory stimulant, hypotensive drug, and sedative Tetramethylpyrazine, the active constituent extracted from *L wallichii*, inhibits platelet aggregation in vitro and lowers blood pressure by vasodilation in dogs. With its actions independent of the endothelium, tetramethylpyrazine's vasodilatory effect is mediated by calcium channel antagonism and nonselective antagonism of α-adrenergic receptors. Some evidence suggests that tetramethylpyrazine acts on the pulmonary vasculature. Currently, there is insufficient information to evaluate the safety and efficacy of this herbal medicinal.

Uncaria rhynchophylla is sometimes used in traditional Chinese medicine to treat hypertension. Its indole alkaloids, rhynchophylline and hirsutine, are thought to be the active principles of *U rhynchophylla's* vasodilatory effect. The mechanism of *U rhynchophylla's* actions is unclear. Some studies point to an alteration in calcium ion flux in response to activation, whereas others point to hirsutine's inhibition of nicotine-induced dopamine release. One in vitro study has shown *U rhynchophylla* extract relaxes norepinephrine - precontracted rat aorta through endothelium - dependent and - independent mechanisms. For the endothelium-dependent component, *U rhynchophylla* extract appears to stimulate endothelium-derived relaxing factor and/or nitric oxide release without involving muscarinic receptors. Also, in vitro and in vivo studies have shown that rhynchophylline can inhibit platelet aggregation and reduce platelet thromboses induced with collagen or adenosine diphosphate plus epinephrine.[31] Safety and efficacy cannot be evaluated at this time because of a lack of clinical data.

Veratrum (hellebore) is a perennial herb grown in many parts of the world. Varieties include *Veratrumviride* from Canada and the eastern United States, *Veratrumcalifornicum* from the western United States, *Veratrumalbum* from

Alaska and Europe, and *Veratrum japonicum* from Asia. All *Veratrum* plants contain poisonous alkaloids known to cause vomiting, bradycardia, and hypotension. Most cases of *Veratrum* poisonings are due to misidentification with other plants. Although once a treatment for hypertension, the use of *Veratrum* alkaloids has lost favor owing to a low therapeutic index and unacceptable toxicity, as well as the introduction of safer antihypertensive drug alternatives. *Veratrum* alkaloids enhance nerve and muscle excitability by increasing sodium ion conductivity. They act on the posterior wall of the left ventricle and the coronary sinus baroreceptors, causing reflex hypotension and bradycardia via the vagus nerve (Bezold-Jarisch reflex). Nausea and vomiting are secondary to the alkaloids' actions on the nodose ganglion. The diagnosis of *Veratrum* toxicity is established by history, identification of the plant, and strong clinical suspicion. Clinical symptoms usually occur quickly, often within 30 minutes. Treatment is mainly supportive and directed at controlling bradycardia and hypotension. *Veratrum*-induced bradycardia usually responds to treatment with atropine; however, the blood pressure response to atropine is more variable and requires the addition of pressors. Other electrocardiographic changes, such as atrioventricular dissociation, may also be reversible with atropine. Seizures are a rare complication and may be treated with conventional anticonvulsants. For patients with preexisting cardiac disease, the use of β-agonists or pacing may be necessary. Nausea may be controlled with phenothiazine antiemetics. Recovery usually occurs within 24 to 48 hours. *Evodia rutaecarpa* (wu-chu-yu) is a Chinese herbal drug that has been used as a treatment for hypertension. It contains an active vasorelaxant component called rutaecarpine that can cause endothelium-dependent vasodilation in experimental models.

Angina Pectoris

Crataegus hawthorn, a name encompassing many *Crataegus* species (such as *Crataegus oxyacantha* and *Crataegus monogyna* in the West and *Crataegus pinnatifida* in China) has acquired the reputation in modern herbal literature as an important tonic for the cardiovascular system that is particularly useful for angina. *Crataegus* leaves, flowers, and fruits contain a number of biologically active substances, such as oligomeric procyanins, flavonoids, and catechins. From current studies, *Crataegus* extract appears to have antioxidant properties and can inhibit the formation of thromboxane as well. Also, *Crataegus* extract antagonizes the increases in cholesterol, triglyceride, and phospholipid levels in low-density lipoprotein (LDL) and very low-density lipoprotein in rats fed a hyperlipidemic diet; thus, it may inhibit the progression of atherosclerosis. This hypocholesterolemic action may be due to an up-regulation of hepatic LDL receptors resulting in greater influx of plasma cholesterol into the liver. *Crataegus* also prevents cholesterol accumulation in the liver by enhancing cholesterol degradation to bile acids, as well as suppressing cholesterol biosynthesis.

According to another study, *Crataegus* extract, in high concentrations, has a cardio protective effect on ischemic-reperfused hearts without causing an increase in coronary blood flow. On the other hand, oral and parenteral administration of oligomeric procyanins of *Crataegus* has been shown to lead to an increase in coronary blood flow in both cats and dogs. Double-blind clinical trials have demonstrated simultaneous cardiotropic and vasodilatory actions of *Crataegus*. In essence, *Crataegus* increases coronary perfusion, has a mild hypotensive effect, antagonizes atherogenesis, and has positive inotropic and negative chronotropic actions. In a recent multicenter, placebo - controlled, double-blind study, an extract of *Crataegus*was shown to clearly improve the cardiac performance of patients with New York Heart Association class II heart failure. In this study, the primary parameter analyzed was the heart rate product (systolic blood pressure × heart rate) Recent studies have suggested that the mechanism of cardiac action for *Crataegus* species may be due to the inhibition of the 3', 5'- cyclic adenosine monophosphate phosphodiesterase

Hawthorn is relatively devoid of adverse effects. In fact, in comparison with other inotropic drugs such as epinephrine, amrinone, milrinone, and digoxin, *Crataegus* has a potentially reduced arrhythmogenic risk because of its ability to prolong the effective refractory period, while the other drugs mentioned previously all shorten this parameter. Also, it should be noted that concomitant use of hawthorn with digitalis can markedly enhance the activity of digitalis Undoubtedly, more studies are needed to show that hawthorn can be used safely and effectively.

Because of its resemblance to *Panax ginseng* (Asian ginseng), *Panax notoginseng* has acquired the common name of pseudoginseng, especially since it is often an adulterant of *P ginseng* preparations. In traditional Chinese medicine, the root of *P notoginseng* is used for analgesia and hemostasis. It is also often used in the treatment of patients with angina and coronary artery disease. *Panax notoginseng* has been described as a calcium ion channel antagonist in vascular tissue. More specifically, its pharmacological action may be as a novel and selective calcium ion antagonist that does not interact with the L-type calcium ion channel but rather may interact with the receptor-operated calcium ion channel.

Although clinical trials are lacking, in vitro studies using *P notoginseng* suggest possible cardiovascular effects. One study that used purified notoginsenoside R1, extracted from *P notoginseng*, on human left umbilical vein endothelial cells showed a dose- and time-dependent synthesis of tissue-type plasminogen activating factor without affecting the synthesis of plasminogen activating inhibitor. Thus, fibrinolytic parameters were enhanced. Another study suggests that *P notoginseng* saponins may inhibit atherogenesis by interfering with the proliferation of smooth muscle cells. In vitro and in vivo studies using rats and rabbits demonstrate that *P notoginseng* may be useful as an antianginal drug, since it dilates coronary arteries in all concentrations. The role of *P notoginseng* in the treatment of hypertension is less certain, since *P notoginseng* causes vasodilation or vasoconstriction depending on the concentration and target vessel. The results of these in vitro and in vivo studies are encouraging; however, clinical trials will be necessary to make a more informed decision regarding the use of *P notoginseng*.

Salvia miltiorrhiza (dan-shen), a relative of the Western sage *Salvia officinalis*, is native to China. In traditional Chinese medicine, the root of *S miltiorrhiza* is used as a circulatory stimulant, sedative, and cooling drug .*Salvia miltiorrhiza* may be useful as an antianginal drug because it has been shown to dilate coronary arteries in all concentrations, similar to *P notoginseng*. Also, *S miltiorrhiza* has variable action on other vessels depending on its concentration, so it may not be as helpful in treating hypertension. In vitro, *S miltiorrhiza*, in a dose-dependent fashion, inhibits platelet aggregation and serotonin release induced by either adenosine diphosphate or epinephrine, which is thought to be mediated by an increase in platelet cyclic adenosine monophosphate caused by *S miltiorrhiza's* inhibition of cyclic adenosine monophosphate phosphodiesterase. *Salvia miltiorrhiza* appears to have a protective action on ischemic myocardium, enhancing the recovery of contractile force on reoxygenation. More recently, *S miltiorrhiza* has been shown to protect myocardial mitochondrial membranes from ischemia-reperfusion injury and lipid peroxidation because of its free radical–scavenging effects. Qualitatively and quantitatively, a decoction of *S miltiorrhiza* was as efficacious as the more expensive isolated tanshinones.

Clinical trials will be necessary to evaluate the safety and efficacy of ***S miltiorrhiza.*** Of note, it has been observed clinically that when *S miltiorrhiza* and warfarin sodium are coadministered, there is an increased incidence in warfarin-related adverse effects; in rats *S miltiorrhiza* was shown to increase the plasma concentrations of warfarin as well as the prothrombin time.

Atherosclerosis

In addition to its use in the culinary arts, garlic (*Allium sativum*) has been valued for centuries for its medicinal properties. Garlic is one of the herbal medicines that has been examined more closely by the scientific community. In recent decades, research has focused on garlic's use in preventing atherosclerosis. Garlic, like many of the other herbal medicines discussed previously, has demonstrated multiple beneficial cardiovascular effects. A number of studies have demonstrated these effects that include lowering blood pressure, inhibiting platelet aggregation, enhancing fibrinolytic activity, reducing serum cholesterol and triglyceride levels, and protecting the elastic properties of the aorta.

Consumption of large quantities of fresh garlic (0.25 to 1.0 g/kg or about 5-20 average sized 4-g cloves in a person weighing 78.7 kg) has been shown to produce the beneficial effects mentioned earlier. In support of this, a recent double-blind cross-over study was conducted on moderately hypercholesterolemic men that compared the effects of 7.2 g of aged garlic extract with placebo on blood lipid levels. This study found that there was a maximal reduction of 6.1% in total serum cholesterol levels and 4.6% in LDL cholesterol levels with garlic compared with placebo. However, despite positive evidence from numerous trials, some investigators have been hesitant to outright endorse the routine use of garlic for cardiovascular disease because many of the published studies had methodological shortcomings, perhaps because constituent trials were small, lacking statistical power. Also, inappropriate methods of randomization, lack of dietary run-in period, short duration, or failure to undertake intention-to-treat analysis may explain the cautious acceptance of previous meta-analyses. In fact, one recent study found no demonstrable effect of garlic ingestion on lipid and lipoprotein levels. This study used a cross-over design protected by a washout period to reduce between-subject variability as well as close assessment and reporting of dietary behavior, which had been lacking in previous trials.

Another study found no effect of garlic on cholesterol absorption, cholesterol synthesis, or cholesterol metabolism. As is evident, the precise extent of garlic's impact on atherosclerosis remains controversial; larger, more rigorously designed trials may be necessary to better determine its utility in preventing cardiovascular disease. Garlic has also been studied in hypertensive patients as a blood pressure–lowering agent. Similar to its lipid effects, no conclusive studies have been conducted and many methodological shortcomings exist in study designs. The results of one meta-analysis that considered

8 different trials suggest some clinical use for patients with mild hypertension, but there is insufficient evidence to recommend its use as routine clinical therapy. Garlic has also been shown to possess antiplatelet activity. In the past, this action was mostly documented in vitro. A new study examined the effect of the consumption of a fresh clove of garlic on platelet thromboxane production and showed that after 26 weeks, serum thromboxane levels were reduced about 80%. This may prove to be beneficial in the prevention of thrombosis in the future. Recently, the effect of long-term garlic intake on the elastic properties of the aorta was also studied. Participants in the trial (limited to those aged 50-80 years) consumed 300 mg/d of standardized garlic powder for more than 2 years. The results showed that the pulse-wave velocity and standardized elastic vascular resistance of the aorta were lower in the garlic group than in the control group. Consequently, long-term garlic powder intake may have a protective effect on the elastic properties of the aorta related to aging. In these ways, garlic has shown numerous beneficial cardiovascular effects that need to be investigated further to determine its therapeutic utility.

Intact cells of garlic bulbs include an odorless, sulfur-containing amino acid known as *allinin*. When garlic is crushed, allinin comes into contact with allinase, which converts allinin to allicin. Allicin has potent antibacterial properties, but it is also highly odoriferous and unstable. Ajoenes, self-condensation products of allicin, appear to be responsible for garlic's antithrombotic activity. Most authorities now agree that allicin and its derivatives are the active constituents of garlic's physiological activity. Fresh garlic releases allicin in the mouth during the chewing process. Dried garlic preparations lack allicin but contain allinin and allinase. Since allinase is inactivated in the stomach, dried garlic preparations should be coated with enteric so that they pass through the stomach into the small intestine where allinin can be enzymatically converted to allicin. Few commercial garlic preparations are standardized for their allicin yield based on allinin content, hence making their effectiveness less certain.[5]However, one double-blind, placebo-controlled study involving 261 patients for 4 months using one 800-mg tablet of garlic powder daily, standardized to 1.3% allinin content, demonstrated significant reductions in total cholesterol (12%) and triglyceride levels (17%)

Aside from a garlic odor on the breath and body, moderate garlic consumption causes few adverse effects. However, consumption in excess of 5 cloves daily may result in heartburn, flatulence, and other gastrointestinaldisturbances. Some people have reported allergic reactions to garlic, most commonly allergic contact dermatitis. Patchtesting with 1% diallyl disulfide is recommended when garlic allergy is suspected. Because of its antithrombotic activity, garlic should be used with caution in people taking oral anticoagulants concomitantly.

The resin of *Commiphora mukul* (gugulipid), a small, thorny tree native to India, has long been used in Ayurvedic medicine to treat lipid disorders. The primary mechanism of action of gugulipid is through an increase in the uptake and metabolism of LDL cholesterol by the liver. In a double-blind, cross-over study completed in 125 patients taking gugulipid compared with 108 patients taking clofibrate, the average decrease in serum cholesterol and triglyceride levels was 11% and 16.8%, respectively, with gugulipid compared with 10% and 21.6%, respectively, with clofibrate. In general, hypercholesterolemic patients responded more favorably to gugulipid therapy than hypertriglyceridemic patients. Moreover, it was shown in another randomized, double-blind trial that C mukul also decreased LDL cholesterol levels by 12.5% and the total cholesterol–high-density lipoprotein cholesterol ratio by 11.1%, whereas the levels were unchanged in the placebo group.

Besides being potentially as effective in lowering blood lipid levels as modern hyperlipidemic drugs, gugulipid may even be safer. In the trial mentioned previously, compliance was greater than 96%, with only the adverse effects of headache, mild nausea, and hiccups noted. However, it has been shown that gugulipid may affect the bioavailability of other cardiovascular drugs, namely, propranolol hydrochloride and diltiazem hydrochloride. Gugulipid significantly reduced the peak plasma concentration and area under the curve of both these drugs, which may lead to diminished efficacy or nonresponsiveness. Undoubtedly, gugulipid is a natural lipid-lowering drug with potential for therapeutic use, but rigorous, larger clinical trials will be necessary to further evaluate its safety and efficacy before it can be endorsed as an alternative therapy for hyperlipidemia and prevention of atherosclerosis.

Maharishi amrit kalash-4 and *Maharishi amrit kalash*-5 are 2 complex herbal mixtures with significant antioxidant properties that have been shown to inhibit LDL oxidation in patients with hyperlipidemia. In experimental studies, the herbal mixtures have also been shown to inhibit enzymatic- and nonenzymatic-induced microsomal lipid peroxidation and platelet aggregation

Cerebral and Peripheral Vascular Disease

Having existed for more than 200 million years, Ginkgo biloba (maidenhair tree) was apparently saved from extinction by human intervention, surviving in Far Eastern temple gardens while disappearing for centuries in the West. It was reintroduced to Europe in 1730 and became a favorite ornamental tree. Although the root and kernels of G biloba have long been used in traditional Chinese medicine, the tree gained attention in the West during the 20th century for its medicinal value after a concentrated extract of G biloba leaves was developed in the 1960s. At least 2 groups of substances within G biloba extract (GBE) demonstrate beneficial pharmacological actions. The flavonoids reduce capillary permeability as well as fragility and serve as free radical scavengers. The terpenes (ie, ginkgolides) inhibit platelet-activating factor, decrease vascular resistance, and improve circulatory flow without appreciably affecting blood pressure. Continuing research appears to support the primary use of GBE for treating cerebral insufficiency and its secondary effects on vertigo, tinnitus, memory, and mood; also, GBE appears to be useful for treating peripheral vascular disease, including diabetic retinopathy and intermittent claudication.

In a randomized, placebo-controlled, double-blind study, EGb 761, which is a standardized extract of G biloba with respect to its flavonol glycoside and terpene lactone content, was shown to significantly decrease the areas of ischemia as measured by transcutaneous partial pressure of oxygen during exercise. Because of its rapid anti-ischemic action, EGb 761 may be valuable in the treatment of intermittent claudication and peripheral artery disease in general.

Also, studies have been examining the cardioprotective efficacy of EGb 761 in regard to its anti–free radical action in myocardial ischemia–reperfusion injury. In vitro studies with animal models have shown that this compound may exert such an effect. A clinical study of 15 patients undergoing coronary bypass surgery demonstrated that oral EGb 761 therapy may limit free radical–induced oxidative stress occurring in the systemic circulation and at the level of the myocardium during these operations. It remains to be studied whether extracts of G biloba may be used as pharmacological adjuvants to limit tissue damage and metabolic alterations following coronary bypass surgery, coronary angioplasty for acute myocardial infarctions, or even in managing coronary thrombosis.

Although approved as a drug in Europe, Ginkgo is not approved in the United States and is instead marketed as a food supplement, usually supplied as 40-mg tablets of extract. Since most of the investigations examining the efficacy of GBEs used preparations such as EGb 761 or LI 1370, the bioequivalence of other GBE products has not been established. The recommended dosage in Europe is one 40-mg tablet taken 3 times daily with meals (120 mg/d). Adverse effects due to GBE are rare but can include gastrointestinal disturbances, headache, and allergic skin rash.

Known mostly as a culinary spice and flavoring agent, Rosmarinus officinalis (rosemary) is listed in many herbal sources as a tonic and all-around stimulant. Traditionally, rosemary leaves are said to enhance circulation, aid digestion, elevate mood, and boost energy. When applied externally, the volatile oils are supposedly useful for arthritic conditions and baldness.

Although research on rosemary is scant, some studies have focused on antioxidant effects of diterpenoids, especially carnosic acid and carnosol, isolated from rosemary leaves. In addition to having antineoplastic effects, antioxidants in rosemary have been credited with stabilizing erythrocyte membranes and inhibiting superoxide generation and lipid peroxidation. Essential oils of rosemary have demonstrated antimicrobial, hyperglycemic, and insulin-inhibiting properties. Rosemary leaves contain high amounts of salicylates, and its flavonoid pigment diosmin is reported to decrease capillary permeability and fragility.

Despite the conclusions derived from in vitro and animal studies, the therapeutic use of rosemary for cardiovascular disorders remains questionable, because few, if any, clinical trials have been conducted using rosemary. Because of the lack of studies, no conclusions can be reached regarding the use of the antioxidants of rosemary in inhibiting atherosclerosis. Although external application may cause cutaneous vasodilation from the counterirritant properties of rosemary's essential oils, there is no evidence to support any prolonged improvement in peripheral circulation. While rosemary does have some carminative properties, it may also cause gastrointestinal and kidney disturbances in large doses. Until more studies are done, rosemary should probably be limited to its use as a culinary spice and flavoring agent rather than as a medicine.

Venous Insufficiency

The seeds of horse chestnut, Aesculus hippocastanum, have long been used in Europe to treat venous disorders such as varicose veins. The saponin glycoside aescin from horse chestnut extract (HCE) inhibits the activity of lysosomal enzymes thought to contribute to varicose veins by weakening vessel walls and increasing permeability, which result in dilated veins and edema. In fact, recent research has shown that A hippocastanum inhibits only against hyaluronidase but not elastase, and this activity is linked mainly to the saponin escin. In animal studies, HCE, in a dose-dependent fashion, increases venous tone, venous flow, and lymphatic flow. It also antagonizes capillary hyperpermeability induced by histamine, serotonin, or chloroform. This extract has been shown to decrease edema formation of lymphatic and inflammatory origin. Horse chestnut extract has antiexudative properties, suppressing experimentally induced pleurisy and peritonitis by inhibiting plasma extravasation and leukocyte emigration, and its dose-dependent antioxidant properties can inhibit in vitro lipid peroxidation. Randomized, double-blind, placebo-controlled trials with HCE show are eduction in edema, measured using plethysmography.

In another recent randomized, placebo-controlled study, the efficacy and safety of class 2 compression stockings and dried HCE were compared. Both HCE and the compression stockings decreased lower leg edema after 12 weeks of therapy; the results showed an average 43.8-mL reduction with HCE and 46.7-mL with compression stockings, while the placebo group showed an increase of 9.8 mL. Both HCE and compression therapy were well tolerated, with no serious adverse effects. This study may indicate that both of these modalities are reasonable alternatives for the effective treatment of patients with chronic venous insufficiency. Also, HCE has been shown to markedly improve other symptoms associated with chronic venous insufficiency, such as pain, tiredness, itching, and tension in the swollen leg, in a case-observation study. Aside from effects on venous insufficiency, prophylactic use of HCE has been thought to decrease the incidence of thromboembolic complications of gynecological surgery. However, since this issue is still controversial, this does not appear to be the case.

Standardized HCE is prepared as an aqueous alcohol extract of 16% to 21% of triterpene glycosides, calculated as aescin. The usual initial dosage is 90 to 150 mg/d of aescin, which may be reduced to 35 to 70 mg/d if clinical benefit is seen. Standardized HCE preparations are not available in the United States, but nonstandardized products may be available.

Some manufacturers promote the use of topical preparations of HCE for treatment of varicose veins as well as hemorrhoids; however, at least one study has demonstrated poor aescin distribution at sites other than the skin and muscle tissues underlying the application site. Moreover, the involvement of arterioles and veins in the pathophysiology of hemorrhoids makes the effectiveness of HCE doubtful, since HCE has no known effects on the arterial circulation. For now, research studies have yet to confirm any clinical effectiveness of topical HCE preparations.Although adverse effects are uncommon, HCE may cause gastrointestinal irritation.

Parenteral aescin has produced isolated cases of anaphylactic reactions, as well as hepatic and renal toxic effects. In the event of toxicity, aescin can be eliminated via dialysis, with elimination dependent on protein-binding. Horse chestnut extract is also one of the components of venocuran, a drug marketed as a treatment for venous disorders. In 1975, venocuran was determined to cause a pseudolupus syndrome characterized by recurrent fever, myalgia, arthralgia, pleuritis, pulmonary infiltrates, pericarditis, myocarditis, and mitochondrial antibodies in the absence of nuclear antibodies after prolonged treatment. Venocuran has since been withdrawn from the market; however, the nature of its pathophysiologic action is still unknown.

Like A hippocastanum, Ruscus aculeatus (butcher's broom) is also known for its use in treating venous insufficiency. Ruscus aculeatus is a short evergreen shrub found commonly in the Mediterranean region. Two steroidal saponins, ruscogenin and neurogenin, extracted from the rhizomes of R aculeatus are thought to be its active components. In vivo studies on hamster cheek pouch reveal that topical Ruscus extract dose dependently antagonizes histamine-induced increases in vascular permeability. Moreover, topical Ruscus extract causes dose-dependent constriction of venules without appreciably affecting arterioles. Topical Ruscus extract's vascular effects are also temperature dependent and appear to counter the sympathetic nervous system's temperature-sensitive vascular regulation : venules dilate at a lower temperature (25°C), constrict at near physiologic temperatures (36.5°C), and further constrict at higher temperatures (40°C); arterioles dilate at 25°C, are unaffected at 36.5°C, and remain unaffected or constrict at 40°C, depending on Ruscus concentration. Based on the influence of prazosin, diltiazem, and rauwolscine, the peripheral vascular effects of Ruscus extract appear to be selectively mediated by effects on calcium channels and α1-adrenergic receptors with less activity at α2-adrenergic receptors. Also, R aculeatus exhibits strong antielastase activity and has little effect on hyaluronidase in direct contrast to A hippocastanum. This activity may contribute to their efficacy in the treatment of venous insufficiency since these enzyme systems are involved in the turnover of the main components of the perivascular amorphous substance.

Several small clinical trials using topical Ruscus extract support its role in treating venous insufficiency. One randomized, double-blind, placebo-controlled trial involving 18 volunteers showed a beneficial decrease in femoral vein diameter (median decrease, 1.25 mm) using duplex B-scan ultrasonography. The decrease was measured 2.5 hours after applying 4 to 6 g of a cream containing

64 to 96 mg of Ruscusextract.120 In another small trial (N = 18) it was shown that topical Ruscus extract may be helpful in reducing venous dilation during pregnancy. Oral agents may be useful as topical drugs for venous insufficiency, although the evidence is less convincing. Although capsule, tablet, ointment, and suppository (for hemorrhoids) preparations of Ruscus extract are available in Europe, only capsules are available in the United States. These capsules contain 75 mg of Ruscus extract and 2 mg of rosemary oil. Aside from occasional nausea and gastritis, adverse effects from using R aculeatus have rarely been reported, even in high doses Nevertheless, one should be wary of any drug that has not been thoroughly tested. Although there is ample evidence to support the pharmacological activity of R aculeatus, there is still a relative deficiency of clinical data to establish its actual safety and efficacy. Until more studies are completed, no recommendations regarding dosage can be offered.

Arrhythmia

In traditional Chinese medicine, arrhythmias are categorized by the characteristic symptoms of palpitations and abnormal pulse. Numerous Chinese herbal medicines are identified to have antiarrhythmic effects, such as xin bao, ci zhu wan, bu xin dan, and several others. However, few clinical trials have been conducted to study their effects and safety. Xin bao is one agent that has begun to be examined. The mechanism of action of xin bao is thought to be through its stimulation and increased excitability of the sinuatrial node. In one observational study, the effects of xin bao were documented in 87 patients with sick sinus syndrome. Xin bao was administered orally 2 to 3 times per day for 2 months. Patients with major symptoms of sick sinus syndrome, which included dizziness, palpitations, and chest pressure, improved significantly after treatment. No serious adverse effects were noted. This study suggests a possible role of xin bao in the treatment of sick sinus syndrome. However, more scientific research on xin bao and other antiarrhythmic Chinese herbs mentioned previously are necessary before any recommendations can be made for their routine use in patients with sick sinus syndrome or other arrhythmias.

Possible Negative Cardiovascular Effects Caused by Herbal Medications

In addition to those mentioned earlier, other herbal medications used for treatment of noncardiovascular conditions may raise relevant cardiovascular concerns. For example, bitter orange, which is commonly used as a dietary supplement for weight loss and as an appetite suppressant, contains synephrine, an alkaloid with adrenergic properties.

Synephrine has been shown in clinical studies to cause tachycardia, tachyarrhythmia, QT prolongation, ischemic stroke, angina, and myocardial infarction. Ephedra, a product that contains ephedrine and used to be widely used for weight loss, was banned from the market in 2004 by the FDA because of a high risk of cardiovascular events, in particular arrhythmias, heart failure, myocardial infarction, changes in blood pressure, and death. Between 1995 and 1997, the FDA received more than 900 reports of possible side effects related to this product, including stroke, myocardial infarction, and sudden death. Herbal medications can also interact with cardiovascular drugs by altering the pharmacokinetics of cardiovascular medications, thus influencing their distribution and metabolism. For example, Salvia miltiorrhiza has been shown to significantly decrease the binding of warfarin to serum albumin, increasing free drug concentrations in vivo, leading to an increased risk of bleeding . Goldenseal, a product used as an antimicrobial agent to prevent common colds and upper respiratory tract infections, significantly inhibits CYP2D6 and CYP3A4, leading to an increase in the concentration of drugs, including atorvastatin, simvastatin, warfarin, diltiazem, verapamil, and propranolol, metabolized by these CYPs .

Cranberries, which are used to prevent urinary tract infections in women, and Asian ginseng might inhibit the activity of CYP2C9, the primary isoenzyme involved in the metabolism of warfarin, causing elevation of the international normalized ratio and increased risk of bleeding. In contrast, St. John's wort, which has been shown in clinical studies to be effective in the treatment of depression, can induce CYP3A4 and CYP2C9 activity, reducing the efficacy of medications metabolized by these enzymes. St. John's wort can also induce the activity of P-glycoprotein, 1 of the most clinically important transmembrane transporters in humans, influencing plasma concentrations of known P-glycoprotein substrates, such as digoxin. Herbal medications may antagonize the effect of cardiovascular drugs. For example, green tea contains small amounts of vitamin K, and therefore can antagonize the effect of warfarin . However, the effects of cardiovascular medications might be potentiated by concomitant use of herbal medications. For example, ginkgo and garlic might reduce platelet function, possibly leading to an increased risk of bleeding if taken together with aspirin or anticoagulant agents ; hawthorn might increase the blood concentration of digoxin, raising the risk of arrhythmias; and European elder might potentiate the effect of diuretic agents. A final concern relates to the concomitant use of licorice and loop or thiazides diuretic agents because of an increased risk of hypokalemia

Table 33.2: *Most Relevant Interactions Between Herbal Medications (Used Both for the Treatment of Cardiovascular Diseases and for Other Conditions) and Cardiovascular Medications*

Herbal Medication (Ref. #)	Interacting Cardiovascular Medication(s)	Mechanism of Action	Potential Side Effect
Asian ginseng	Warfarin	Inhibition of CYP2C9	↑ Risk of bleeding
Cranberry	Warfarin	Inhibition of CYP2C9	↑ Risk of bleeding
European elder	Diuretics	Additive diuretic effect	↑ Diuresis
Garlic	Aspirin and anticoagulant agents	Reduction of platelet function	↑ Risk of bleeding
Ginkgo	Aspirin and anticoagulant agents	Reduction of platelet function	↑ Risk of bleeding
Goldenseal	Medications metabolized by CYP2D6 and CYP3A4	Inhibition of CYP2D6 and CYP3A4	↑ Effect
Green tea	Warfarin	Contains vitamin K	↓ Effect
Hawthorn	Digoxin	Increased blood concentration of digoxin	Arrhythmias
Licorice root	Loop and thiazide diuretic agents	Mineralocorticoid-like effect	Hypokalemia
Salvia miltiorrhiza	Warfarin	Reduction in binding to albumin	↑ Risk of bleeding
St. John's wort	Medications metabolized by CYP3A4 and CYP2C9	Induction of CYP3A4 and CYP2C9	↓ Effect

CYP = cytochrome.

Table 33.3: *Vitamin and Nutraceutical Supplements That Have Been Used for Prevention or treatment of CVD*

Nutraceutical	Estimated Average Requirement (Adults)	Doses Used in Clinical Studies
Vitamin E	Men: >4 mg/day; women >3 mg/day[g]	100-600 mg/day
Vitamin C	25 mg/day	250-500 mg/day
Thiamin	0.8-1.0 mg/day[f]	
Vitamin B12	1.25 μg/day	
Vitamin D	10 μg/day after 65 years[b]	
Vitamin K	1 μg/kg/day[c]	
Folic acid	150 μg/day	
Pyridoxine (vitamin B6)	Men: 1.4 mg/day; women: 1.2 mg/day[e]	
Niacin (nicotinic acid)	Men: 16 mg/day; women: 12 mg/day[f]	1000-2000 mg single dose
Carotenoids	—d	β-Carotene 20-50 mg/day
Flavonoids	—d	200-1000 mg/day
Alcohol		
Magnesium	Men: 250 mg/day; women: 200 mg/day	800-1000 mg/day
Zinc	Men: 7.3 mg/day; women: 5.5 mg/day	No study
Manganese	1.4 mg/day[a]	
Selenium	Men: 75 μg/day; women: 60 μg/day	
Chromium	25 μg/day[a]	200 μg/day
Molybdenum	50-40 μg/day	No study
Calcium	525 mg/day	
Coenzyme Q10	—d	300 mg/day
L-carnitine	—d	2 g/day
Omega-3 fatty acids	—d	EPA 1500 mg/day

Note: **Estimated average requirement:** Department of Health, United Kingdom. (HMSO 1991)

[a] Considered adequate

[b] Also for those confined indoors

[c] Lack of adequate data—safe intake recommended

[d] No reliable data

[e] Varies with protein intake

[f] Varies with energy intake

[g] Varies with PUFA intake

Bibliography and Acknowledgement

- Bossi M Brambilla G Cavilla A *et al.* Threatening arrhythmia by uncommon digitalic toxicosis [in Italian]. G Ital Cardiol. 1981; **11**, 2254- 2257
- Z'Brun A Ginkgo: myth and reality [in German]. Schweiz Rundsch Med Prax.1995; **84**, 1- 6
- 80. Rose KD Croissant PD Parliament CF Levin MB Spontaneous spinal epidural hematoma with associated liver dysfunction from excessive garlic ingestion: a case report. *Neurosurgery.* 1990; **26**, 880- 882
- Al-Hader AA Hasan ZAAqel MB Hyperglycemic and insulin release inhibitory effects of Rosmarinus officinalis. *J Ethnopharmacol.* 1994; **43**, 217- 221
- Allard M Treatment of the disorders of aging with Ginkgo biloba extract [in French]. Presse Med. 1986; **15**, 1540- 1545
- Ansford AJMorris H Fatal oleander poisoning. *Med J Aust.* 1981; **1**, 360- 361 Google Scholar
- Astin JA Why patients use alternative medicine: results of a national study. JAMA. 1998; **279**, 1548- 1553
- Bagrov AY Roukoyatkina NI Pinaev AG Dmitrieva RI Effects of two endogenous Na+, K(+)-AT Pase inhibitors, marinobufagenin and ouabain, on isolated rat aorta. *Eur J Pharmacol.* 1995; **274**, 151- 158
- Bahorun TTrotin FPommery J *et al.* Antioxidant activities of Crataegus monogyna extracts. *Planta Med.* 1994; **60**, 323- 328
- Berg D Venous constriction by local administration of ruscus extract [in German]. *Fortschr Med.* 1990; **108**, 473- 476
- Berg D Venous tonicity in pregnancy varicose veins [in German]. Fortschr Med.1992; **1**, 1067- 6871- 72
- Bieler CAStiborova MWiessler M *et al.* 32 P-post-labelling analysis of DNA adducts formed by aristolochic acid in tissues from patients with Chinese herbs nephropathy. *Carcinogenesis.* 1997; **18**, 1063- 1067
- Bisler H Pfeifer R Kluken N Pauschinger P Effects of horse chestnut seed extract on transcapillary filtration in chronic venous insufficiency [in German]. Dtsch Med Wochenschr. 1986; **111**, 1321- 1329
- Blesken R Crataegus in cardiology [in German]. *Fortschr Med.*1992; **110**, 290- 292
- Bordia A Verma SK Srivastava KC Effect of garlic on platelet aggregation in humans: a study in healthy subjects and patients with coronary artery disease. Prostaglandins Leukot Essent Fatty Acids. 1996; **55**, 201- 205
- Bouskela E Cyrino F Z Marcelon G Effects of Ruscus extract on the internal diameter of arterioles and venules of the hamster cheek pouch microcirculation. *J Cardiovasc Pharmacol.* 1993; **22**, 221- 224
- Bouskela ECyrino FZMarcelon G Possible mechanisms for the inhibitory effect of Ruscus extract on increased microvascular permeability induced by histamine in hamster cheek pouch. *J Cardiovasc Pharmacol.* 1994; **24**, 281- 285
- Bouskela ECyrino FZMarcelon G Possible mechanisms for the venular constriction elicited by Ruscus extract on hamster cheek pouch. *J Cardiovasc Pharmacol.* 1994; **24**, 165- 170
- Breithaupt-Grogler K Ling M Boudoulas H Beliz GG Protective effect of chronic garlic intake on elastic properties of aorta in the elderly. *Circulation.*1997; 962649-
- Brunton LLAgents affecting gastrointestinal water flux, emesis and antiemetics, bile acids and pancreatic enzymes. Hardman JG Limbird LEMolinoff PB *et al.* eds Goodman and Gilman's The Pharmacological Basis of Therapeutics 9th ed. New York, NY McGraw-Hill Book Co1996; 917- 936
- Chan KLo A C Yeung J H Woo KS The effects of Danshen (Salvia miltiorrhiza) on warfarin pharmacodynamics and pharmacokinetics of warfarin enantiomers in rats. *J Pharm Pharmacol.* 1995; **47**, 402- 406
- Chen ZY Use of Xin Bao in the treatment of 87 patients with sick sinus syndrome. Chung Hsi I Chieh Ho Tsa Chih. 1990; **10**, 529- 531
- Cheung KHinds JADuffy P Detection of poisoning by plant-origin cardiac glycoside with the Abbott Tdx analyzer. *Clin Chem.* 1989; **35**, 295- 297
- Chiou W-FShum AY-CLiao J-FChen C-F Studies of the cellular mechanisms underlying the vasorelaxant effects of rutaecarpine, a bioactive component extracted from an herbal drug. *J Cardiovasc Pharmacol.* 1997; **29**: 490- 498
- Dalvi S S Nayak V K Pohujani S M Desai N K Kshirsagar N A Gupta KC Effect of gugulipid on bioavailability of diltiazem and propranolol. *J Assoc Physicians India.* 1994; **42:** 454- 455
- Delaney T A Donnelley A M Garlic dermatitis. *Australas J Dermatol.*1996; **37**: 109- 110
- derangements. Planta Med. 1989; **55:** 51- 54
- Dickstein ESKunkel FW Foxglove tea poisoning. *Am J Med.* 1980; **69**: 167- 169
- Diehm C Trampisch H J Lange S Schmidt C Comparison of leg compression stocking and oral horse chestnut seed extract therapy in patients with chronic venous insufficiency. *Lancet.* 1996; **347:** 292- 294
- Diehm C Vollbrecht Not Available Amendt K Comberg HU Medical edema protection: clinical benefit in patients with chronic deep vein incompetence: a placebo controlled double-blind study. Vasa. 1992; **211**: 88- 192
- Doly MDroy-Lefaix MTBraquet P Oxidative stress in diabetic retina. EXS.1992; **62**: 299- 307
- Eisenberg DMKessler RCFoster C *et al.* Unconventional medicine in the United States. *N Engl J Med.* 1993; **328**: 246-252
- Ernst E Harmless herbs? a review of the recent literature. *Am J Med.*1998; **104**: 170- 178

- Facino R M Carini M Stefani R Aldini G Saibene L Anti-elastase and anti-hyaluronidase activities of saponins and sapogenins from Hedera helix, Aesculus hippocastanum, and Ruscus aculeatus: factors contributing to their efficacy in the treatment of venous insufficiency. *Arch Pharm* (Weinheim). 1995; **328**: 720- 724
- Grob P J Muller-Schoop J W Hacki M A Joller-Jemelka H I Drug-induced pseudolupus. *Lancet*. 1975; **2**: 144- 148
- Guillaume MPadioleau F Veinotonic effect, vascular protection, antiinflammatory and free radical scavenging properties of horse chestnut extract. *Arzneimittelforschung*. 1994; **44**: 25- 35
- Haraguchi H Saito T Okamura N Yagi A Inhibition of lipid peroxidation and superoxide generation by diterpenoids from Rosmarinus officinalis. *Planta Med*.1995; **61**: 333- 336
- Isaacsohn J L Moser M Stein EA *et al*. Garlic powder and plasma lipids and lipoproteins: a multicenter, randonized, plcebo-controlled trial. *Arch Intern Med*. 1998; **158**: 1189-1194
- Jaffe A M Gephardt D Courtemanche L Poisoning due to ingestion of Veratrum viride (false hellebore). *J Emerg Med*. 1990; **8**: 161- 167
- Kawashima K Hayakawa T Miwa Y et al. Structure and hypotensive activity relationships of tetrandrine derivatives in stroke-prone spontaneously hypertensive rats. Gen Pharmacol. 1990; 21: 343- 347
- Lang W Dialysability of aescin [in German]. Arzneimittelforschung.1984; 34: 221- 223
- Lang W Studies on the percutaneous absorption of 3H-aescin in pigs. Res Exp Med (Berl). 1977; 169: 175- 187
- Lei X L Chiou G C Cardiovascular pharmacology of Panax notoginseng (Burk) FH Chen and Salvia miltiorrhiza. Am J Chin Med. 1986; 14: 145- 152
- Lin S G Zheng X L Chen Q Y Sun JJ Effect of Panax notoginseng saponins on increased proliferation of cultured aortic smooth muscle cells stimulated by hypercholestoremic serum. Chung Kuo Yao Li Hsueh Pao. 1993; 14: 314- 316
- Mader FH Treatment of hyperlipidaemia with garlic powder tablets: evidence from the German Association of General Practitioners' Multicentric Placebo-Controlled Double-Blind Study. Arzneimittelforschung. 1990; 40: 1111- 1116M Thomson M Consumption of a garlic clove a day could be beneficial in preventing thrombosis. Prostaglandins Leukot Essent Fatty Acids.1995; 53: 211- 212
- Nasa Y Hashizume H Hoque A N Abiko Y Protective effect of Crataegus extract on the the cardiac mechanical dysfunction in isolated perfused working rat heart. Arzneimittelforschung. 1993; 43: 945- 949
- Oates JA Antihypertensive agents and the drug therapy of hypertension. Hardman J G Limbird L E Molinoff PB et al. eds Goodman and Gilman's The Pharmacological Basis of Therapeutics. 9th ed. New York, NY McGraw-Hill Book Co 1996; 781- 808Petkov V Plants and hypotensive, antiatheromatous and coronarodilating action. Am J Chin Med. 1979; 7: 197- 236
- Pietri S Seguin J R D'Arbigny P Drieu K Culcasi M Egb 761 pretreatment limits free radical-induced oxidative stress in patients undergoing coronary bypass surgery. Cardiovasc Drugs Ther. 1997; 11: 121- 131

Quatrehomme G Bertrand F Chauvet C Ollier A Intoxication from Veratrum album. Hum Exp Toxicol. 1993; 12: 111- 115

- Radford DJGillies ADHinds JADuffy P Naturally occurring cardiac glycosides. Med J Aust. 1986; 144: 540- 544
- Rothkopf M Vogel G New findings on the efficacy and mode of action of the horse chestnut saponin escin [in German]. Arzneimittelforschung.1976; 26: 225- 235
- Safadi R Levy I Amitai Y Caraco Y Beneficial effect of digoxin-specific Fab antibody fragments in oleander intoxication. Arch Intern Med.1995; 155: 2121- 2125
- Schmeiser H H Bieler C A Wiessler M Van Ypersele D E Strihou C Cosyns J P Detection of DNA adducts formed by aristolochic acid in renal tissue from patients with Chinese herbs nephropathy. Cancer Res. 1996; 56: 2025- 2028
- Sing RBNiaz MAGhosh S Hypolipidemic and antioxidant effects of Commiphora mukul as an adjunct to dietary therapy in patients with hypercholesterolemia. Cardiovasc Drugs Ther. 1994; 8: 659- 664
- Singh V Kaul S Chander R Kapoor N K Stimulation of low density lipoprotein receptor activity in liver membrane of guggulsterone treated rats. Pharmacol Res. 1990; 22: 37- 44
- Steiner M Khan A H Holbert D Lin R I A double-blind cross-over study in hypercholesterolemic men that compared the effect of aged garlic extract and placebo administration on blood lipids. Am J Clin Nutr. 1996; 64: 866- 870
- Takegoshi K Tohyama T Okunda K et al. A case of Venoplant-induced hepatic injury. Gastroenterol Jpn. 1986; 21: 62- 65
- Tyler VE The Honest Herbal: A Sensible Guide to the Use of Herbs and Related Remedies. 3rd ed. New York, NY Pharmaceutical Product Press1993;
- Vanherweghem JL A new form of nephropathy secondary to the absorption of Chinese herbs [in French]. Bull Mem Acad R Med Belg. 1994; 149: 128- 135
- Voigt EJunger H Acute posttraumatic renal failure following therapy with antibiotics and beta-aescin [in German]. Anaesthesist. 1978; 27: 81- 83
- Walli F Grob P J Muller-Schoop J Pseudo-(venocuran-) lupus: a minor episode in the history of medicine [in German]. Schweiz Med Wochenschr.1981; 111: 1398- 1405
- Wu B-NHuang Y-CWu H-MHong S-JChiang L-CChen I-J A highly selective (?1-adrenergic blocker with partial? 2 agonist activity derived from ferulic acid, an active component of Ligusticum wallichii Franch. J Cardiovasc Pharmacol.1998; 31:750- 757
- Yagi A Fujimoto K Tanonaka K et al. Possible active components of tan-shen (Salvia Zhang WWojta JBinder BR Effect of notoginsenoside R1 on the synthesis of tissue-type plasminogen activator and plasminogen activator inhibitor-1 in cultured human umbilical vein endothelial cells. Arterioscler Thromb Vasc Biol.1994; 14: 1040- 1046
- Zhou Z Y Jin HD Clinical Manual of Chinese Herbal Medicine. New York, N Y Churchill Livingstone Inc1997;

A New Management Strategies In Heart Failure. Multiscientic A-Review

Heart failure is an enormous problem with around 20 million people affected worldwide. Initially HF was believed be caused by low Left ventricular ejection fraction i.e. systolic dysfunction.It was then found that nearly 50% of the patients with heart failure had normal ejection fraction. So, heart failure was then effectively classified as HF with reduced EF i.e. HFrEF and HF with preserved ejection fraction i.e. HFpEF.

Echocordiographic and strain and strain rate are the best noninvasive investigative techniques in the categorization of heart failure. These are as follows -

1. Heart failure with preserved Left ventricular ejection fraction i.e. HFpEF, also called as diastolic heart dysfunction.
2. Heart failure with reduced Left ventricular ejection fraction i.e. HFrEF, also called as systolic heart dysfunction.
3. A new HF subcategory(HFmEF)

The recent ESC guidelines have introduced a new category heart failure with mid range ejection fraction HFmEF. The elements required for diagnosis of HFmEF are symptoms with or without signs of HF, LVEF of 40-49%,elevated natriuretic peptides and relevant structural heart disease; LV hypertrophy or left atrial enlargement or diastolic dysfunction. However, the usefulness of this categorization is stll controversial as standard echocardiography is not good enough to categorise this entity. However, strain and strain rate evaluation may be helpful. Most of the older and newer drugs are prescribed according to the types of heart failure as mentioned above.

Etiology:- Although there are numerous causes leading to heart failure but hypertensive and valvular heart diseases remains the leading causes of HFpEF whereas ischemic heart disease and dilated cardiomyopathy were more likely in HFrEF.

Pathophysiological changes:- In patients with HFrEF, the LV is dilated with eccentric remodelling and thus there is an increased LV end -diastolic volume when compared to stroke volume. In patients with HFpEF, the end- diastolic volume is not increased when compared to stroke volume, and there is concentric remodelling of the ventricles. In patients with HFrEF, LV systolic elastance is less and the arterial elastance is high, whereas in HFpEF, LV systolic elastance and arterial elastance both high. Thus,arterial vasodilation is useful in patients with HFrEF, but is of hardly any use in patients with HFpEF

Pharmacotherapy: Emerging Drugs and Concepts

Sacubitril/Valsartan or LCZ696

LCZ696 is a first-in-class angiotensin receptor neprilysin inhibitor (NEPi; ARNi). Although a NEPi was first synthesized in 1980. the initial clinical use of these agents as a single drug class in hypertension was disappointing. However, when NEPi was combined with an angiotensin-converting enzyme inhibitor, or later, with an angiotensin receptor blocker (ARB), the dual actions of the drugs together were more effective than either alone The development of angioedema in many patients given a combination of NEPi and angiotensin-converting enzyme inhibitor facilitated the development of the ARNi class

Circulating natriuretic peptides, which include atrial natriuretic peptide, B-type natriuretic peptide (BNP), and urodilatin, are secreted by the heart, vasculature, kidney, and central nervous system in response to increased cardiac-wall stress and other stimuli, resulting in a potent natriuretic and vasodilatory effect. In addition, the natriuretic peptides inhibit the renin–angiotensin–

aldosterone system, reduce sympathetic drive, and have antiproliferative and antihypertrophic effects as well. The interactive role of natriuretic peptides to influence the development of myocardial fibrosis is being clarified. Natriuretic peptides are cleared through 2 mechanisms : degradation of the enzyme (neprilysin) and a natriuretic peptide receptor–mediated clearance; NEPi results in an increased concentration of natriuretic peptides. Drugs that inhibit the renin–angiotensin–aldosterone system have been foundational to cardiovascular drug therapy for almost 3 decades; the beneficial effects of renin–angiotensin–aldosterone system inhibition seem to be augmented by the enhancement of natriuretic peptide activity

The first randomized clinical trial of LCZ696 in HF was in 301 HF with preserved ejection fraction (HFpEF) patients, the Prospective Comparison of ARNi With ARB on Management of Heart Failure With Preserved Ejection Fraction (*Paramount*) trial. The primary end point, plasma N-terminal pro-BNP (NT-proBNP), was significantly lower at the end of 12 weeks in the LCZ696 group compared with the valsartan (an ARB) patients. By 36 weeks, the patients in the LCZ696 arm had improved New York Heart Association (NYHA) symptoms and smaller left atrial volumes—used as a surrogate for ventricular filling pressures—in comparison with the ARB-treated patients. A larger HFpEF trial is now underway, the Prospective Comparison of LCZ696 With ARB Global Outcome in HF With Preserved Ejection Fraction (Paragon) trial. These encouraging preliminary findings were followed by a trial in HFrEF.

In a Prospective Comparison of ARNI with ACEI to Determine Impact on Global Mortality and Morbidity in Heart Failure (Paradigm-HF) trial, LCZ696 was compared with an enalapril-based, guideline-directed regimen in 8442 symptomatic patients with HFrEF. LCZ696, compared with enalapril, significantly and remarkably reduced the risks of death from any cause, from cardiovascular causes, and the risk of hospitalization for HF. Patients' quality of life, as measured by the Kansas City Cardiomyopathy Questionnaire, was significantly improved as well. Subsequent publications from this same trial revealed that LCZ696 was superior to enalapril in reducing sudden cardiac death and preventing the clinical progression of HF in survivors.

The results of the Paradigm-HF trial generated a wave of enthusiasm for the promise of a new drug class for patients with HFrEF; discussions about the potential to change the guidelines quickly followed. Translating the remarkable statistical results of the trial into a guideline recommendation, however, has triggered some concerns. The trial was stopped early, according to the prespecified metrics of the trial design, after a median follow-up of 27 months, because of the overwhelming benefit seen with LCZ696. Thus, some have voiced concerns about the durability of the drug's effect over many more years and potential adverse effects of long-term use of LCZ696. In addition, patients enrolled in the trial had a several week run-in period to demonstrate their ability to tolerate 10 mg of both LCZ696 and enalapril twice daily. LCZ696 was given initially at a dose of 100 mg twice daily, which was increased to 200 mg twice daily. The ARB component of the 200-mg dose of LCZ696 is equivalent to 160 mg of valsartan. The doses of both the angiotensin-converting enzyme inhibitor and the ARB in the ARNi are higher than many HFrEF patients may tolerate, although are clearly target dosages listed in most HF guidelines. Guideline-writing committees will need to weigh the obvious potential benefit of the drug against the need to carefully describe the typical patient who might be considered for initiation. Finally, this considerable challenge to the long-standing algorithm of care for the patient with HFrEF will be further complicated by the cost of the drug in the United States. Clinicians are already reporting a high frequency of drug denials from payors.

Ivabradine

In April of the same year, ivabradine was approved in the United States to reduce the risk of hospitalization in stable HFrEF patients with a heart rate >70 bpm despite optimal use of β-blocking agents. The drug has been available in Europe since 2005. Ivabradine is a specific inhibitor of the I_f current in the sinoatrial node, and at concentrations used clinically has no other apparent action on the myocardium or vascular system. Mechanistically, it is used exclusively to reduce the heart rate in patients; an intensified interest in the prognostic implications of heart rate reduction has resumed.

In the Systolic Heart Failure Treatment With the I_f Inhibitor Ivabradine Trial (SHIFT) study, 6558 patients with HFrEF in sinus rhythm with a heart rate >70 bpm were randomized to evidence-based treatment with or without ivabradine. The primary end point was the composite of cardiovascular death or hospital admission for worsening HF. There was a significant, 18% decrease in risk of cardiovascular death or admission for HF with ivabradine compared with placebo, primarily fueled by the salutary effect on hospitalization events. The authors suggested that the SHIFT trial was a test of the effect of isolated heart rate reduction on a HFrEF population, as treatment with ivabradine during the trial averaged a reduction of 15 bpm from the baseline heart rate of 80 bpm. Moreover, patients with higher heart rates seemed to benefit more from ivabradine. Skeptics worried that the same magnitude of effect would have been seen if the patients had been given a higher dose of β-blockade. A subsequent publication with additional analyses argued that the magnitude of heart rate reduction by ivabradine beyond what was achieved by a β-blocker, rather than background β-blocker dose, primarily determined the subsequent outcome.

Interestingly, in a previous study in patients with coronary artery disease and low left ventricular ejection fraction (LVEF), ivabradine did not confer a clinical benefit, but the subgroup with a heart rate of ≥70 bpm at baseline despite guideline-based therapy had improved outcomes. Accordingly, the Study Assessing the Morbidity–Mortality Benefits of the I_f Inhibitor Ivabradine in Patients With Coronary Artery Disease (*Signify*) trial was done, involving patients with stable coronary artery disease and no HF symptoms; patients with LVEF <40% were excluded. The primary end point was a composite of death from cardiovascular causes or nonfatal myocardial infarction. The Signify trial showed no clinical benefit with ivabradine in this patient population. Thus, the use of the drug at present should be confined to the specific HFrEF patients with higher heart rates despite maximally tolerated β-blocker therapy.

Aliskiren

Given the enormous benefit of more proximal inhibition of the renin–angiotensin–aldosterone system in the HF syndrome and the known compensatory increase in renin as a consequence of these agents, the development of direct renin inhibitors was a logical step. Aliskiren is an orally active direct renin inhibitor, approved for use in hypertension in the United States in March of 2007. Previous trials in patients with HF suggested a favorable hemodynamic response to the drug; an observed increase in renal blood flow in normal subjects was especially noteworthy. A subsequent trial in patients with symptomatic HF showed that aliskiren decreased BNP levels, plasma renin, and urinary aldosterone more than placebo.

The Aliskiren Trial on Acute Heart Failure Outcomes (*Astronaut*) study was, therefore, designed to evaluate the effect of aliskiren or placebo, added to standard medical therapy, on hospitalized patients with HFrEF. The primary end point was cardiovascular death or HF rehospitalization at 6 months. Studied in >1600 patients, aliskiren had no significant effect on the primary composite end point or on any clinical end point ≤12 months of follow-up. Not unexpectedly, patients who received aliskiren had more hyperkalemia, hypotension, and renal impairment.

A provocative, prespecified subgroup analysis of *Astronaut* revealed a variable outcome in the trial dependent on baseline diabetic status. The risk of all-cause mortality with aliskiren significantly decreased at 12 months in nondiabetic patients; these same patients experienced less adverse events from aliskiren. A similar adverse event profile of aliskiren in diabetic patients was seen in another trial in patients with type 2 diabetes mellitus and chronic kidney disease, cardiovascular disease, or both. These latter investigators concluded that there was no role for aliskiren in patients with type 2 diabetes mellitus; this caveat is likely applicable to the majority of patients with HF and diabetes mellitus as well.

Iron Therapy

It has been recognized for many years that patients with chronic HF are frequently anemic; iron deficiency and disordered iron homeostasis are often found to be important contributors to the anemia. The presence and degree of anemia have functional correlates in patients with symptomatic HF and have been shown to be a determinant of prognosis. Correcting anemia with synthetic erythropoietin was shown to be an ineffective method to improve outcomes for patients with HFrEF in the Reduction of Events by Darbepoetin Alfa in Heart Failure (Red-HF) trial. The Ferric Carboxymaltose Assessment in Patients with Iron Deficiency and Chronic Heart Failure (Fair-HF) study randomized 459 ambulatory HFrEF patients with iron deficiency (with or without anemia) to placebo or intravenous iron formulated as ferric carboxymaltose. The treatment with intravenous iron improved symptoms, functional capacity, and quality of life and was well tolerated. A later analysis of these same patients showed that renal function was enhanced with iron as well.

Despite these persuasive findings, routine screening for iron deficiency did not become a standard practice in most HF programs. Accordingly, the Ferric Carboxymaltose Evaluation on Performance in Patients With Iron Deficiency in Combination With Chronic Heart Failure (Confirm-HF) trial was undertaken to address the sustainability of iron's beneficial effects. T he study enrolled 3 04 ambulatory, symptomatic HFrEF patients with elevated natriuretic peptides and iron deficiency to intravenous ferric carboxymaltose or placebo, in addition to evidenced-based therapy; patients were followed up for 1 year. The iron therapy resulted in a sustained improvement in functional capacity, symptoms, and quality of life. Importantly, a post hoc analysis showed a significant risk reduction of hospitalization for worsening HF in the iron group. Taken together, these data provide a compelling argument for the inclusion of regular screening for iron deficiency in all patients with HFrEF. Unresolved issues surrounding the role of iron supplementation include (1) the optimal formulation of the iron to be used, as both trials referred to above used intravenous ferric carboxymaltose, and (2) whether iron administered orally can be equally effective. The ongoing trial Oral Iron Repletion Effects on Oxygen Uptake in Heart Failure (Ironout) is underway in the National Heart, Lung, and Blood Institute Heart Failure Network to explore the role of oral iron polysaccharide compared with placebo on functional capacity in patients with HFrEF

Phosphodiesterase Type 5 Inhibitor

The phosphodiesterase type 5 (PDE5) inhibitors have become one of the principle classes of therapy for patients with pulmonary arterial hypertension. Because left HF so commonly leads to pulmonary hypertension—World Health Organization group 2 pulmonary hypertension—it seemed appropriate to evaluate the effect of the PDE5 inhibitors in patients with either HFrEF or HFpEF. Kass has elegantly summarized the many potential mechanisms whereby the PDE5 inhibitors might improve cardiovascular function in HF. PDE5 plays an important role in the hydrolysis of cyclic GMP; through its primary signaling kinase, protein kinase G, cyclic GMP can modify stress remodeling in the heart and other vascular beds. As a result, PDE5 inhibition has been shown to restrain cardiac pressure and volume overload, ischemic injury, and cardiotoxicity.

In patients with HF being considered for cardiac transplant or the implantation of left ventricular assist devices (VADs), it becomes critical to reduce elevated pulmonary vascular resistance irreversible pulmonary hypertension leads to right ventricular failure after surgery in the absence of such efforts. The PDE5 inhibitors, primarily sildenafil, are increasingly used to lower abnormal pulmonary pressures in this clinical scenario.

Patients with HFpEF have also been shown to have a steep increase in pulmonary pressures with exertion. Thus, the Phosphodiesterase-5 Inhibition to Improve Clinical Status and Exercise Capacity in Heart Failure With Preserved Ejection Fraction (Relax) trial was developed to compare sildenafil with placebo on exercise capacity in patients with HFpEF. The investigators enrolled 216 stable outpatients with an LVEF ≥50%, elevated NT-proBNP or measured filling pressures, and reduced exercise capacity. Despite a strong physiological rationale, the PDE5 inhibitor had no effect on any aspect of exercise capacity, clinical status, quality of life, diastolic function parameters, or pulmonary pressures. Biomarkers increased more with sildenafil, and renal function worsened more than placebo. Further investigation into the cardiovascular adverse effects observed in the trial revealed a negative inotropic action of sildenafil. A trial of PDE5 inhibition in HFrEF had been planned but has been delayed for unclear reasons.

Glucagon-Like Peptide-1 Receptor Agonists

A second class of drugs, glucagon-like peptide-1 receptor (GLP-1) agonists, currently used for diabetes mellitus, has also been repurposed for HF. The effect of diabetes mellitus on the outcome and pathophysiology of HF is an area of great investigative interest. GLP-1 is a naturally occurring incretin peptide released from the intestine that enhances cellular glucose uptake by stimulating insulin secretion and enhancing insulin sensitivity. GLP-1 receptors have been identified in the heart, kidneys, and blood vessels; GLP-1 stimulation has a salutary effect on endothelial function, sodium excretion, recovery from ischemic injury, and myocardial function in animals. It has been argued that GLP-1 agonists have the potential to augment cardiac function by providing fuel for the energy-starved failing heart. Accordingly, the Functional Impact of GLP-1 for Heart Failure Treatment (Fight) study was designed by the National Heart, Lung, and Blood Institute Heart Failure Network to explore the use of a GLP-1 agonist or placebo in high-risk, hospitalized patients with HFrEF, both with and without diabetes mellitus. Results from the study were presented as a Late Breaking Clinical Trial at the 2015 Scientific Sessions of the American Heart Association. The investigators found that the GLP-1 agonist liraglutide did not seem to improve posthospitalization clinical stability in patients with advanced HF.

Nevertheless, the metabolic pathways linking diabetes mellitus and HF will undoubtedly lead to additional, novel pharmacological approaches. Empagliflozin, an inhibitor of sodium-glucose cotransporter-2, was able to reduce the risk of the primary composite end point (cardiovascular death, nonfatal myocardial infarction, or nonfatal stroke), as well as some secondary end points, including all-cause death, cardiovascular death, and hospitalization for HF in diabetic patients at high cardiovascular risk.

Cardiac Devices

Unlike pharmacotherapy, device therapy for HF is invasive, expensive, and mostly irreversible, highlighting the need for accurate prediction of who will benefit before implantation. Devices in HF are typically considered after a background of optimal medical therapy has been implemented and include cardiac resynchronization therapy (CRT), implantable cardioverter-defibrillators (ICD), and VADs.

CRT and Beyond

CRT improves symptoms, survival, and quality of life in addition to salutary effects on cardiac function and structure. Patients who derive the most benefit include those with persistent NYHA functional class II–III symptoms despite optimal medical therapy, sinus rhythm with wide QRS complex, and severe left ventricular dysfunction. It is reported in the literature that up to one third of patients do not respond to CRT therapy. Debate continues on how to identify nonresponders, with most data focusing on QRS duration and morphology, NYHA functional class, and LVEF as reflected in the guidelines. A recent prespecified subgroup analysis of the Echocardiography Guided Cardiac Resynchronization Therapy (EchoCRT) study reported no benefit of CRT and possible harm with QRS <130 ms. A novel measure of electric dyssynchrony, the sum absolute QRST integral, was tested retrospectively in the Smart Delay Determined AV Optimization : A Comparison to Other AV Delay Methods Used in Cardiac Resynchronization Therapy (Smart-AV) study. Importantly, the sum absolute QRST integral can be measured from a standard 12-lead ECG and is a simplified measurement of action potential heterogeneity in the heart. In theory, multipolarity of electric activation correlates with electric dyssynchrony. In this study, the sum absolute QRST integral was independently associated with CRT response.

Often, implantation of a CRT device is accompanied by implantation of a defibrillator. A recent meta-analysis suggests that recovery of LVEF after CRT is associated with significantly reduced appropriate ICD therapy, particularly in a subset of patients with improvement in LVEF to ≥45% and ICD implanted as primary prevention. This study raises the question of whether continued ICD therapy is warranted in this group of patients who are at relatively low risk of ventricular tachyarrhythmias.

When we are able to accurately predict response to CRT before implantation, those who are in the subset of likely nonresponders will be prime targets for an alternative therapy. Cardiac contractility modulation has been proposed to fill this niche. Cardiac contractility modulation signals are nonexcitatory electric signals delivered during the absolute refractory period that serve to enhance cardiac contraction. The mechanism of action may affect regulation of calcium cycling. A randomized controlled trial evaluating safety and efficacy of this therapy is underway (Evaluate Safety and Efficacy of the Optimizer® System in Subjects With Moderate-to-Severe Heart Failure [FIX-HF-5C] study), and results are forthcoming. Interestingly, this study included patients with normal QRS duration and LVEF from 25% to 45% with NYHA class III–IV symptoms. There are many devices being actively investigated to modulate the autonomic nervous system in patients with HF, including stimulation of the vagus nerve, carotid body, spinal cord, and renal denervation. The concept of rebalancing the sympathetic and parasympathetic nervous systems in chronic HF is intriguing; results of the Increase of Vagal Tone in Heart Failure (Inovate-HF) study are anticipated in the next few years.

Ventricular Assist Devices

Mechanical circulatory support with VADs for end-stage HF was first shown to be a life-saving therapy in 2001. During the past several years, the first generation pulsatile flow VADs have been replaced for the most part with continuous flow devices that are smaller and more durable. The Heartmate II left VAD (Thoratec, Inc) and HeartWare VAD (HeartWare, Inc) are the most commonly implanted second generation VADs presently. A recently completed but not yet published trial called a Prospective, Randomized, Controlled, Un-blinded, Multi-Center Clinical Trial to Evaluate the HeartWare Ventricular Assist System (VAS) for Destination Therapy of Advanced Heart Failure (Endurance) was presented at the 35th International Society for Heart and Lung Transplantation Annual Meeting in 2015, reporting noninferiority of HeartWare VAD to Heartmate II in destination therapy patients. However, in a multi-institution pooled analysis, a trend was found for higher incidence of driveline infections in patients with Heartmate II, and a higher incidence of stroke was found in patients treated with the HeartWare VAD. We continue to struggle to decide when to implant a VAD in the less sick cohort of patients with ambulatory severe HF, especially those who are not yet on inotropes. The recently published Risk Assessment and Comparative Effectiveness of Left Ventricular Assist Device and Medical Management in Ambulatory Heart Failure Patients (Roadmap) observational study suggested benefit in terms of survival and quality of life despite increase in adverse events in patients who received a VAD compared with those treated with medical therapy. It is important to note that this study was observational and that the patients who received a VAD were sicker than those who received medical therapy.

Despite advances in technology, continuous flow VADs have considerable complications, including arteriovenous malformations, leading to gastrointestinal bleeding, hemorrhagic strokes, hemolysis, pump thrombosis, aortic valve insufficiency, and valve fusion There is debate on how much diminished flow pulsatility and lower arterial pressure contribute to these complications. For example, a recent study investigating the effect of nonpulsatile and pulsatile flow on cerebral perfusion found that the magnitude of oscillation in arterial pressure and cerebral blood flow was greater in patients with continuous flow VADs compared with normal patients or those with pulsatile flow VADs. However, autoregulation of cerebral flow was preserved in both device types. Another intriguing study using a transparent replica of the HeartMate II left VAD (Thoratec, Inc) at different flow rates showed that pulsatility imposed on the system (in theory by the native heart) may induce disturbance to an otherwise stable flow field with possibly prothrombotic effects. This study is particularly interesting as a newly designed VAD, the HeartMate III (Thoratec Corporation, Pleasanton, CA), which is in clinical trials currently, aims to intermittently introduce pulsatility to a centrifugal pump system.

There was considerable excitement in the potential for recovering myocardial function with VAD support in conjunction with pharmacological therapy, including the β2-agonist clenbuterol. However, enthusiasm has been tempered during the past several years by evidence of recovery on a cellular and molecular level without sustainable recovery on a macroscopic or organ level. Hence, a paradigm shift is underway, from a goal of myocardial recovery to one of the remodeling sufficiently to allow for sustainable explantation of the device even if cardiomyopathy remains. Neurohormonal blockade remains a cornerstone of management in conjunction with mechanical support to unload a failing heart and promote positive remodeling. The use of mesenchymal precursor cells may be a promising adjunctive therapy in this regard as recent data from Ascheim *et al* support.

Predicting the Course of the HF Syndrome and Monitoring for Intervention

Monitoring Devices

Hospitalization for HF is demoralizing for patients and contributes to their poor quality of life; it is an enormous component of the rising cost that many countries sustain to care for HF Likewise, the repeated episodes of acute HF decompensation are thought to be a major source of progressive myocardial dysfunction via repeated subendocardial injury. Thus, a reasonable target for many clinical trials has been to show that an intervention reduces HF hospitalizations. Moreover, implantable devices have been designed to help detect the onset of HF instability before the development of the fully manifest decompensated HF syndrome. The hypothesis has been that such early detection systems might prevent HF admissions and reduce mortality.

For many years, ICDs and CRT with and without ICDs have incorporated software that includes HF diagnostic data, such as hemodynamics (pressure or fluid index derived from intrathoracic impedance), correlates of physical activity, or autonomics to predict HF events. Some clinicians and trials have found the addition of this information to be helpful in the assessment of patients with HF, but HF clinical practice guidelines have not considered their value highly. Rather than relying on a single parameter, Program to Access and Review Trending Information and Evaluate Correlation to Symptoms in Patients With Heart Failure (Partners HF) evaluated the utility of combining several diagnostic modalities into an algorithm : long atrial fibrillation duration, rapid ventricular rate during atrial fibrillation, a high fluid index using the thoracic impedance methodology, low patient activity (using implanted device methodology), abnormal autonomics (high night heart rate or low heart rate variability), or notable device therapy (low CRT pacing or ICD shocks), or if they only had a very high fluid index In the 694 patients studied for almost 12 months, a monthly review of HF device diagnostic data identified patients at a 5-fold higher risk of HF hospitalization in the subsequent month. Subsequently, 1562 patients were evaluated on the day of hospital discharge using a similar diagnostic algorithm. The investigators found that the device-derived data accurately predicted those patients at the highest risk of 30-day readmission. The algorithm has now been validated in a prospective fashion. Streamlining the collection of data and applying it in real time to focus resources on the most vulnerable patients are the presumed next steps.

A wireless hemodynamic monitor implanted in the pulmonary artery continuously measures pulmonary pressures in patients with HF and can provide the data quickly and repeatedly over months to years. The Cardio MEMS Heart Sensor Allows Monitoring of Pressure to Improve Outcomes in NYHA Class III Heart Failure Patients (Champion) trial evaluated the role of this device in 550 randomized HF patients with NYHA class III and any LVEF. The investigators were able to demonstrate a significant and clinically meaningful reduction in hospitalization for patients who were managed with the implantable hemodynamic monitoring system; this was true even for patients with HFpEF. Incorporating the information derived from the device into a busy clinical practice with suitable cost accounting remains a challenge. In addition, clinicians need to learn the appropriate management steps in response to rising pulmonary pressures that will keep patients out of the hospital, rather than sending patients to hospital for care.

Biomarkers and Risk Prediction Models

The more accurate and reproducible diagnosis of myocardial infarction, initially with the analysis of the isoenzyme of creatine kinase and later with various forms of troponin, taught clinicians the remarkable utility of using biomarkers to buttress a clinical evaluation. As a result, there was tremendous enthusiasm for the potential of HF biomarkers after the ground-breaking publication showing the applicability of BNP to improve the diagnostic accuracy of HF in the emergency department. Since that time, there has been an explosion of investigations into a myriad of biomarkers. Biomarkers can be grouped into the physiological domains that they reflect, for example, inflammation or fibrosis, renal function, myocardial wall stress, or infection. More recently, micro-RNAs have been proposed as an even more precise biomarker, in 1 example to predict the response to CRT. The ultimate test, however, of any biomarker is to show that clinical knowledge of the same, and an appropriate intervention based on that knowledge, will change clinical outcomes when compared with the gold standard.

The biomarkers that are used most often in the clinical arena include the natriuretic peptides, BNP or NTpro-BNP, which reflect myocardial stress or stretch. A systematic analysis of the incremental value of BNP or NTpro-BNP in predictive models of acute HF concluded that the literature was limited to 7 studies evaluating only mortality outcomes; all had moderate risk of bias. Nevertheless, they acknowledged that there was consistency in the added value to the measurement of natriuretic peptide in patients with acute HF. A more recent meta-analysis had a stronger conclusion : introduction of natriuretic peptide measurement in the investigation of patients with suspected acute HF has the potential to allow rapid and accurate exclusion of the diagnosis. A similar analysis concluded that the addition of NTpro-BNP to predictive models in chronic HF likewise improved accuracy. Indeed, clinicians worldwide use BNP or NTproBNP as a valuable tool to aid in the diagnosis of HF and to identify patients at higher risk of HF complications. A definitive trial demonstrating that the use of natriuretic peptides to guide HF therapy is significantly better than standard management algorithms alone has been more elusive.

One important trial, the St Vincent's Screening to Prevent Heart Failure Study (Stop-HF), proved that a BNP-based screening of patients at risk of HF, combined with subsequent collaborative care, reduced the combined rates of cardiac remodeling (either with respect to systolic or diastolic dysfunction) and HF. The following year, an individual patient meta-analysis of natriuretic peptide–guided HF therapy revealed that all-cause mortality was significantly reduced in patients aged <75 years and overall reduced HF and cardiovascular hospitalizations. Another meta-analyses of individual patient data sought to investigate the interactions between age, comorbidities, or type of HF (preserved or reduced LVEF) and treatment response in the randomized trials of (NT-pro) BNP–guided therapy in HF. These authors concluded that the benefits of therapy guided by (NT-pro) BNP were present in HFrEF only. However, most investigators agree that the ongoing Guiding Evidence Based Therapy Using Biomarker Intensified Treatment in Heart Failure (Guide-IT) trial will help clarify this important question. Guide-IT is designed to determine the safety, efficacy, and cost-effectiveness of a strategy of adjusting HF therapy with the goal of achieving and maintaining a target NT-proBNP level of <1000 pg/mL, compared with usual care in high-risk patients with HFrEF.

Other biomarkers are under active investigation in smaller pilot trials but have yet to be incorporated into clinical practice guidelines as necessary for optimal management of patients with HF. Soluble ST2 is a marker that evokes several mechanistic aspects of HF, including myocardial strain, remodeling, and fibrosis; soluble ST2 belongs to the interleukin-1 receptor family. This marker has been shown to have strong prognostic value for both acute and chronic HF, especially when the combination of ST2 and the natriuretic peptides is used. Cystatin C is a cysteine protease inhibitor that is produced continuously at a constant rate, freely filtered in the kidney, and not secreted in renal tubules; cystatin C is an accurate measure of glomerular filtration rate. During the past decade, cystatin C has been used extensively as a research tool for understanding how kidney function affects health outcomes. Galectin-3 is a member of the β-galactoside–binding lectin family found in many cell types, including fibroblasts and macrophages. This marker also has potential prognostic information, additive to NT-proBNP. Disappointingly, in a recent analysis of the prognostic role of galectin-3 in a trial of patients with HFpEF, galectin-3 levels were found to be associated with age and severity of renal dysfunction, but after adjusting for age, sex, or cystatin-C, galectin-3 was not associated with biomarkers of neurohumoral activation, fibrosis, inflammation or myocardial necrosis, congestion or quality-of-life impairment, cardiac remodeling or dysfunction, or exercise intolerance.

When 1 biomarker adds to a diagnostic algorithm, the use of a multimarker strategy might be more impactful. For example, an intriguing study demonstrated that early increases in multiple biomarkers predicted subsequent cardiotoxicity in patients with breast cancer treated with doxorubicin, taxanes, and trastuzumab. Likewise, combining biomarkers that measure myocardial wall stress and infection allows, for example, an assessment of the breathless patient to exclude HF and consider a bronchitis—an approach that substantially alters treatment. The enthusiasm for this methodology must be tempered with careful outcome trials to justify the additional cost of serial biomarkers.

HF is associated with high mortality, but the risk of death in an individual patient is not easily predictable. Accordingly, many risk models have been developed to help clinicians guide patients toward more advanced therapy or to make end-of-life decisions. A complete list of the currently used risk models is beyond the scope of this review. Two models are increasingly being used in both the clinical setting and incorporated into clinical trials : the Seattle Heart Failure Model and the Meta-Analysis Global Group in Chronic Heart Failure (Maggic) score. Using either score is predicated on the assumption that the variables used are easily obtained during a typical HF evaluation. The Seattle Heart Failure Model is frequently used in the United States as a method to assess risk or need for heart transplant or VAD surgery; critics have suggested that further validation of the score in this population might be needed. The Maggic score, developed in Europe, is currently used to raise awareness of the poor prognosis of patients with HF who appear well compensated. There have been many analyses comparing one risk score with another in a variety of HF patient populations. Inevitably, information from biomarkers and other diagnostic testing have been added to the risk scores to examine the resultant change in predictive capability. This has prompted a cautionary note suggesting that the marginal benefit of complex prognostic evaluations must be balanced against potential patient discomfort and cost escalation. Current HF guidelines suggest that risk profiling may be helpful to inform patient decision making and guide clinical management.

Exercise Training

It is well recognized that regular physical activity or exercise training contributes substantially to the prevention and treatment of cardiovascular disease. For many years, patients with chronic HF were urged to perform regular aerobic activity. Cardiac rehabilitation has been convincingly shown to be effective in improving functional capacity and quality of life and to reduce HF hospitalizations in both patients with HFrEF and HFpEF. Indeed, the US Centers for Medicare and Medicaid Services has approved coverage for cardiac rehabilitation for stable outpatients with HFrEF. Sadly, only a small fraction of eligible patients are referred to cardiac rehabilitation efforts are underway to ensure that exercise training becomes more routine.

Both the European and the American clinical practice guidelines are in the process of being updated to reflect some of the trials summarized above. A reasonable, stepped approach to the patient with HFrEF is depicted in (personal communication.

Problem of the Patient With HFpEF

Most of the major advances in HF management during the past 20 years have been for the patient with HFrEF. Yet, ≈50% of patients hospitalized with HF have a preserved LVEF. This journal has recently published 2 excellent reviews on the mechanistic aspects of HFpEF; HFpEF seems to be a different syndrome from HFrEF. Paulus and Tschöpe have sought to translate the observation that patients with HFpEF have multiple comorbidities into a novel pathophysiologic explanation of the disease. They hypothesize that the comorbidities that typically include diabetes mellitus, hypertension, and obesity lead to a systemic proinflammatory state, which in turn leads to microvascular endothelial inflammation. The vascular inflammation reduces nitric oxide bioavailability, cyclic GMP content, and protein kinase G activity in adjacent cardiomyocytes. The resulting low protein kinase G activity favors hypertrophy development and increases myocardial resting tension because of hypophosphorylation of titin. The attractive nature of this hypothesis is that many potential new targets for treatment can be imagined. This is critically needed, as the current landscape of HFpEF trials has been littered with neutral or negative outcomes.

Cause of Cardiomyopathy: Role of Deep Phenotyping and Precision Medicine

Cardiovascular disease emerges from the background of an individual's unique genetic make-up with subsequent imposition of environmental factors. It has long been recognized that patients with HFrEF and coronary artery disease have, in general, a worse prognosis than those patients with nonischemic dilated cardiomyopathy. It is now increasingly important to elucidate more carefully the various types of dilated cardiomyopathies. The burgeoning field of precision medicine aims to target care based on stratification of disease into subclasses, which share a common biological basis. Personalizing the management of cardiac disease will first require a more sophisticated and integrated approach to phenotyping than is common in current practice. One such nosology, the Moge(S) (morphofunctional characteristic, organ involvement, genetic or familial inheritance pattern, explicit etiological annotation, functional status) classification, was proposed in 2014 Although cumbersome at first glance, this scheme incorporates not only the standard morphofunctional attributes of cardiomyopathy but also the increasingly important pathologic (genetic, environmental, etc) and spectrum of functional status, including preclinical disease (genotype positive and phenotype negative). A classification scheme that provides a common language among clinicians and scientists promotes collaboration and discovery, as illustrated in a recent study by Hazebroek *et al*.

An important example highlighting the need for deep phenotyping is the rapidly unfolding pathophysiology of arrhythmogenic right ventricular cardiomyopathy (ARVC). The presence of cardiotropic viruses was documented in patients with ARVC by Bowles *et al* in 2002; however, the pathophysiologic role was unknown. During the past decade, genetic testing for ARVC has demonstrated a pathogenic mutation in desmosomal or nondesmosomal genes in >50% of patients. Groundbreaking work by Kim *et al* in 2013 using patient-specific, induced pluripotent stem cells demonstrated the requirement of both pathological genotype and metabolic derangement to recapitulate the ARVC disease state in an in vitro model. A zebra fish model of ARVC with cardiac myocyte–specific expression of the human 2057del2 mutation in the gene-encoding plakoglobin was developed by Asimaki *et al*, allowing for a platform of high throughput screening. This study identified a small molecule that rescues the phenotype, moving ever closer to a therapeutic target in humans that addresses the molecular basis of disease. An intriguing recent finding by the Lopez-Ayala *et al* circles back to the role of myocarditis in ARVC, notably reporting an association between acute episodes of myocarditis and the progression of underlying disease. Furthermore, it may be the case that certain mutations increase susceptibility to an environmental insult, such as viral myocarditis.

The theme of abnormal genotypic backdrop and subsequent environmental insult triggering presentation or progression of phenotype is likely to be common among many forms of cardiomyopathy on further investigation. Certainly, there are emerging associations reclassifying peripartum cardiomyopathy as part of familial dilated cardiomyopathy. Although not yet properly investigated, it is conceivable that genetic mutations that predispose to dilated cardiomyopathy may also increase the risk of developing anthracycline-associated cardiomyopathy. Increasing availability of high throughput, affordable next generation sequencing platforms will promote investigation of these theories with subsequent testing of newly discovered genes/mutations in patient-specific models. The therapeutic implications of being able to deeply phenotype and target research and subsequent pharmacological therapy to at-risk individuals or those in early stages of disease will be an exciting frontier of investigation and treatment in the coming years.

Comorbidities and Mortality:- Higher rates of atrial fibrillation has been noted in patients with HFpEF when compared to HFrEF. The increase in mortality rates is comparable in both patients with HFrEF and HFpEF, but the cause of deaths are mostly non-cardiovascular in patients with HFpEF.

Drug Treatment:- Though the treatment aspect is quite clear for patients with HFrEF (systolic dysfunction), the evidence regarding HFpEF (diastolic dysfunction) treatment is still limited. The rationale for treatment of HFpEF presently involves blocking of renin-angiotension system and thus reducing organ damage and myocardial stiffness. Calcium channel blockers and anticoagulants are usually recommended in patients with HFpEF.

Many large randomized controlled trials have found that drugs such as an angiotension –converting enzyme inhibitors, beta-adrenergic blockers, angiotension 11 receptor blockers,aldosterone blockers and cardiac resynchronization with biventricular pacing are useful for decreasing morbidity and mortality in patients with HFrEF but not with HFpEF.

Bibliography and acknowledgement

- AbouEzzeddine of, Haines P, Stevens S, Nativi-Nicolau J, Felker GM, Borlaug BA, Chen HH, Tracy RP, Braunwald E, Redfield MM.Galectin-3 in heart failure with preserved ejection fraction. A Relax trial substudy (phosphodiesterase-5 inhibition to improve clinical status and exercise capacity in diastolic heart failure). JACC *Heart Fail.* 2015; **3**:245–252.
- Abraham WT, Adamson PB, Bourge RC, Aaron MF, Costanzo MR, Stevenson LW, Strickland W, Neelagaru S, Raval N, Krueger S, Weiner S, Shavelle D, Jeffries B, Yadav JS; Champion Trial Study Group. Wireless pulmonary artery haemodynamic monitoring in chronic heart failure: a randomised controlled trial. *Lancet.* 2011; **377**:658–666.
- Abraham WT, Lindenfeld J, Reddy VY, Hasenfuss G, Kuck KH, Boscardin J, Gibbons R, Burkhoff D; FIX-HF-5C Investigators and Coordinators. A randomized controlled trial to evaluate the safety and efficacy of cardiac contractility modulation in patients with moderately reduced left ventricular ejection fraction and a narrow QRS duration: study rationale and design.*J Card Fail.* 2015; **21**:16–23.
- Abraham WT, Stough WG, Piña IL, Linde C, Borer JS, De Ferrari GM, Mehran R, Stein KM, Vincent A, Yadav JS, Anker SD, Zannad F.Trials of implantable monitoring devices in heart failure: which design is optimal? *Nat Rev Cardiol.* 2014; **11**:576–585.

- Bavishi C, Messerli FH, Kadosh B, Ruilope LM, Kario K. Role of neprilysin inhibitor combinations in hypertension: insights from hypertension and heart failure trials. *Eur Heart J.* 2015; **36**:1967–1973.
- Chatterjee NA, Roka A, Lubitz SA, Gold MR, Daubert C, Linde C, Steffel J, Singh JP, Mela T.Reduced appropriate implantable cardioverter-defibrillator therapy after cardiac resynchronization therapy-induced left ventricular function recovery: a meta-analysis and systematic review. *Eur Heart J.* 2015; **36**:2780–2789.
- Dei Cas A, Khan SS, Butler J, Mentz RJ, Bonow RO, Avogaro A, Tschoepe D, Doehner W, Greene SJ, Senni M, Gheorghiade M, Fonarow GC. Impact of diabetes on epidemiology, treatment, and outcomes of patients with heart failure. *JACC Heart Fail.* 2015; **3**:136–145.
- Edelmann F, Wachter R, Schmidt AG, *et al.*; Aldo-DHF Investigators. Effect of spironolactone on diastolic function and exercise capacity in patients with heart failure with preserved ejection fraction: the Aldo-DHF randomized controlled trial. *JAMA*. 2013; *309*:781–791.
- Felker GM, Ahmad T, Anstrom KJ, *et al.* Rationale and design of the GUIDE-IT study: guiding evidence based therapy using biomarker intensified treatment in heart failure. *JACC Heart Fail.* 2014; **2**:457–465.
- Hauptman PJ, Schwartz PJ, Gold MR, Borggrefe M, Van Veldhuisen DJ, Starling RC, Mann DL. Rationale and study design of the increase of vagal tone in heart failure study: Inovate-HF. *Am Heart J.* 2012; **163**:954–962.
- Jain P, Massie BM, Gattis WA, Klein L, Gheorghiade M.Current medical treatment for the exacerbation of chronic heart failure resulting in hospitalization. Am Heart J. 2003; 145:S3–S17.
- Kass DA.Cardiac role of cyclic-GMP hydrolyzing phosphodiesterase type 5: from experimental models to clinical trials. Curr Heart Fail Rep. 2012; 9:192–199.
- Lavie CJ, Arena R, Swift DL, Johannsen NM, Sui X, Lee DC, Earnest CP, Church TS, O'Keefe JH, Milani RV, Blair SN.Exercise and the cardiovascular system: Clinical Science and Cardiovascular Outcomes. Circ Res. 2015; 117:207–219.
- Maisel AS, Krishnaswamy P, Nowak RM, et al. Breathing Not Properly Multinational Study Investigators. Rapid measurement of B-type natriuretic peptide in the emergency diagnosis of heart failure. N Engl J Med. 2002; 347:161–167.
- Nanas JN, Matsouka C, Karageorgopoulos D, Leonti A, Tsolakis E, Drakos SG, Tsagalou EP, Maroulidis GD, Alexopoulos GP, Kanakakis JE, Anastasiou-Nana MI. Etiology of anemia in patients with advanced heart failure. J Am Coll Cardiol. 2006; 48:2485–2489.
- O'Connor CM, Whellan DJ, Lee KL, et al. HF-ACTION Investigators. Efficacy and safety of exercise training in patients with chronic heart failure: HF-ACTION randomized controlled trial. JAMA. 2009; 301:1439–1450.
- Packer M, McMurray JJ, Desai AS, et al.; Paradigm-HF Investigators and Coordinators. Angiotensin receptor neprilysin inhibition compared with enalapril on the risk of clinical progression in surviving patients with heart failure. Circulation. 2015; 131:54–61.
- Redfield MM, Anstrom KJ, Levine JA, *et al.* NHLBI Heart Failure Clinical Research Network. Isosorbide mononitrate in heart failure with preserved ejection fraction. *N Engl J Med.* 2015; **373**:2314–2324.
- Sacks CA, Jarcho JA, Curfman GD. Paradigm shifts in heart-failure therapy–a timeline. *N Engl J Med.* 2014; **371**:989–991.
- Steffel J, Robertson M, Singh JP, Abraham WT, Bax JJ, Borer JS, Dickstein K, Ford I, Gorcsan J, Gras D, Krum H, Sogaard P, Holzmeister J, Brugada J, Ruschitzka F.The effect of QRS duration on cardiac resynchronization therapy in patients with a narrow QRS complex: a subgroup analysis of the EchoCRT trial. Eur Heart J. 2015; 36:1983–1989.
- Tedford RJ, Hemnes AR, Russell SD, Wittstein IS, Mahmud M, Zaiman AL, Mathai SC, Thiemann DR, Hassoun PM, Girgis RE, Orens JB, Shah AS, Yuh D, Conte JV, Champion HC. PDE5A inhibitor treatment of persistent pulmonary hypertension after mechanical circulatory support.Circ Heart Fail. 2008; 1:213–219
- van Spaendonck-Zwarts KY, Posafalvi A, van den Berg MP, Hilfiker-Kleiner D, Bollen IA, Sliwa K, Alders M, Almomani R, van Langen IM, van der Meer P, Sinke RJ, van der Velden J, Van Veldhuisen DJ, van Tintelen JP, Jongbloed JD.Titin gene mutations are common in families with both peripartum cardiomyopathy and dilated cardiomyopathy. Eur Heart J. 2014; 35:2165–2173.
- Wasielewski M, van Spaendonck-Zwarts KY, Westerink ND, Jongbloed JD, Postma A, Gietema JA, van Tintelen JP, van den Berg MP. Potential genetic predisposition for anthracycline-associated cardiomyopathy in families with dilated cardiomyopathy. Open Heart. 2014; 1:e000116.
- Yamamoto K, Origasa H, Hori M; J-DHF Investigators. Effects of carvedilol on heart failure with preserved ejection fraction: the Japanese Diastolic Heart Failure Study (J-DHF). Eur J Heart Fail. 2013; 15:110–118.
- Yang F, Kormos RL, Antaki JF. High-speed visualization of disturbed pathlines in axial flow ventricular assist device under pulsatile conditions. J Thorac Cardiovasc Surg. 2015; 150:938–944.
- Zinman B, Wanner C, Lachin JM, Fitchett D, Bluhmki E, Hantel S, Mattheus M, Devins T, Johansen OE, Woerle HJ, Broedl UC, Inzucchi SE; EMPA-REG Outcome Investigators. Empagliflozin, cardiovascular outcomes, and mortality in type 2 diabetes. N Engl J Med. 2015; 373:2117–2128.

Role of Kumbhaka & Nisshesha Rechaka (intermittent hypoxia) In Chronic Debilitating Ailments

Pranayama is an ancient Indian yogic technique of regulation of breath included in the daily routine of the yogis .It involves gradual training of the respiratory apparatus for prolonging the breathhold time. The aspirant is required to practice every day and advance very slowly over several days to months for perfection. In the yogic literature there are more than 8 types of *Pranayama*, which involve breathing through one or the other nostril, or through the rolled tongue made like a tube; and holding the breath in inspiration, expiration, or somewhere between the two.

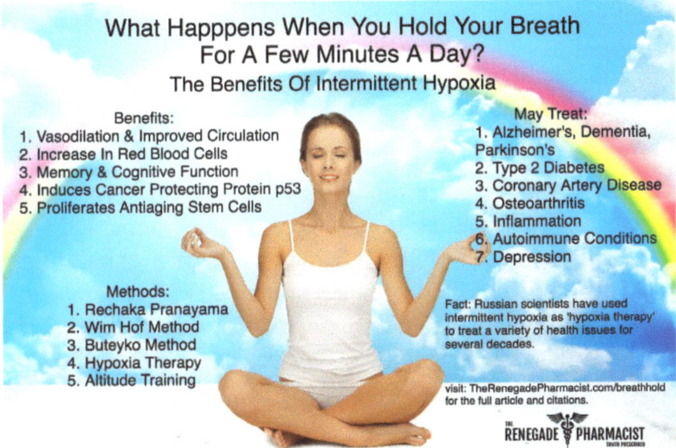

Fig. 35.1: *Benefits of Indian yogic technique of intermittent hypoxemia .*

In the last few years, *Yoga* is gradually getting established as a therapy. In the recent edition of the ancient text H.P. published by Kaivalyadhama, a chapter has been added that contains a very useful method of yogic treatment of various disorders .It is called the "*Nisshesha rechaka*" (The literal translation is "full exhalation with no residual air," and the physiological translation is "breathholding at RV").

Pranayama is being taught to millions of people via the television channels by the Yoga Gurus, and it is commonly adorned as "providing extra oxygen to the system." This explanation comes to them most naturally but does not convince the medical professionals who have 100% oxygen available at their disposal and know that it cannot cure all ills. The truth is that while extra oxygen cannot cure all ills, *intermittent hypoxia can.* The yoga gurus are so far unaware of the beneficial effects of brief, intermittent hypoxia, and little do they realize that of the 8 varieties of *Pranayama*, only Nisshesha Rechaka leads to hypoxia

What is Kumbhak? (Breath retention)

Raise your arms to the level of your chest. Press your left palm with the fist of your right hand.

You will see the more force you want to create, the more you hold your breath. The same goes for lifting weight, jumping, pushing, pulling or even mental focus. Whenever you do any of these, the breath gets held. *Therefore, we can see that without holding your breath one cannot create any effort or strength.* All physical and mental effort or strength is created by holding breath. This hold of breath is called as Kumbhak. When this hold is used in a certain way for a certain period of time then it can empower a particular functioning of an organ. Doing specialized breath hold is known as Kumbhak Therapies.

How does Kumbhak work?

The human body responds to the triggers it gets. These triggers can be natural like the natural food, sunlight, air, environment etc. The unnatural triggers include man made conveniences like air-conditioning, processed food, education, medicine, quality of fabrics for clothes, etc. Kumbhak is the most natural and powerful trigger that the body or the human system uses to create physical and mental strength. When you lift a heavy weight, push or pull someone, get up from a chair, jump up or down or if you focus on something, the breath gets held. Without the breath-hold, the required strength for doing the same is not possible.In Kumbhak, we use the breath-hold (in a certain way, over certain time) to give a natural trigger to the body or the human system. The purpose of this trigger is to build the strength on any weakened aspect of the human system.

Historical Background

The yoga scholar Andrea Jain states that while pranayama in modern yoga as exercise consists of synchronising the breath with movements (between asanas), in ancient texts like the Bhagavad Gita and the Yoga Sutras of Patanjali, pranayama meant "complete cessation of breathing", for which she cites Bronkhorst The Yoga Sutras state. Distractions act as barriers to stillness. One can subdue these distractions by pausing after breath flows in or out. Yoga Sutras, translated by Chip Hartranft with effort relaxing, the flow of inhalation and exhalation can be brought to a standstill; this is called breath regulation. Yoga Sutras, 2:49, translated by Chip Hartranft. According to the scholar-practitioner of yoga Theos Bernard, the ultimate aim of pranayama is the suspension of breathing, "causing the mind to swoon". Swami Yogananda writes, "The real meaning of Pranayama, according to Patanjali, the founder of Yoga philosophy, is the gradual cessation of breathing, the discontinuance of inhalation and exhalation"

1. Puraka (inhalation)
2. 2.Kumbhaka (retention)
3. 3 Rechaka (exhalation).

Lithograph "'breath-control' or Pr nay ma" by Day & Son from artwork by Sophie Charlotte Belnos in The Sundhya or the Daily Prayers of the Brahmins The yoga scholars James Mallinson and Mark Singleton write that "pure breath-retention" (without inhalation or exhalation) is the ultimate pranayama practice in later hatha yoga texts. They give as an example the account in the 13th century Datt treyayoga stra of kevala kumbhaka (breath retention unaccompanied by breathing). They note that this is "the only advanced technique" of breath-control in that text, stating that in it the breath can be held "for as long as one wishes". The Datt treyayoga stra states that kevala kumbhaka gives magical powers, allowing the practitioner to do anything:Once unaccompanied [kevala] breath-retention,free from exhalation and inhalation, is mastered,

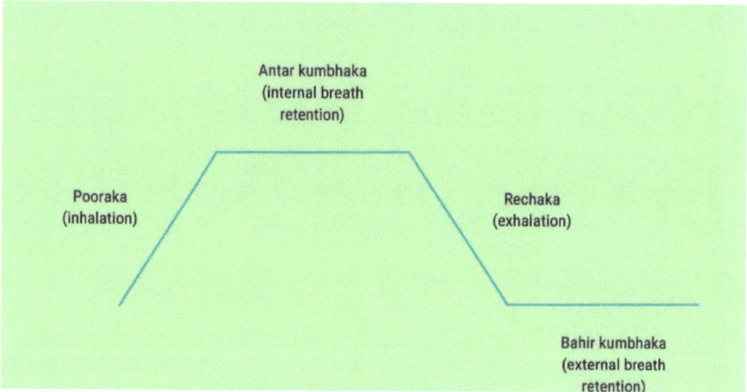

Fig. 35.2: *Kumbhaka terminology of breath retention in pranayama (courtesy by Ian Alexande r5th august 2019)*

there is nothing in the three worlds that is unattainable. —Datt treyayoga stra The 15th century Hatha Yoga Pradipika states that the kumbhakas force the breath into the central sushumna channel (allowing kundalini to rise and cause liberation

The 18th century Gheranda Samhita states that death is impossible when the breath is held in the body

Mallinson and Singleton note that sahita kumbhaka, the intermediate state which is still accompanied (the meaning of sahita) by breathing, was described in detail. They write that the Goraksha Sataka describes four sahita kumbhakas, and that the Hatha Yoga Pradipika describes another four. They point out, however, that these supposed kumbhakas differ in their styles of breathing, giving the example of the buzzing noise made while breathing in bhramari.

Kumbhaka is the retention of the breath in the hatha yoga practice of pranayama. It has two types, accompanied (by breathing) whether after inhalation or after exhalation, and, the ultimate aim, unaccompanied. That state is *kevala kumbhaka*, the complete suspension of the breath for as long as the practitioner wishes.

Types of Kumbhaka: Types of Kumbhaka are eight in number.

They are Surya Bhedan, Ujjayi, Sitkari, Sitali, Bhastrika, Bhramari, Murchha, and Plavini.

The different kinds of Kumbhaka are an extension of the basic breathing exercise. While doing

Surya bhedana air should be drawn in slowly, through the right nostril. Thereafter it should be let out through the left nostril. This asana cleans forehead, removes disorders of Vata as well as worms. While performing

Ujjayi air should be drawn in such a way that it goes touching from the throat to the chest thereby making noise while passing. It should be controlled and then let out through the left nostril. This removes phlegm in the throat as well as increases the appetite. The defects of nadi are destroyed.

Sitkari is performed by drawing air through the mouth and the tongue is between the lips. It is believed that the practitioner becomes the destroyer of creation. They are not affected by hunger, thirst sleep or laziness.

In Sitali the tongue is slightly protruding out of lips when the air is drawn inwards. It goes out through nostrils. This is effective in curing enlarging spleen, fever, disorders of bile, hunger and thirst.

In Bhastrika first one needs to sit in Padma asana posture after which the feet is crossed and placed on both thighs. The mouth is closed so that the air passes through the nostrils. It should be filled up to the lotus of the heart, making noise and touching the throat, the chest and the head. It should be expelled again and filled again and again. The air should be drawn through the right nostril by pressing the thumb against the left side of the nose, thereby closing the left nostril; and when it is filled it should be closed with the fourth finger and kept confined. This should go out through the left nostril. Bhastrika destroys Vata, pitta and phlegm and increases the digestive power.

In Bhramari the air is filled with force and making a peculiar noise and expel it slowly, making noise in the same way.

The Murchha is a process that involves closing the passages with Jalandhar Bandha firmly at the end of Puraka, and drive out the air slowly that gives the mind great comfort.

In Plavini the belly is filled with air and the inside of the body is filled with air, the body floats on the deepest water, like a leaf of a lotus.

Kumbhaka (Breath retention)

The name kumbhaka is from Sanskrit कुम्भ kumbha, a pot, comparing the torso to a vessel full of air.

Kumbhaka is the retention of the breath in pranayama, either after inhalation, the inner or Antara Kumbhaka, or after exhalation, the outer or Bahya Kumbhaka (also called Bahir Kumbhaka.

According to B.K.S. Iyengar in Light on Yoga, kumbhaka is the "retention or holding the breath, a state where there is no inhalation or exhalation".

Sahit or Sahaja Kumbhaka is an intermediate state, when breath retention becomes natural, at the stage of withdrawal of the senses.

Pratyahara, the fifth of the eight limbs of yoga.

Kevala Kumbhaka, when inhalation and exhalation can be suspended at will, is the extreme stage of **Kumbhaka** **"parallel"** with the state of Samadhi or union with the divine, the last of the eight limbs of yoga, attained only by continuous long term pranayama and kumbhaka exercises. The 18th century Joga Pradipika states that the highest breath control, which it defines as inhaling to a count (mātrā) of 8, holding to a count of 19, and exhaling to a count of 9, confers liberation and Samadhi.

The Yoga Institute recommends sitting in a meditative posture such as Sukhasana for Kumbhaka practice. After a full inhalation for 5 seconds, it suggests retaining the air for 10 seconds, exhaling smoothly, and then taking several ordinary breaths. It recommends five such rounds per pranayama session, increasing the time of retention as far as is comfortable by one second each week of practice.

How to Practice kumbhaka

Starting position

1. Do preliminary conditioning in *Sukhasana* or any other meditative posture.
2. If not possible to sit on the floor, sit on a firm chair with an erect backrest.
3. Keep the body above the waist straight and the spine erect. Keep eyes closed.

Sequence of steps in performing Kumbhaka Pranayama

1. Make a short exhalation and then start inhaling – slowly and rhythmically in one long and unbroken inspiration.
2. Continue inhaling until a sense of fullness is experienced in the chest.
3. Retain the inhaled air for a period of 10 seconds (preferably double the period of inspiration).
4. Ensure: No exaggerated movement of the abdomen.
5. While sitting spine, head and neck is maintained erect.
6. Ensure facial muscles relaxed and nose is unconstricted.
7. Inhalation is slow and rhythmic – long, unbroken and without jerks.
8. Now exhale as naturally as possible – gradually, avoiding jerky or hasty movements
9. Take few normal breaths and relax.

Recommended practice:

- Practice daily, 5 rounds/session, with pause in-between rounds.
- Begin with a count of 5 seconds inhalation and 10 seconds retention. Gradually increase it by 1 sec/ every week, when practised daily.

- Practice without strain to a count as per individual comfort

Limitations /Contraindications

Children under 12 years should not practice.

- Not recommended in serious cardiac and hypertension cases.

Benefits of Kumbhaka Pranayama:

1. Hygienic effect on dead space air or residual air and alveolar air.
2. Better ventilation of air happens.
3. Favourable effect on intra-thoracic and intra-pulmonary air pressures.
4. Increase in carbon dioxide level (due to retention) activates respiratory centre in brain leading to greater interchange of oxygen.
5. Better oxygenation – improves health and concentration.
6. Reduces strain on circulatory system.
7. Recombinant biological molecules, such as Erythropoietin (EPO) and Vascular Endothelial Growth Factor (VEGF) are finding increasing use as therapeutic agents for various disease conditions.
8. Injectable Recombinant Human Erythropoietin is already in use for anemia associated with chronic renal failure and to stimulate erythropoiesis for autologous blood transfusion; and efforts are on to use it to stimulate nerve growth after mechanical nerve injury in peripheral neuropathies associated with diabetes mellitus, and in autonomic neuropathies. Recombinant VEGF is waiting to find clinical use in revascularization in diseased coronary and other vascular beds as an alternative to angioplasty and bypass grafting.
9. At the same time, the stem cells–related research is looking forward to find a cure for a number of as-yet incurable diseases. Embryonic stem cells (ESC) obtained from umbilical cord blood have already been effectively used in the treatment of sickle cell anemia, leukemia, non-Hodgkin's lymphoma, other forms of cancer, life-threatening anemias, and autoimmune diseases. Stem cells may hold the key to replacing cells lost in situations, such as spinal cord injury and many progressive, devastating diseases, such as Parkinson's disease, multiple sclerosis, Alzheimer's disease, diabetes, chronic heart failure, end-stage renal disease, liver failure and cancer. Lately stem cell use has been tried in the treatment of burns, infertility, lupus, and deafness.

   Stem cells survival and self-renewal has been found to be better at low tissue oxygen levels. In other words, stem cells are kind of a minority of anerobic cells in the multimillion populations of aerobic cells of the body. It is therefore these cells which are most susceptible to oxidative injury. Yogic di*et al*lows for huge amounts of antioxidants in the diet.

   Mobilization of stem cells from the bone marrow can come to use in the therapy of a number of degenerative diseases, including type-2 diabetes mellitus and Idiopathic Parkinson's disease and Osteoarthritis. Indeed this is the frontier area of research these days.

   Scientists are trying to harvest stem cells from the bone marrow, suitably multiply them, and then plant them at the place of need. Transportation of stem cells from the bone marrow to the tissues can be hindered at the oxygen levels prevalent in the bloodstream. It can be facilitated by brief, episodic hypoxia. Intermittent hypoxia therapy has been tried, developed, and practiced by Russian scientists for the last 50 years.
10. Studies done at the Antar Prakash Centre for Yoga, Haridwar, have shown that *Nisshesha rechaka*, a type of *Pranayama* described in Hatha Pradeepika (H.P.) is the easiest way to produce brief, intermittent hypoxia. According to H.P., it can work on any organ on which the practitioner wants it to work by focusing the mind on that organ while performing the *rechaka*.

Oxygen and hypoxia

Oxygen has been considered essential for life since its discovery in the late 18th century. Earliest experiments showed a rat dying when enclosed under a bell jar, further, if a burning candle was also enclosed under a bell jar it would get extinguished and the remaining air would not support life. These experiments established the role of oxygen as essential for our life, and hypoxia, or lack of oxygen has been considered as injurious underlying serious diseases, such as ischemic strokes and myocardial infarctions. That a whole world of anaerobic organisms exists was not known till that time—this discovery came much later. However, lately we have started realizing the multifold benefits of episodic, brief intermittent hypoxia. It is now well recognized that episodic hypoxia leads to adaptive responses in the tissues which protect them from ischemic and other injuries. In the former USSR this knowledge has come to develop into a full-fledged therapy.

Hypoxia therapy

In the erstwhile USSR, for the last 50 years research was being carried out on finding uses of and ways to produce hypoxia .Initially the scientists simulated the hypoxic conditions of high altitudes in the plains to train the pilots of small fighter aircrafts and the mountaineers. Thereafter, it took the form of a training tool for athletes, and ultimately developed into a full-fledged therapeutic modality. At that time the Russian scientific community was completely cut off from the rest of the world and these studies were not available elsewhere. It is only recently that some English translations of the studies have come out.

The Russian scientists have used several different techniques to produce hypoxia. They include the following:

- Hypobaric chambers
- Quick ascent to high altitudes for short durations.
- Normobaric hypoxic gas mixtures. To deliver such gas mixtures, there they have commercially available "Hypoxicators "that is, instruments that deliver a hypoxic gas mixture containing 10% oxygen. This mixture is called "HGM-10."
- Intermittent hypoxia is defined as repeated episodes of hypoxia with intervening periods of normoxia. The actual durations used in different experimental studies vary widely, with hypoxia periods ranging from 3 to 90 min.

Beneficial Effects of Intermittent Hypoxia

All the effects of hypoxia are generated through the now well-documented "Hypoxia-Inducible-Factor-1" (HIF-1) Its molecular structure has been studied in great detail. In various tissues, the HIF-1 produces different chemicals, such as the EPO in the kidney and the VEGF in several other tissues.

- Hypoxia has been shown to increase hemoglobin levels through the formation of EPO.
- In ischemic tissues, hypoxia leads to the formation of growth factors, such as the VEGF, and this leads to formation of new blood vessels (angiogenesis). In ischemic myocardium this can lead to the formation of coronary collaterals.
- Hypoxia induces the enzyme Nitric Oxide Synthase (NOS). Nitric oxide has been assigned different roles in different tissues. Widely, it is one of the defense mechanisms against oxidative damage. Thus more of nitric oxide is able to protect the tissues better. Nitric oxide contributes to dilatation of coronary arteries when needed. It is also involved in the quick vasodilatation required for the erection of penis and intermittent hypoxia can be an effective treatment for erectile dysfunction.
- Hypoxia has been shown to increase resistance of tissues to various insults and injuries, including radiation injuries and aging.
- Hypoxia induces p53 "Guardian of the genome." p53 is a transcription regulation factor. It has a protective role in DNA damage. It is well known that during the process of normal cell division some DNA damage does occur. There are in-built processes for the repair of such damage. If the damage goes beyond repair, then p53 is involved in activating the apoptosis program.
- Stem cells only survive in hypoxia .Stem cells are abundant in fetal circulation where the partial pressure of oxygen (pO_2) is low. They disappear from the circulation soon after birth. They survive in various locations (Niches) in the body in adulthood. A young individual has an abundance of these stem cells. Old age is when the stem cell population reduces. It is possible that stem cells from the bone marrow migrate to various tissues, and such migration may be facilitated by even a few minutes of hypoxia every day. Thus hypoxia can be of benefit in a host of the so-called degenerative disorders, including Idiopathic Parkinson's disease, Alzheimer's disease, and Osteoarthritis, which is also called as "Joint Failure."

Hypoxia and stem cell life cycle

Stem cells are in one of the frontier areas of research these years. Stem cells are those wonderful cells that have enormous capacity to differentiate into virtually any kind of cell in our body. This knowledge has become the foundation stone of regenerative medicine, whereby we dream of being able to produce any lost or damaged organ. In the mother's womb the fetus develops from a single cell, the zygote, which is formed by fusion of the ovum of the mother and the sperm of the father. This single cell gives rise to the vast diversity of tissues in the developed human body. During embryonic life, differentiation goes on at a very fast pace. By about the third month of intrauterine life the development of all the organs is nearly complete.

The mother's womb provides the fetus a protected environment. The watery amniotic fluid protects it from mechanical shocks and provides a constant ambient temperature. All its nutritional requirements are met through the umbilical cord, which also serves to take away the waste products.

The mother's womb also provides a further valuable gift that commonly goes unsung: A hypoxic environment. The embryo breathes in a very low partial pressure of oxygen, about equal to that present at the Mount Everest. It is this hypoxic environment that is so important for

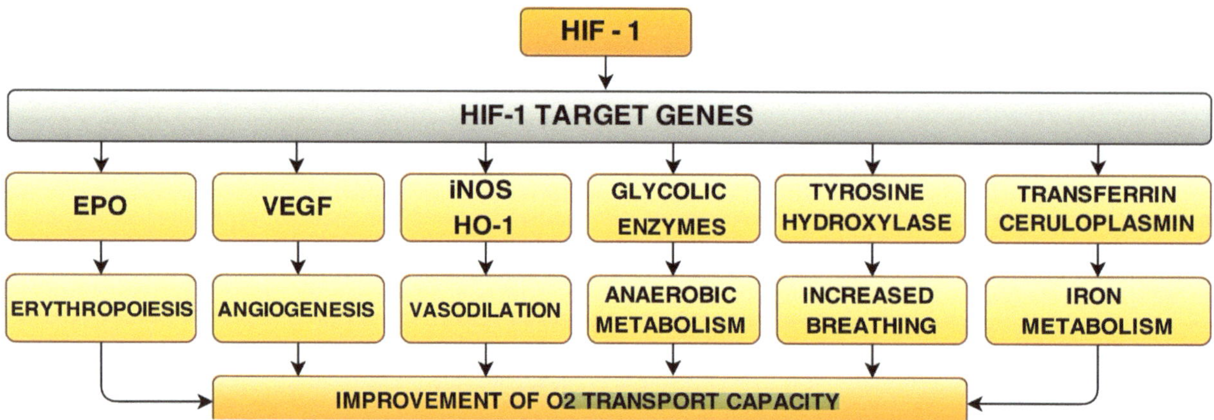

Fig. 35.3 *The above diagram shows some of the science associated with Intermittent Hypoxic Training (IHT). One of the main aspects of Intermittent Hypoxic training is the stimulation of HIF-1, also known as Hypoxia Inducible Factor-1. HIF-1 is an extremely important growth factor. HIFs are transcription factors (factors that directly affect various genes) that respond to decreases in available oxygen (hypoxia) in the cellular environment. Hypoxia-inducible factors (HIFs) are key molecules that regulate cellular responses to inflammation and hypoxia. These responses are essential for the normal cell function and survival. In hypoxic conditions, HIF-1 serves as a transcription factor that regulates over 100 genes essential for survival in oxygen-deprived conditions. The next diagram shows how cell biology comes into play with hypoxia compared to Normoxia (normal oxygen concentration and pressure found at sea level at sea-level).*

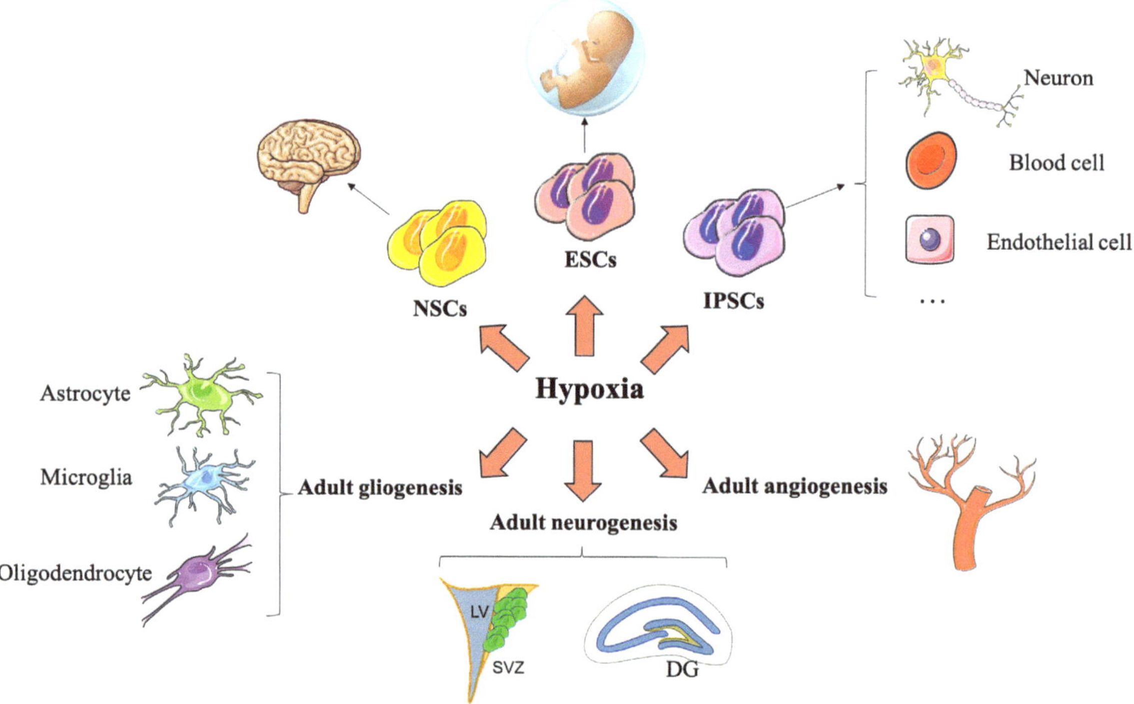

Fig. 35.4 *Hypoxia promotes stem cell proliferation, differentiation, and survival. Hypoxia promotes the pluripotency, proliferation, and directed differentiation of embryonic stem cells (ESCs) and neural stem cells (NSCs) and helps induced pluripotent stem cells (iPSCs) to develop into different types of cells in vitro. Hypoxia is also involved in adult neurogenesis, angiogenesis, and gliogenesis. DG, dentate gyrus; LV, lateral ventricle; SVZ, subventricular zone*

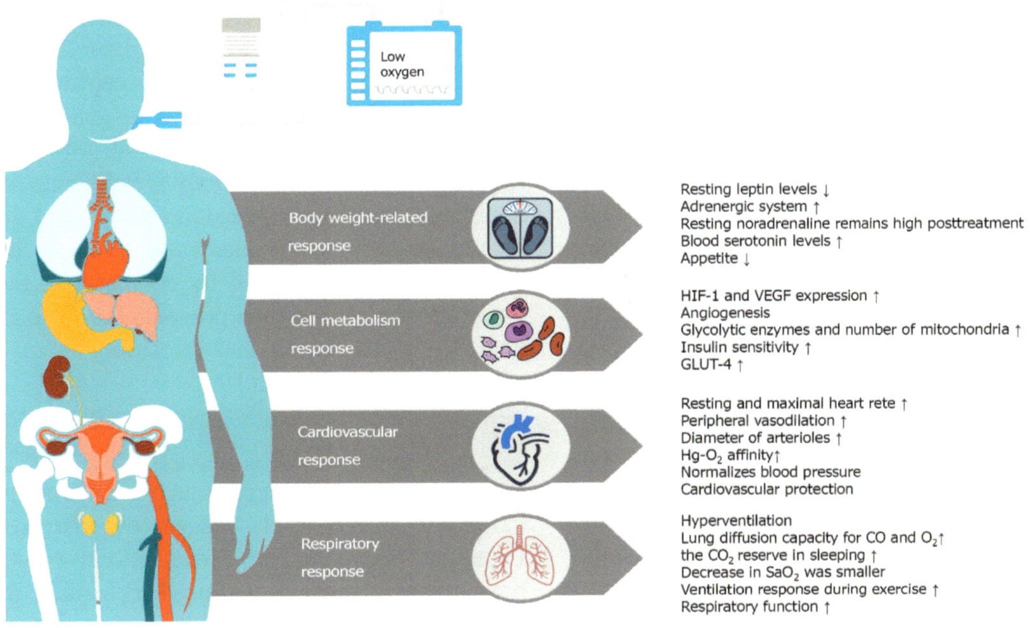

Fig. 35.5 *The illustration demonstrates tthat there are a number of other influences hypoxic conditions have on our health .One of the above responses is how intermittent hypoxia can affect body weight One of these mechanisms is the reduction of appetite. Another one is the reduction of Leptin levels. Leptin is a hypoxia-inducible hormone released from fat cells in adipose tissue. Leptin acts upon the brain, in particular to an area called the hypothalamus. Leptin does not affect food intake from meal to meal but, instead, acts to alter food intake and control energy expenditure over the long term. Leptin has a more profound effect when we lose weight and levels of the hormone fall. This stimulates a huge appetite and increased food intake. The hormone helps us to maintain our normal weight and unfortunately for dieters, makes it hard to lose those extra pounds! HIT increases Leptin. In the next illustration we see some of the methods hypoxia training affects weight loss. The studies have shown that the weight loss benefits are multifaceted and include aspects that have already been mentioned such as decreased Leptin levels which can then suppress appetite. Another response mentioned above is cell metabolism. The cell metabolism is affected on a number of different levels. One such effect includes an increase sensitivity to insulin by the body. Typically, when one has diabetes the insulin sensitivity is much lower and thus more insulin is needed to do the job. In addition to promoting O2 delivery, HIF-1 also activates the transcription of genes encoding enzymes, transporters, and mitochondrial proteins that decrease O2 utilization. Thus, HIF functions as a master regulator to switch cells from oxidative metabolism to glycolytic metabolism. One condition in the body which can be favorably affected by hypoxia training is the health of our mitochondria. This is probably the most piece of all. As science is now discovering, the health of our mitochondria typically will determine out health. Many diseases have their roots in mitochondrial dysfunction. Many studies suggest that hypoxic gas mixtures may be useful in treating or preventing mitochondrial disorders. This approach is seemingly counterintuitive, since oxygen is a key substrate for the respiratory chain which produces the body's energy currency ATP. However, hypoxia activates an adaptive program that allows us to cope with limiting oxygen levels. This program decreases our reliance on mitochondrial oxidative metabolism, more commonly known as the Krebs cycle. Such adaptive programs are not necessarily triggered by mitochondrial disease given the fact the hypoxic signal is absent.*

the multiplication and growth of the stem cells, with differentiation being the natural consequence. The number of stem cells in the circulating blood is maximum during fetal life. In the laboratory, embryonic stem cells are obtained from the umbilical cord blood samples just after birth. Currently, the practice to store the umbilical cord blood for future use is being popularized.

Just after birth, when the newborn is exposed to the atmospheric air containing high pO_2 and as the pO_2 of the arterial blood rises, the stem cells soon disappear from the blood circulation. In the adult they survive only in certain locations called "niches." One such location is the bone marrow where the blood circulation is sluggish, oxygen extraction is more, and there is relative hypoxia. In addition, anatomically the niche allows the cells to remain in clusters where the stem cells stay in the center, surrounded by more differentiated cells, which consume a large amount of oxygen, thus creating a hypoxic zone for the stem cells. In other words, the stem cells and more mature cells are distributed along an *oxygen gradient*—primitive stem cells residing in the most *hypoxic areas* of the bone marrow where oxygen content is low. It has been shown in rats that the number of Mesenchymal Stem Cells (MSC) in the peripheral blood increases by as much as 15 folds by hypoxia. Hypoxia enhances proliferation of mouse embryonic stem cell–derived neural cells.Since cells cannot circulate in clusters, it is understandable what difficulty the marrow stem cells would encounter had they had to circulate in the blood. That probably explains why some of us are not able to regenerate lost tissues and suffer from such diseases as diabetes mellitus, osteoarthritis of the knees, and idiopathic Parkinson's disease.

It may be of interest to note that the prevalence of osteoarthritis of the knees has been found to be less in hilly areas. Although some scientists believe this difference may be due the fact that the residents of hills get more exercise having to walk up and down the hills; there may be something more to it. The hypoxic environment of the hills may contribute to the persistence of stem cells in the articular cartilages, or their migration from niches like the bone marrow.

That the stem cells survive better when cultured in hypoxic environment is now well recognized. Artificial culture of stem cells in different environmental conditions showed that stem cells retain their self-renewing character if cultured under hypoxic conditions, in 2% oxygen as compared with the 20% present in air.

However, the direction of regenerative medicine appears misguided. The scientists are trying to capture stem cells from the bone marrow, cultivate them, and then inject them at the site of desired organogenesis or organ repair. This may be a little out of place; given the wisdom of the body. The way we do not need to capture, cultivate, and re-inject the bone marrow cells to generate more *blood* cells, we should not need to do the same for any other organ, because the whole body is well connected through a meticulous network of blood vessels, and the stem cells should be able to circulate and relocate themselves at the place of need guided by chemotactic factors as yet unrecognized. What then prevents the bone marrow stem cells from circulating and relocating themselves to the place of need? – Oxygen!

Oxidative stress and injuries

It is now well recognized that oxidative stress is a great damaging force that causes degenerative diseases. Diseases believed to result from oxidative injuries include osteoarthritis and Idiopathic Parkinson's disease. The bone marrow stem cells and the mesenchymal stem cells are poor in number of mitochondria, that is, they are adapted to anaerobic survival. From the discussion in the previous paragraphs it must be clear that the cells most likely to suffer damage from excess of oxygen are the stem cells.

Conditions where self-administered brief intermittent hypoxia can be useful

Type-2 Diabetes mellitus

Type-2 Diabetes mellitus has acquired epidemic proportions. A patient affected with Type-2 Diabetes Mellitus (T2DM) gradually loses the β-cell mass. The current therapeutic strategies include stimulating insulin release from the β cells by sulfonylureas, stimulating peripheral utilization of glucose by biguanides, and reducing insulin resistance using thiazolidinedione derivatives. These drugs need to be taken continuously; and over the years their effect vanishes. Incretin mimetics, such as GLP-1 analogs (eg, Exenatide) hold promise as they stimulate the proliferation and inhibit the apoptosis of β cells. Drugs inhibiting breakdown of endogenous GLP-1, for example, vildagliptine are other agents used for the treatment of T2DM.

Human embryonic stem cells can be directed to differentiate into cells that produce insulin. The adult body is endowed with a population of adult stem cells, which by definition are capable of self-renewal as well as differentiation in any one of several different types of adult tissues.

It is wise to expect that nature must have provided for the regeneration of β cells through the use of stem cells. Mice have been seen to regenerate β-cell mass after ablation of 70%–80% of it. In them the source of new beta cells is the adult, differentiated beta cell. The capacity of hemopoietic stem cells to differentiate to insulin-producing cells has been at the center of debate for the past 5 years and it now seems that their role could more likely be that of helper cells able to facilitate survival or stimulate proliferation of endogenous β cells.

Coronary artery disease

In addition to the existing therapies with drugs, stents, and bypasses, the scientists are keen to find other ways to regenerate the blocked coronary arteries in a more natural way. Stimulating the formation of coronary collaterals "Natural Bypasses" has been pointed out to be a neglected field.

The major disease affecting the coronary arteries is atherosclerosis, which is the underlying cause for angina pectoris and myocardial infarction. When the narrowing of the coronary artery is gradual, it is associated with the development of collateral channels. The mechanism involved is thought to be tissue hypoxia leading to formation of VEGF. Physical exercise also must offer relief in coronary artery disease through generating brief hypoxia. Coincidentally, patients with sleep apnea and hypoxic spells have been found to have developed better coronary collaterals!

Osteoarthritis

Osteoarthritis, rightly named "Joint Failure" is a degenerative disease, thereby meaning a disease of old age caused by progressive damage to the joint cartilage at a rate the body is not able to repair. The factors that lead to destruction of the joint cartilage are the same over all the ages, but in children as well as young adults the cartilage that gets damaged due to wear and tear gets completely repaired by the body's regenerative process on a day-to-day basis. It is when either the rate of destruction increases or the rate of repair lags behind that the problem manifests clinically. The destructive forces are wear and tear, and with the weight-bearing joints, such as the knees, the damage increases in proportion to the body weight. It is important to understand the role of oxidative damage to the regenerative tissues so that the use of antioxidants in the diet can be promoted. Natural reparative process is largely carried out by the chondrocytes, which secrete the extracellular matrix. Cellular damage to the chondrocytes is made good by chondroblasts and deficiency of chondroblasts can be made good by stem cells present in the near vicinity. With insufficiency of stem cells more stem cells can be mobilized from the bone marrow, which serves as the storehouse. This process occurs under the influence of chemotactic factors. Some of such factors may be inhibited by the Non Steroidal Anti-Inflammatory Drugs (NSAIDs). Scientists are trying to harness stem cells from the bone marrow, suitably multiply them in culture and then plant them at the site of injury to replenish the cartilage.Infrapatellar fat pad (IPFP) is a possible source of stem cells for the repair of articular cartilage defects. Hypoxic conditions increase hypoxia-inducible transcription factor HIF-2α and enhance chondrogenesis in stem cells from the infrapatellar fat pad of osteoarthritis patients.

Parkinson's disease

Parkinson's disease (PD) affects around 3% of people aged over 65 years. It occurs as a result of the loss of dopamine-producing brain cells in specific location called the substantia nigra. Symptoms of PD are tremor, or trembling in hands, arms, legs, jaw, and face; rigidity, or stiffness of the limbs and trunk; bradykinesia, or slowness of movement; paucity of facial expression and postural instability, that is, impaired balance and coordination. These symptoms are gradually progressive and some patients may have difficulty walking, talking, or performing simple day-to-day tasks. PD usually affects people over the age of 50 years. At present, there is no cure for PD. Bradykinesia and rigidity respond best to treatment with levodopa, whereas tremors respond better to anticholinergics, such as trihexyphenydyl. Other drugs, such as bromocriptine mimic the role of dopamine in the brain.

The possible approach of taking stem cells, growing them into new brain cells and transplanting these into the patient is currently being discussed. Jaslok Hospital, Mumbai, is trying to study the safety and efficacy of bone marrow–derived mesenchymal stem cells transplant in Parkinson's disease.

Chronic renal failure

In developed as well as developing countries, Chronic Renal Failure (CRF) is a great public health problem. In the developing countries, people commonly cannot afford the cost of dialysis and the average life span of a patient after diagnosis is short, up to 3 years. For the treatment of anemia of CRF, injections of recombinant Human Erythropoietin are commonly employed whether the patient is on dialysis or not. However, researches have shown that the diseased kidney still has intact capacity to secrete EPO. Acute hypoxic stress is associated with increased levels of EPO. Hence it is thought that the EPO deficiency of chronic renal failure is a result of a functional disturbance.Hypoxia induced by breath holding in full expiration (*Nisshesha rechaka pranayama*) as described can greatly help patients by increasing endogenous EPO production, thus cutting down expenditure on EPO injections and reducing cost of treatment.

Erectile dysfunction

Erectile dysfunction (ED) occurs in about 5% of 40-year-old men and in 15%–25% of 65-year-old men. It is defined as an inability to achieve penile erection sufficient for satisfactory sexual activity. The penis contains two elongated structures called the corpora cavernosa, consisting of spongy tissue, which run the length of the organ. The corpora cavernosa are surrounded by a membrane, called the tunica albuginea. Erection begins with sensory or mental stimulation, or both. The tunica albuginea helps trap the blood in the corpora cavernosa, thereby sustaining erection. This requires a quick vasodilatation, which is mediated by some neurotransmitters, such as the vasoactive intestinal peptide (VIP) released from the supplying nerves. Nitric oxide plays a very important role in the quick vasodilatation. Nitric oxide is produced by vascular endothelium and diffuses into the smooth muscle cells of the arteries where it leads to the release of cyclic GMP. Drugs such as sildenafil act by inhibiting the metabolizing enzyme phosphodiesterase-5 (PDE5), thus inhibiting the breakdown and prolonging the effect of the endogenous cyclic GMP. Brief intermittent hypoxia induces Nitric Oxide Synthase (NOS) thereby facilitating the quick vasodilatation in the penile arteries thus enabling quick and hard erection.

Thyroid Dysfunctions

Thyroid disorder has indeed become a household name these days, close behind hypertension and diabetes. According to the American Thyroid Association (ATA), around 20 million people in the US have some form of thyroid disorder, and at least 60% of those who do are not even aware of it. Also, the prevalence of the condition is believed to be higher in women than men. One of the leading causes of thyroid disorders is believed to be the stressful lifestyle we are leading. Even though there is increasing prevalence of thyroid disorders today, there are numerous treatment options available to patients. Of course, every treatment would take time to show results, but in the meantime, you have something to cheer about. Yoga and meditation can help treat thyroid naturally. A few minutes of yoga practice daily helps reduce stress and also make your life smoother and happier. The followings are the yogic techniques in the treatment of thyroid disorders:

For hypothyroidism

- Suryabhedan Pranayama with Kumbhak (10 minutes)
- Bhastrika Pranayama with Kumbhak (10 minutes)

For hyperthyroidism

- Sheetali Pranayama with Kumbhak (10 minutes)
- Sitakari Pranayama with kumbhak (10 minutes)

Benefits in cancer patients.

pure *pranayama* intervention in a population of patients with cancer successfully demonstrated that yoga breathing is feasible and can be safely recommended for patients with cancer receiving chemotherapy. Any increase in the yoga breathing practice was correlated with improvements in both cancer chemotherapy associated symptoms and QOL. *Pranayama* may be helpful for improving sleep disturbance, anxiety, and mental QOL among patients undergoing chemotherapy. Definitive conclusions on efficacy await further study.

Bibliography and Acknowledgement

An WG, Kanekal M, Simon MC. Stabilization of wild-type p53 by hypoxia-inducible factor 1 alpha. Nature. 1998;392:405–8. [PubMed]

Burnett A. Nitric Oxide in the Penis: Physiology and Pathology. J Urol. 1997;157:320–4. [PubMed]

Burnett AL. The role of nitric oxide in erectile dysfunction: Implications for medical therapy. J Clin Hypertens (Greenwich) 2006;8(12 Suppl 4):53–62. [PubMed]

Cao G1, Shukitt-Hale B, Bickford PC, Joseph JA, McEwen J, Prior RL. Hyperoxia-induced changes in antioxidant capacity and the effect of dietary antioxidants. [PubMed]

Digambaraji S, Kokaje RS, editors. Ha hapradipika of Swatmarama. Lonavala, Dist. Pune, India: S.M.Y.M.Samiti; 1970. ISBN:81-89485-12-1.

Koerselman , van der Graaf Y, de Jaegere PP, Grobbee DE. Coronary collaterals: An important and underexposed aspect of coronary artery disease. Circulation. 2003;107:2507–11. [PubMed]

Kurtz A, Eckardt KU. Erythropoietin production in chronic renal disease before and after transplantation. Contrib Nephrol. 1990;87:15–25. [PubMed]

Parkes M . Breath-holding and its breakpoint. Exp Physiol. 2006;91:1–15. [PubMed]

Rodrigues CA, Diogo MM, da Silva CL, Cabral JM. Hypoxia enhances proliferation of mouse embryonic stem cell-derived neural stem cells. Biotechnol Bioeng. 2010;106:260–70. [PubMed]

Sordi V, Piemonti L. The contribution of hematopoietic stem cells to beta-cell replacement. Curr Diab Rep. 2009;9:119–24. [PubMed]

Steiner S. Occurrence of coronary collateral vessels in patients with sleep apnea and total coronary occlusion. Chest. 2010;137:516–20. [PubMed]

Yin ZS, Zhang H, Gao W. Erythropoietin promotes functional recovery and enhances nerve regeneration after peripheral nerve injury in rats. Am J Neuroradiol. 2010;31:509–15. [PubMed]

Nadi Shodhan Pranayama &Hath Yoga in Maintaining Health Wellness

Nadis form part of the subtle anatomy as defined by Yoga. The Hatha Yoga Pradipika states there are 72,000 Nadis, and The Shiva Samhita says there are 350,00. The term Nadi is defined as a channel for *Prana* to flow. *Nadis* congregate and intersect at several locations forming Chakras, or plexuses of subtle energy, just as nerves accumulate and become nerve plexuses at major locations in the gross body.

Relationship Between Nadis, Chakras and Nervous System

The Central Nervous System (CNS) is the bodies communications structure. Information from the senses is sent to the brain, and the brain then delivers the data out to the body back through the CNS

Autonomic Nervous System

The Autonomic nervous system (ANS) a section of the CNS is responsible for the bodies involuntary functions. The ANS is subdivided into the sympathetic nervous system, or Pingala Nadi and the Parasympathetic nervous system, or Ida Nadi

Hypothalamus

The Sympathetic nervous system is controlled the Hypothalamus, with the nerves spreading on both sides of the spinal cord, connecting to nerve plexuses and correspondingly to Chakras.

- Cervical Plexus – Vishuddhi Chakra
- Cardiac Plexus – Anahata Chakra
- Enteric Plexus – Manipura Charkra
- Lumbar Plexus – Swadhistana Chakra
- Pelvic Plexus – Muladhara Chakra

The Sympathetic nervous system is our fight and flight response. If a threat exists the Hypothalamus sends signals throughout the Sympathetic system preparing for action. The heart rate and blood pressure increases, blood Glucose is generated and the air passages open Sympathetic system preparing for action.

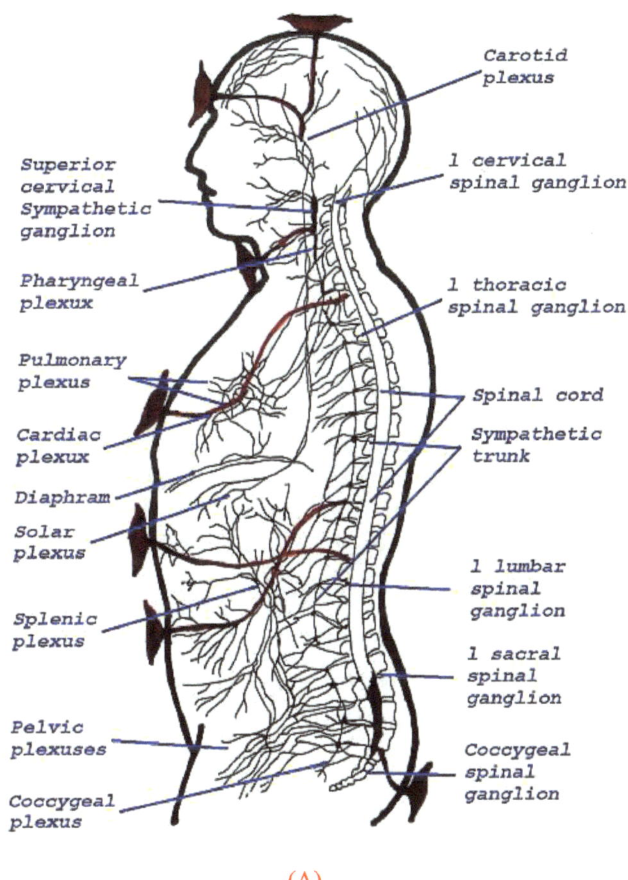

(A)

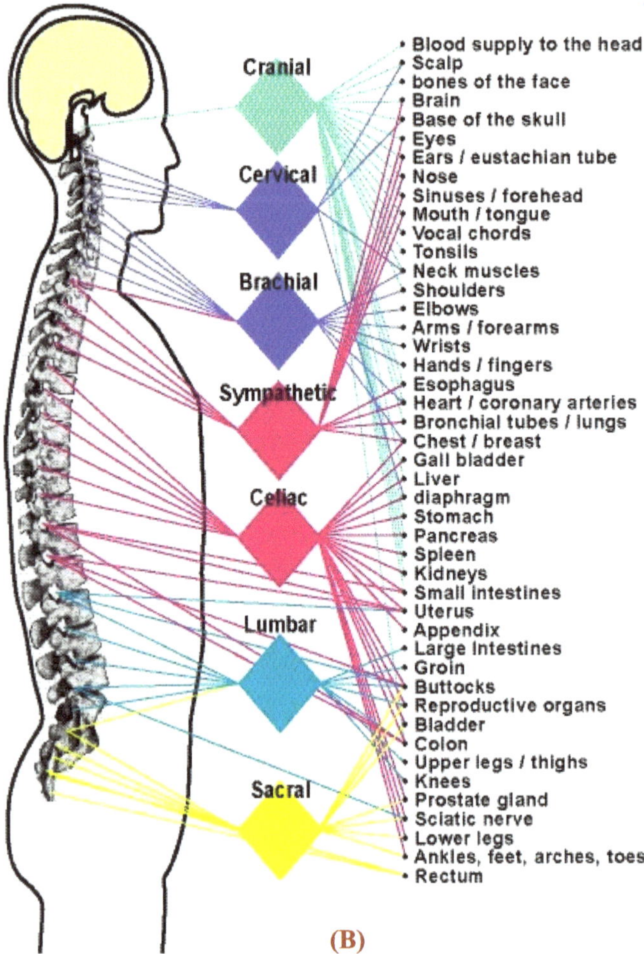

Fig. 36.1: *A. Showing chakras and the nervous system B. Different organs supplied by nerve plexus from head to bottom*

The heart rate and blood pressure increases, blood Glucose is generated and the air passages open Sympathetic system preparing for action. The heart rate and blood pressure increases, blood Glucose is generated and the air passages open.

Vagus Nerve

The **Parasympathetic nervous system** runs along the Vagus nerve, descending from the brain stem through the neck, chest, stomach and connects organ to organ. The Parasympathetic nervous system is our rest and relax response. The heart rate and blood pressure drops, and the airways are constricted. The Parasympathetic nervous system restores the body back to a normal state.

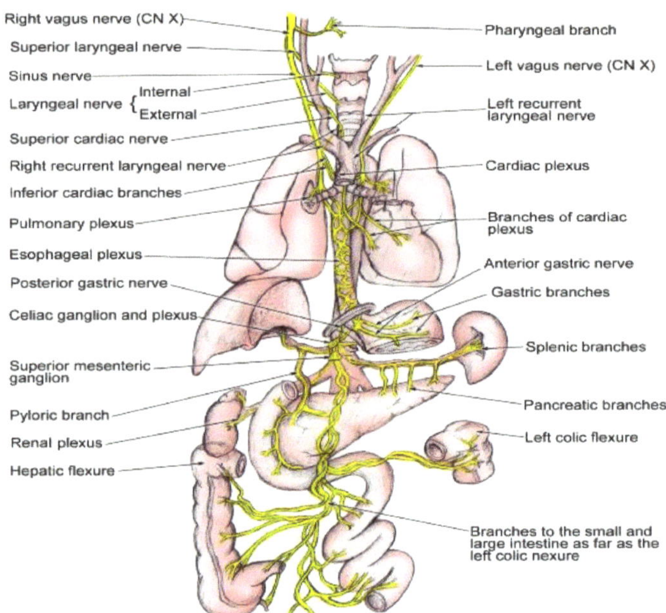

Fig. 36.2: *The vagus nerve has a larger distribution than any other cranial nerve. Originating in the medulla, the vagus nerve innervates structures in the neck, thorax, and abdomen and has influence over cardiac and digestive functions. As the vagus nerve travels from the brain stem to the abdomen, it gives off many branches. Two branches of great importance are the superior and recurrent laryngeal nerves. The vagus nerve carries five different fiber types : general somatic afferent, general visceral afferent, special visceral afferent, general visceral efferent, and special visceral efferent fibers. A neurological exam and, if necessary, imaging and electrophysiological testing, are useful in diagnosing and localizing pathology of the vagus nerve.*

Brain Hemispheres

The brain is divided into left and right hemispheres. The right side of the brain is in control of the Parasympathetic nervous system and the left side the Sympathetic nervous system. Yoga places the regulating and controlling of the two opposite sides very highly, and prescribes Pranayama as a tool for this task. Yoga says the right side of the brain is linked to Ida Pingala, and the left nostril, and the left side of the brain is linked to the right nostril and *Pingala Nadi*. During the course of the day, the nostrils alternate so that at any given time one nostril will be more open that the other. This is said to be because the nostrils share the load, as the nostrils have different scent receptors, and the Cilia are rested during the closed. This means over the course of a 24 hour period, we will swing between the two opposite poles of Ida and Pingala. The Pranayama practice of Nadi Shodhana, or alternate nostril breathing is said to bring balance between the two channels.

Nadis-IDA & Pingala

Yoga describes three main energy channels, or Nadis, which transcend and traverse the spinal column around the Chakras

Ida Nadi: left channel – left nostril – right brain – Parasympathetic nervous system – rest & relax

Pingala Nadi: right channel – right nostril – left brain

Sympathetic nervous system – fight & flight

Shushumna Nadi – both channels – both brains – neutral

Shushumna Nadi

When Ida and Pingala Nadis are harmonised, Shushumna Nadi opens. Prana rises through the central Nadi facilitating meditation. Shushmna Nadi is said to be composed of layers of subtle energy containing the three qualities of Tamas, Rajas and Sattva. Shushumna Nadi becomes more refined until at the core it is beyond the qualities

The out layer is said to represent Tamas as it is dormant. Inside the outer layer is Vajrana Nadi, which is Rajasic in nature. Within this is Chittra Nadi, equating to Sattva. Beneath all is Brahma Nadi, or the gateway to Brahman

What are the main energy channels of human body?

There are three main Nadis (Ida, Pingala, and Sushumna) Nadis convey the life force. The Hatha Yoga tradition says that there are about 72,000 nadis (subtle channels of prana [energy]) that convey the life force in a human being. Ida, pingala, and sushumna are known to be the three principal nadis. The ending point of the three main nadis is brahmarandhra (the "*Brahmic aperture*"), at the crown of the head. In the state of nirvikalpa samadhi, an important part of the energies passing through these three channels is absorbed in the single para or amrita nadi

- Each organ-mother, which should not be confused with the organ known in Western anatomo-physiology, is attached to a more general functional aspect, including the body, the psyche and the unconscious part of the Being, the ancestral energies which modulate our behavior and our reactions to the outside.
- At the intersection of 21 nadis is formed a main chakra.
- At the intersection of 14 nadis a secondary chakra is formed.
- At the intersection of 7 nadis is formed a tertiary chakra or acupuncture point, located on the path of the meridians.

Ida Nadi—The Passive Channel (Feminine and Creative Principle)

Functions:

Yin energy channel, it governs mental strength, psychic and extrasensory perceptions. Stimulates creative, artistic activities, processes information and controls orientation in space. Represents our subconscious, frees fears and feelings of guilt. Ida corresponds to the moon. It represents the feminine element, which symbolizes the Woman. Ida is the feminine side of the personality and all the forces and functions connected with it, the mother, the influence that she represents and the relationship with her, whether it is the inheritance that she has transmitted, the relation to she, the principles according to which she participated in our education and our structuration. His energy is cold, ascending and blue in color. Ida is in relation with the elements earth and water

Journey:

Ida starts from the base of the spine, at the right end of the coccyx (perineal region), and ends in the left nostril. It carries Prâna lunar and ascendant (Prâna).

Qualities:

Ida influences the parasympathetic nervous system which transmits the impulses to the organs to stimulate their functioning. Through her right brain irrigation, Ida is responsible for psychic and extrasensory perceptions. It stimulates creative, artistic activities, processes information and controls orientation in space. Its cold energy helps to lower the body temperature. In her harmonious function, Ida, who represents our subconscious, frees fears and feelings of guilt.

Imbalances:

We encounter ignorance, laziness, a passive mind turned towards the past, as well as all the negative emotional aspects. To shut oneself up in silence, to doubt without being able to take action, to remain dependent on family, social or personal conditioning. All these states reflect the imbalance of the Ida channel. His pathology is manifested by psychic and mental disorders such as certain depressions, certain forms of epilepsy, senility considered as the culmination of a long imbalance. It should be known that any excessive physical or mental activity, paralyze the emotional side, so Ida, which can cause serious diseases.

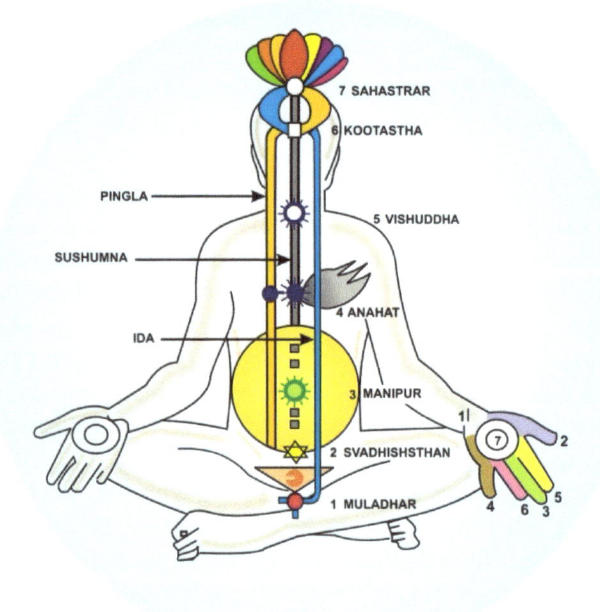

Fig. 36.3: *A simplified view of the subtle body of Indian philosophy, showing the three major nadis or channels, the Ida Sushumna and Pingala), and seven kundalini chakras which run vertically in the body.*

Pingala Nadi—The Active Channel Pingala (Masculine and Analytical Principle)

Functions:

Plots of Nadis and chakras, used in Egyptian-Essenian therapy

Pingala is the Yang energy channel, it governs physical strength. In relation to the sympathetic nervous system, it stimulates the muscular activity (releasing adrenaline). Pingala controls the heartbeat, activates the physical body and directs consciousness to the outside world. Pingala is the sun. It represents the masculine principle, the symbol of Man, of the father, of the hereditary and educational influences coming from him and all that he can represent in our development. Stimulates muscle activity (releasing adrenaline) Controls the heart rate, activates the physical body and directs the consciousness to the outside world Its energy is solar, hot, dynamic, downy and red. The elements concerned by Pingala are Fire and Air.

Journey:

Pingala starts from the right nostril and ends at the base of the spine (perineal region) at the left end of the coccyx. He carries solar and descending Prana (Apana).

Qualities:

Connected to the left hemisphere, Pingala is responsible for reasoning, analysis and logic. Its warm energy allows to increase the heat of the body and controls the digestive energy. Pingala governs the energy through which we work and act.

Imbalances:

On the physical plane, we encounter hot-type diseases. So essentially acute inflammatory diseases and some heart and digestive disorders. These disorders can translate an excess of the EGO to the detriment of the SOI. On a psychological level, Pingala imbalances engender a domineering, selfish, angry, aggressive and materialistic spirit. Treacherous, unscrupulous people live in excess on this nadis.

Sushumna Nadi—The Central Channel (Gracious Principle)

Functions:

Represents the unconscious, it constitutes the supra mental, the abolition of the dualities, the awakening. Awakening of intellectual and spiritual faculties. Nadis resulting, it is on him that are located the 7 main chakras. If the other two are our first references, our components, our bases, only Sushumna represents the result, represents us. Its progressive construction is our personal development.

Journey:

Sushumna is centrally located, equidistant from the other two, in the axial canal in front of the spine. The axis that can grow right only in harmony and balance of influences of the other two. This central nadis is located inside the spine and corresponds to the spinal cord. Allowing the relationship of the chakras between them, it starts from the end of the coccyx and ends in the cervical cavity, at the Brahma hole. Sushumna is the most important channel Its energy is neutral : it is the axis of Life and Sensibility. Without confusing it with the central nervous system or cerebrospinal system, it would be in relation with this one. It is through him that the Kundalini - that is, the latent spiritual energy, or divine power - rises in the form of a coiled snake.

The Kundalini, which is in each individual, can be awakened or animated by breathing exercises, by the evolution of consciousness, or by various energetic techniques. The techniques (of Tantric origin) of breath control (Swara Yoga) or dynamics of the breath (Pranayama) allow to activate this channel and to awaken the intellectual and spiritual faculties. But in Swara Yoga, the adepts are warned : Indeed, if the spiritual faculties wake up, the criminal tendencies can also manifest themselves. So Sushumna can be active both among yogis in deep meditation and among terrorists and criminals!

Like the Caduceus of Hermes, the two lateral nadis (Ida and Pingala) thus surround Sushumna, straight up from the earth to the sky, from their spiral and intertwine in particular at the level of each of the main chakras where the nodes are that the energy must dissolve during its ascent. They are located on the path of the spine and the head and represent the subtle counterpart of ganglia of the sympathetic nervous system.

This spiral progression, such as caduceus, is the representation of man built, harmonized, perfect channel of energies, accomplished, having grown progressively, patiently, in total harmony between his masculine and feminine references, between father and mother, taking advantage qualities and possibilities of one and the other. These possibilities are of several orders : hereditary, physical, psychic, and also all the archives stored in the unconscious bequeathed by our parents and the lineages that preceded them. I must point out that in all well-interpreted traditions, the snake, far from being a hideous and demonic animal, represents the symbol of consciousness, consciousness, lunar, intuitive and symbolic in Ida Nadi, solar, inductive and conceptual in Pingala Nadi. Our harmony results from the judicious and balanced use of both.

Vitality and purification of nadis.

In the vast majority of humans, only a small fraction of the available energy flows in these three nadis and the seven major chakras. To awaken this subtle energy by breathing, by the evolution of consciousness, or by various energetic techniques (Reiki, Qi Gong, Yoga, Essene Care...) allows its current to flow into these centers by activating them. The purification of nadis is essential since it ensures the circulation of Prana. Indeed, any blocking of the vital energy in the nadis, or meridians, can result in organic and mental diseases. If the circulation is weakened or blocked, the individual experiences the abandonment, the anguish, the fear and searches in the outside world what is in him. Specific energy treatments, such as those taught in the Essene or Egyptian-Essene Care approach, are very effective in revitalizing and toning nadis. The purification of nadis by specific breaths is the first and most important exercise for yogis. It regulates the whole life and balances the human being. Also yoga exercises work, in the same way as acupuncture, in the direction of purification and strengthening of nadis. Pranayamas, breathing techniquesof yoga, help the circulation and balance of energy. As a result, he increases the blockage of the chakras, inhibits his emotions and compensates for his frustrations by an exaggerated flight into activities or negative behavior. Remember that unresolved emotional experiences are stored in physical death and manifest themselves in a subsequent incarnation. They will partly determine the circumstances in which we re-born.

The Prana

The *Prana* connects man to the cosmos : it is the subtle substance, or vital energy, which exists within each thing and which penetrates in it mainly by the breaths and secondarily by the food. He travels along the nadis, which lead him : in the chakras he is going to vivify, in the organs of the senses that he is going to feed (each of them having a nadis connecting him to the brain and the subtle body with which he is related). This penetration into the subtle bodies is by the two nostrils for Ida and Pingala, by the cervical cavity for Sushumna. These energies thus penetrate the human being, feeding the two chakras of the head first, then traveling along the subtle channels, from top to bottom and from bottom to top, and feeding in turn the chakras on the path of the spine and the relay chakras that activate the main organs of the body as a whole. In the usual time, the polarized energy borrows the two lateral paths Ida and Pingala, each carrying a Prana differently polarized : negative on the left (*Ida*) and positive on the right (*Pingala*). Ida and Pingala do not communicate with each other but when they neutralize each other in the Muladhara root chakra, the energy can no longer circulate in the sideways, it will have to take the middle way of Sushumna... and it will be along from the Sushumna ride that the Kundalini fires will go up and down when the follower reaches a certain degree of purity and awakening. These 3 major nadis will therefore have to be cleansed of karmic residues before the Akashic current of Sushumna can serve as a channel for life in its totality, welcoming both the influx of descending Spiritual Life and the already existing and static Life. To obtain the release of the Ida Lunar Canal, the beginner must purify his blood by a healthy diet and a strict lifestyle. He will also have to discipline his emotional body, his body of desire and sensation. To obtain the release of the Solar Canal Pingala, he will have to purify his thoughts and actions. He will thus discipline his mental body.

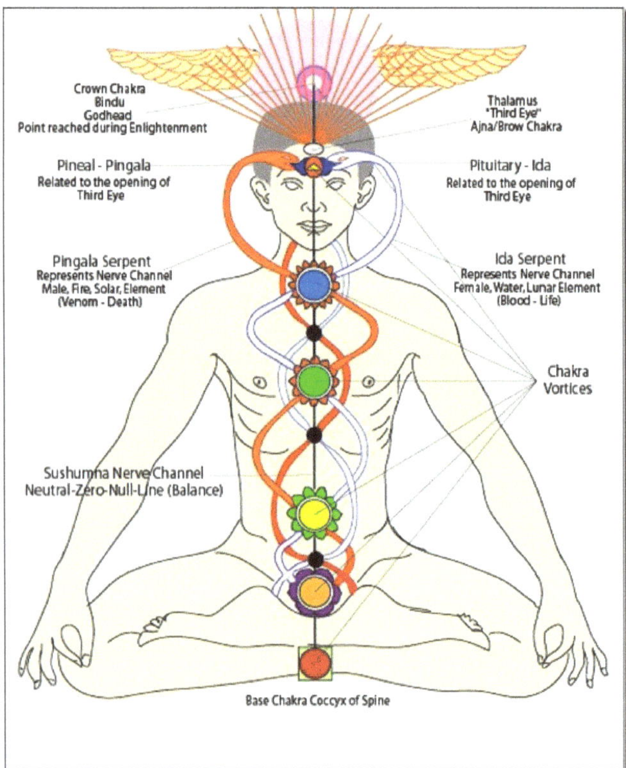

Fig. 36.4: *shows localization of three nadis and seven chakras from Base chakra coccyx spine to ajna at the top. Energy is flowing in a spiral fashion from bottom to the head.*

The practices of yoga work together to force prana into the central Sushumna channel, allowing kundalini to rise, leading to moksha, liberation. The shatkarmas purify the nadis, while the mudras trap prana, and other practices (not shown) force the prana out of the Ida and Pingala channels.

Balancing Sun and Moon, or pingala and ida, facilitates the awakening and rising of kundalini shakti through sushumna nadi and, thus, the awakening of higher consciousness. Some yoga teachings hold that as long as either ida or pingala predominates, sushumna stays closed and the power of kundalini lies dormant. In yoga, we endeavor to make prana (*life force energy*) run in sushumna nadi, which is also known as brahma nadi. When energy flows predominantly through sushumna for long periods of time, we become *"dead to the world,"* and enter into samadhi. Symbolically, sushumna is associated with the Fire element (*tejas tattva*) and it is considered sattvic (*harmonious*) in nature. According to the Lalita Sahasranama (a Tantric text devoted to the Goddess), fiery-red sushumna has within it both the lustrous vajra nadi (which is of the nature of the Sun) and the pale nectar-dropping chitra nadi (which is of the nature of the Moon). Chitra (or *chitrini*) nadi is responsible for dreams, hallucinations, and visions.Yoga involves physical exercises (*asana*), breathing techniques (*Pranayama*) and meditation. All of these have their own benefits either for physical or mental health. There are numerous yoga breathing techniques for boosting immunity. Breathing technique in yoga is called as *'Pranayama'*. *'Prana'* refers to breathe or the vital energy and *'yama'* means *'flow'*. Thus Pranayama is 'yoga breathing techniques which improves the flow of vital energy and life force in body.' This effectively improves the blood oxygenation by utilizing the maximum of lung capacity. Better oxygenation and blood circulation as well as it rejuvenates body and boosts immunity.

Research indicates that yogic breathing is effective way to improve pulmonary functions. Slow breathing at 6 breaths/min effectively increases vital capacity (VC). Moreover, the yogic breathing techniques are beneficial for respiratory system and indicate a positive change in the respiratory physiology. Another study reveals the positive effect of yoga on a person's physical as well as psychological well-being. It suggests that Yoga can effectively reverse the expression of inflammatory mediators and to maintain homeostasis. Consequently, it improves the physiological functions of various other systems that are associated to immune system responses. Yoga techniques down-regulate the expression of inflammatory cytokines such as NF-κB and subsequently reduce the expression of pro-inflammatory cytokines in various chronic stress-induced diseases. Thus, yoga interventions are effective to boost immunity and maintaining overall health.

It is possible to go even further in the globalization of nadis. It is the step taken by Ayurvedic and Tibetan medicine that consider 3 important nadis, directly related to the 7 main chakras : The two lateral nadis : Ida and Pingala thus surround Sushumna and intersect each other at the level of each of the main chakras, where are the nodes that the energy must dissolve during its ascent. They are located on the path of the spine and the head and represent the subtle counterpart of ganglia of the sympathetic nervous system. To understand the energy functioning of the human being, it is necessary to know these 3 important nadis.

What happens when Ida and Pingala are balanced?

The regulation of the Ida and Pingala brings harmony, balance, health and well-being to the life system. The Pingala Nadi, associated with the right nostril and the left hemisphere of the brain, aligns with the Yang, extroverted, male, Solar, vital, Shiva energy, and it warms, activates and enlivens.

How to activate Ida Pingala and Sushumna?

You may have guessed what to do if you are in need of warmth and activation. To increase the activity of the Pingala Nadi inhale from your right nostril and exhale from the left for 8 – 12 breath or until you feel a shift. The Sushumna Nadi runs along the spine. It goes through all the major Chakras.

What happens when Sushumna Nadi is activated?

When kundalini shakti awakens it passes through sushumna nadi. The moment awakening takes place in mooladhara chakra, the energy makes headway through sushumna up to ajna chakra. Then this generated energy is pushed upward by a negative pressure and forced up to ajna chakra

What is sushumna awakening?

Sushumna nadi is regarded as a hollow tube in which there are three more concentric tubes, each being progressively more subtle than the previous one. The moment awakening takes place in mooladhara chakra, the energy makes headway through sushumna up to ajna chakra. Mooladhara chakra is just like a powerful generator

What happens when Nadis are purified?

Swami Sivananda says in his book "*The Science of Pranayama*", when the nadis are purified there is a "lightness of the body, brilliancy in complexion, increase of the gastric fire, leanness of the body, and the absence of restlessness"

How do I know if my Nadi is active?

If Sushumna nadi is active there is a balance between your sympathetic and parasympathetic systems. When you go to sleep by 9 or 10 O'clock at night, observe the right nostril switch to the left. If you get sufficient amount of sleep, your right nostril will automatically be predominant first thing in the morning.

How can I activate Pingala Nadi?

To activate Pingala nadi (right nostril) sleep on the left side. In 1 or 2 minutes, this activity turns on the right nostril (and suppresses left). To activate ida nadi (left nostril) - sleep on the right side. In 1 or 2 minutes, this activity turns on the left nostril (and suppresses right).

How many Nadis or channels are cleansed by pranayama

Nadis Sodhana Pranayama, also known as alternate nostril breathing, is a great way to lead into your morning meditation practice. It is a controlled breathing practice designed to purify the nadis (energy channels). There are over 72,000 nadis in the body.

How do I purify my Nadis?

Performing Samanu Purification Inhale through left nostril repeating the Vayu Bija Mantra for 16 times.

Later the breath should be restrained for a period of 64 repetitions of the Mantra. Exhalation of the breath should be done through the right nostril slowly by repeating the Bija Mantra for 32 times.

What is Vajra Nadi?

Vajra Nadi is located within Sushumna Nadi. It initiates at the level of the Sacral Chakra and rises up from that point. Vajra Nadi is responsible for the movement of the Astral Body (pranic movement)

How do you strengthen Nadis?

Ways to clear the nadis and balance your energy

1. Right Intention – Your energy flows where your attention goes, so *Mind Your Mind*!
2. Hatha Yoga – Yoga helps to free stagnant energy and balance two of the main nadis that we have through the chakras : Ida & Pingala, the female (lunar) energy & male (solar) energy.

Which is Surya Nadi?

In yoga, surya nadi is one of the three primary sources of energy in the body. The term comes from the Sanskrit, surya, signifying "*sun,*" and nadi, signifying "*channel*" or "*stream.*" Surya nadi, otherwise called *pingala nadi*, is so-named on the grounds that it is identified with sun powered energy.

At which chakra the Union of Ida and Pingala Nadi takes place?

Finally, ida, pingala and sushumna meet in the pineal gland – ajna chakra. When the left nostril is open, it is the lunar energy or ida nadi which is flowing. When the right nostril is free, the solar energy or pingala nadi is flowing.

Which pranayama is the best?

Yoga Breathing Exercise: Top 5 Pranayama Exercises You Must Start Doing

1. Bhastrika Pranayama (Breath of fire)

2. Kumbhaka Pranayama (Breath retention)
3. Simhasana (Lion's Breath)
4. Mrigi Mudra Pranayam (Deer seal breathing)
5. Kapalabhati Pranayam (Skull shining)

How many Nadi Shodhana are there?

Nadi Shodhana - Alternate Nostril Breathing. There are over 72,000 nadis or subtle energy channels in our body where prana moves. If the nadis are blocked, prana can't move freely through the body, consciousness is inhibited and it's difficult to attain meaning from our daily lives

Which side of your nose goes to your brain?

Although the olfactory bulbs on each side are connected, anatomical studies have shown that information from smells entering the left nostril goes predominantly to the left side of the brain, and information from the right nostril goes mainly to the right side of the brain.

Can Anulom Vilom cure nerve damage?

Pranayama maintains the blood pressure and purifies the veins and nerves in the entire body. It can also cure ailments associated with BP, such as heart blockages and diabetes

What is the difference between prana and kundalini?

Prana has been translated as the "*vital breath*" and "*bio-energetic motility*"; it is associated with maintaining the functioning of the mind and body. Kundalini, in its form as prana-kundalini, is identical to prana; however, Kundalini also has a manifestations as consciousness and a as a unifying cosmic energy.

Which process purifies the mind and body?

It is Shaucha and is translated as "*cleanliness or purity*" and it is a yogic technique to cleanse the mind, speech, and body. Purification is a central aim of all the yogic practices and Shaucha is the first principle of Niyama, the eight moral observances in Patanjali's Yoga Sutras.

Nadi Shodhan Pranayama (Alternate nostril breathing)

What is Nadi Shodhana

Nadi = subtle energy channel;
Shodhan = cleaning, purification;
Pranayama = breathing technique.

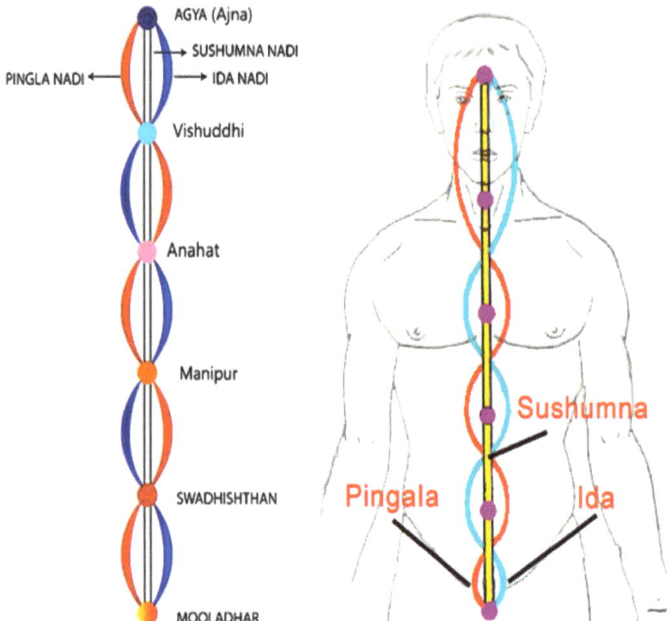

Fig. 36.5: *(Left) shows seven Kundalis and three nadis (right) The serpentile configuration of two nadis ie left sided Ida and right sided pingla where as sushumna remains centeral*

Nadi = subtle energy channel;
Shodhan = cleaning, purification;
Pranayama = breathing technique.

Nadis are subtle energy channels in the human body that can get blocked due to various reasons. The Nadi Shodhan pranayama is a breathing technique that helps clear these blocked energy channels, thus calming the mind. This technique is also known as Anulom Vilom pranayama. Alternate nostril breathing improves responsiveness and sensitivity to the breath in the nostrils. This breathing technique is ideal for reliving obstructions in respiratory tract. As we know that human brain is divided into left and right hemispheres. Alternate nostril breathing stimulates and invigorate both these hemispheres respectively.

Causes of Obstruction in the Nadis:

- Nadis can get blocked on account of stress
- Toxicity in the physical body also leads to blockage of nadis
- Nadis can get blocked due to physical and mental trauma
- Unhealthy lifestyle

What Happens When these Nadis are Blocked?

Pingala and Sushumna are three of the most important nadis in the human body. When the Ida nadi is not functioning smoothly or is blocked, one experiences cold, depression, low mental energy and sluggish digestion, blocked left nostril. Whereas when the Pingala nadi is not smoothly functioning or is blocked, one will experience heat, quick temper and irritation, itching body, dry skin and throat, excessive appetite, excessive physical or sexual energy, and blocked right nostril. The left nostril (right brain) breathing cools excess fire and calms anger and frustration with its lunar energy. It is good for sensitive skin types, Pitta conditions, or simply to cool down the physiology on a hot day. Right nostril (left brain) breathing, on the other hand, stimulates the mind with its solar energy and warms up the body on a cold day. Alternate nostril breathing relieves Vata conditions such as stress, worry, and fear.

Reasons why you should practice Nadi Shodhan Pranayama

1. Nadi Shodhan pranayama helps relax the mind and prepares it to enter a meditative state.
2. Practicing it for just a few minutes every day helps keep the mind calm, happy and peaceful.
3. It helps in releasing accumulated tension and fatigue.

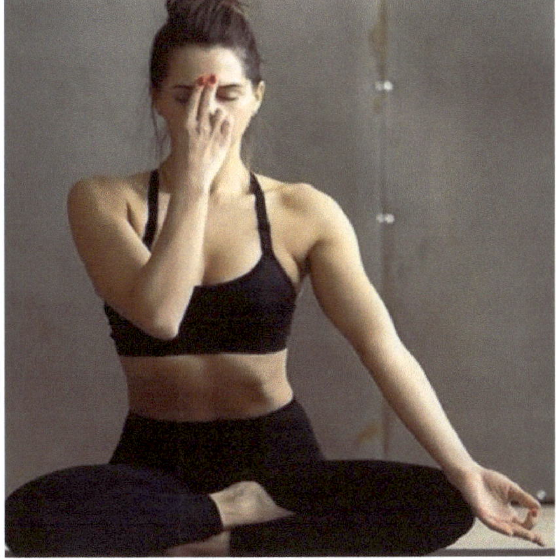

Fig. 36.6: *Pose (A). in Nadi Shodhan Pranayama* **Step**

1: Sit cross-l egged in an upright position.

- You should sit in a clean room, preferably on a mat or carpeted surface.
- Try to get comfortable.
- Keep a gentle smile on your face.
- Close your eyes. Keep your spine straight, shoulders relaxed and concentrate on your normal breath for about three to five minutes
- Place your left hand on the left knee, and palms open to the sky or in Chin Mudra (thumb and index finger gently touching at the tips).

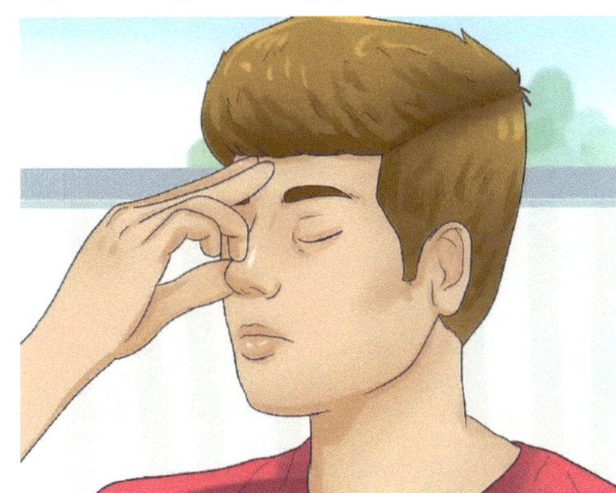

Fig. 36.7: *Pose (B.) in Nadi Shodhan Pranayama*

Step 2: Close your right nostril. Bring your right hand to your face.[3] Using your right thumb, press gently but firmly on your right nostril to prevent air from flowing into or out of it.

- Some practitioners like to bring their middle and index fingers up to rest on their foreheads or on a point between their eyes. Others simply keep their other four fingers curled into the palm.

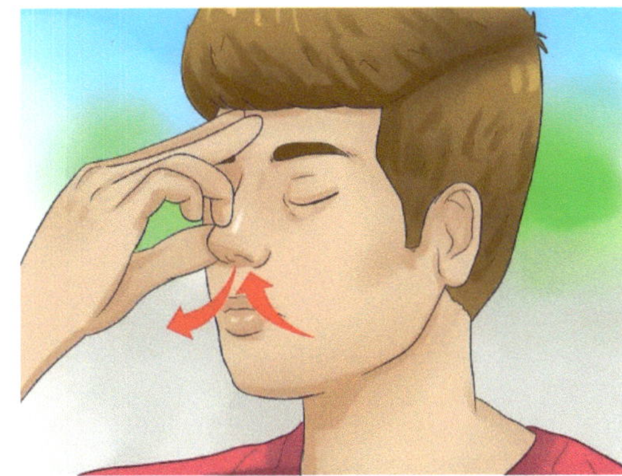

Fig. 36.8: *Pose (C) in Nadi Shodhan Pranayama*

Step 3: Breathe in deeply through your left nostril. With your right nostril covered, take a long, slow breath in through your nose. When you've reached maximum lung capacity, hold your breath for a length of time equal to the time it took you to breathe in.

- Release your breath in a slow exhalation that is also equal to the amount of time it took you to breathe in.
- Once you've fully exhaled, uncover your right nostril and return your right hand to your thigh.

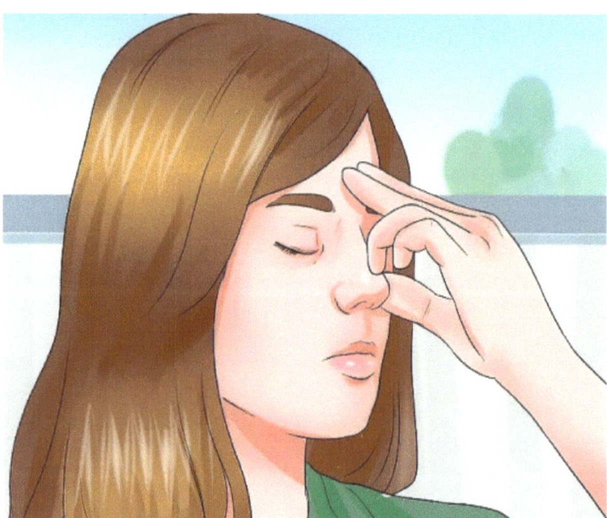

Fig. 36.9: *Pose (D) in Nadi Shodhan Pranayama*

Step 4: Close your left nostril. Bring your left hand to your face. Use your left thumb to close your left nostril by pressing it gently but firmly into the side of your nose. The process should replicate the way you closed your right nostril, but on the opposite side.

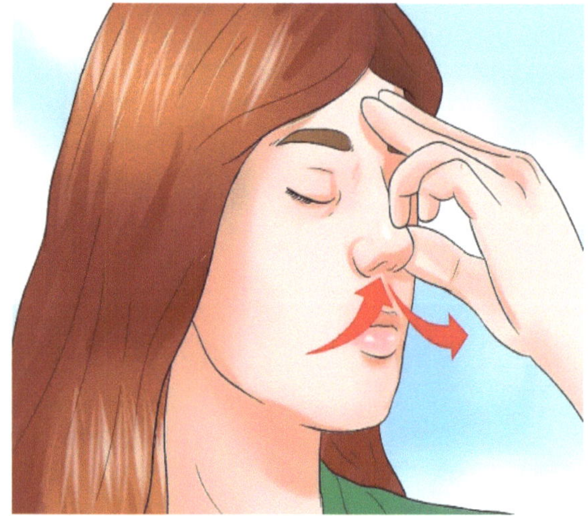

Fig. 36.10: *Pose (E). in Nadi Shodhan Pranayama*

Step 5: Breathe in deeply through your right nostril. Just as you did when you had your right nostril closed, breathe in deeply through your single open nostril. At the top of your inhalation, hold your breath for as long as it took you to inhale. Then, breathe out in a smooth motion. Remove your left thumb from your nose.

Alterrnative Technique in nostril breathing (Other name: Nadi Shodhana Pranayam.)

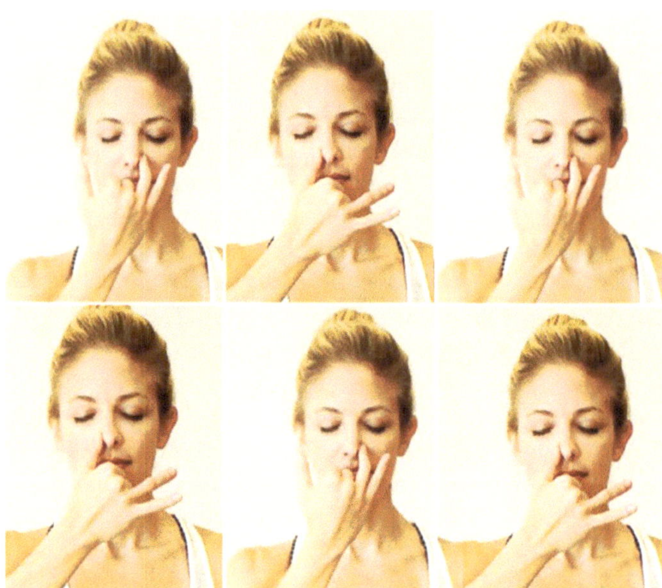

Fig.36.11: *(from left –right) Different Steps in alternative breathing exercises (Nadi Shodhana Pranayam)*

Steps

1. Sit comfortably. Take a long and deep breath.
2. Block the right nostril using your thumb. Breathe 5 times through the left nostril.
3. Then unblock the right nostril. Take a deep breath through both nostrils.
4. Now block the left nostril with your thumb. Breathe 5 times through right nostril.
5. At the end of practice, breathe deeply through both nostrils five times.
6. Breathe in from the right nostril and exhale from the left. You have now completed one round of Nadi Shodhan pranayama.
7. Continue inhaling and exhaling from alternate nostrils.
8. Complete 9 such rounds by alternately breathing through both the nostrils. After every exhalation, remember to breathe in from the same nostril from which you exhaled. Keep your eyes closed throughout and continue taking long, deep, smooth breaths without any force or effort.

Cautions to be Taken While Practicing Nadi Shodhan Pranayama (Alternate Nostril Breathing Technique)

1. Do not force the breathing, and keep the flow gentle and natural. Do not breathe from the mouth or make any sound while breathing.
2. Do not use the Ujjayi breath.

3. Place the fingers very lightly on the forehead and nose. There is no need to apply any pressure.
4. In case you feel dull and are yawning after practicing Nadi Shodhan pranayama, check the time you take to inhale and exhale. Your exhalation should be longer than inhalation.
5. This breathing technique is not suitable for those having asthma or cardiovascular diseases.
6. Practice yoga postures after consulting a doctor and Yoga teacher.

Tips While Doing Nadi Shodhan Pranayama

- It is a good idea to do a short meditation after doing Nadi Shodhan pranayama.
- This breathing technique can also be practiced as part of the Padma Sadhana sequence.

Benefits of Nadi Shodhan Pranayama (Alternate Nostril Breathing Technique)

1. Excellent breathing technique to calm and center the mind.
2. Our mind has a tendency to keep regretting or glorifying the past and getting anxious about the future. Nadi Shodhan pranayama helps to bring the mind back to the present moment.
3. Works therapeutically for most circulatory and respiratory problems.
4. Releases accumulated stress in the mind and body effectively and helps to relax.
5. Helps harmonize the left and right hemispheres of the brain, which correlates to the logical and emotional sides of our personality.
6. Helps purify and balance the nadis - the subtle energy channels, thereby ensuring a smooth flow of prana (life force) through the body.
7. Maintains body temperature.

Contraindication : **None.**

After you have learnt this breathing technique from iYoga teacher, you can practice this pranayama on an empty stomach, 2-3 times a day. Yoga practice helps develop the body and mind bringing a lot of health benefits yet is not a substitute for medicine. It is important to learn and practice yoga postures under the supervision of a trained teacher. In case of any medical condition,approach medical expert.

Hatha Yogza

The human body boasts as many as 72,000 *nadis? As if this were not enough, yoga texts disagree on the number! **Shiva Samhita quotes a whopping 3,50,000 nadis arising from the navel center. While Hatha Yoga Pradipika and Goraksha Samhita speak of 72,000 nadis, each branching off into another 72,000 nadis. In Kundalini yoga there are three main nadis. The Ida, Pingala and Sushumna. The Ida and Pingala symbolize the basic duality of existence. Ida spirals up the left side of the spine ending at the left nostril. Pingala is a mirror image of Ida, ending up at the right nostril. Lunar energy is aligned with Ida. Solar energy with Pingala. Ida is cool, comforting, introverted, feminine, governs the intellect. Pingala on the other hand, is warm, challenging, extroverted, masculine, in control of vital processes like digestion. *A nadi is a pathway or channel of subtle energy. It cannot be seen upon dissection of the human body.

What is hatha yoga?

The word *'ha'* means Sun, *'tha'* means Moon. Hatha means to balance the Sun and Moon energies in you. *Hatha yoga* is the science of harmonizing *Pingala* and *Ida*; or the solar and lunar energies within us so as to prod our higher consciousness to life. It is the science of activating the third, central nadi- Sushumna - which is the path to enlightenment. Hatha also means being adamant, making an effort. Sri Sri Ravi Shankar says, "Hatha yoga is stretching your boundaries a little bit. We define our boundaries and stay there. Hatha yoga says, okay stretch a little bit. Extend your boundary, little by little." Hatha yoga begins with exertion. Your body may say, "That's it, I can do no more." Or your mind may groan, "Yoga? Oh no not again!" But you stay determined. You just do it. Every time you raise the bar just a tad, step out of your comfort zone a little further.

The Rationale Behind Hatha Yoga

Traditionally you would work with the body first by diligently doing yoga asanas. Next comes the breath. You would practice pranayamas like Nadi Shodhan. Finally you would move on to the mind with meditation. In its true classical sense, Hatha yoga is practiced to bridge the gap between your body and higher states of consciousness. Let's look at the physical aspect of meditation as an example. In order to meditate effectively, you need to sit comfortably with spine erect and unsupported for long periods. This requires a strong back, a flexible groin and well-toned legs. Knees, ankles and feet need to be healthy. Hatha yoga prepares your body. And ensures that meditation is a blissful experience - not a painful one.

Hatha Yoga Asanas and Benefits

Before you start your Hatha yoga practice, check out which nostril is more active. If it is the left nostril, Ida is more dominant. Time to do asanas like standing poses, back bends, twists and inversions. If the right nostril is more switched on, Pingala is more energized. Seated postures and forward bends will cool you down.

- Hatha yoga boosts overall health.
- Tones the spine.
- Improves flexibility.
- Strengthens muscles.
- Enhances balance.
- Revs up blood circulation.
- Increases immunity.
- Relieves stress.
- Helps with focus and concentration.
- Balances the flow of energy.
- Makes you happy.
- Hatha yoga also balances the three gunas or qualities inherent in you. Tamas, the quality of inertia and delusion; and rajas the quality of activity and selfishness will be tempered. While Sattva, the quality of harmony and goodness will prevail.
- With regular practice of Hatha yoga, you will not just exist in this world, you will live. With enthusiasm, spirituality and a strong sense of divinity.
- Hatha yoga helps develop the body and mind, bringing a lot of health benefits. Even so, it is not a substitute for medicine. It is important to learn and practice yoga postures under the supervision of a trained yoga teacher. In case of any medical condition, practice yoga postures after consulting a doctor, and a Yoga teacher.

What is Hatha Yoga?

The Sanskrit term "*Hatha*" literally means "*forcibly*". Hatha yoga uses bodily posture in the vigorous form to control the physical self in relation to the mind. Along with physical postures, hatha yoga comprises different breathing exercises, cleansing techniques (*shatkarma*), mudras & bandhas for channelizing energy in the body & mind. The concept of hatha yoga poses came in the first place when ancient yogis realized mental and psychic aspects of humans can't be controlled unless the physical body is disciplined by various means

Childs Pose (Balasana)

Also known as Balasana, child's pose is a great starting to begin your hatha yoga practice. It's a relaxing posture and doesn't require any sort of flexibility, instead, performing it will give you a nice stretch to open your body in the first place. Also, come into this pose to relax the body for a while in between poses.

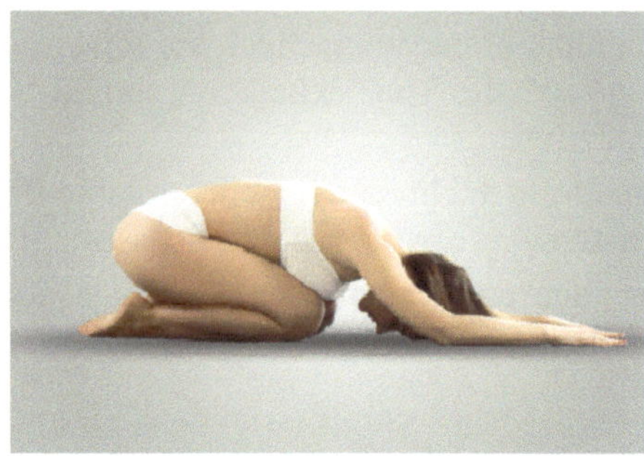

Fig. 36.12: *Showing physical features in Child's Pose*

How to Perform

- Begin by sitting on your heels, knees together, and straighten your trunk.
- Open your knees equal to the width of the mat.
- Now slowly walk forward with your hand, start bending your trunk in space between open knees.
- Reach forward so that your forehead touches the ground. Rest your forearms on the ground, shoulder away from your ears, relax the whole body.
- Stay in this position for 30 seconds before beginning the next pose.

Benefits: Child's pose reduces fatigue, it promotes blood circulation throughout the body. It calms down the nerves and relieves stress. Practicing this pose helps stretch the muscles and ligaments around the knee area.

Downward-facing Dog Pose

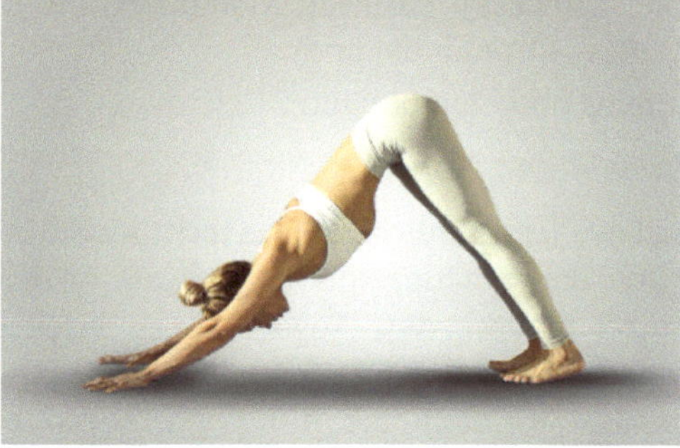

Fig. 36.13: *Showing physical features in Downward-facing Dog Pose*

How to Perform

- Downward-facing dog is one of the foundational hatha yoga postures. Here, the body is stretched bringing the upper body into an inversion as a dog stretches itself. People also refer to it as adho mukha svanasana.

- Form a table-like structure using your arms and legs and your back posture should be like the top of the table.
- Straighten your elbows and knees.
- Form an inverted V-shape. Place your hands shoulder-width apart and feet at hip-width apart.
- Press your hands firmly on the ground and keep your face downwards and your gaze should be at your navel.

Benefits - Down dog pose helps improve blood flow to our brain. It strengthens the arms and improves body posture. It also stretches the ankles, the back of the body, the calves, and the whole spine.

Cat-Cow Pose

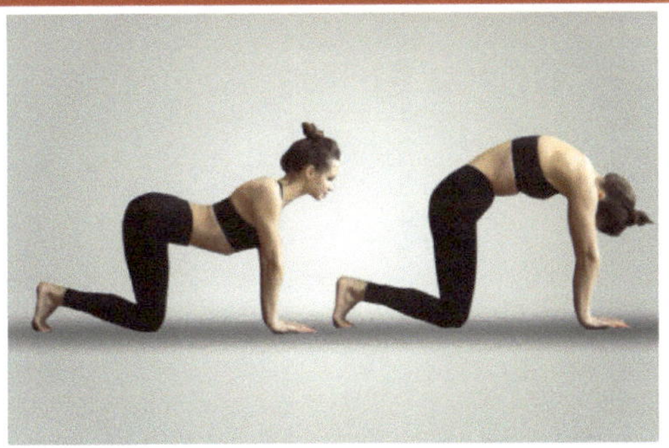

Fig. 36.14: *Showing physical features in Cat-Cow Pose*

How to Perform

- The cat-cow pose is a body warm-up practice involving a gentle stretching sequence. It stretches the muscles by fusing forward bend and back arch where body posture mimics cat and cow respectively. It is also known as *Bitilasana Marjaryasana*.
- Come to your all fours (hands and knees) to attain the table-top position.
- Pressing the palms on the floor sink your belly to the floor and raise your tailbone.
- Lift your head and move your shoulders away from the ears.
- Lower your head towards the floor by rounding the spine outwards.
- Repeat this flexion and extension of the spine for about 5-7 rounds.

Benefits: Cat-cow pose is great for increasing spinal flexibility and curing back pain. It also tones the core muscles and facilitates better digestion. This pose acts as a chest opener which is beneficial to both lungs and heart.

Standing Forward Bend (Aka uttanasana)

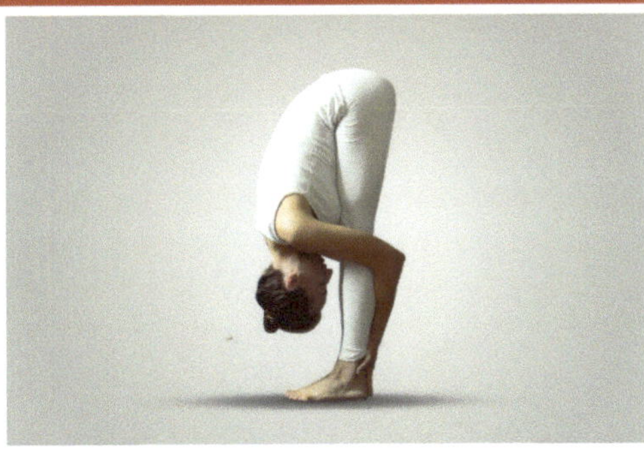

Fig. 36.15: *Showing physical features in Standing Forward Bend ((aka uttanasana)*

How to Perform

Standing forward fold pose aka uttanasana is beginner level practice of Hath yoga which involves inversion of the upper body. It is practiced as a restorative asana while exercising other standing poses.

- It begins with standing erect in tadasana for a few deep breaths.
- Then, bend the upper body forward at the hips keeping the spine erect.
- Keep bending until the head touches the knees and palms are placed on the floor beside the feet.
- Hold the position for about 30-60 seconds with slow deep breaths.
- Beginner's tips:
- Beginners can keep the feet separated apart to easily reach the floor with the palms and gradually decrease the distance between the feet.
- To bend forward without losing the integrity of the back, try pushing the hips backward. Also, practicing it with slightly bent knees is quite helpful to avoid any strain in the knees.

Benefits: Standing forward fold acts as a stress buster pose by enhancing the supply of blood and oxygen to the brain. It improves the overall flexibility of the body and tones the abdominal organs. This even helps in getting rid of infertility and alleviating menopausal symptoms.

Mountain Pose (Aka tadasana)

How to Perform

Mountain pose aka tadasana is a standing pose that can be performed by standing on the bases of your big toes. This is one of the basic standing poses of Hatha Yoga practice that serves as a foundational pose for all standing poses.

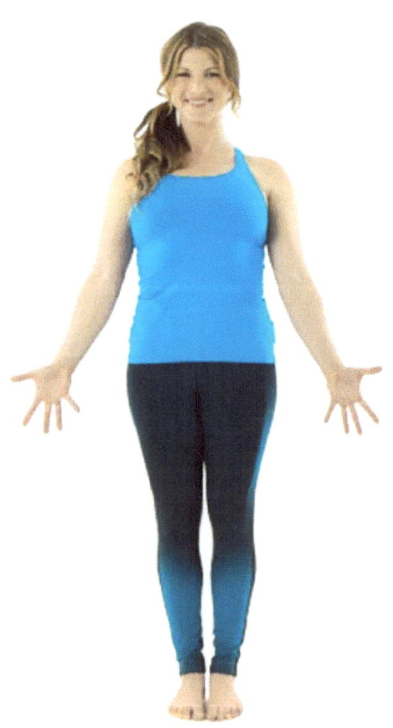

Fig. 36.16: *Showing physical features in Mountain Pose (Aka tadasana)*

- Lift your toes and press them firmly on the ground. Place your heels little apart from each other.
- Place your feet slowly down on the floor. Move back and side to side.
- Keep your thigh muscles firm and lift your ankles
- Push your shoulder blades slightly towards back and release them down by widening your collar bones a little.

Benefits: Mountain Pose helps in improving body posture, strengthens your knees and thighs, and firms your hips and abdomen

Tree Pose (Vrikshasana)

How to Perform

Tree pose is done to improve your ability to balance the body just like the tree balances itself being rooted in the ground. This is one of the easiest Asanas of Hatha Yoga practice. This pose is basically a standing pose where the body posture resembles a tree.

- Stand straight. Put your right foot on the inside of your left thigh. Place the heel firmly on the root of the thigh. Keep the left leg straight.
- Balance your body and raise your hands over your head while breathing. Join the hands so that they form a Namaste Mudra.
- Look straight at a single point in order to improve balance and concentration.
- Staying in this position for a few seconds (30-60 secs) slowly bring your hands down and relax by putting your legs in your original position.
- Repeat the same position with the other leg.

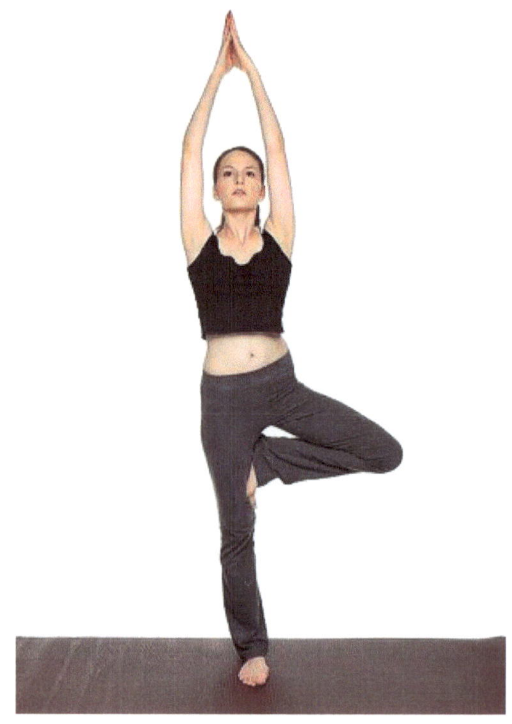

Fig. 36.17: *Showing physical features in Tree Pose (Vrikshasana)*

Bene its: Vrikshasana improves the flexibility of the body and strength of the spine. It helps in maintaining calmness in the body. It also tones the muscles of hips and helps in preventing the pain caused due to sciatic nerve weakness.

Triangle Pose (trikonasana)

How to Perform

Triangle pose is an asymmetrical standing posture practiced by stretching the upper body into a side bend. Due to the resemblance of the body with a triangle in this asana, it is widely known as trikonasana.

- Stand with separating the legs 2 feet apart and spreading the arms at the shoulder level.
- Rotate the leading foot (say right) outwards at 90° and bend the upper body at the waist towards the right foot.

- Hold the right ankle with the right hand and left arm is extended upward.
- The neck muscles are also turned to gaze towards the thumb of left hand.
- Releasing in the reverse order continue the same steps to bend towards the left side.

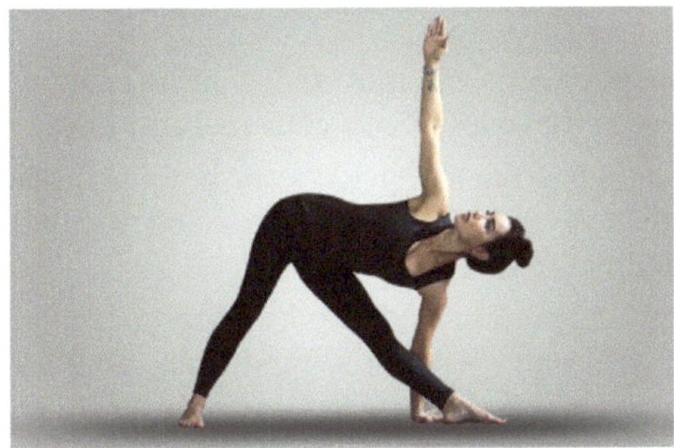

Fig. 36.18: *Showing physical features in Triangle Pose (trikonasana)*

Bene its: Triangle pose enhances the legs, hips, core, shoulders, and back muscles. It acts as a therapeutic pose for curing sciatica, flat feet, and psychological issues like stress, depression, etc.

Cobra Pose (Bhujangasana)

How to Perform

Cobra pose is a reclining posture that involves back-bending by throwing the head back like a serpent (cobra) raises its hood. It is also known as Bhujangasana that has been derived from the Sanskrit word Bhujanga (meaning Snake).

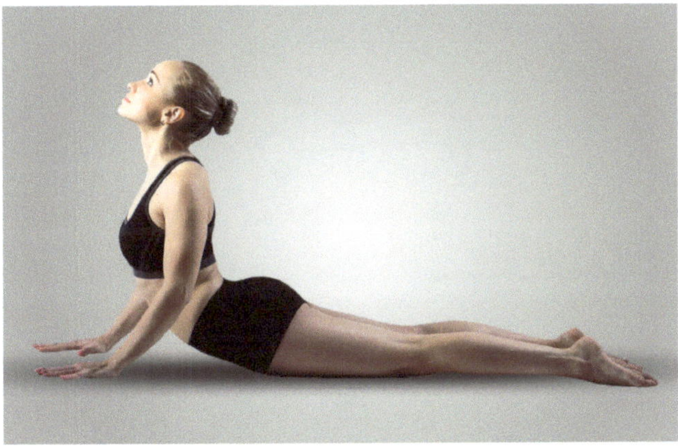

Fig.36.19:*Showing physical features in Cobra Pose (Bhujangasana)*

- Lie on your stomach and rest your forehead on the ground.
- Press your top portion of your feet on the ground.
- Gradually place your palms below your shoulders so that your palms can support while lifting your shoulders.
- Breath in and lift your head and chest off the ground with the support of your palms.
- Stay in this pose for 30 seconds.

Benefits: Bhujangasana helps in strengthening the spine and stimulates abdominal organs. It helps relieve stress. It is also helpful for asthma. Bhujangasana also helps reduce belly fat.

Thunderbolt Pose (Vajrasana)

How to Perform

Thunderbolt pose is one of the classical hatha yoga poses for digestion after having a meal. In Sanskrit, it is known as Vajrasana. Since, '*Vajra*' is a weapon of Lord Indra, known for its integrity and power, similar are the effects of this pose on the practitioner.

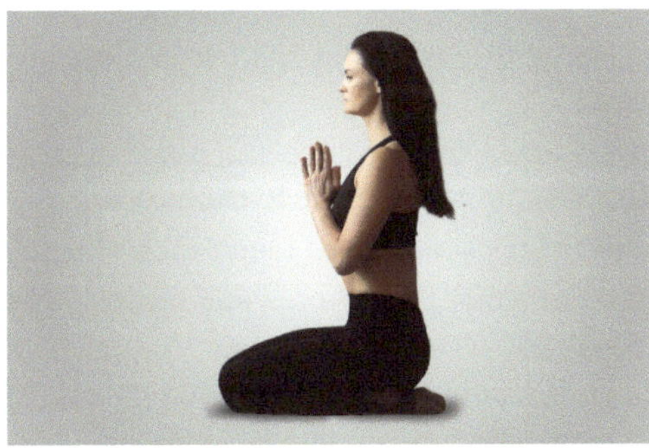

Fig. 36.20: *Showing physical features in Thunderbolt Pose (Vajrasana)*

- Sit on your knees and then sit on the ankles to shift the weight from your knees.
- Place your hands on the respective knees. Your palms should face downwards.
- You can place your hands at your back in Namaste Mudra also.

Benefits: Thunderbolt pose improves the memory and cures backache. It improves our concentration level and strengthens the thighs and knees. Vajrasana also helps in improving our digestion.

Gracious Pose (Bhadrasana)

How to Perform

Gracious pose is a basic sitting posture and can be held for longer periods comfortably, hence serves as an ideal meditative pose. It's one of 15 original hatha yoga asanas mentioned in hatha yoga pradipika. Sanskrit term for '*gracious*' is '*Bhadra'*, hence also referred to as *Bhadrasana*

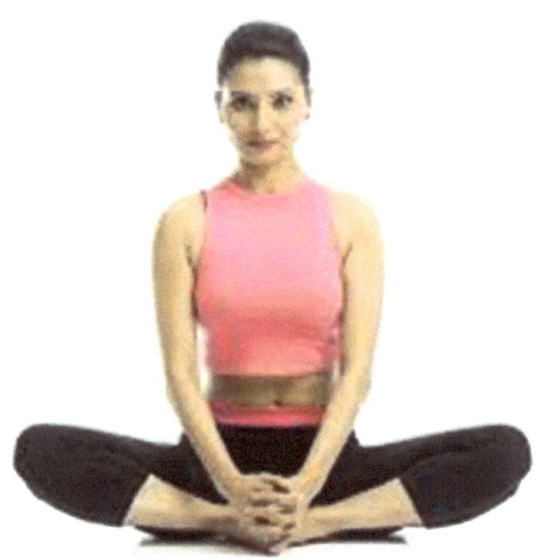

Fig. 36.21: *Showing physical features in Gracious Pose (Bhadrasana)*

- To perform this pose, sit with legs stretching them outwards.
- Bend the legs from the knee and place them such that the feet should be put close to each other.
- The sole of the feet should touch each other.
- Gently put your thighs on your calves. Keep your spine straight and relaxed.
- Place your hands on your respective knees. Maintain this position for a few seconds.

Benefits: Bhadrasana has several benefits like strengthening the knee and hip joints and it helps reduce the stress around the abdominal area. It improves our meditation and hence helps relieve stress. It also strengthens our spine and has a positive impact on both body and mind.

Corpse Pose (savasana)

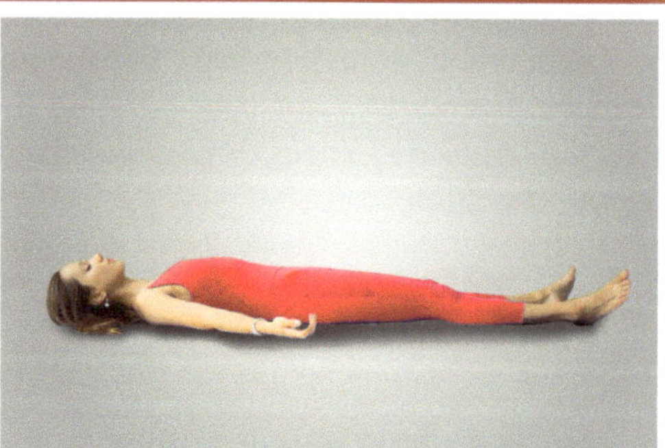

Fig.36.22:*Showing physical features in Corpse Pose (savasana)*

How to Perform

Corpse pose is the ending relaxing pose of hatha yoga performed in laying down position. This is a very relaxing posture and can also be done in between different yoga poses to relax the muscles.

- Lie flat with the support of your back and close your eyes.
- Keep your legs straight and a little apart with toes facing to the sides. Keep your feet and knees relaxed
- Place your arms alongside your body and place them a little away from the body while keeping palms open in an upward direction.
- Slowly relax your body by keeping your attention on your different body parts. First bring your awareness to your right foot, then to your right knee, and move your attention towards the other leg. Then Move your Awareness towards your head.
- Breath slowly and deeply and stay in this position for 10-20 minutes, roll onto your right side and be in this position for another one minute. Gently sit up with the support of your right hand.
- Take deep breaths keeping your eyes closed. Gradually come to an awareness of the environment.

Benefits: In Sanskrit, '*dead body*' is translated as '*shava*' and '*pose*' as '*asana*', hence it is commonly known as Shavasana. It relaxes your body and mind and provides you a deep meditative state of rest by releasing stress. This also helps reduce blood pressure, anxiety, and problems of sleeplessness.

Natrajasana (Lord of the Dance Pose)

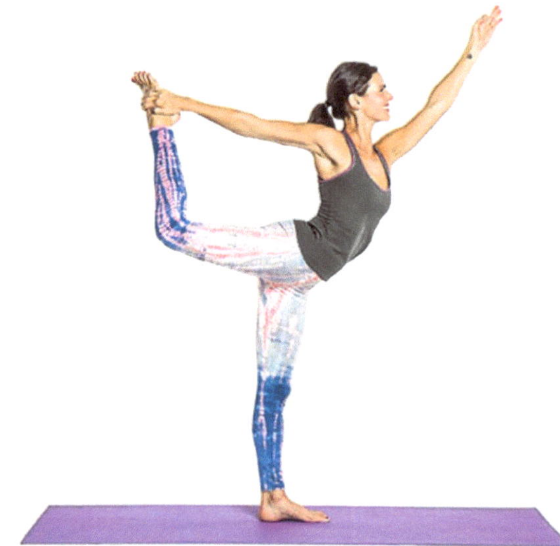

Fig. 36.23: *Showing physical features in Natrajasana (Lord of the Dance Pose)*

How to Perform

- Stand in Tadasana (or Mountain Pose)
- Shift your weight on the right leg and carefully lift the left leg backward while slightly tilting the upper body toward the front in order to gently support this movement.
- Hold the left leg with the left hand for balancing the pose.
- Raise the right arm parallel to the floor with your gaze fixed on the front.

Benefits: An excellent yoga asana for deeply stretching the shoulder muscles, chest, thighs, and abdominal muscles. Ideal for strengthening the legs and feet while improving the balance and posture.

Contraindications: This is a safe yoga pose. However, extreme precaution must be taken while performing it as the practitioner may lose balance resulting in heavy injury. People suffering from soreness or injury anywhere in the body should avoid this pose.

Padma Mayurasasna (Peacock Pose Variation)

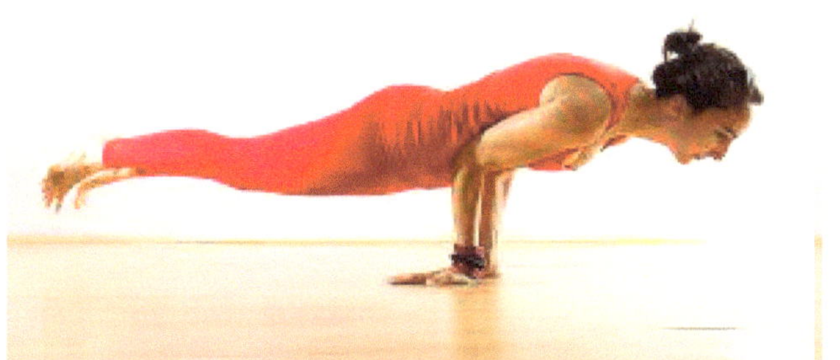

Fig.36.24: *Showing physical features in Padma Mayurasasna (Peacock Pose Variation)*

How to Perform

- Sit in Padmasana (Lotus Pose).
- Bend your torso forward to let the head touch the floor.
- Twist your wrist outwards and bend your elbows in the crease of your waistline.
- Support the torso weight on the palms facing the floor.

Benefits: This yogasana provides an excellent tone to the abdomen and the forearms. It is ideal for the strengthening of wrists, forearms, torso, hamstrings, and thighs.

Contraindications: People suffering from any kind of strain or injury in the wrist or elbow are advised against performing this pose.

Anantasana (Side-Reclining Leg Lift)

How to Perform

- Lie on your right side, spine aligned with the hips, legs straight and aligned on top of each other.
- Bend the elbow of the right arm to support the head.
- Now, slowly lift the left leg high in the air until it is perpendicular to the groin
- Raise your left arm high in the air to touch the toes of the raised left leg. Feel stretch in the side abdomen and the thighs as you do it.
- Grab the toe of the left foot between the thumb and the forefinger of your hand. Hold the pose for 30 seconds.

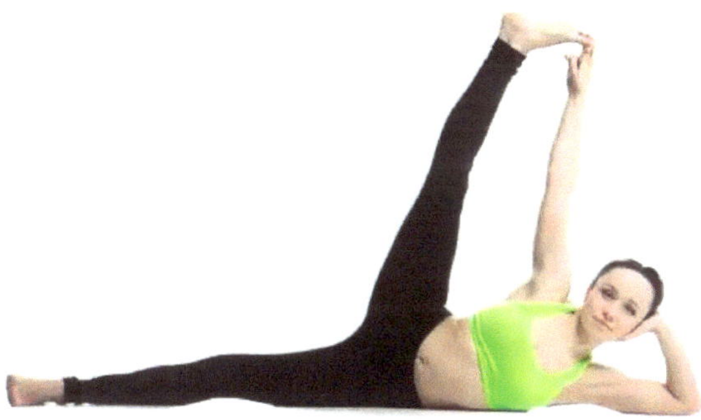

Fig.36.25: *Showing physical features in 14. Anantasana (Side-Reclining Leg Lift)*

Bene its: The pose provides complete stretch to the hamstrings and oblique muscles while toning the abdomen.

Contraindications: This is a relatively safe yoga asana. People suffering from sciatica, spinal injury, lower back injury or slipped disc issues are not advised to perform this asana.

Ardha Matsyendrasana

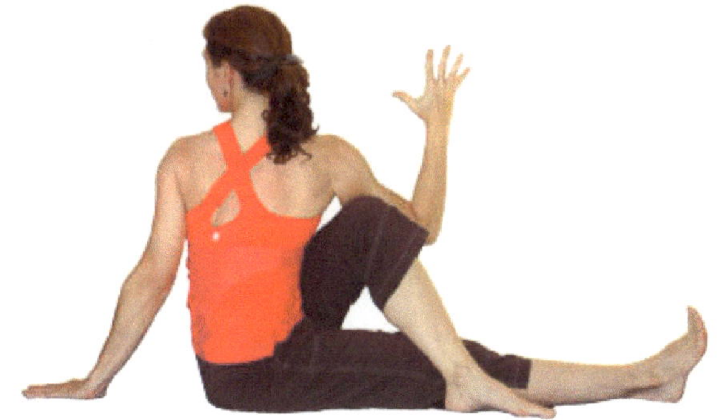

Fig.36.26: *Showing physical features in Ardha Matsyendrasana*

How to Perform

- Inhale, begin seated with legs extended.
- Exhale, bending right knee and crossing over left placing right foot flat or choose a variation.
- Inhale, twisting toward right leg, place right hand on floor behind back.
- Exhale, place left elbow on outside of right knee.
- Inhale, slowly rotating head towards the right.
- Exhale, using core and elbow finding full twist, keeping spine extended.
- Hold pose 3 to 5 breaths or as long as comfortable.
- Repeat on other side.

Benefits:

1. Tones and strengthens abs and obliques.
2. Stretches and energizes the spine.
3. Open the shoulders, neck, and hips.
4. Increases flexibility, especially in hips and spine.
5. Cleanses the internal organs.
6. Improves digestion and elimination of wastes.

Setu Bandhasana

How to Perform:

Lie flat on your back, and bend your legs at the knees. Lift your hips and back off the floor. Be gentle. Now, straighten your shoulders and stretch out your arms as they rest on the floor such that they reach your feet. Take a few deep breaths as you hold the pose for a few seconds, and release.

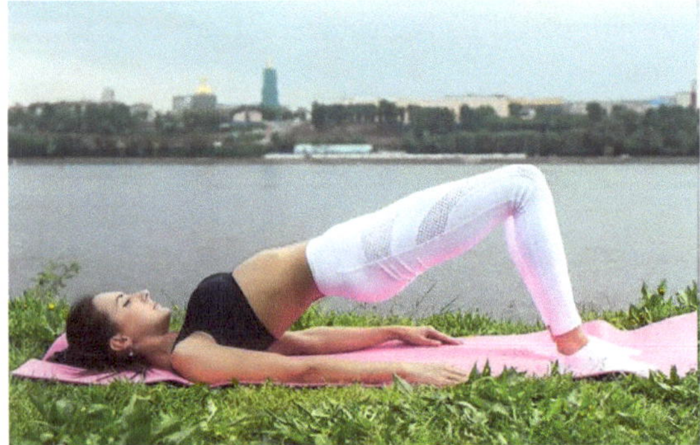

Fig. 36.27: *Showing physical features in Setu Bandhasana*

Benefits: T his asana works on straightening and strengthening the back. It also helps to open up the chest and reduce thyroid problems. It is an excellent asana for women as it strengthens their reproductive system. It also aids digestion. This asana works wonders for those suffering from insomnia, anxiety, and high blood pressure. The Setu Bandhasana calms the brain and relaxes the body.

Handstand Pose (Adho Mukha Vrksasana)

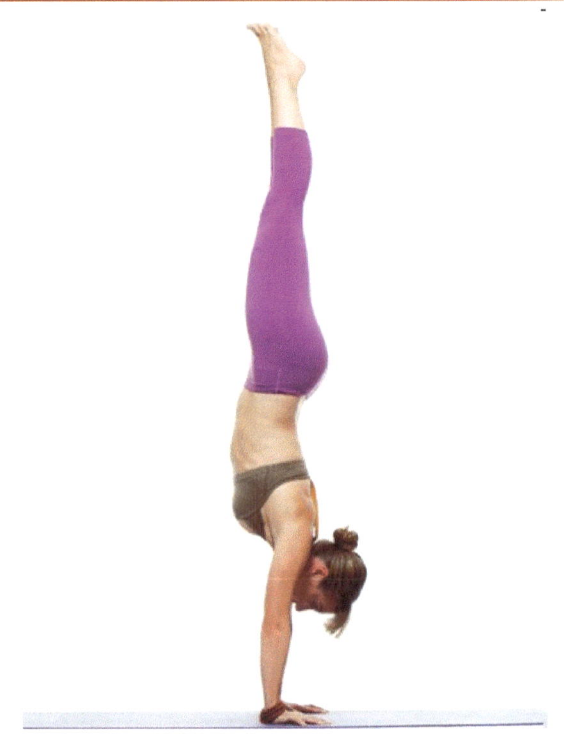

Fig. 36.28: *Showing physical features in Handstand Pose (Adho Mukha Vrksasana)*

Step-by-Step Instructions

- Come into Downward Facing Dog with your hands about 6 inches away from the wall.
- Walk your feet in closer to your hands, bringing the shoulders over your wrists and, if possible, your hips over your shoulders.
- Keep your right foot on the ground lifting onto the ball of it and begin to bend at the knee. Lift the other foot off the floor straightening the lifted leg behind you. Take a few hops here, jumping off from the bent leg and lifting the straight leg toward vertical. Flex your lifted food the entire time for engagement.
- Try bringing both heels to the wall. Keep your head down between your upper arms and breathe deeply.
- Practice taking the heels off the wall and balancing, remembering to keep your feet flexed. You will need to strongly engage your legs and reach up through your heels. You can also start to work on bringing your gaze to the floor.
- Bring one leg down at a time and rest before trying to kick up with the opposite leg for balance.

Benefits

- Handstand builds strength in your shoulders, arms, and core. The psoas muscle also gets a workout in keeping your spine stabilized while creating more flexibility through the hamstrings in order to kick up into the pose.
- As an inversion, it sends blood to your head, which can both be energizing and conversely help to calm you. Handstand also helps you improve your sense of balance.
- Like all poses that are difficult, it's fun to accomplish something that you doubted your ability to do.

Twisted Floor Bow Pose (Dhanurasana)

Steps

- You can perform Bow Pose on a yoga mat or carpeted floor. No equipment is necessary, but a yoga towel is optional.
- Lie flat on your stomach. Keep your chin on the mat and your hands at your sides. Your hands should be palm up.
- Exhale while you bend your knees. Bring your heels as close as you can to your buttocks. Your knees should be hip-width apart.

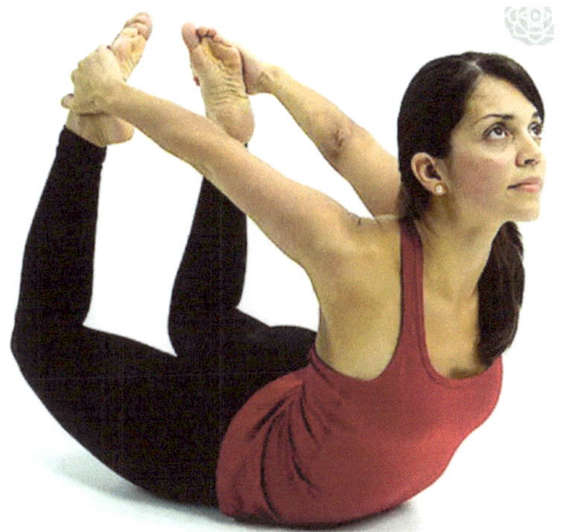

Fig. 36.29: *Showing physical features in Twisted Floor Bow Pose (Dhanurasana)*

- Lift your hands and take hold of your ankles. Be sure to grab the ankle and not the top part of the feet. Your fingers should wrap around the ankles, but your thumb does not. Keep your toes pointed.
- Inhale and lift the heels away from the buttocks, keeping a hold of your ankles. Simultaneously, lift your head, chest, and thighs away from the mat. As you lift, rotate your shoulders safely and comfortably. At this point, only your core should touch the mat, while the rest of your body is lifted towards the ceiling.
- Draw your tailbone into the mat to deepen the stretch. You should feel the stretch in your back as the weight and balance shifts to your core. Your chest and shoulders should feel open.
- Look straight ahead and hold the pose for about 15 seconds while you focus on stretching, breathing, and balancing.
- Exhale and release the pose. Lower your head, chest, thighs, and feet back towards the mat. Let go of your ankles and return to your hands to your side. Relax for a few seconds and repeat the pose as needed or continue to your next pose

Benefits

- Bow Pose primarily benefits the chest and back. It's natural for the body to bend backward, but this is rarely a position we find ourselves in.
- Bow Pose can be used to open up the chest and stretch out the back, which is especially beneficial for people who sit or stand for long periods of time.
- This yoga pose also opens up the neck, shoulders, and abdomen. It improves flexibility in the back and encourages balance in the core and chest.
- If you have a stiff back, Bow Pose may be beneficial. For people with a desk job, Bow Pose can help improve posture and alleviate the discomfort that slouching may cause.

Crane Pose (Bakasana)

Steps

- Begin by standing in Mountain Pose (Tadasana) with your arms at your sides. Breathe steadily throughout this pose.
- Bend your knees slightly so that you can bring your palms flat on the floor about shoulder's distance apart.
- Plant your palms firmly on the mat about a foot in front of your feet. Spread your fingers wide and press into the top joint of each finger.
- Bend your elbows straight back. Don't bend them into full Chaturanga arms, but head in that direction.
- Come up onto the balls of your feet and open your knees so that they line up with your upper arms.
- Place your knees on the backs of your upper arms.
- Begin to bring your weight forward into your hands, lifting your head as you go.

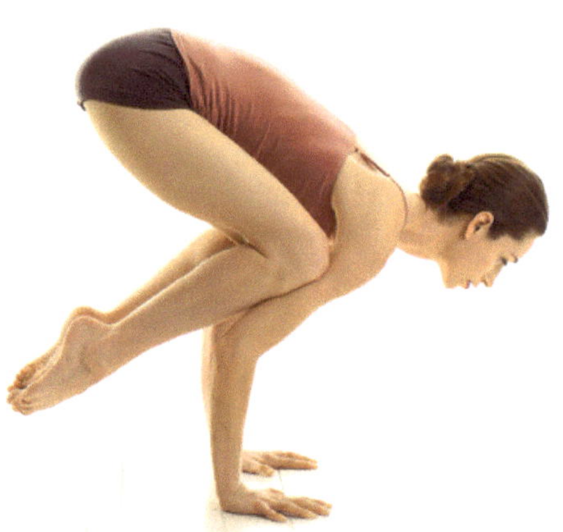

Fig.36.30:*Showing physical features in Crane Pose (Bakasana)*

- Come up onto your tiptoes, then lift one foot and then the other off the floor.
- Engage the inner thighs for support while keeping the knees on the arms.
- Hug your feet toward your butt.
- Focus on the feeling of the body lifting. Avoid sinking into the pose, which can dump weight into the shoulders.
- To come out, exhale and transfer your weight back until your feet come back to the floor.

Benefits

- Crow Pose strengthens the wrist, forearms, and abdomen while stretching your upper back.
- It improves balance and core strength. Mastering Crow builds your yoga confidence and opens the door to many more poses involving arm balance.
- You will improve your awareness of where your body is in space and enhance your body control.

Split Pose (Hanumanasana)

Splits Pose Steps:

Given below are the step-by-step instructions to follow for the practice of Hanumanasana (Splits Pose):

- Follow the instructions as explained in Ardha Hanumanasana to begin with the practice and warm up the legs.
- From Ardha Hanumanasana, stretch the left leg in front with the toes still pulled upwards and facing you.
- The, exhaling stretch the right leg behind taking support from the hands placed on the sides on the floor.
- While moving the right leg towards the floor, ensure the front left leg stays strong balancing on the heels.
- Exhale completely once the back right leg rests on the ground settling the right knee, right upper foot, right lower thighs on the ground.

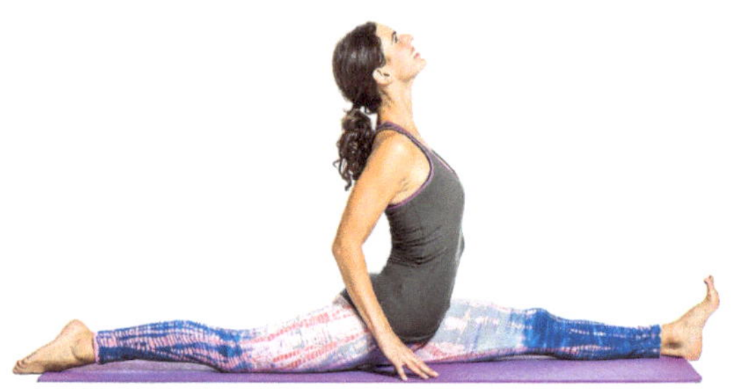

Fig. 36.31 *Showing physical features in Split Pose (Hanumanasana)*

- Stretch the back leg completely until the perineum is closer to the floor (it may not rest at first, but with practice it will).
- Inhale, stretch the spine, point the toes up of the left leg, push the palms towards the ground to get fully comfortable, lift the chest, push the hips towards the ground, and breathe naturally.
- Then, once comfortable, raise release the hands from the floor and bring the hands to Anjali Mudra and stay here for about 3-4 breaths.
- Then, inhale and slowly raise the arms above your head gently going in a backbend and looking up.
- Stretch the chest and shoulders to stay here for about 3-4 breaths, initially.
- Breath naturally and feel the connections to the ground.
- To release, bring the hands back to the floor at the sides, inhale, lift yourself up and bring the front left leg behind and come to rest in Adho Mukha Svanasana (Downward Facing Dog Pose).
- Repeat with the other leg, taking the right leg in front and stretching the left leg behind and stay following the instructions for about 3-4 breaths. Release and relax.

Splits Pose Benefits:

1. Hanumanasana is a deep hip opener that challenges the strength and flexibility of the leg muscles and hip flexors. Mastery over this pose comes with a lot of benefits, which are explained below:
2. Follow the benefits as explained in Ardha Hanumanasana (Half Split Pose).

3. Stretches the leg muscles, strengthening and toning them. The lengthening of the leg muscles also helps to bring stability in the hips.
4. Better circulation of blood in the hip girdle and the legs. There is fresh flow of blood towards the legs right after being released from the posture, and this helps in rejuvenating the muscles, tissues, ligaments and tendons.
5. In most seated poses the weight of the body is on the hips and the sit bones, but in Hanumanasana (Splits Pose) it is on the pelvic girdle, engaging the pelvic floor muscles. Thus, it works on strengthening these muscles, improving blood supply, the coccygeal region (tailbone) is stretched which helps since it connects to perineum and the spine.
6. With the stretch in the groin area, groin muscles, psoas muscles, and abdominal muscles are strengthened helping in keeping the hips stable.
7. With the practice of Splits Pose, there is scope for bringing balance and stability to the hips and pelvic girdle. With the opposite movement of the hip flexors and the legs, students can learn to neutralize the rotation of the hips. With better hip stability, mastering advance poses that require deeper hip opening can be achieved.
8. Awareness and Alignment plays an important role with the practice of Hanumanasana (Splits Pose). With the awareness, students should work on the alignment of the body to ensure achieving the best from the practice as well as avoid injury. Hence, for perfect alignment, using blocks where needed, should be encouraged.
9. The practice of Hanumanasana teaches students to be patient along with endurance. Since it is a challenging pose most students would give up going further and may not even come back to this practice. But being patient, understanding the requirements of the body strength, going step-by-step into the practice are all essential to master this posture. But it is believed that if students master this posture they should learn to let go and practice meditation seated here, taking the practice towards the spiritual level.

One-Legged King Pigeon Pose (Eka Pada Rajakapotasana)

Step-by-Step Instructions

Step 1

Begin on all fours, with your knees directly below your hips, and your hands slightly ahead of your shoulders. Slide your right knee forward to the back of your right wrist; at the same time angle your right shin under your torso and bring your right foot to the front of your left knee. The outside of your right shin will now rest on the floor. Slowly slide your left leg back, straightening the knee and descending the front of the thigh to the floor. Lower the outside of your right buttock to the floor. Position the right heel just in front of the left hip.

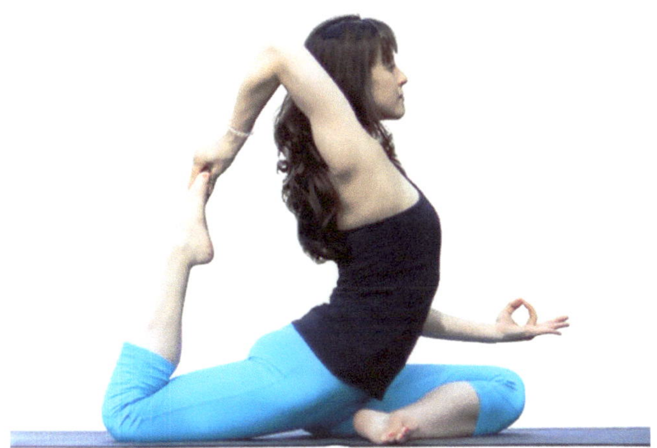

Fig. 36.32: *Showing physical features in One-Legged King Pigeon Pose (Eka Pada Rajakapotasana)*

Step 2

The right knee can angle slightly to the right, outside the line of the hip. Look back at your left leg. It should extend straight out of the hip (and not be angled off to the left), and rotated slightly inwardly, so its midline presses against the floor. Exhale and lay your torso down on the inner right thigh for a few breaths. Stretch your arms forward.

Step 3

Then slide your hands back toward the front shin and push your fingertips firmly to the floor. Lift your torso away from the thigh. Lengthen the lower back by pressing your tailbone down and forward; at the same time, and lift your pubis toward the navel. Roll your left hip point toward the right heel, and lengthen the left front groin.

Step 4

If you can maintain the upright position of your pelvis without the support of your hands on the floor, bring your hands to the top rim of your pelvis. Push heavily down. Against this pressure, lift the lower rim of your rib cage. The back ribs should lift a little faster than the front. Without shortening the back of your neck, drop your head back. To lift your chest, push the top of your sternum (at the manubrium) straight up toward the ceiling.

Step 5

Stay in this position for a minute. Then, with your hands back on the floor, carefully slide the left knee forward, then exhale and lift up and back into Adho Mukha Svanasana (Downward Facing Dog Pose). Take a few breaths, drop the knees to all-fours on another exhalation, and repeat with the legs reversed for the same length of time.

Benefits

- Stretches the thighs, groins and psoas, abdomen, chest and shoulders, and neck
- Stimulates the abdominal organs
- Opens the shoulders and chest

Contraindications and Cautions

- Sacroiliac injury
- Ankle injury
- Knee injury
- Tight hips or thighs

Forearm Hollow Back Pose (Pincha Mayurasana)

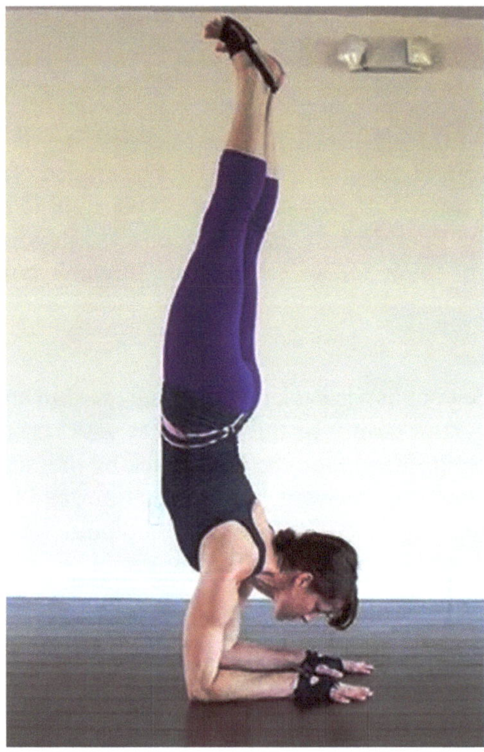

Fig.36.33: *Showing physical features in Forearm Hollow Back Pose (Pincha Mayurasana)*

Steps in (Pincha Mayurasana)

- As with other inversions, it's helpful to learn this pose at the wall and with the help of a skilled teacher. If you're more experienced and able to work on balancing in the posture, you're welcome to follow the same instructions while in the milddle of the room.
- Set up facing a wall.
- Place your forearms on the floor with your elbows shoulder-width apart. Your forearms should be parallel to each other and your palms should face down. Adjust your distance from the wall so that the wall is just barely beyond the reach of your fingertips.
- There are many different ways to use a block in this pose and I'm an advocate for all of them! For the purpose of this blog, I'm simply going to suggest that you place a block between your hands.
- More specifically, look at your fingers and place the block so that your index fingers touch the sides of the block and your thumbs touch the bottom of the block.
- Bring your shoulders forward so that they're direclty above your elbows. Step one foot half way to your elbow and bend your knee. Choose whichever leg feels the most natural.
- Root down through the base of each finger and thumb.
- Look at the floor in between your hands. Take a slow, deep breath. Don't freak out.
- As you exhale, bend the knee that you brought forward more deeply and strongly push the floor away. As this leg jumps, simultaneously swing the back leg toward the wall. Keep the knee of your "swinging" leg straight.
- As one leg swings toward the wall and the other leg jumps, draw your navel toward your spine to recruit your core muscles and create greater lift.
- You need to use enough strength and momentum to get your hips over your shoulders. Once your hips are above your shoulders, your "swinging" leg will make it to the wall and stay there. At this point, you can bring your second leg (your "jumping" leg to the wall).
- Now that you're in the pose, you can refine it by using the infographic above!
- Hold the pose for a few seconds before slowly lowering one of your feet toward the floor. As you lower one leg, the second will follow shortly thereafter.
- Spend a few moments in Child's Pose or Standing Forward Bend.

Benefits

- The Funky Forearm Stand Pose (Funky Pincha Mayurasana) is an inversion with primary focus of the muscles of the upper body. Hence all the benefits of inversion and the upper body position strength are listed below:
- **Inversion and Benefits:** Although Funky Pincha Mayurasana is a creative way to balance the body, yet all the qualities of an inversion are present in this posture. Hence, the general benefits of all inversion will apply to this pose, which are explained here.
- **Balance and Equilibrium:** The Funky Forearm Stand Pose is definitely a test to the body's strength and balance. One has to maintain balance not only while attempting to get into the pose, but also to hold the pose and breathe normally. The asymmetrical position of the arms is what makes it so challenging, but once mastered this pose helps improve one's balance, equilibrium of the body and focus.
- **Shoulder Strengthening:** An immense amount of upper body strength is required to perform the Funky Forearm Stand Pose. It is more challenging for the shoulders than the traditional Feathered Peacock Pose (Pincha Mayurasana). The student may tend to put more weight on the forearm, causing the body to tilt. However, with practice the student will not only gain strength in the shoulders and arms, but also get a better understanding of the body's center of gravity and find the pose to be attainable.
- **Core Engagement:** The Funky Forearm Stand Pose requires core engagement in order to find the center of gravity. This is what will counter the asymmetrical position of the arms, and help one hold the pose for a longer duration. It engages and works the deep core muscles, which one will need to access for other inversions like Adho Mukha Vrksasana.
- **Energizing:** Initially the breathing in this pose may be shallow, but with practice, as the body gets used to the position, the nervous system relaxes and allows the body to breath normally. Due to the increased blood circulation in the head and torso, the spine experiences a flow of prana, which helps one feel energized. It also helps one build confidence in the capabilities of their body.
- **Preparatory Pose:** Funky Pincha Mayurasana (Funky Forearm Balance Pose) is included in advanced yoga poses. As part of upper back yoga poses, this practice helps to strengthen the shoulders and abs and core, preparing the body for poses like Eka Hasta Vrksasana (One Handed Tree Pose).

Contraindications

Funky Forearm Balance Pose is a advanced level yoga pose that is performed in prone position. Funky Forearm Balance Pose additionally involves inversion, Forward-Bend, Stretch, Strength, Balance.Need Funky Forearm Balance Pose contraindications? Please sign-up to request contraindications of Funky Forearm Balance Pose and we will notify you as soon as your request has been completed.

Conclusion

Hatha Yoga poses are very beneficial even if you perform them using certain props or support. Beginners can easily incorporate themselves in these body postures as simple techniques are used to perform these poses. With regular practice, it can make your muscles flexible and provide you ample motivation to increase the duration of performing poses. Once you master these poses you can easily perform the next level yoga poses comfortably and avail many health benefits of practicing yoga. Hatha yoga is regarded as a great yoga for relaxation and improving the awareness of the mind. Hatha Yoga practice itself adopts the techniques of slowing down, putting the focus on static body postures, and shifting from one pose to the next with ease. There is a myth that beginners will have difficulty in performing Hatha Yoga as they do not possess the flexibility of muscles. But the fact is the regular practice of some easy hatha yoga poses improves the flexibility of muscles; hence it is best for beginners who lack muscular flexibility

Yogic Breath of Fire (Bhastrika Pranayama)

(Other name: Bhastrika Paranayma) Bhastrika is Sanskrit word which means 'roar'. This breathing technique involves deep inhalation and forceful exhalation which sounds like bellow. The vigorous breathing technique enhances the flow of breath into the lungs. Furthermore, it develops internal warmth on a physical and subtle level. This technique strengthens lung capacity. That is why this technique is very effective for relieving cough, flu, breathing problems, allergies, etc.

Steps to perform

- Sit in a comfortable position. Inhale deeply. Exhale vigorously or powerfully through nose.
- Again inhale with same force. Remember you should expand the abdominal muscles to full capacity.
- Observe the movements of diaphragm. It moves downward during inhalation and upwards during exhalation. Try to improve both movements.

- For beginners, 5 rounds of breathing are recommended.

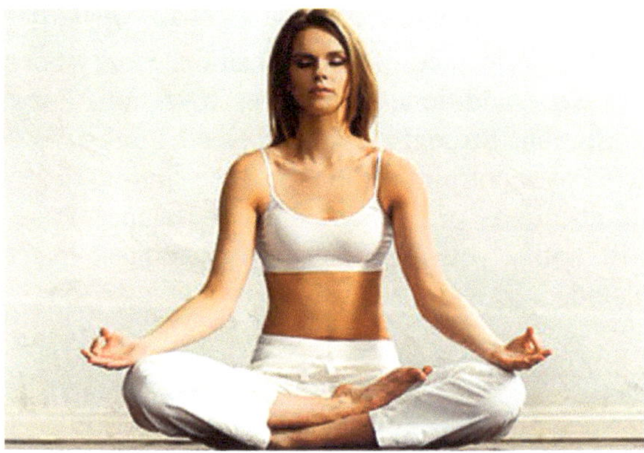

Fig. 36.34: *A young lady is practicing Bhastrika Paranayma*

Precautions:

This breathing technique is not suitable for elderly, pregnant women in the first trimester of pregnancy and asthma patients. Moreover, if your feel nausea or excessive sweating, it indicates something wrong with your practice. Therefore, its better to consult some expert in such case.

Forehead Shining Breathing

(Other name: *Kapalbhati Pranayama* or Kapalshodhana.) The Sanskrit meaning of this breathing techqnuie is 'which brings light and awareness to brain'. The breathing practice is believed to be effective for improving lung capacity and to relive respiratory obstructions.

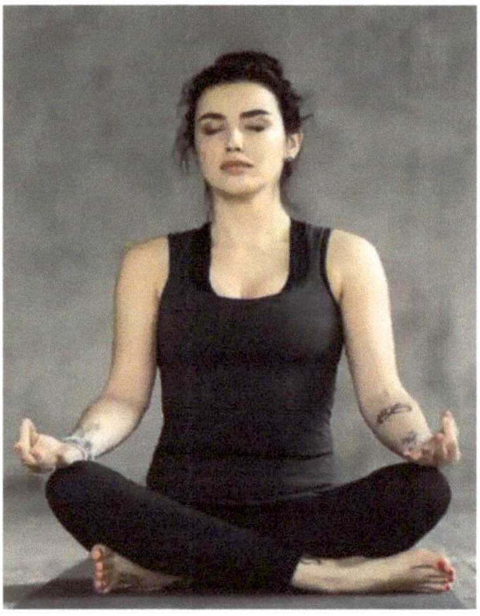

Fig. 36.35: *A young lady is practicing Kapalbhati Pranayama or Kapalshodhana*

Steps in Kapalbhati Pranayama

1. Sit comfortably.
2. Inhale a long and deep breath.
3. Exhale through both nostrils with strong and forceful contraction of the diaphragm/ abdominal muscles.
4. Again inhale deeply but no strain. keep the abdominal muscles relaxed.
5. Exhalation should be forceful.
6. Practice 5-10 rounds and then take a deep and relaxed breath.

Precautions:

This breathing technique is not suitable for pregnant women in their first trimester, patients of asthma and cardiovascular diseases and high blood pressure.

Health Benefits

Yoga breathing techniques are effective for removing obstructions in respiratory system. These techniques improve the lung capacity, blood oxygenation, blood circulation. Research reveals the effectiveness of these techniques for boosting immunity and overall health.

Kundalini Awakening: What Is It and How To Awaken It

Kundalini yoga is a deeply spiritual practice. In fact, many say that the Kundalini process can lead to a spiritual awakening. And while spiritual enlightenment sounds like a really good thing, it can come with a whole lot of intense experiences. The way that yoga talks about this spiritual experience is through the Kundalini process, where prana (life force energy) moves through the subtle body until it reaches the Sahasrara Chakra to awaken Kundalini. Before you go chasing the Kundalini experience (like I did), take some time to get acquainted with the Kundalini awakening process. There are a few things you should know about awakened Kundalini, first. And then I'll share my tips on how to use this ancient practice to achieve your own spiritual awakening too. So buckle up. We are about to embark on a spiritual journey.

What is Kundalini Awakening?

Kundalini Awakening is a remarkably powerful spiritual experience. In the yoga world, it is spiritual enlightenment. It is something that devoted yogis and practitioners spend many years preparing for and working towards. So what happens when we awaken our dormant Kundalini energy? Well, consider that Kundalini is our spiritual energy. A Kundalini practice uses the physical body to move the spiritual energy along our central channel.

In essence, it's waking up the divine feminine life force energy, known as the Kundalini serpent, that lies coiled and locked at the base of our spine.Once this energy is woken and able to flow freely up and down our centerline, it makes its way up to penetrate the seventh chakra where it meets the divine masculine forces.Where our divine feminine energy represents creation, our divine masculine energy is higher consciousness.And with this meeting comes a shift into a broadened state of awareness. There, in the seventh chakra, a spiritual awakening can occur.This is what we call Kundalini Awakening. It is an experience that will move you to your core and bring all into light.

Is Kundalini awakening rare?

Kundalini awakening is somewhat common in the spiritual world. But generally speaking, it's rare. It's a total transformation that will open your mind, body and soul to a whole new magnitude. And the thing is, you really have no control over when or if Kundalini will awaken. (Hello, spontaneous awakening) While we can work faithfully with Kundalini energy to summon her rising in the end, it is she who decides when she is ready. For some, reaching awakening can take a lifetime to achieve and there's absolutely nothing wrong with that because it's all about the process.

And everything happens in the divine way that it should.

What triggers Kundalini awakening?

Awakening Kundalini can go two ways.

1. Kundalini awakens through many years of hard work and dedication.
2. Kundalini awakens spontaneously.

You are not actively working to achieve awakening nor are you mentally preparing yourself but somehow, awakening is triggered. Though we can take the steps to awaken dormant Kundalini energy, there is truly no rhyme or reason to when and how Kundalini will awaken. I know, it sounds discouraging and quite like a mystical experience. But that's because it is and it has a lot to do with Karma, from this life and many lives before. After all, our spiritual journey begins long before we enter this physical body. And a dedicated yoga practice can help us get closer to the spiritual path. Intentional or not, some things that can trigger awakening are:

1. Meditation

Meditation in general is a wonderful practice and tool for preparing and awakening Kundalini.

In particular, practicing extended meditation within a short time period, such as in a retreat setting, can be a trigger for awakening to occur.

2. Yoga Asana

Both Kundalini Yoga and Hatha Yoga can trigger awakening through activating and clearing the energy centers through specific chakra-aligned postures. Other spiritual postural practices like Qi-gong can be a trigger too.

3. Breathwork

Working with the breath and certain pranayama exercises can trigger awakening as you guide your life force to flow up and down the energy line within.

4. Prayer

Much of awakening stems from intention. Therefore, intense prayer and deep devotion to connection with the divine can trigger awakening.

5. Energy Healing

Chakra work, Reiki, hypnosis, trauma therapy, and so on, can be a big trigger for awakening Kundalini as you are working intently to clear blockages in the subtle body, making space for Kundalini energy to flow.

6. Physical Trauma

Awakening can be triggered through working to heal physical trauma and injury, especially in the lower back or spine area as that where she lays.

7. Emotional Trauma and Depression or Grief

Losing someone close to you whether it be through death, a break-up, or physical separation can be a strong trigger for awakening as well as suffering from depression or experiencing great grief.

8. Near-Death Experience

Kundalini is a life force within the sublet body. Sometimes, Kundalini energy will awaken in an attempt to sustain life in a near-death experience.

9. Love

Falling in love can trigger awakening by opening up the Anahata chakra in the heart center.

10. Childbirth

Giving birth to a child can trigger Kundalini Awakening as new life passes through the Muladhara chakra.

Working to awaken Kundalini energy is a safe practice in itself. However, there are some dangers to it. You must be aware that awakening Kundalini unleashes tremendous force. And with great power comes great responsibility.

Think of Kundalini as a fierce and powerful goddess. Her presence is strong and intense. Waking the goddess is an ancient and sacred art form that must be handled with care, grace and intention.

Where the danger lies is in not being prepared.

If you are not prepared for Kundalini energy to awaken, the experience can be quite frightening. There will be a lot of confusion, discomfort and resistance as the ego begins to dissolve and we are confronted with truth. This can feel like a bad drug trip or even psychotic break with reality.

In order to be able to merge graciously with Kundalini energy, a person must go through a period of careful purification and strengthening of their entire system first. This means that practicing under the guidance of a trusted and knowledgeable teacher or guru is pretty much always necessary. While the energy of the divine force is loving, nurturing and healing in its essence, the sudden shift in perception can be extremely overwhelming if we're not ready.

Not only will allowing a teacher to guide you will help you understand how to manage the power that Kundalini brings forth but also your teacher can guide you through practices and techniques based on what is right for you and your particular make-up Awakening the divine feminine force inside brings great change and transition. It's not a process that should be rushed and it's not always smooth sailing either. It can be rocky waters that bring us to the depths of our soul too. So, be willing and ready to do the work and embark on the journey if awakening Kundalini calls to you.

Methods to Awaken Kundalini Shakti

Awakening of the Kundalini is a major event in the evolution of the soul. There are various methods to awaken kundalini. In fact, most spiritual practices, eventually culminate in the awakening of the kundalini Shakti. Most of these methods have to be learned from a qualified master. Not all methods suite everyone. Practitioners can be classified based on percentage of Tamas (inertness or dullness), Rajas (active and restless) or Sattva (purity and clarity) inherent in them. Everyone is a combination of these qualities. Based on one's nature and practices done in the past, one will be attracted towards a certain type of spiritual practice. Kundalini practice should be done strictly under the guidance of a master.

Kundalini awakening through Mantra Yoga

Mantra practice is the first method to awaken kundalini. Mantra is a sacred syllable, word or words that can unleash the spiritual potential in man. These mantras were discovered by ancient seers or Rishis and has been passed on for generations through the master disciple tradition. Kundalini Shakti can be awakened by the practice of *Mantra Japa*, which is daily repetition of a mantra certain number of times. To awaken the kundalini, the master has to initiate the disciple with the intention or *Sankalpa* of awakening the inner dormant power. It also depends on the quality or state of evolution of the master. If the Guru has an awakened kundalini, then it is easy for the disciple to get awakening through initiation. Else, it can take a long time and many repetitions of the mantra. Awakening by mantra is an easy and relatively safe method.

Kundalini Awakening through Music

Music, consisting of the seven notes or *Sapta Svaras*, can alter the state of consciousness. The seven notes or frequencies have effect on the brain and the energy channels in the body. Awakening through music may happen spontaneously without the knowledge of the person. But, after awakening, if the kundalini is not taken up towards the crown chakra, it can create side effects. The person may not know, that it is caused by the awakening process. Such persons should approach a kundalini master to balance his energies and safely guide the kundalini upwards.

Kundalini Awakening through Pranayama

Awakening through pranayama is a quick and direct method to awaken kundalini, but requires ample preparations. Practitioner has to prepare the body through proper diet and cleaning techniques called *Shatkarma*. Pranayama purifies the energy channels or *Nadis*, particularly the three main channels *Ida*, *Pingala* and *Sushumna*. The central channel *Sushumna* has to be clear for the energy to go up. Pranayama creates heat in the body, which when directed properly, will awaken the kundalini Shakti. For this practice of the three Bandhas *Mula Bandha* (Root lock), *Uddhiyana Bandha* (Abdominal lock) and *Jalandhara Bandha* (Chin lock) has to be practiced to direct the energy upwards. Once awakened, the Kundalini tries to enter the *Sushumna* at the base of the spine and goes up.

Awakening through pranayama can be very quick and can bring many experiences. The practitioner should be well prepared to handle the experiences. It is always advisable to do this under the guidance of a master.

Kundalini Awakening through Herbs

Another method to awaken Kundalini is by consumption of certain chemicals. Herbs or medicines (*Aushadhi*) can be used to activate the *Nadis* or energy channels and for awakening the kundalini. Such knowledge is not readily available and is shrouded in secrecy. Awakening through herbs is also dangerous as it can lead to wild awakening with many side effects including madness, hallucinations and physical ailments, unless it is done under proper guidance. This method is shrouded in mystery and not available to everyone.

Kundalini Awakening through Tapas or austerity

The word *Tapas* in *Sanskrit* comes from the root word *Tapah*, meaning heat. Tapas or austerity is undertaken to purify the body, mind and emotions. During Tapas, our latent impressions in the mind will come to the surface and cause many emotional and mental imbalances. One has to go through these with a witness attitude and understand it as a cleansing process. Tapas helps to weaken our *Vasanas* or inherent tendencies and increases our will power. Awakening of Kundalini can happen during the process due to the churning of the subconscious and unconscious mind. The awakening by *Tapas* can be violent and may be difficult to handle. You may get many visions and experiences, thrown up from your latent unconscious mind. One may even develop some siddhis or supernatural powers. Presence of a teacher is essential during such times so that the practitioner can handle these side effects.

Kundalini Awakening through Raja Yoga

Raja yoga comes from *Ashtanga yoga* and primarily deals with *Dharana* (concentration), *Dhyana* (meditation) and *Samadhi* (Superconscious awareness). Raja yoga is not for everyone. It requires a very *Sattvic* or pure mind. Prolonged practice of *Hatha yoga* is recommended to make a practitioner fit for *Raja Yoga*. Raja yoga can be taken up only after purifying the mind through *Karma Yoga* (Yoga of action or work), *Bhakti Yoga* (Yoga of devotion) along with *Hatha Yoga* practices.

In Raja Yoga, the method of awakening kundalini is slow and steady.

Kundalini Awakening through Kriya Yoga

Kriya Yoga is another slow, safe and steady method to awaken Kundalini. Most people today do not have the pure *Sattvic* mind to take up meditational practices of Raja Yoga. Most practitioners today are *Rajasic* in nature, nor do they have the patience to take up rigorous practices. *Kriya yoga* is a good method for them as the awakening happens slowly and safely over a period of time. The experiences during *Kriya yoga* is usually mild and can be handled by most practitioners. There are many systems of *Kriya yoga* being practiced today. Most systems use the process of rotation of breath along the different chakras leading to activation of *Chakras*, *Nadis* and finally the *Kundalini Shakti* itself. One has to find a master with an authentic lineage to get initiated into this practice.

Kundalini Awakening through Shaktipat

Shaktipat is transferring of energy or power from Guru to disciple either by touch, sight or by mere thought. It can be done in the physical presence of the master or over a distance. It can be transmitted even by an object given by the Guru to the disciple. The awakening happens instantly, but may not be permanent. For this student has to be sufficiently ready for the master to transfer his energy to awaken the disciple. The disciple may have many experiences during the awakening which will subside slowly. The guru chooses the disciple for *Shaktipat*. The disciple cannot prepare for this process. It just happens at the right moment.

Kundalini Awakening through Tantric Initiation

Kundalini awakening through Tantric initiation is an esoteric subject shrouded in secrecy. The practitioner has to understand the principle of Shiva and Shakti. Males predominantly manifest the Shiva principle and females predominantly manifest the Shakti principle. When there is a coming together of these two forces, there can be an explosion and awakening can happen. This path is for people who have transcended the passions and desires to a good extend. Purity of mind is required. It is not a path for pleasure lovers. Guidance from a guru is essential.

Kundalini Awakening through Bhakti Yoga

Bhakti or devotion is pure love for God. This love is not born of passion or attachment as in worldly love. Here the main feature is *Saranagathi* or Self-Surrender. The devotee surrenders his life to his *Ishta Devata* or the form of God that he likes and worships. This path is based on total faith and surrender. Kundalini awakening can happen without any particular practice via surrender.

Kundalini awakening from Birth

Some rare persons can have kundalini awakened from birth. This can happen because of the spiritual practices done in previous births. Such children may grow up as geniuses, prodigies, people influential in worldly affairs of politics, military, finance, arts and sciences, etc. or may even become spiritual leaders.

Such individuals too, may need the help of a kundalini master to guide their energy upwards to prevent any side effects and utilise the energy for the good of the world.

Thus, the methods of awakening the kundalini Shakti are many. But one has to choose their spiritual practices according to one's own inclination. You have to find a master who will initiate you into that particular method of your choice

What Are The Signs of Kundalini Awakening?

"*Kundalini*" simply means '*that which is coiled*', and it can also be interpreted as '*coiling like a snake*' or '*coiled up*'. Kundalini is represented as a serpent coiled around the Root or Muladhara Chakra, the first of 7 chakras at the base of the spine. Kundalini lies in the nervous system and is regenerated through each breath, it is a life force energy. The main purpose of Kundalini awakening is to awaken one's higher ability and the potential that each individual possesses within oneself. Kundalini symbolizes the divinity of feminism and can be deeply related to Shaktism in most of the aspects. Everyone has a Kundalini but it has to be awakened and should be activated as it tends to stay inactive in the base of our spine, Root Chakra (Muladhara). It is said that if one's Kundalini does not awaken, their energy stays coiled at the base of their spine. For those whose Kundalini is awakened, each of their chakras is activated and they achieve enlightenment.

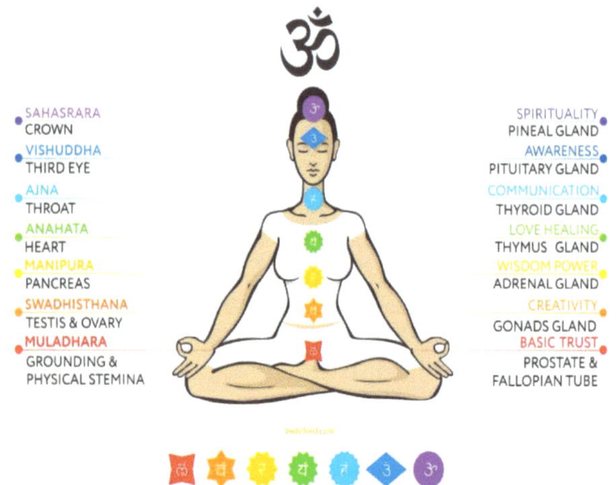

Fig. 36.36: *showing (left) localization of different body organs in relation to seven chakras. (Right) shows human behaviors in relation to body organs*

Kundalini awakening process can be one of the most traumatizing and confused and equally dangerous phases of your life. It is a deep purification process and one experiences a lot of changes during this phase. The awakening of Kundalini symbolizes the pinnacle of spiritual progress or the samadhi. The process of awakening of Kundalini has to be done very cautiously as it comes up with side effects when not done properly. The awakening of Kundalini can be performed with different ways and methods. A lot of systems of yoga focus majorly on awakening kundalini with the different meditation techniques, pranayama breathing, the practice of asana, and the chanting of mantras. Kundalini Yoga is highly influenced by Tantra schools of Hinduism and Shaktism.

Signs and Symptoms to Know if Your Kundalini is Awakening:

1. You find yourself going through the process of emotional turmoil evaluating through all the past experiences, mourning about things that you longer have, wishing for certain things to happen and feeling sad about things that you had to go through in the first place.
2. The past has a huge impact when the Kundalini awakens. Meaning, you analyze a lot about the incidents that happened in the past. You go through self-realization and try to analyze things that you did in the past. You revisit your experiences and wish if they had a different turn rather than what actually happened. This is a time to find peace within past thoughts and release them.
3. If your Kundalini is in the process of awakening, you may also experience some physical symptoms, for instance, waking up at random hours at the night, sweating a lot, crying or even sensing an intense rush of energy passing through your spine.
4. You get determined to make radical changes in your life, be it your diet or job choices or choice of people you want to spend time with. You concentrate on fixing your life and a sense of realization of what's not working hits you.
5. The phase of Kundalini awakening is a phase of self-realization in a wider picture. You keep your happiness in the topmost priority and let go of your ego. You come to realize that your mind is the ultimate force of holding back from presence and happiness. Moreover, you try to take a grip on your happiness.
6. You strengthen your empathetic abilities meaning, you tend to feel and think exactly what a certain person is experiencing at a certain period of time. This is the sign that your third eye is opening and you become acquainted with your true nature, which is connectedness.
7. You feel a strong sense of connection towards nature and want to stay outside as often as possible. Looking at the sky, hills, rivers excite you and you try to invest most of the time outside.

8. You begin to question the existence of systems and structures that you see around. You begin to look at and analyze religion, tradition, and politics like never before, trying to identify the purpose they serve in human beings.
9. You get an urge to filter your life in all the ways possible- broken relationships, old habits, you need to let them go as to achieve peace.
10. You feel the need to serve others. You understand that we all are one and that devotion for others' aide is the noblest and the most wonderful thing you can do.

Awakening kundalini needs proper guidance from the expert, if you are experiencing these symptoms without the help of a teacher, you should stop exploring yourself. Please find an expert and seek help.

Note: In the end, awakening Kundalini is a process. A journey of deep devotion, purification, patience and training.So please, move slowly and with ease.Be kind to yourself and the divine feminine energy that resides within.Each step should be embraced fully with love, presence and joy

Bibliography and Acknowledgement

- Aiyar, K. N., translator, 1914. Thirty minor Upanishads, including the Yoga Upanishads. Madras, 280 pages.
- *Āraṇya, Hariharānanda* (1983). *Yoga Philosophy of Patanjali. State University of New York Press.* ISBN 978-0873957281.
- Bal BS (2010). Effect of anulom vilom and bhastrika pranayama on the vital capacity and maximal ventilatory volume. *J. Phy. Educ. Sport Manage.*, **1**(1): 11-15.
- Bal BS, Singh K (2010) Effects of 4-week rope mallakhamb training on respiratory indices in adolescent girls. *Biomed. Hum. Kinetics*, **2**: 70- 73.
- Beck, Guy L. (1995). Sonic Theology: Hinduism and Sacred Sound. Motilal Banarsidass. ISBN 978-81-208-1261-1.
- Bhargava R, Gogate MG, Mascarenhas JF (1988). Autonomic responses to breath holding and its variations following pranayama. *Indian J. Physiol. Pharmacol.*, **32**: 257-264.
- Birch, Jason (2011). "The Meaning of Haṭha in Early Haṭhayoga". *Journal of the American Oriental Society*. **131** (4 (October-December 2011)): 527–558. JSTOR 41440511.
- Burley, Mikel (2000). Haṭha-Yoga: Its Context, Theory, and Practice. Motilal Banarsidass. ISBN 978-81-208-1706-7.
- Chhina CS (1974). The voluntary control of autonomic responses in Yogis. *Proc Int. Union Physiol. Sci.*, **10**: 103-104.
- Daniélou, Alain (1955). Yoga: the method of re-integration. University Books. ISBN 978-0766133143.
- De Michelis, Elizabeth (2007). "A Preliminary Survey of Modern Yoga Studies". Asian Medicine. Brill Academic Publishers. **3** (1): 1–19. doi:10.1163/157342107x207182.
- Deussen, Paul. 1980. Sixty Upanishads of the Veda - Part 2. Translated by V. M. B edekar, G. B. Palsule. First ed. 2 vols. Vol. 2. Delhi: Motilal Banarsidas, 544-1095 pages.
- Deussen, Paul. 1980. Sixty Upanishads of the Veda - Part I. Translated by V. M. B edekar, G. B. Palsule. First ed. 2 vols. Vol. 1. Delhi: Motilal Banarsidas,543 pages.
- Eliade, Mircea Elde (2009). Yoga: Immortality and Freedom. Princeton University Press. ISBN 978-0-691-14203-6.
- Florence V, Melody Y, Pierre B, Yves J (2005). Training to yoga respiration selectively increases respiratory sensation in healthy man, *Respir. Physiol. Neurobiol.*, **146**(1): 85-96.
- Gopal KS, Bhatnagar OP, Subramaniam N, Nishits SD (1973). Effects of Yogasanas & Pranayamas on blood pressure, pulse rate and some respiratory functions. *Indian J. Physiol. Pharmacol.*, **17**: 273- 276.
- Guyton AC (1996). Textbook of Medical Physiology, 9th edition. Philadelphia: W.B. Saunders, pp. 161- 169. Hadi N (2007) Effects of hatha yoga on well-being in healthy adults in Shiraz, *Islamic Republic of Iran. East. Mediterr. Health J.*, **13**: 829- 837.
- Harinath K, Malhotra AS, Pal K, Prasad R, Kumar R, Kain TC, Rail L, Sawhney RC (2004). Effects of hatha yoga and omkar meditation on cardiorespiratory performance, psychological profile, and melatonin secretion. *J. Altern. Complement. Med.* **10**: 261-268.
- Jacobsen, Knut A. (2011). Yoga Powers: Extraordinary Capacities Attained Through Meditation and Concentration. Brill. ISBN 978-90-04-21431-6.
- Joshi LN, Joshi VD, Gokhale LV (1992). Effect of short-term 'pranayama' practice on breathing rate and ventilatory functions of lung. *Indian J. Physiol. Pharmacol.*, **36**: 105-108.
- Joshi, K. S. (2005). Speaking of Yoga and Nature-Cure Therapy. Sterling Publishers. ISBN 978-1-84557-045-3.
- Kriyananda, Goswami. 1993. The Kriya Yoga Upanishad and the Mystical Upanishads. Fourth ed. Chicago: The Temple of Kriya Yoga, 99 pages.
- Larson, Gerald James; Bhattacharya, Ram Shankar; Potter, Karl H. (2008). Yoga: India's Philosophy of Meditation. Motilal Banarsidass. ISBN 978-81-208-3349-4.
- Malhotra V, Singh S (2002). Study of yoga asanas in assessment of pulmonary function in NIDDM patients. *Indian J. Physiol. Pharmacol.*, **46**: 313-320.
- Mallinson, James (2004). The Gheranda Samhita: The Original Sanskrit and an English Translation. Yoga Vidya. ISBN 978-0971646636.
- Mallinson, James (2007). The Shiva Samhita: A Critical Edition. Yoga Vidya. ISBN 978-0-9716466-5-0.
- Mallinson, James (2008). The Khecarividya of Adinatha: A Critical Edition and Annotated Translation of an Early Text of Hathayoga. Routledge. ISBN 978-1-134-16642-8.
- Mallinson, James (2011). "Yoga: Haṭha Yoga". In Basu, Helene; Jacobsen, Knut A.; Malinar, Angelika; Narayanan, Vasudha (eds.). Brill's Encyclopedia of Hinduism. 3. Leiden: Brill Publishers. pp. 770–781. doi:10.1163/2212-5019_BEH_

COM_000354. ISBN 978-90-04-17641-6. ISSN 2212-5019 – via Academia.edu.

- Mallinson, James (2011b). Knut Jacobsen (ed.). Siddhi and Mahāsiddhi in Early Haṭhayoga in Yoga Powers: Extraordinary Capacities Attained Through Meditation and Concentration. Brill Academic. pp. 327–344. ISBN 978-90-04-21214-5.
- Mallinson, James (March 2012). M. Moses; E. Stern (eds.). "Yoga and Yogis". Namarupa. 3 (15): 1–27
- Nayar HS, Mathur RM, Sampath Kumar R (1975). Effects of Yogic exercises on human physical efficiency. *Indian J. Med. Res.,* **63**: 1369-137.
- Pathale JD, Mehrotra PP, Joshi SD, Shah AH (1978). Aplea for Pranayam for elderly. *Ind. J. Pharmacol.*, **22**(4 Suppl): 77
- Raghuraj P, Ramakrishnan AG, Nagendra HR, Telles S (1998). Effect of two selected yogic breathing techniques on heart rate variability. *Indian J. Physiol. Pharmacol.*, **42**: 467-472.
- Ross A, Thomas SJ (2010). The health benefits of yoga and exercise: a Review of Comparison Studies. *J. Altern. Complement. Med.*, **16**: 3- 12.
- Sandeep B, Pandey US, Verma NS (2002). Improvement in oxidative status with yogic breathing in young healthy males. *Indian J. Physiol. Pharmacol*., **46**: 349-354.
- Sastri, A. Mahadeva, ed. 1968. The Yoga Upanishads. Adyar: Adyar LIbrary and Research Center, 984 pages. (In Sanskrit)
- Selvamurthy W, Nayar HS, Joseph NT, Joseph S. (1983). Physiological effects of yogic practice. *NIMHANS J.*, **1**: 71-80.
- Sjoman, Norman (1999) [1996]. The Yoga Tradition of the Mysore Palace (2nd ed.). Abhinav Publications. ISBN 81-7017-389-2.
- Svatarama. 1972. The Hathayogapradipika of Svatmarama. Translated by Radha Burnier and Tookaram Tatya. Adyar, Madras: The Adyar Library and Research Center, 106 pages.
- Svatmarama. 1970. The Hatha Yoga Pradipika. Translated by Swami Digambarji and Raghunathashastri Kokaje. First ed. Lonavla, Maharashtra: Kaivalyadhama,230 pages.
- Svatmarama. 1984. The Hatha Yoga Pradipika. Translated by Pancham Sinh. First ed. Delhi: Shri Satguru Publications,63 pages.
- Svatmarama. 1985. The Hatha Yoga Pradipika. Translated by Swami Muktibodhananda Saraswati. First ed. Munger, Bihar: Bihar School of Yoga,106 pages.
- Svatmarama; Akers, Brian (translator) (2002). The Haṭha yoga Pradipika. Yoga Vidya. ISBN 978-0-9899966-4-8.
- Telles S, Desiraju T (1993). Autonomic changes in Brahmakumaris Raja Yoga meditation. *Int. J. Psychophysiol.*, **15**: 147-152,
- Udupa KN, Singh RH, Settiwar RM. (1975). Studies on the effect of some yogic breathing exercise (pranayama) in normal persons. *Indian J. Med. Res.,* **63**: 1062-1065,
- Udupa KN, Singh RH. (1972). The scientific basis of Yoga. *JAMA*, 220: 1365
- Upadhyay DK, Malhotra V, Sarkar D, Prajapati R (2008) Effect of alternate nostril breathing exercise on cardiorespiratory functions. *Nepal Med. Coll. J.*, **10**: 25-27.
- Varenne, Jean. 1989. Yoga and the Hindu Tradition. Translated from French by Derek Coltman. Delhi: Motilal Banarsidas,253 pages. (Contains translation of the Darshana Upanishad)
- Veenhof, Douglas (2011). White Lama: The Life of Tantric Yogi Theos Bernard, Tibet's Emissary to the New World. Harmony Books. ISBN 978-0385514323.
- Wernicke-Olesen, Bjarne (2015). Goddess Traditions in Tantric Hinduism: History, Practice and Doctrine. Taylor & Francis. ISBN 978-1317585213.
- White, David Gordon (2011). Yoga in Practice. Princeton University Press. ISBN 978-1-4008-3993-3.
- White, David Gordon (2012). The Alchemical Body: Siddha Traditions in Medieval India. University of Chicago Press. ISBN 978-0-226-14934-9.
- Yeshe, Thubten (2005). The Bliss of Inner Fire: Heart Practice of the Six Yogas of Naropa. Wisdom Publications. ISBN 978-0861719785

Role of Vedic Astrology On Our Daily Life & Health Wellness

Vedic Astrology or Jyotish Shastra is perhaps one of the oldest astrology in the world. It is much more than a simple divination system. It is a great Vidya (Spiritual Science), which is deeply embedded in a profound philosophy of life. It is also known as Vedic astrology or Hindu Astrology. Jyotish means 'the science of light or heavenly body' and Shastra means the 'knowledge on the particular field'. *Jyotish Shastra* is the knowledge of the future, which is an important limb of the Vedas. Thus, it is a fascinating subject with many interesting facts.

The Father of Vedic Astrology

Maharshi Parashara is a well-known Vedic Sage who is regarded as the father of Jyotish Shastra or Vedic Astrology. He is accredited as the author of Vishnu Purana, the first of 18 Puranas of Hindu Literature compiled by his son Veda Vyasa. Parashara Rishi was the son of Shakti Muni and Adrishyanti and a disciple of Bashkal and Yajnavalkya.

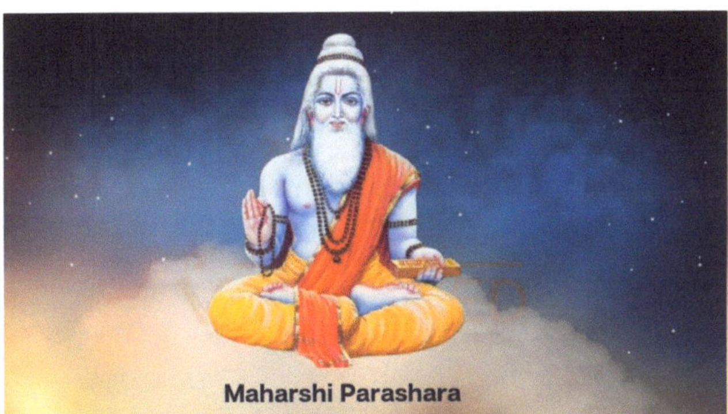

Fig. 37.1: *Photograph of Maharshi Parashara*

Birth of Rishi Parashara

Sage Parashara was actually raised by his grandfather, *Rishi Vasishtha*, one of the Saptarishi. It is because his father Shakti Muni had died before his birth and there is an interesting story behind the birth of Sage Parashara involving the death of his father Shakti Muni.

Curse of Sakti Muni to Veerasha, Prince of Ayodhya

Once when Shakti Muni was crossing the bridge, there came the prince of Ayodha named Veersah. *Veersah* was the son of King Sudaas and grandson of *King Rituparan* belonging to the Ikshavaku Dynasty. Veersah was riding on his chariot so that there was no enough space left for Shakti Muni to move forward. Shakti Muni politely requested Veersah, but the king did not pull back his chariot. They both remained stuck on the matter. When Veersah did not compromise, Shakti Muni became very angry and cursed Veersha to become a Rakshasa. Soon the king turned into a monster. Then the Rakshasa killed the sons of Rishi Vasishtha along with Shakti Muni. When the sage Vashistha came to know of this incident, he got frustrated with extreme sorrow. Distracted Rishi also decided to give up his life. But he could not succeed even after trying many times. Then went to the Himalayas with his family. One day, suddenly the recite of the Veda started to be heard and he started looking around in amazement. But he did not see anyone who was reciting the Vedas. Then Shakti Muni's wife told him that she was pregnant and the child in the womb was pronouncing Vedas for over 12 years. Rishi Vashistha got happy and discarded the idea to give up his life. The child was Parashara.

Parashar Rishi and Satyavati

Satyavati, also named *Matsyagandha* because her organs smelled like fish, used to work as a sailor. Her work was to take people across the river Yamuna in her boat. One day Rishi Parashara got in her boat in course of crossing the river and fell attracted to her beauty. Rishi Parashara then expressed his desire to have a relationship with her. But she refused to have an immoral relationship. However, Parashara kept on pleading her and at last, Satyavati agreed under three conditions:

No one should see what they were doing. So, the sage Parashara spreads dense fog all around with his yogic power and makes peace with Satyavati. Her virginity should not be dissolved under any circumstances. Parashara then assured her that she would get her virginity back after she gave birth.

She wanted the fishy odor that came from her body to be transformed into an aroma. Then the sage made an atmosphere of fragrance. After this, both of them made a relationship and a son was born from Satyavati named Krishnadvaipayan. Later Krishnadvaipayan was popularly known as Veda Vyasa, a compiler of Four Vedas.

Revenge of Rishi Parashara

When sage Parashara grew up, he came to know that his father was killed by a Rakshasa. Then he decided to take revenge that he would end all Rakshasa clan from the earth. So, he started a Yajna named, Rakshasa Satra Yajna. As a result, all the Rakshasas in the world including the blameless ones started turning into ashes one by one.

Maharishi Pulastya

Maharishi Pulastya (Grandfather of Ravana) approached Parashara Rishi and requested him to stop this Yajna and he also preached non-violence. He explained that it is unfair to kill all Rakshasa without any fault. After the prayers and sermons of Pulastya and Vyasa, he stopped this by giving the complete sacrifice of the demon-session yajna. Being pleased with it, Maharishi Pulstya gave him many blessings and also told a prediction in the future composition of the Purana Samhita. Later on, he composed many scriptures including Purana Samhita.

Compositions of Parashara

The sage Parashara had acquired knowledge of many disciplines and given them to the world. Parashara has many verses in the Rigveda. The Vishnu Purana, Parashara Samhita, Videharaj Janaka referred to as Gita (Parashara Geeta), Brihat Parashara Sanhita, etc. are compositions of Parashara.

Parashara Gita

In the dialogue of Bhishma and Yudhishthira in the Shanti Parva of Mahabharata, Bhishma reveals the conversation between Raja Janak and Parashara to Yudhishthira. This conversation is known as '*Parashara Gita*'. There are talks of knowledge related to religion and action. In fact, in Shanti Parva, a detailed description of the answers to all kinds of philosophy and religion questions is available.

Parashara's Astrology

Parashara Rishi composed many texts out of which his texts written about astrology are very important. Astrology of ancient and present is based on the rules laid down by Parashara. Rishi Parashara has written the Brihat Parashara Hora Shastra, *Laghu Parasharai* (Astrology).

10 Basic Facts about Jyotish Shastra or Vedic Astrology

1. The Origin of Jyotish Shastra

Jyotish Shastra emerged in the context of the Vedas, the ancient holy book of Hindus. According to Veda, Joytisha means (the shining world of light). It basically complemented this worldview in its attempt to shine the divine light on the individual's life. So it endeavours to dispel the darkness of illusion and assist the person to understand the purpose of the soul's present incarnation.

2. Modern Astrology

The credit for modernization of Vedic astrology goes to Rishi Parashara and Rishi Jaimini. It was Rishi Parashara who wrote Jyotish Shastra, a book which describes the rules and regulations to make astrological predictions. Further, Rishi Jaimini, who was a student of Ved Vyasa, compiled some important notes on Vedic astrology.

3. It's Difference with Western Astrology

One thing that is very peculiar about Jyotish Shastra is the fact that it has a considerable difference in its principles and logic from the western astrology. The Vedic birth chart differs from the traditional Western horoscope in several ways. Most importantly, Vedic astrologers use what is termed the sidereal zodiac rather than the tropical zodiac. The sidereal zodiac is based upon the actual positions of the 12 signs of the zodiac in the sky. The tropical zodiac is based upon the position of the Sun as it rises at the spring equinox.

4. The Precision of Birth Chart

The most important aspect of Jyotish Shastra is the fact that it takes into account the place, time and date of birth of a person while building his or her birth chart. Even little error in these three details leads to an extremely big error while creating the chart.

5. Planets or The Grahas

The most important elements in the individuals' charts are the planets, which were in ancient times identified with lesser deities. Planets are termed Graha, that which possesses a person, hence the planets are seen as symbolic of the illusions (Maya) of earthly existence that obscure the individual's divine nature. Each planet has acquired a set of associations and its particular placement in the chart indicates a variety of strengths and weaknesses. Generally, only the ancient visible planets are utilized by Vedic astrologers and thus one will not find Uranus, Neptune, or Pluto.

6. Movement of The Moon

Vedic astrology not only divides the zodiac into the 12 signs, but it also divides it into 27 lunar mansions roughly defined by the movement of the Moon around the earth every 27 days. The planetary periods relate to the lunar mansions very much as houses relate to the traditional signs. The planetary periods are of varying lengths as they are related to the different planets. The place of the newborn in the cycle of periods is determined by the position of the Moon in Kundali – the natal chart. The recognition of these periods provides Vedic astrologers with an additional level of interpretation of the person's life.

7. Movement of The Stars

Jyotish Shastra is known for widely using the stars and different constellations that one sees in the sky. As per Jyotish Shastra, the movement of stars plays a very important role in the life of an individual and decides on the important phases in his or her life, such as marriage, career, death, happiness, etc.

8. A Spiritual Subject

Vedic astrology is not a mundane subject like mathematics and other subjects. For its believers, it is a divine subject. Vedic astrologers are required to be spiritually aware and observe some ethics.

9. Vedic Astrology Is More Accurate Than The Western System

Vedic astrology is based on the sidereal zodiac, that is it is based on observing the fixed position of constellations in the sky. Meanwhile, western astrology is based on the tropical zodiac or the observation of the constellations in relation to the movement of the sun. The movement of the earth has changed by 23 degrees after thousands of years of its revolution and rotation. As Vedic astrology is based on the sidereal zodiac system, hence, it is considered to be more accurate than the western system.

10. Everything is Linked

Jyotish Shastra revolves around one basic principle. That is that all things in the universe are linked to one another. The fortune and destiny of an individual is linked to some cosmic design and is highly influenced by it. The life of a person is, in fact, the incarnation of the soul and reflects the greater whole inside the body of which he or she is a part. This is the crux of Jyotisha Shastra

Positive and Negative Traits of 12 Zodiac Signs

Rashi – Zodiac is a twelve-fold division of the Sun's apparent path along the ecliptic. Twelve segments of the sky have been given names and certain constellations are associated with each. The constellations form imaginary figures which are associated with special influences flowing through their area. An understanding of these influences is derived from the characteristics suggested by these signs of the Rashis. Positive and Negative traits of 12 Zodiac Signs or Rashi according to Vedic Astrology. The traits of the zodiac signs are merely suggestive and have influences on one's character and personality in many ways.

Mesha Rashi – Aries

Positive traits: People under *Aries Rashi,* are ambitious, courageous, and vigilant for self-respect. They shape their own destiny by dint of struggle and hard work. They are straightforward, generous and lovers of freedom. They are practical at work and work for welfare in many areas of the social fabric.

Negative Traits: They have the weakness of exaggerating things. Often short-sighted in their approach, they are inclined to lose patience too fast. They may speak falsehood for the sake of selfish motives. Lack of self-control and headstrong tendencies are likely. They enjoy the personal glory. But tend to dominate others.

Vrisha Rashi – Taurus

Positive traits: People under *Taurus Rashi*, have regulated habits and possess remarkable tolerance power. They are devotees of respectable people and are obedient to their parents. They acquire riches and develop good qualities. They love to travel and have an aptitude for the purchase and selection of things. They have a worry-free nature. They feel happy in every situation to which they adapt themselves easily.

Negative Traits: They are inclined to be egotistical and domineering. They much prefer actions to settle to allowing things to settle on their own. They tend to get angry quickly.

Mithun Rashi – Gemini

Positive traits: People under *Gemini Rashi,* have an effective personality, depicting their intelligence, judicious, and humane nature. Their nature is versatile, imaginative, pleasant, thoughtful, and adaptable. They are generally soft-spoken, with the good power of oration. They are learned people with good command of the language.

Negative Traits: They are short-tempered but cool down quite easily. They lack concentration and quick decisions. They should not give themselves up to petty strife. They should give up curious traits hastening others Advice.

Kark Rashi – Cancer

Positive traits: People under *Cancer Rashi,* are of a fertile imagination, sentimental, and sympathetic. They have strong emotional nature and are romantic. They are secretive, impressionable, and magnetic. They have a deep interest in traveling. They have a secret and concealing nature. They can master many languages.

Negative Traits: They hover over details which often kill their time. They have eyes for little things this way they un-notice happy moments that pass by them. Their temper is changeable which needs to be corrected.

Simha Rashi – Leo

Positive traits: The people born under *Leo Rashi* have a kingly personality, magnanimity, and lion-hearted nature. They always forgive others and forget the mistakes, sins, and errors of others, Very independent in their views, have excellent organizing powers, they are constructive, inventive, magnanimous, and ingenious. They possess a magnetic personality.

Negative Traits: Leo has argumentative nature. Altercations and actions in them annoy their superiors. They should not be hasty and get irritated. They should avoid forcing their desires and opinions on others. They should remain more detached from their feelings.

Kanya Rashi – Virgo

Positive traits: People under *Virgo Rashi,* are very practical. They are chaste, pure, and refined. Sociable and friendly in nature, they show up occasional shyness also. Well informed and scholarly personality. They show interest in the occult and ancient sciences. They have a strong sense of justice.

Negative Traits: They are worrisome and sometimes perceived to be fussy. Fussing over others can sometimes be harmful. They should learn to let others make their own decisions. It is very difficult to make them content.

Tula Rashi – Libra

Positive traits: People under *Libra Rashi,* are affectionate, kind, generous, and compassionate. Since the Rashi is symbolic of balance, equilibrium and justice are its keynotes. Weighing both sides of every problem is in their character. They have a slightly detached temperament and gentle manners. They are interested in gaining knowledge and tend to be eloquent. They have a spiritual bend of mind and remain God-fearing.

Negative Traits: They should control their emotional nature. They should not be extravagant, be decisive, and avoid copying mannerisms from others. Being of liberal nature, they should develop the habit of forgiving others.

Vrischika Rashi – Scorpio

Positive traits: People under *Scorpio Rashi* are quick, keen, shrewd, critical of penetrating the mind, and keen judgment. They are self-reliant, bold, and of fixed views having this fixed sign. They cannot remain idle while facing obstacles and hindrances. They are at their best talents and never surrender but fight to the last end.

Negative Traits: They lose their temper quickly and get irritated. They are cunning but very true, loyal, faithful, and reliable. But in case others misbehave or become unfaithful etc. they become revengeful, relentless, and selfish. Revengeful nature must be avoided. They should learn to be patient and wait for the results of their efforts.

Dhanus Rashi – Sagittarius

Positive traits: People under this *Sagittarius Rashi*, are very friendly and cheerful in nature. They are of deep thinking and of high intellect. They show great interest in outdoor sports. They are quite independent in nature. These people can handle men and matter very well. They are good-humored. They are frank, fearless, demonstrative, outspoken, nervously energetic, ambitious, sincere, and quick.

Negative Traits: Exaggerating things without truth, false promises, insulting, or hurting others are their basic traits of Sagittarius people. They have inconsiderate behavior at times. They have the nature of disturbing others in an unnecessary way and they change their opinion often which needs correction.

Makara Rashi – Capricorn

Positive traits: People under *Capricorn Rashi,* have deep common sense. Their aspirations are very high, from a humble beginning they rise to greater heights. Adamant by nature, persons of Makara Rasi will not be inclined to take advice from others. They are calculative and business-minded persons.

Negative Traits: Capricorn born people keep suspecting others and mistrust others. They should be more careful not to indulge in sinful deeds which will affect their mental peace. They should not overwork and exert too much but also take rest to maintain their health.

Kumbha Rashi – Aquarius

Positive traits: People under *Aquarius Rashi*, are serious, quiet, thoughtful, and of contemplative nature. They are generally idealistic. The materialistic property of these people is linked to their spiritual nature. They are very social but very choosy about friends. They do all the things which are morally right. They have their own individuality and specialty.

Negative Traits: If Aquarius lacks spirituality, they are bound to become self-centered. The native will be lazy and lethargic, and hence they should cultivate activity, promptness, etc. They should avoid solitude. They should not be worried, become gloomy, and pessimistic.

Meena Rashi – Pisces

Positive traits: People under *Pisces Rashi* are a strong, kind, loving, truthful, and sympathetic nature. They are philosophical and lead a romantic life. They are quick in understanding. They are inspirational, versatile, and easy-going. They have great love and affection towards their friends and relatives. They have more compassion and desire to help others who suffer.

Negative Traits: They have fluctuating moods. At times they are over anxious and become disheartened, indecisive, and lacking in life and energy. They should avoid suspicious nature and varying moods

Gemstones according to Vedic Astrology — Rashi Ratna

Gemstones, also known as a Ratnas are believed to have powers that may influence one's life when they wear it as a ring or in the neck chain. These Ratnas are stones that have a profound impact on human life and destiny. However, the selection of suitable gemstones according to Rashi is important; else it is believed that negative energy may be produced against the individual who wears the wrong stone. And wearing the accurate gemstone according to one's Horoscope will have positive effects on their life.

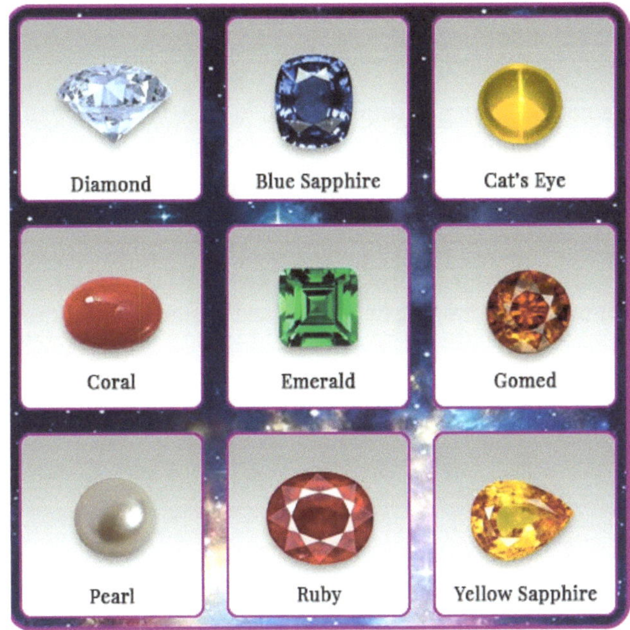

Fig. 37.2 *Illustration showing various Gemstones used in Astrology*

Vedic astrology suggests that we should wear gemstones according to our Rashi to dispel tide over troubles. Wearing the gemstone as per Horoscope speeds up the fructification of the good results promised in a birth chart of a person. If one wants good results in a particular area of life, we may wear favourable stones as per our relevant divisional chart.

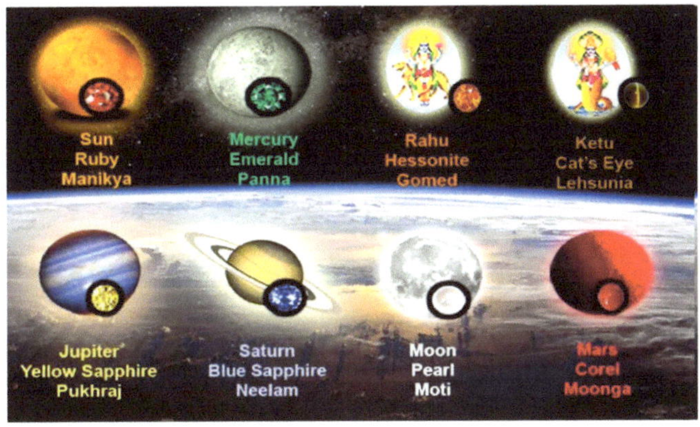

Fig. 37.3: *Gemstones based on Horoscope*

1. Mesha Rashi – Aries

The appropriate gemstones for Aries are *Ruby, Diamond, and Onyx*. These stones reduce the evil effects of Kuja Dosha. The suitable time for wearing it is Tuesday. Coral is also beneficial to the person belonging to this Rashi. The metal to be used is either copper or silver. After the ring is made, it has to be cleaned with pure milk.

2. Vrisha Rashi – Taurus

Persons belonging to Taurus Rashi have to wear *Diamond and their sub gemstone is Opel.* The colour of the Diamond is white and very shining. It reduces the evil effects of Sukra. They will possess financial and domestic happiness after wearing stones. The suitable day for wearing the ring is Friday. The gem has to be purified with milk and the ring has to be made of gold metal only.

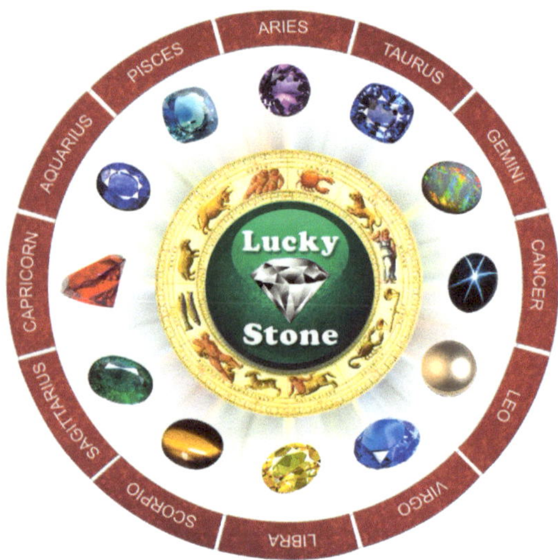

Fig. 37.4. *Gemstones according to various Rashies*

3. Mithun Rashi – Gemini

The major gemstone for Gemini Rashi is *Emerald and sub gems are Firoz and Onyx.* The gem is greenish in colour. It reduces the negative effects of Budh. It helps for the development of business, peace of mind and guards the health. The suitable day for wearing the Gem is Wednesday at the time of sunrise. Before wearing, the stone has to be purified with milk and water and it should be made of gold metal only.

4. Kark – Cancer

The person belonging to *Cancer Rashi* has to mainly wear *Pearl* as its major gemstone. It is white in colour. It reduces the negative effects of Chandra Graha. It produces peace of mind and controls mental tension. The pearl has to be purified with pure milk and the ring has to be made of silver only. The suitable day for wearing the ring is Monday at the time of sunrise.

5. Simha – Leo

Ruby is the prime gemstone of Leo Rashi. It reduces the negative effects of Ravi Graha Dasa. It produces financial gain from father and safeguards the health of the natives' father. It produces good health. Ruby after purifying with milk and pure water, the Gem has to be made of the ring with silver metal only and has to be worn on the ring finger on Sunday at sunrise time.

6. Kanya – Virgo

People of Virgo Rashi have to wear genuine *Green Sapphire* and their sub gems are Emerald or Nix. The colour of the stone is green. It reduces the negative effects of Budha and develops financial improvement and guards' health. The Gem before making into the ring has to be purified with milk and water and the best metal is gold. The suitable day for wearing the ring is Wednesday at Sunrise time to the little finger.

7. Tula – Libra

The key gemstone for Libra Rashi is *Diamond* and sub Gem is Opel. As it is white in colour, it reduces the negative effects of Sukra Graha Dasha. It invokes good health and immense wealth. The diamond has to be purified with milk and water and the ring has to be made of gold metal only. The suitable day for wearing the gem is Friday at the time of Sunrise.

8. Vrischika – Scorpio

Coral is the right gemstone for Scorpio Rashi, which is of reddish in colour and the sub gem is Loc Onyx. It reduces Kuja Dasa. It drives away any negative vibrations that may come to the wearer. The *Coral* has to be purified with milk and water and the ring has to be made of silver. The best day for wearing the gem is Tuesday at the sunrise time and one should wear it to ring finger only.

9. Dhanush – Sagittarius

People of Sagittarius Rashi should wear *Yellow Sapphire* and their sub gem is *Topaz.* It is in yellow color. It reduces the Guru Graha Dasa and helps the wearer to increase finance and good progress in education. The gem has to be purified with milk and the ring has to be made of gold metal only. The suitable day for wearing the gem is Thursday early hours to the pointing finger only.

10. Makara – Capricorn

Blue Sapphire is the major gemstone for Capricorn Rashi and the sub gem is *Blue Spinal*. It reduces the Saturn negative effects and guards' health and wealth and increases longevity. The gem has to be purified with milk and water and the best metal for making the ring is silver. The best day for wearing the ring is Saturday sunrise time and to be worn on the left-hand second finger.

11. Kumbha – Aquarius

People belonging to this Aquarius Rashi should go for *Turquoise and Cats eye*. Turquoise is sea blue in colour and Cat's eye is greyish in colour. It overall helps to dispel the negativity bestowed by the adverse planetary transits, get rid of negatives thoughts, evil eye and improve finical crisis and help from common diseases. The gem has to be purified with milk and water and the best metal for making the ring is silver. The best day for wearing the ring is Saturday sunrise time and to be worn on the left hand in the second finger.

12. Meena – Pisces

As per Jyotish Shastra, *Yellow Sapphire* is the most important gemstone for Meena Rashi. Their sub gems are Topaz or Citrine. It is in yellow colour. It reduces the negative effects of Guru Graha Dasa. It usually increases well in business, education and spiritual affairs. The gem has to be purified with milk and water and the metal to be used to make a ring is only gold. The suitable day for wearing the gemstones is Thursday at Sunrise time and it should be worn on point finger.

The 4 Elements of Astrology — Fire, Water, Earth & Air Signs

Astrology is vast as it holds not only the 12 zodiac signs or rashis but also the four elements or tattvas. The four elements in astrology are Agni (fire), Jal (water), Prithvi (earth), and Vayu (air). These elements are the building blocks of a cosmos, and each of them possesses unique qualities and forces (energy). The four elements of Astrology, govern the three zodiac signs each. And, 12 zodiacs are classified under these elements based on the qualities they depict. Astrological elements represent the feminine and muscular features of a zodiac. Like water and earth, signs represent femininity, whereas air and fire signs signify masculinity. Altogether, water, air, earth, and fire are known as the elemental signs of astrology.

Knowing the elements ruling on a zodiac allows one to fully understand one's true nature. Also, one can analyze the compatibility of a particular element with another when establishing a relationship. The appearance of elements in an astrological birth chart helps to figure out one's personality and behavior.

The Elements of Astrology

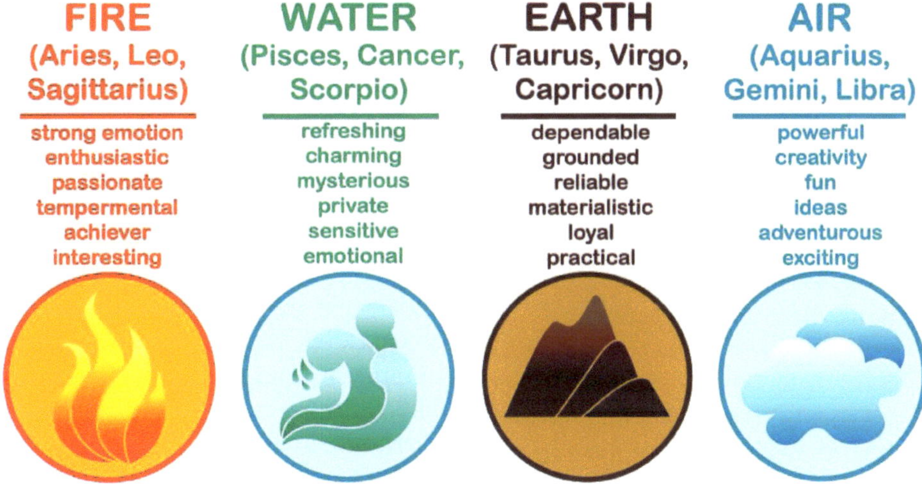

Fig. 37.5: *Illustration showing four elements of Astrology*

An In-Depth Explanation of How Earth's Elements Affect Each and Every One of Us Every element has three modalities – cardinal, mutable, and fixed. These four life forces of the cosmos help to describe the 12 zodiacs they ruled on. Here's a detailed explanation of zodiac elements with their functions and signs they rule.

Did you know that Astrology correlates to the four seasons? Each sign corresponds to the four elements, and lasts three months in each element. Each of these three-month-long seasons consists of a beginning, a middle, and an end. You probably already know your zodiac sun sign, but do you know which element dominates your personality?

What is a Quality / Modality?

A quality assigns the signs into quadruplicities. A *quadruplicity* simply means a group of four. In astrological terms this often means the groups of cardinal, fixed and mutable signs, each being a group of four signs. For example, the four signs : Aries, Cancer, Libra and Capricorn equals the cardinal quadruplicity.

- **Cardinal:** associated with initiation, creativity and Leadership. They are the 1st (Aries), 4th (Cancer), 7th (Libra) and 10th (Capricorn).
- **Fixed:** associated with the stabilisation, determination and persistence. They are the 2nd (Taurus), 5th (Leo), 8th (Scorpio), and 11th (Aquarius) signs.
- **Mutable:** associated with adaptability, self providing and expansion. They are the 3rd (Gemini), 6th (Virgo), 9th (Sagittarius), and 12th (Pisces).

What is an element?

Seeing the world in terms of elements is a tradition that dates back many generations and spread out through many different cultures. Each element represents a basic principle of life. The elements that appear in your chart represents our underlying qualities, "the stuff we are made of." The universe is made up of four elements : fire, earth, air, and water. The zodiac divides the signs into four elements of nature relevant for our deeper understanding. Western Astrology uses four elements, while Eastern Chinese Astrology and Feng Shui, on the other hand, work with five elements.

- Fire signs are Aries, Leo and Sagittarius
- Air signs are Aquarius, Gemini, and Libra
- Water signs are Pisces, Cancer and Scorpio
- Earth signs are Taurus, Virgo and Capricorn

The Meaning of Each Element

The 12 zodiac signs are coupled into four groups of four elements, which make up the existence and form of the world.

Fire: energy and passion, bossy... Known for having a desire for life, the will to be and become. Tends to be spontaneous, enthusiastic and impulsive. *Fire* can "burn itself out" if it lacks a practical outlet for its high voltage energy. If expressed negatively, there is an over expression of outward self expression without considering others feelings resulting in egotism and selfishness. Inspire is lacking in someone's chart to cultivate courage passion and self confidence.

Air: thoughtful and smart... Represents the mind and communication. Tends to be the net workers of the zodiac, often connecting with diverse people, sharing new ideas and information. Typically intellectual, objective and socially inclined. Bringing the gift of detachment and perspective, having the ability to detach and step back from a situation and weigh the good and the bad, while seeing it from all angles with neutrality. If expressing negatively, there's a tendency of becoming cold and aloof. When are lacks in someone's chart, they are forced to develop another person's perspective and learn the ability to think logically.

Water: emotional and intuitive... Known for representing the realm of emotions. Extremely sensitive to the environment and are the feelers of the zodiac. in touch with not only their deep feelings, but with everyone else's and may even be psychic. Typically nurturing, compassionate, intuitive and resourceful. If expressed negatively they absorb other people's emotions point of feeling overwhelmed. Those who lacks water in their chart may have a hard time accessing their emotions and be insensitive to others feelings.

Earth: well-grounded and practical... Known for having their feet planted firmly and being the builders and producers of the zodiac, with an innate gift of bringing dreams into reality. The what are the structures and systems to establish comfort and security. If expressed negatively an unbalanced Earth signs will lean towards fear, materialism, stagnation, greed, and over indulgence. those who lack Earth in their chart may have to work harder in order to bring their ideas into their reality.

Water Signs

Water Signs has a heart as deep as an ocean. People born under the water signs are known for their emotions. They understand and analyze things and connects to people on a deep level. Unlike other elements, water signs believe in intuition, thus makes them more into spiritual aspects. The three zodiacs that fall under the water signs are Cancer, Scorpio, and Pisces. Each one of the zodiacs in water signs possesses specific traits. But the qualities that bring them together are empathy and sensitivity. Water sign has a great potential to become an extraordinary artist as they have extensive power of imagination.

Cancer is a cardinal, Scorpio is a fixed, and Pisces is a mutable sign in Water signs. Cancer is all about caring and nurturing loved ones whereas, Scorpio understands things at a much deeper level. Finally, Pisces are the most artistic and one of the most empathetic zodiacs in astrology.

Earth Signs

When it comes to being realistic and practical, Earth signs outshine other elements. People having earth as an element in their zodiac birth chart are grounded and lives in a materialistic world. Earth signs are the builders in astrology as they prefer to do work that is needed and complete with excellent stability and honesty. The Earth signs' zodiacs are Taurus, Virgo, and Capricorn. The attributes that link all the zodiacs in earth signs are their down-to-earth, hardworking and pragmatic nature. They believe in doing things that make sense rather than doing in emotion, pressure, and overthinking. Capricorn is a cardinal sign, Virgo is a mutable sign, and Taurus is a fixed sign. Taurus is one of the most dependable zodiacs and believes in stability and patience. Virgo is the logical reasoner and presumed to be practical and sensible. Lastly, Capricorn is independent, laborious, and has faith in old traditions, making them very conservative.

Air Signs

Air signs zodiac are winds of changes, trends, and communication. The element air deals with analytical reasoning, ideas, information, actions, and socialization. Air signs take a systematic and critical approach to analyze situations and make decisions based on that rather than emotions. Gemini, Libra, and Aquarius are the zodiac of air signs. All of the zodiacs in air signs have a great sense of communicating and thinking. They can analyze problems from every perspective and come to the conclusion that offers justice. Libra is a cardinal sign, Gemini is a mutable sign, and Aquarius is a fixed sign. Gemini is the most versatile as it can adapt to new circumstances. Libra believes in justice, communication, and taking action. Aquarius is all about being original and visionary. Besides, Aquarius has an extraordinary sense of examining situations or problems from a long distance.

Fire Signs

The fire element is an energy of creation, devotion, confidence, and fierce. Individuals born under the fire element are very passionate, brave, optimistic, and always ready to take action. Fire can be impulsive sometimes, which may lead them to difficult situations. Aries, Leo, and Sagittarius belong to fire signs. They let their passion drive them rather than emotions and thoughts. In Fire signs, Aries is a cardinal sign, Sagittarius is a mutable sign, and Leo is a fixed sign. Aries, ruled by Mars – the god of war, ultimately makes it courageous and risk-takers. Sagittarius possesses the qualities like independence, kind and brilliant. Leo has the personality of liberality, self-confidence, willpower, and leadership.

Elements Compatibility

Air with other elements

Air signs can make an excellent connection to all elements to some extent. They can be benefitted from Air signs traits like critical and logical thinking, socialization, and adaptability.

Fire with other elements

Fire signs can teach other elements to be more fierce, confident, and optimistic. In return, fire signs can inherit traits like artistic, creativity, flexibility, and honesty from the air, water, and earth signs.

Water with other elements

Water signs make a great match to the earth signs. As water signs can add some emotions and artistic quality to them, the earth can teach water signs to be more practical and grounded. Water signs are incompatible with Fire signs. There will be a clash of emotions between water and fire signs as both are the opposite. Water signs can have a partial connection to Air signs as both have different approaches for analyzing situations. Air makes decisions based on logic, whereas water makes on emotions.

Earth with other elements

Earth signs make a perfect match with water signs as both of them balance each other very well. With Air and Fire, Earth signs make a good bond. Air signs provide ideas while Earth signs execute them practically. Fire signs can teach Earth signs to take risks and do things with a fierce attitude, while Earth signs provide groundedness and patience to Fire signs.

Birth Element by Month

Earth Element

- 20th April to 20th May (Taurus)
- 23rd August to 22nd September (Virgo)
- 22nd December to 19th January (Capricorn)

Water Element

- 22nd June to 22nd July (Cancer)
- 23rd October to 21st November (Scorpio)
- 19th February to 20th March (Pisces)

Fire Element

- 21st March to 19th April (Aries)
- 21st July to 22nd August (Leo)
- 22nd November to 21st December (Sagittarius)

Air Element

- 21th May to 21st June (Gemini)
- 23rd September to 23rd October (Libra)
- 20th January to 18th February (Aquarius)

Astrological benefits of Gemstones

Astrological benefits of Gemstones. Gems and precious stones contain healing energies that can be activated by wearing them as ornaments, such as rings or necklaces, or by placing them in water overnight and drinking the water the following day. Gems enliven the vital energy centers in the body (the chakras) and have a direct influence on vats, pitta, and kapha. They may be used to pacify or activate specific organs of the body, or to enhance or neutralize the effects of particular planets in the person's astrological birth chart. Before we go into the effects of specific gems and stones, here are a few important general points.

- Gems tend to absorb the qualities and energy vibrations of their owners. It is beneficial to purify any stone before using it. Soaking it for two days in saltwater or milk should be sufficient. This will not harm the stone.
- When you wear a gemstone, it should touch the skin through a small window in the setting, so that the subtle energies of the stone can interact directly with the energies of the body.

Ayurveda generally recommends that rings be worn on the right hand, though in the West, if someone wants to wear their wedding ring on the left hand to conform with tradition, that is all right.

- Processed or chemically treated stones may not have the same healing energy. It is best to get authentic, unprocessed, clean stones without a flaw or crack. When you are considering buying a stone be sure to use a magnifying glass to examine it for cracks or imperfections.
- Unless you are knowledgeable both in stones and in Vedic astrology (jyotish), it is wise to consult an expert before investing in a stone. The wrong gem for you, or one worn on the wrong part of the body, can have a negative influence. Here are some of the characteristics of main gems and stones.

Ruby: Astrologically, the ruby represents the sun. It is a life-protecting stone that promotes longevity, especially for vata and kapha individuals, and brings prosperity. This gem strengthens concentration and bestows mental power. It also strengthens the heart. Rubies pacify vats and kapha but may elevate pitta. Garnets have the same vibration as rubies; they are the poor man's ruby. Wear both Rubies and garnets either in a ring on the ring finger, or in a necklace

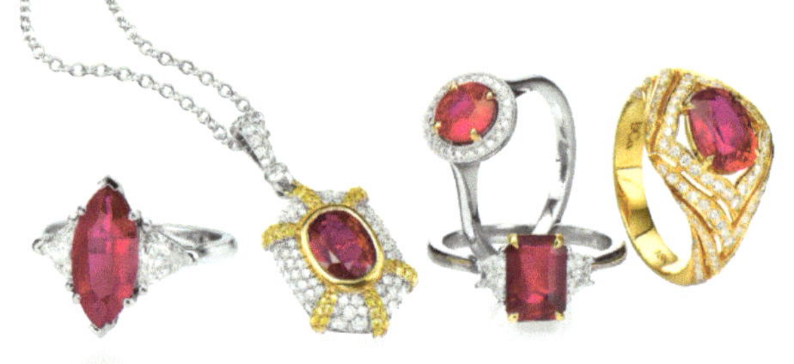

Fig. 37.6: *Showing physical feature of Ruby and its application in different ornaments*

Pearl: As rubies represent the sun, pearls symbolize the moon. They have a cooling effect and a calming, healing vibration. Pearls are balancing to all the doshas, though their cooling action is particularly good for pitta. Pearls confer mental peace and tranquillity. Pearl ash is used internally to effectively treat many ailments. You can gain many of the strengthening effects of pearls by making pearl water. Place 4 or 5 pearls in a glass of water; let it stand overnight, and drink the water in the morning.

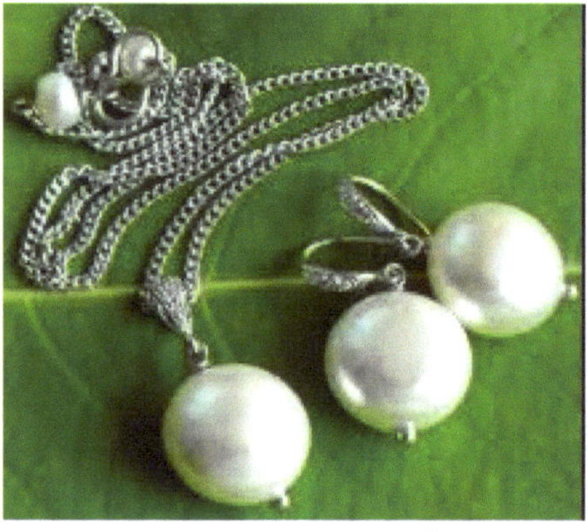

Fig. 37.7: *Showing physical feature of Pearl and its application in a ornament*

Yellow Sapphire: This precious stone, which represents Jupiter, brings groundedness, stability, and wisdom. It helps to calm both vata and pitta and may slightly increase kapha qualities. It strengthens the heart and also builds lung and kidney energy. Yellow sapphire should always be worn on the index finger, the finger of Jupiter. Yellow topaz, the poor man's sapphire, has many of the same qualities and produces similar benefits.

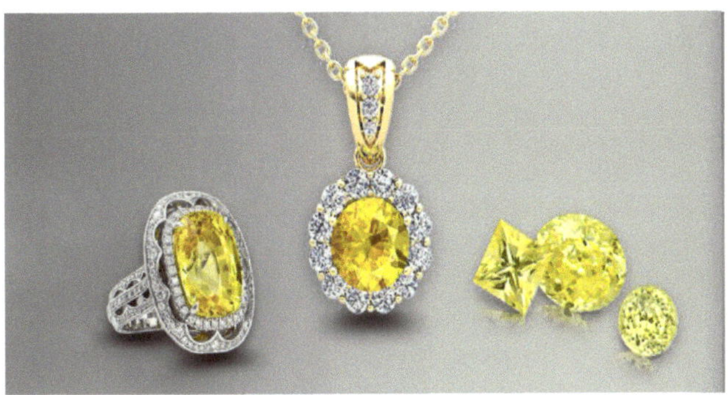

Fig. 37.8: *Showing physical feature of Yellow sapphire and its application in different ornaments*

Blue Sapphire: This beautiful precious stone represents Saturn and brings the benefits of that very spiritual planet. Saturn, a deity of earth and iron, confers enlightenment. Blue sapphire calms vata and kapha and may stimulate pitta. it builds up muscles and the skeletal system and helps to heal arthritis. Wear blue sapphire on the right middle finger, preferably in a silver setting. Do not wear it with diamonds; this will create disharmony.

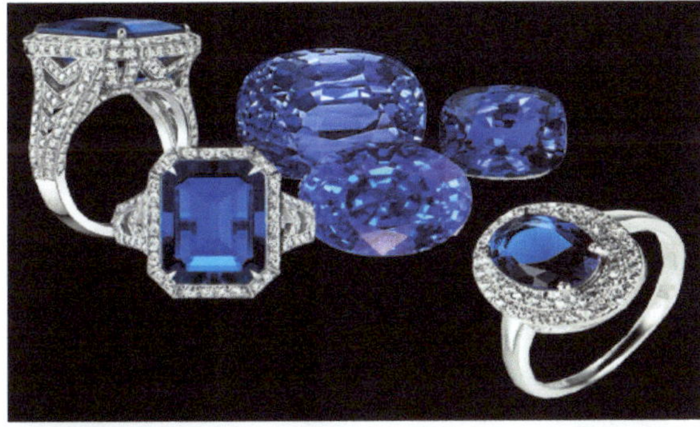

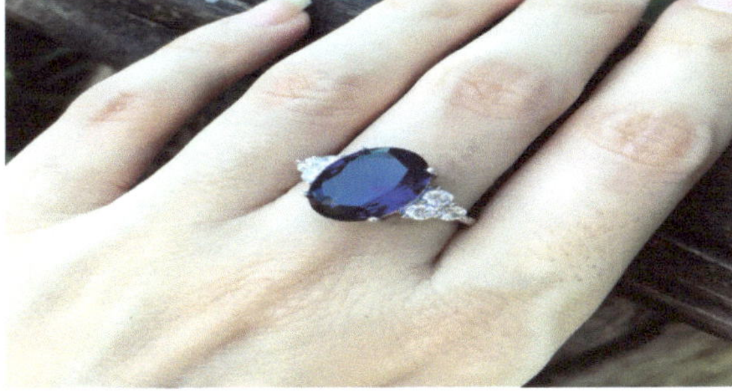

Fig. 37.9: *Showing physical feature of blue sapphire(top) and its application in different ornaments(bottom)*

Emerald: This powerful precious stone brings prosperity and spiritual awakening. It calms vata and pitta, settles the nervous system, and relieves nervousness. Symbolic of the planet Mercury, emeralds improve writing skills, enhance the power of speech, and promote intelligence. They are best set in gold and worn on the little finger.

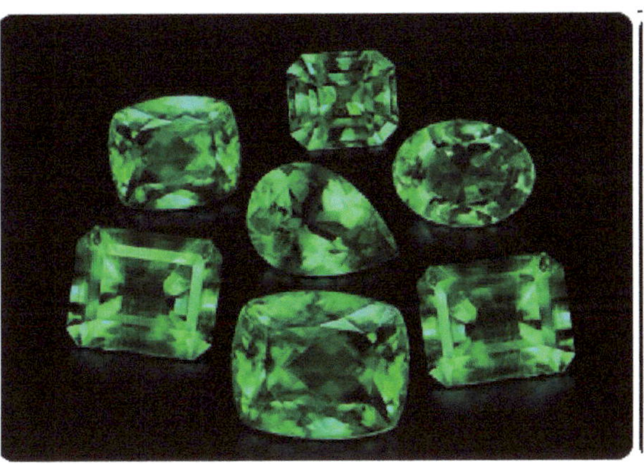

Fig. 37.10: *Showing physical feature of Emeralds*

White Sapphire: This powerful gemstone combates premature aging, enhances the span of life, and strengthens immunity. Its energy brings subtle energy vibrations to the heart, brain, and deeper bodily tissues. It is the best stone for rejuvenation. It brings prosperity and is spiritually uplifting. Symbolic of the planet Venus, white sapphire actually do help to create a close bond in relationships and are rightfully associated with marriage. These stones stimulate shukra, the body's reproductive tissue. Art, music, romance, and sex all go together with this stone. Wear your white sapphire set in silver, either as a pendant or as a ring on the ring finger. But note : white sapphire of low quality may have negative effects upon the body. One should also pray to lord Venus chant Mantra "*Om Shun Shukraye Namah*" 108 times to attain best results.

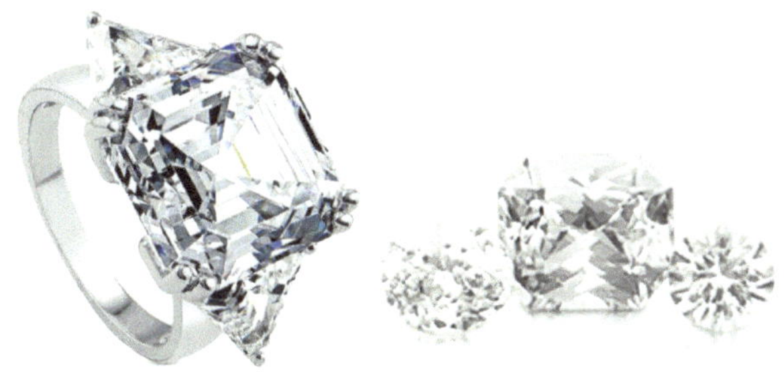

Fig. 37.11: *Showing physical feature of white sapphire and its application in different ornamental sets*

Cat's -Eye: This stone is good for allergies, repeated colds and congestion and allergic asthma. It pacifies kapha and vata while slightly increasing pitta. It aids in healing kidney dysfunction. Cat's-eye enhances awareness and helps a person not get caught up in emotions. People working in psychological healing should wear this stone in a gold setting on their ring or little finger; it will help protect them from negative influences.

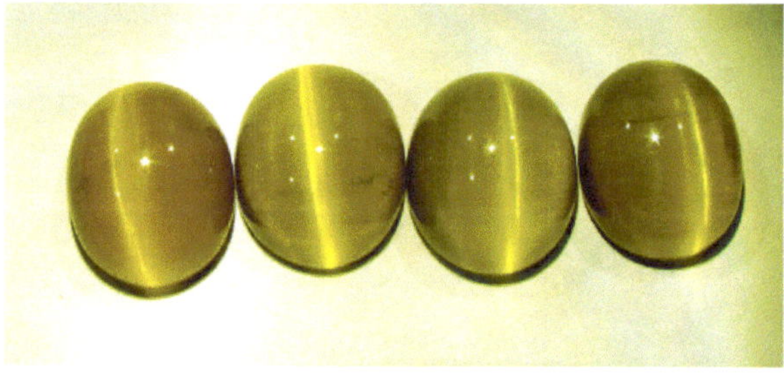

Fig. 37.12 *Showing physical feature of Cat's-eye*

Opal: This semiprecious stone represents the planet Neptune. It strengthens majja dhatu (bone marrow and nerves) as well as shukra dhatu (reproductive tissue). It improves vision, relieves fever, calms pitta, and is good for migraine headaches. Opals enhance spiritual feelings, increase devotion, and help to unfold intuition. This gem is particularly beneficial for individuals with Neptune in their third, fourth, sixth, tenth, or twelfth astrological house. It should be set in gold or silver and worn on the ring finger.

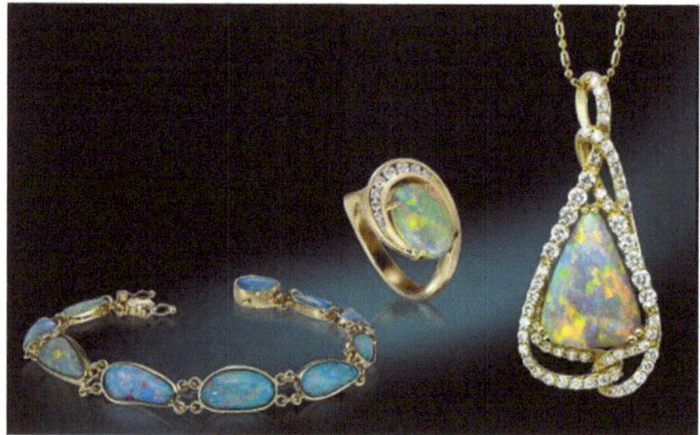

Fig. 37.13:*Showing physical feature of Opal and its application in different ornamental sets*

Amethyst: Amethyst is a stone for the crown chakra and is good for mental clarity. To bring prosperity, it should be set in gold. You can also wear it around the neck on a gold necklace. A person with neuromuscular weakness can be helped by wearing amethysts and by putting them at the four corners of the bed. Some amethysts have a darker color, which gives them a Saturn-like energy similar to blue sapphire. Amethysts bestow dignity, love, compassion, and hope. This gem helps the individual to control emotions and is good for vata and pitta imbalance.

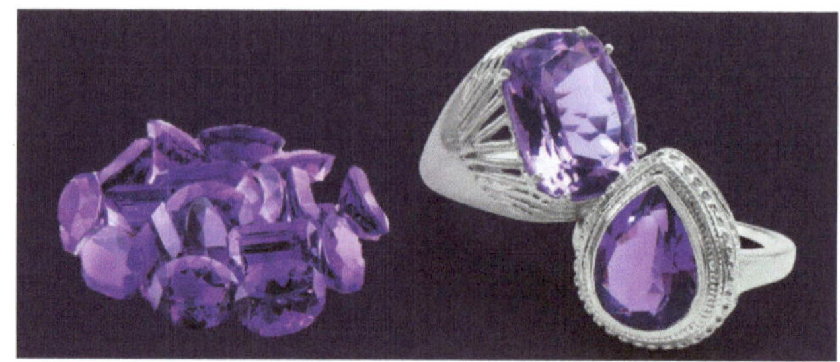

Fig. 37.14: *Showing physical feature of Amethyst and its application in ornamental set*

Aquamarine: A substitute for emerald, which symbolizes Mercury, aquamarine reduces dullness of mind, promotes happiness and intelligence, enhances the power of speech, and improves memory. This stone also has Venus-like qualities; it is good for married couples to wear aquamarine to enhance love in their relation-ship. Aquamarine should be set in silver and worn on the little finger. Remember that in all these cases, simply wearing the correct stone is not enough to take care of a doshic imbalance; you need to watch your diet, meditate, do appropriate exercise and yoga postures, and consciously and conscientiously look after your day-to-day and moment-to-moment health.

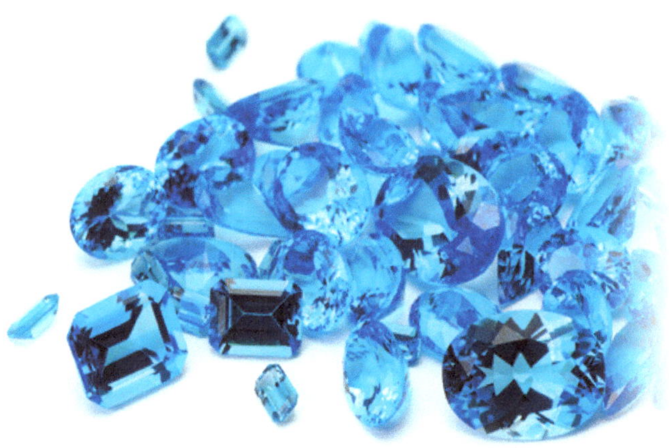

Fig. 37.15: *Showing physical feature of Aquamarine*

Red Coral: This gemstone from the sea represents the planet Mars. It calms pitta and helps one to control anger, hatred, and jealousy. Coral gives energy to the liver, spleen, and pericardium. Wear your red coral as a necklace or as a ring set in copper (preferably), silver, or white gold and worn on the ring finger. Red coral is strength-giving and imparts gracefulness.

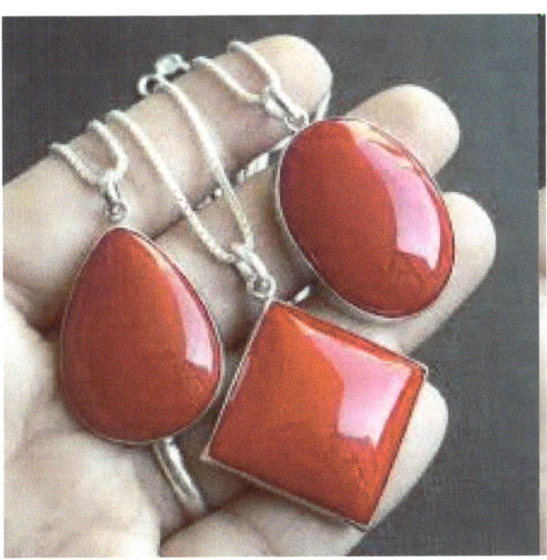

Fig.37.16:*Showing physical feature of Red coral in different shapes and sizes according to its use in ornamental sets*

Lapis Lazuli: This stone, which has Saturn-like energy, is heavenly and sacred. It gives strength to the body, mind, and consciousness, and it sensitizes the wearer to higher spiritual vibrations. It strengthens the eyes, calms vata and pitta, and is helpful for anxiety, fear, and weakness of the heart. It is also good for the liver and for skin diseases. Lapis Lazuli should be set in gold and worn on the little finger, or worn as a necklace.

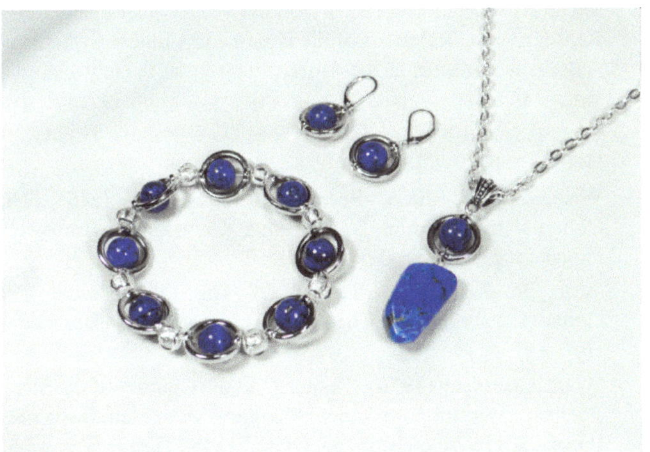

Fig. 37.17: *Showing physical feature of Lapis Lazuli and its application in different ornamental sets*

Bibliography and Acknowledgement

- Artificial treatment of gemstones. Dictionary of Gems and Gemology. Berlin, Heidelberg: Springer Berlin Heidelberg. 2009. pp. 50. doi:10.1007/978-3-540-72816-0_1308. ISBN 9783540727958.
- A complete guide to Gemstones". Jewellery Monthly. 2015-04-02. Archived from the original on 2017-08-28.
- Alden, Nancy (2009). Simply Gemstones: Designs for Creating Beaded Gemstone Jewelry. New York, NY: Random House. p. 136. ISBN 978-0-307-45135-4.
- AskOxford.com Concise Oxford English dictionary online. [full citation needed]
- Barton, Tamsyn (1994). Ancient Astrology. Routledge. ISBN 978-0-415-11029-7.
- Bauer, Max (1968). Precious Stones. Dover Publications. p. 2. ISBN 9780486219103.
- Burgess, Ebenezer (1866). "On the Origin of the Lunar Division of the Zodiac represented in the Nakshatra System of the Hindus". *Journal of the American Oriental Society*.
- Burnham, S.M. (1868). Precious Stones in Nature, Art and Literature. Bradlee Whidden. Page 251 URL: Helen of Troy and star corundum Archived 2010-10-13 at the Wayback Machine
- Campion, Nicholas (1982). An Introduction to the History of Astrology. ISCWA.
- Chandra, Satish (2002). "Religion and State in India and Search for Rationality". Social Scientist
- Church, A.H. (1905). "Definition of Precious Stones". Precious Stones considered in their scientific and artistic relations. His Majesty's Stationery Office, Wyman & Sons. p. 11. Archived from the original on 2007-09-29 – via Farlang.com.
- Desirable diamonds: The world's most famous gem. by Sarah Todd.[full citation needed]
- Frangoulis, George (18 April 2015). GEM HUNTER. Lulu. com. ISBN 9781329075634.[self-published source]
- Gemstone. Lexico. Oxford University Press.
- New process promises bigger, better diamond crystals. Carnegie Institution for Science. Archived from the original on 1 December 2010. Retrieved 7 January 2011.
- Padparadscha Sapphires: 10 Tips On Judging The Rare Gem. The Natural Sapphire Company Blog. 2015-04-06. Retrieved 2018-01-19.
- Rapaport report of ICA Gemstone Conference in Dubai. Diamonds.net. 2007-05-16. Archived from the original on 2011-07-26. Retrieved 2010-07-30.
- Tanzanite heating – the science. Archived from the original on 20 June 2016.
- The Gem and Jewelry Institute of Thailand (Public Organization). Bangkok Post.
- Fleet, John F. (1911). "Hindu Chronology". In Chisholm, Hugh (ed.). Encyclopædia Britannica. 13 (11th ed.). Cambridge University Press. pp. 491–501.
- Folkard, Claire; Freshfield, Jackie; Masson, Carla; Dimery, Rob (12 December 2017). Guinness World Records 2005. Guinness World Records Limited. ISBN 9780851121925.
- Frawley, David (2000). Astrology of the Seers: A Guide to Vedic (Hindu) Astrology. Twin Lakes Wisconsin: Lotus Press. ISBN 0-914955-89-6
- Frawley, David (2005). Ayurvedic Astrology: Self-Healing Through the Stars. Twin Lakes Wisconsin: Lotus Press. ISBN 0-940985-88-8

- Gemstone Enhancement: History, Science and State of the Art by Kurt Nassau
- Hainschwang, Thomas; Notari, Franck; Massi, Laurent; Armbruster, Thomas; Rondeau, Benjamin; Fritsch, Emmanuel; Nagashima, Mariko (Summer 2010). "Hibonite: A New Gem Mineral" (PDF). Gems & Gemology. 46 (2): 135–138. doi:10.5741/GEMS.46.2.135.
- Holden, James Herschel (2006). A History of Horoscopic Astrology (2nd ed.). AFA. ISBN 978-0-86690-463-6.
- Jain, Sanat K. "Astrology a science or myth", New Delhi, Atlasntic Publishers 2005 - highlighting how every principle like sign lord, aspect, friendship-enmity, exalted-debilitated, Mool trikon, dasha, Rahu-Ketu, etc. were framed on the basis of the ancient concept that Sun is nearer than the Moon from the Earth, etc.
- Jewelers' circular-keystone: JCK. Chilton Company. 1994.[full citation needed]
- Katz, Michael (2005). Gemstone Energy Medicine: Healing Body, Mind and Spirit. Natural Healing Press. ISBN 9780924700248. Retrieved 2020-04-06.
- Kay, Richard (1994). Dante's Christian Astrology. Middle Ages Series. University of Pennsylvania Press.
- Kraus, Pansy D. (2007). Introduction to Lapidary. Krause Publications. ISBN 9780801972669.
- Long, A.A. (2005). "6: Astrology: arguments pro and contra". In Barnes, Jonathan; Brunschwig, J. (eds.). Science and Speculation. Studies in Hellenistic theory and practice. Cambridge University Press. pp. 165–191.
- Wayback Machine
- Most Precious Stones". HowStuffWorks.com. 2009-11-09. Archived from the original on 2014-11-06.
- Maurice Winternitz (1963). History of Indian Literature, Volume 1. Motilal Banarsidass. ISBN 978-81-208-0056-4.
- Nassau, Kurt (1994). Gem Enhancements. Butterworth Heineman.
- Parker, Derek; Parker, Julia (1983). A history of astrology. Deutsch. ISBN 978-0-233-97576-4.
- Pingree, David (1963). "Astronomy and Astrology in India and Iran". Isis – *Journal of The History of Science Society*. pp. 229–246.
- Pingree, David (1973). "The Mesopotamian Origin of Early Indian Mathematical Astronomy". Journal for the History of Astronomy. SAGE. 4 (1): 1–12. Bibcode:1973JHA.....4....1P. doi:10.1177/002182867300400102. S2CID 125228353.
- Pingree, David (1981). Jyotiḥśāstra in J. Gonda (ed.) A History of Indian Literature. Vol VI. Fasc 4. Wiesbaden: Otto Harrassowitz.
- Pingree, David (1981). Jyotihśāstra : Astral and Mathematical Literature. Otto Harrassowitz. ISBN 978-3447021654.
- Pingree, David and Gilbert, Robert (2008). "Astrology; Astrology In India; Astrology in modern times". Encyclopædia Britannica. online ed.
- Plofker, Kim (2009). Mathematics in India. Princeton University Press. ISBN 978-0-691-12067-6.
- Plofker, Kim. (2008). "South Asian mathematics; The role of astronomy and astrology". Encyclopædia Britannica, online ed.
- Raman, BV (1992). Planetary Influences on Human Affairs. South Asian Books. ISBN 978-8185273907.
- Robbins, Frank E., ed. (1940). Ptolemy Tetrabiblos. Harvard University Press (Loeb Classical Library). ISBN 978-0-674-99479-9.
- Secrets of the Gem Trade; The Connoisseur's Guide to Precious Gemstones, Richard W Wise, Brunswick House Press, Lenox, Massachusetts., 2003
- Sutton, Komilla (1999). The Essentials of Vedic Astrology. The Wessex Astrologer, Ltd.: Great Britain. ISBN 1902405064
- Tester, S. J. (1999). A History of Western Astrology. Boydell & Brewer.
- Vargas, Glenn; Vargas, Martha (2002). Faceting For Amateurs. ISBN 9780917646096.
- Veenstra, J.R. (1997). Magic and Divination at the Courts of Burgundy and France: Text and Context of Laurens Pignon's "Contre les Devineurs" (1411). Brill. ISBN 978-90-04-10925-4.
- Wedel, Theodore Otto (1920). The Medieval Attitude Toward Astrology: Particularly in England. Yale University Press.
- Whitney, William D. (1866). "On the Views of Biot and Weber Respecting the Relations of the Hindu and Chinese Systems of Asterisms", Journal of the American Oriental Society
- Wise, R. W., 2006, Secrets Of The Gem Trade, The Connoisseur's Guide To Precious Gemstones, Brunswick House Pr, pp. 3–8 ISBN 0-9728223-8-0
- Wise, R. W., 2006, Secrets of The Gem Trade, The Connoisseur's Guide To Precious Gemstones, Brunswick House Pr, p.36 ISBN 0-9728223-8-0
- Wise, R. W., 2006, Secrets Of The Gem Trade, The Connoisseur's Guide To Precious Gemstones, Brunswick House Pr, p. 15
- Wood, Chauncey (1970). Chaucer and the Country of the Stars: Poetical Uses of Astrological Imagery. Princeton University Press. ISBN 9780691061726. OCLC 1148223228.
- Yukio Ohashi (1993). "Development of Astronomical Observations in Vedic and post-Vedic India". Indian Journal of History of Science. 28 (3).
- Yukio Ohashi (1999). Johannes Andersen (ed.). Highlights of Astronomy, Volume 11B. Springer Science. ISBN 978-0-7923-5556-4.

Rudraksha In Health Wellness Including Cardiovascular Ailments

Rudraksha is a seed of the Elaeocarpus ganitrus tree, and it not only plays a significant role in a spiritual seeker's life, but it has proven scientific benefits of wearing this bead. Rudra that is another name for Lord Shiva, and Aksha that means teardrops. Hence, *Rudraksha* means tears of Lord Shiva. Legends are that the origin of this bead is the eyes of Lord Shiva in the form of tears, which landed on earth and formed the tree.

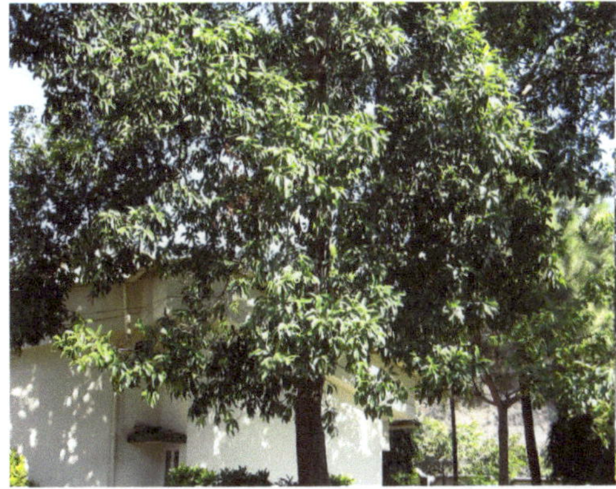

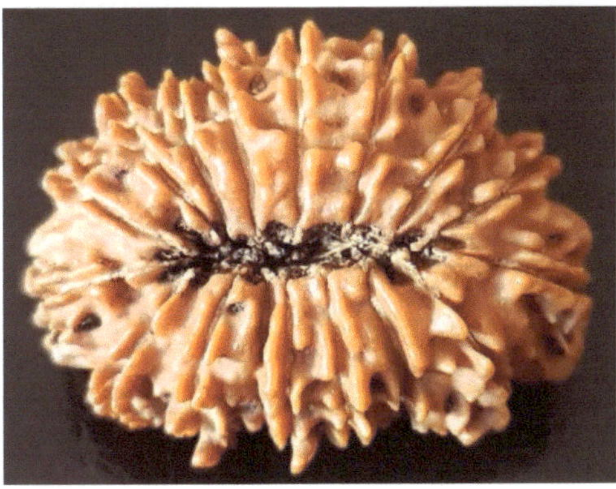

Fig.38.1: *showing Rudraksha tree (top) and features of 17 mukhi Rudraksha (bottom)*

Rudraksha tree grows mostly in the Himalayan regions of India, Nepal, Java, Sumatra, Myanmar, and Indonesia. Though, you can find different types of Rudraksha beads growing. The number of faces or mukh in a Rudraksha bead depends on the vertical rows seen rolling down on the surface. These rows are known as Mukhi or in other words the clefts or furrows on the surface. This different Mukhi Rudraksha usually ranges between 1 and 21 faces. Though there are some rare types of Rudraksha with more than 22 clefts, and their properties are yet unknown. On the other hand, 1 to 14 Mukhi Rudraksha is common.

Why did Shiva weep?

Some say that Shiva shed tears of ecstasy during meditation and these tears sprouted into the rudraksha trees when they touched the ground. Others believe that Shiva opened his eyes after several years of mediation and saw humanity suffering. Tears of compassion welled up in the divine eyes and wherever these tears fell, there budded the Rudraksha trees. Still, others maintain that these are tears of unimaginable grief, shed when Sati, Shiva's beloved consort, was consumed in the ceremonial fire. Another story links the tears of Shiva to the intense meditation he undertook to destroy three demons, the *Tripurasuras.* These demons lived in three floating Purams or cities and were protected by a boon from Brahma. They could only be destroyed when their cities came into a single axis, which happened once in a thousand years. Shiva destroyed the demons and liberated them with a single arrow. May be it was the intense concentration with which he focussed as he readied himself to aim at the cities that his half-closed eyes (Ardha Nimeelita neetra) watered and that created the rudraksha. Ecstasy, compassion, grief or destruction for liberation, whatever be the cause of those tears, the rudraksha is considered to be imbued with energies that are physically curative and spiritually uplifting. It has a special place in Indian mythology. People wear it as a necklace, a bracelet, as earrings, use it like a rosary or *japamala* to count their prayers or just treasure the fact that they own one.

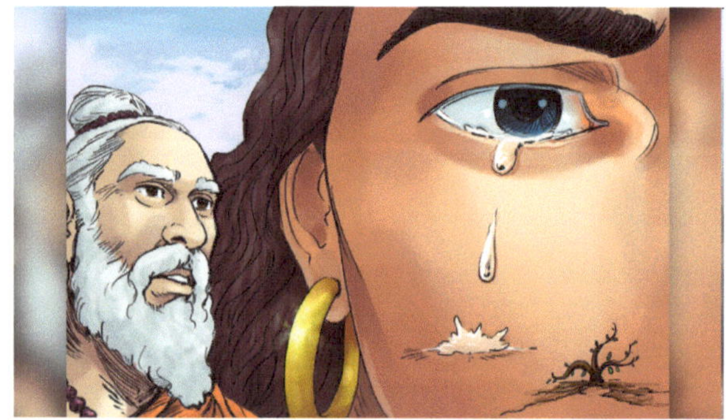

Fig. 38.2: *Illustration showing tears flowing through the eyes of Lord Shiva*

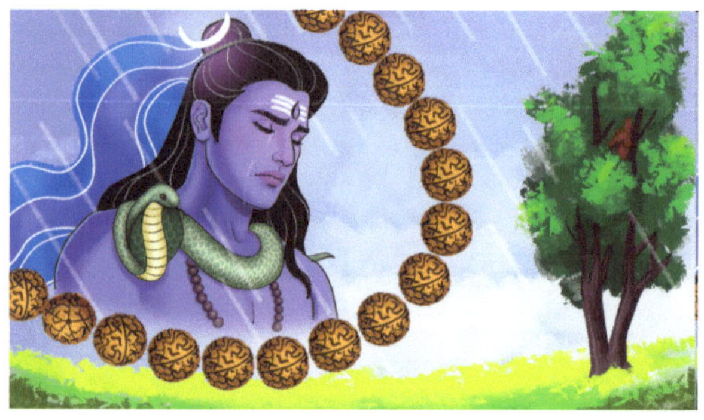

Fig. 38.3: *The teares of Lord Shiva attained the shape of a tree which later produced Rudraksha seeds.*

Biomedical/Biological Properties of Rudraksha

The beneficial powers of Rudraksha are by virtue of its Electrical and Magnetic Biological Properties

1. Electric Biological Properties

Rudraksha beads act as dielectric (i.e.) as a storage of electrical energy. This property of Rudraksha makes it capable in stabilizing and anchoring the *Bioelectric current*. The values are measured in units of Farad. This property is very helpful in controlling hyperactivity, palpitations of heart, streamlining heartbeat etc. Due to stress when there is increased physical activity heart beats faster and the overall activity of hormones and nervous system increases. This causes increased energy levels or increase in potential difference. As a result of this the magnitude of the Bioelectric Current increases.

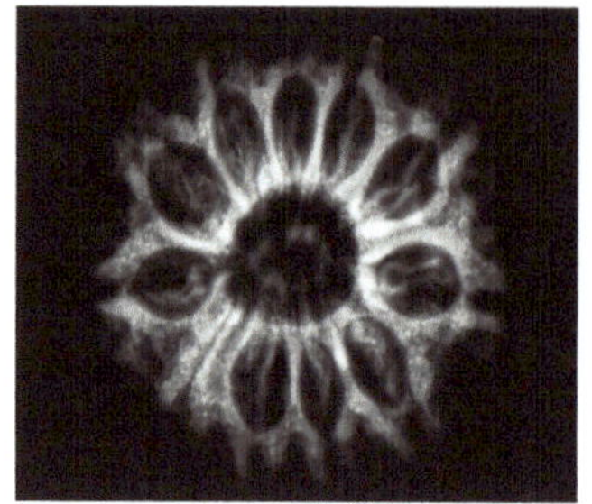

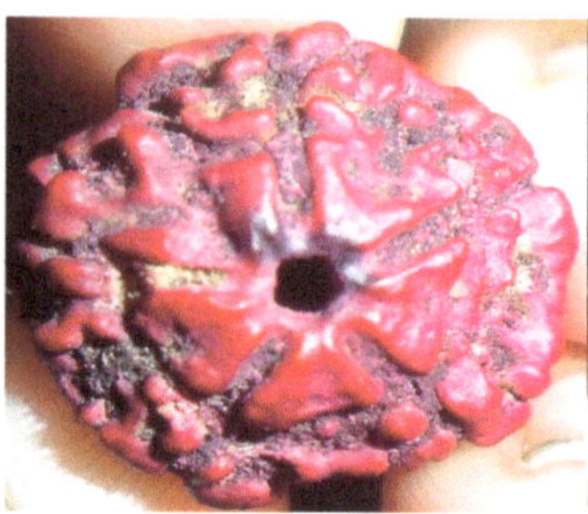

Fig. 38.4: *(left) X-ray of 10 mukhi Rudraksha reveals 10 seeds storing chambers and one central chamber(Right)) showing colored features of panch mukhi Rudraksha*

Rudraksha beads acting as Dielectric stores this excess Bioelectric Energy, thereby streamlining the overall activity to Normalcy. There is a third element to the Body and Brain that is Bio Electronic circuit Interface, that of the mind. Any activity that can produce stress or maladjustment can throw the streamlined activity, the Electronic circuit of the Body & Mind out of gear. Human beings and all living beings are prone to stress continuously in the continuous fight for survival and prosperity and resistance. Rudraksha beads of particular Mukhis or Facets have a definitive Factor of Resistance. It is measured in Ohms.

When these beads resist the flow of bioelectrical impulses to a specific or a particular brain chemical, thereby by effecting specific positive changes in personality. It is well proven that the state of mind and our personality is governed almost completely by the Brain; it's functioning and that of Central Nervous System. There is continuous and subtle flow of bioelectrical signal throughout the body due to potential difference between parts of the Body. When these beads resist the flow of bioelectrical impulses a specific ampere of current flow is generated depending on the factor of resistance. This acts in tandem with heartbeat, streamlining it and sending out specific impulses to brain. These impulses stimulate certain positive brain chemicals. Making us feel better, more confidents, poised and more energetic.

2. Capacitance or the Dielectric Biological Properties

Rudraksha beads act as dielectric (i.e.) as a storage of electrical energy. This property of Rudraksha makes it capable in stabilizing and anchoring the Bioelectric current. The values are measured in units of Farad. This property is very helpful in controlling hyperactivity, palpitations of heart, streamlining heartbeat etc. Due to stress when there is increased physical activity heart beats faster and the overall activity of hormones and nervous system increases. This causes increased energy levels or increase in potential difference. As a result of this the magnitude of the Bioelectric Current increases and Rudraksha beads act as *Dielect.* In modern age with intense competition the Stress levels have increased tremendously. Almost every individual has problems of Stress and Stress related ailments like insomnia, alcoholism, depression, Maladjustments, heart diseases, skin diseases etc. Any Doctor will confirm that almost 95% of the ailments are Psychosomatic or Stress related (i.e.) originating from Mind. When there is Stress or Maladjustment corresponding Stress signals are sent to the Central Nervous systems, there is an increased activity or abnormality of Neurons and Neuro transmitters. The magnitude of change will depend on the cause and specific case. When such a thing occurs and it occurs continuously, streamlined flow of electrical signals throughout the Mind-Body interface is disrupted and it makes us feel uncomfortable and we are not able to act with our full efficiency. Our Blood circulation becomes Non-ideal and we feel various illnesses. Unfortunately this happens all the time. As long as the flow of Bioelectricity is smooth the body functions normally and we have the feeling of being in control. As long as the flow of Bioelectricity is smooth the body functions normally and we have the feeling of being in control

3. Inductance

Rudraksha beads by it have permanent magnetic biological properties. They have been observed to send out Inductive vibrations with frequencies measured in units of Henry (Volt Seconds/Ampere). This perhaps is the reason why people have felt better even when Rudraksha beads do not touch them physically.

Magnetic biological properties: Rudraksha beads have both paramagnetic and diamagnetic with the most important property of dynamic polarity. We all are most probably aware of the beneficial healing biological properties of magnets. Magnetic healing is becoming extremely popular off late and everyone who have been using magnets for healing have been getting the benefits and found overall betterment and rejuvenation. Rudraksha beads retain most of the biological properties of magnets but it is unparallel in one aspect, that of the ability to change it's polarity or the property of dynamic polarity. The basic way of healing is based on the fact that when the passage of arteries and veins which carry blood to and from heart to all the parts of the body is blocked or reduced due to variety of reasons, various illnesses creep. Blood carries oxygen and energy to various parts of the body and cleanses it off waste materials. Any disruption of the smooth flow of blood circulation is bound to cause illnesses. As long as the flow of Bioelectricity is smooth the body functions normally and we have the feeling of being in control.

4. Rudraksha beads act as a Stabilizing Anchor

Every one experiences pain and uneasiness due to improper blood circulation. Every cell in the blood as well as the Arteries and veins are charged either positively or negatively. Magnets have the poles Positive (+) and Negative (-). When magnets are passed on various parts of the body the opposite poles of the magnets and that of cells get attracted and there is an expansion of the passage .The Arteries and veins open up to facilitate streamlined blood circulation. When there is a streamlining of blood circulation most of the illnesses get automatically healed and we feel better and rejuvenated But with magnets the polarity is fixed. When magnets are brought near a particular part of the body it opens up only those sections of veins and arteries where there is a matching of polarities hence complete healing and streamlining of blood circulation cannot be ensured. We experience healing and feel better but we can still go much further with dynamic polarity of Rudraksha beads. Rudraksha has the ability to Change its polarity-The property of dynamic polarity. This in turn is by virtue of its property, diamagnetism. *Diamagnetism* is termed as the ability of any material to acquire temporary magnetic property in presence of an external magnetic field. The polarity of the charge induced is opposite to that of the external field inducing the charge. Blood circulation and heart beat automatically induces a magnetic field around the body and particularly the heart Region. Bioelectricity automatically gives raise to biomagnetism Depending on the polarity of the Induced magnetic field. Rudraksha bead acquires a polarity that is opposite of the inducing field. As a result of this the opening up the passages of Arteries and Veins are far better than that of magnets. Much better healing and rejuvenation is experienced.

Various Literatures mention of powerful anti ageing biological properties of Rudraksha beads This is mainly because of the Dynamic Polarity of the Rudraksha bead thus the healing powers of Rudraksha are far superior to that of Magnets. In some sense Rudraksha beads can be termed to have some additional life or Intelligence as against Magnets The wearer of Rudraksha not only makes Lord Shiva happy but pleases Lord Brahma and Lord Vishnu, Ganesh, Kaartikey, Durga, Indra, Aditya and the ruling deities of the nine planets. No men, seers and scholars are tired of describing the importance of

Rudraksha. Rudraksha is very much dear to Lord Shiva. No body can imagine the image of Lord Shiva without Rudraksha. Seeing, chanting and worshipping Rudraksha burns all the sins to ashes. A man can feel unlimited pleasure only by seeing Rudraksha. The wishers of devotion and salvation should wear it after purifying themselves. Mainly the devotees of *Lord Shiva* must wear it because it removes their numerous pains, sorrows, and calamities. Rudraksha fulfills all the wishes. It is the dearest ornament to Lord Shiva. If an innocent,un devoted and immoral man wears Rudraksha with love and faith, he gets rid of all sins and attains the supreme goal. As long as a man keeps wearing Rudraksha, he does not fear untimely death. He cannot die without completing his span of life. At the time of death he gets the true knowledge of Lord Shivaand His abode too. One should wear Rudraksha by all bits of efforts. Rudraksha Beads have been worn by mankind for thousands of years for good health, religious attainment through Japa and Shakti (power) and for the fearless life

Dos and Don'ts of wearing any Rudraksha

- After buying ten Mukhi Rudraksha bead wash it with clean fresh water and dip it in the cow's milk for one day before wearing.
- Worship it every day.
- Always keep trust on it.
- Don't flaunt ten Mukhi Rudraksha bead to anyone.
- Don't wear a broken bead.
- Don't give your bead to anyone.
- Don't use chemical soap after wearing it.
- Don't eat non-veg food after wearing it.
- Don't drink alcohol after wearing it.
- Don't go any dead or childbirth house wearing it.
- Remove it before going to funeral service.
- Don't do any Sex with wearing it.
- Remove it before sleeping and place it where you worship God.

Chemical Formation of Rudraksha

Natural *Rudraksha beads* are plant product that contains Carbon, Oxygen, Hydrogen, Nitrogen, and other trace elements in a fused form. The gaseous elements are present in the proportion : 50.031% Carbon, 30.53% Oxygen, 17.897% Hydrogen, 0.95% Nitrogen. Other components present in lesser quantities are Aluminum, Chlorine, Copper, Calcium, Nickel, Iron, Cobalt, Manganese, Phosphorous, Sodium, Potassium, Zinc, Magnesium, and Silicon Oxide. A Rudraksha bead takes around 15 to 16 years to mature.

Types of Rudraksha Beads & Benefits

With the advancement of modern science, we can find various pieces of research that support the ancient belief of the importance of Rudraksha. Hinduism, especially Shaivism, and Buddhism recognize these beads for their divine power and how they play a significant role in practicing spiritualism. But there is a concern that we often come across, can rudraksha be worn by anyone? Yes, there is no restriction in wearing or keeping Rudraksha. Anyone of any religion, creed, caste, nationality, or gender can wear Rudraksha to attain excellent physical and spiritual benefits. Every type of rudraksha has a different purpose, and it's better being aware of rudraksha how much Mukhi and all their distinct properties. Wearing the wrong sort of Rudraksha bead can upset one's life.

How Does Rudraksha Work?

In this modern era, the constant shift regarding lifestyle choices has created various mental and physical issues. Diseases like angina, high blood pressure, migraine, diabetes, stress, hypertension, and other psychological problems are affecting the well-being of individuals. To fit definite social norms, one takes up a temporary refugee in smoking, consuming alcohol, drugs, etc. Eventually manifesting the body with harmful chemicals and lower life expectancy. Our ancient scriptures have uplifting and fascinating remedies for naturally removing such toxic physical-mental-emotional imbalances. Rudraksha is one such way. It is a sacred seed of the tree Rudraksha which has unique properties that aid in wholesome effect. These Rudraksha beads come in a variety of faces, mainly in 1 to 21 Mukhi Rudraksha, which has tremendous power that can eliminate any imbalances from one's life and bring divine grace. Each *Rudraksha Mukhi* has specific benefits, but before getting hands-on with these holy beads, one must consider Rudraksha where to buy. One must at all cost buy a genuine bead because the imitated Rudraksha won't be beneficial. Remember to buy certified Rudraksha.

Health Benefits of Rudraksha

- Ayurveda considers rudraksha a great medicine. It is warm and nonacid tic as well as humid in temperament; some persons regard it cold also. It tastes bitter. It is used not only to wear on different parts of the body, but it can also be used as Oral medicine and for besmearing externally. Many doctors, Vaidyas, scientists and ascetics use it

- It destroys worms and it gives brilliancy to the body. It cures tri dosha namely Vaat (air), Pitta (bile) and cough automatically.
- Rudraksha is a good medicine for skin diseases. In leprosy of both the kinds it can be used. It effects as a medicine to cure sores, ringworm, pimples, boils and it is useful in burns also. It is also useful for women in pregnancy
- Rudraksha is the most useful for the persons having blood pressure. It does not let it go up or down. It keeps the B.P. normal. For this Rudraksha rosary should be worn so close that it should touch the heart. It is sure that its wearer can never fall prey to a sudden heart attack, shrinking of heart or brain hemorrhage.The patient of blood pressure should keep the five faced Rudraksha in water filled in a glass vessel throughout the night and should drink it as soon as he gets up in the morning. By doing so the person would have normal Blood pressure. Put a rudraksha in a copper pot filled with water at night to drink in the morning to benefit against heart troubles and constipation. It cures ulcers if applied in paste made after scrubbing in water
- The children, who are mostly sick with fever, should wear three faced Rudraksha. In Chechak (typhus) Rudraksha and black pepper having equal weight should be ground and sieved through a cloth-sieve. This powder should be drunk with stale water to cure chechak Cough is cured fully if the powder of ten faced Rudraksha is rubbed and licked with milk thrice a day.
- Hysteria, Coma, Leucorrhoea and female diseases related to genital organs can be cured bywearing 3 (three) beads of six faced Rudraksha. All the diseases relating to the mind and brain are cured by drinking milk that is boiled with four faced Rudraksha. It helps enhance the memory also. It is useful in all phlegm and wind related disorders.

How To Wear Rudraksha: Rudraksha Wearing Rules

Now can Rudraksha be worn by anyone? Yes. Anyone, irrespective of culture, gender, religion, or ethnic ground can wear Rudraksha. A person at any point or stage of life, irrespective of physical and mental condition, can wear Rudraksha, by students, children to elderly for attaining its benefits.

But why rudraksha is good and why rudraksha is powerful? You may also be wondering how does rudraksha work? Well, let's take a look:

Some desire to come out of their unwanted habits and while others want to live a pure life. Wearing this mala may find one to free and achieve what they desired off after wearing it. Rudraksha is more powerful than any ordinary Yantra, Tantra, or mantra, even gems. In general, the worshipper and wearer of Rudraksha are blessed with good health, peace, and prosperity.

Yet there are a few precautions one needs to take to avoid attempting sins such as:

- Rudraksha must be worn only after Siddhi, the method of purification with chanting Mantras.
- Rudraksha Mantra must be chanted 9 times a day while wearing it in the morning and removing it before going to bed. Can rudraksha be worn while sleeping? No, otherwise you may gain sin.
- Can rudraksha be worn while bathing - While before taking a bath, it must not be touched? One should always clean his hands properly after using the restroom.
- It must not be taken to funerals or cremation grounds and also while visiting a newborn baby.
- Can rudraksha be worn during intercourse - Never wear these holy beads while consummating a relationship.
- Can rudraksha be worn during menstruation - women shouldn't wear this bead during their cycle.

Rudraksha How To Clean

Always try to keep your Rudraksha clean. Dirt and dust can settle in the bead pores, so cleaning them as frequently as possible is necessary. If the worn thread becomes worn out or dirty, change it. After cleaning, wash the Rudraksha with holy water. It will help in maintaining its purity.

Rudraksha Where To Buy

Many get confused about where to buy authentic rudraksha. One should not worry about it. You can buy authentic beads from anyone who certified rudraksha. You have to carefully notice whether the Mukhi is well defined, the contours and corns, with no cracks near the central hole.

Rudraksha is known to possess immense power to heal all the ills and misfortunes in one's life. It is worn for good luck, good health, prosperity and spirituality.

Table:38.1 *The list of Rudraksha as per Zodiac Sign (Rashi)*

Zodiac Sign (Rashi)	Suitable Rudraksha
Aries (Mesh)	3 Mukhi
Taurus (Vrish)	6 Mukhi
Gemini (Mithun)	4 Mukhi
Cancer (Kark)	2 Mukhi
Leo (Singh)	1 Mukhi and 12 Mukhi

Virgo (Kanya)	4 Mukhi
Libra (Tula)	6 Mukhi
Scorpio (Vrishchika)	3 Mukhi
Sagittarius (Dhanu)	5 Mukhi
Capricorn (Makar)	7 Mukhi & 14 Mukhi
Aquarius (Kumbh)	7 Mukhi & 14 mukhi
Pisces (Meen)	5 Mukhi

Rudraksha for Zodiac Signs

Rudraksha For Aries Ascendant: ruled by Mars, this Three Mukhi Rudraksha is best-fitted for Aries.

Rudraksha For Taurus Ascendant: ruled by Venus, this Six Mukhi Rudraksha is suitable for Taurus.

Rudraksha For Gemini Ascendant: ruled Mercury, Gemini ascendants can get benefit from Four Mukhi Rudraksha.

Rudraksha For Cancer Ascendant: ruled by Moon, the Two Mukhi Rudraksha is beneficial and suitable for Cancerians.

Rudraksha For Leo Ascendant: ruled by Sun, Leo can benefit from One Mukhi and Barah Mukhi Rudraksha.

Rudraksha For Virgo Ascendant: ruled by Mercury, the Four Mukhi Rudraksha is profitable for Virgo.

Rudraksha For Libra Ascendant: ruled by Venus, Libras can benefit and best-suited for Six Mukhi Rudraksha and Thirteen Mukhi Rudraksha.

Rudraksha For Scorpio Ascendant: ruled by Mars, Three Mukhi Rudraksha is best-suited for Scorpions.

Rudraksha For Sagittarius Ascendant: ruled by Jupiter, Five Mukhi Rudraksha is beneficial for Sagittarians.

Rudraksha For Capricorn Ascendant: ruled by Saturn, Capricorn can benefit from Seven Mukhi and Fourteen Mukhi Rudraksha.

Rudraksha For Aquarius Ascendant: ruled by Saturn, Seven and Fourteen Mukhi Rudraksha are considered suitable for Aquarians.

Rudraksha For Pisces Ascendant: ruled by Jupiter, Pisces benefits from Five Mukhi Rudraksha.

As per Ayurveda rudraksha is known to be the powerhouse of many medicinal qualities, from treating mental health issues to heart, it is a much revered dark berry. Dr. Ranganayakulu explains the place of prayer beads in Ayurveda folklore. There are several species of trees in the Elacorpus genus, which yield Rudraksha beads. The seeds of Elacorpus genitus or E. spereacorpus are more popular as holy beads. This tree grows in the Ganges delta, sub-Himalayan terrain, and southeast Asia. These are also known as Dark Berries when they are unripe.

In what formulation of Rudraksha be used in Different Diseases?

Ayurveda considered them with dolce flavor, hot potency, and very helpful in the growth of nerve tissue, improve heart function, and overall health. It is an ingredient in several Ayurvedic medicines like *Gorochanadi Vati, Dhanvanthari gutka*, *Mruthasanjeevani gutika*, etc. Here is a list of few useful preparations with Rudraksha.

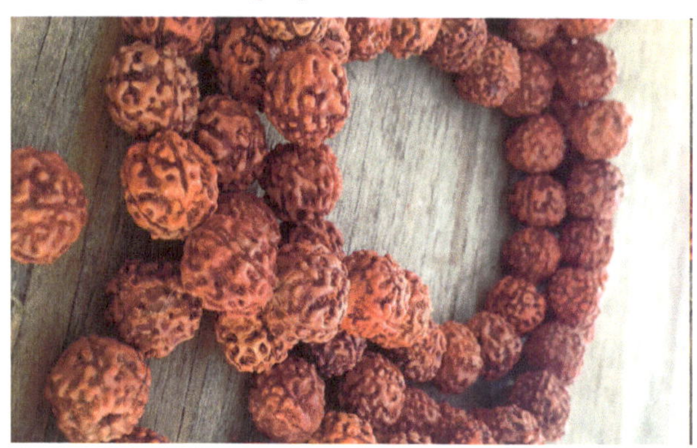

Fig. 38.5: *showing Rudraksha mala to wear it around the neck or chanting the Name of any Deity*

- Prayer bead is effective in Epilepsy – Rudraksha powder is mixed with Brahmi and administered orally.
- Boil Rudraksha in milk and drink once a day to reduce cholesterol.
- Keep a Rudraksha in rose water overnight. This liquid is useful as eye drops in eye infections.
- Wearing a Rudraksha bracelet or neck chain reduces anxiety.
- Soak Rudraksha in a copper vessel with water and drink the water in the morning. It helps reduce symptoms of diabetes.
- Rudraksha powder mixed with Indian madder (manjishta) is a good face pack.
- One part Rudraksha and three parts Shathavari ghrutha (Satavari ghee) help women to maintain good hormonal balance and reproductive health.
- Rudraksha and sandalwood combined is a good coolant.
- Regular use of rudraksha internally and externally has a positive effect as anti-aging
- Rudraksha oil can heal the symptoms of eczema, ringworm, acne, and pimples.
- Experiments on animals proved that its consumption can reduce hypertension and bronchial asthma.

Dr. Ranganayakulu further advises that all the medicines should be taken as per the ayurvedic physician's advice only.

Special Properties of Rudraksha

Rudraksha contains calcium oxalate, *gallic acid*, *tannins*, *flavonoids*, and many other molecules that scavenge free radicals and even prevent gene mutations. Owing to excellent medicinal benefits the prayer bead has made a niche in medicine and religion. Whatever that prevents gene mutations either within the cells or prevents the molecules that potentially alter the gene coding is known as gene repair molecules. Rudraksha is one of them. Rudraksha is formed by association of two words, "*Rudra*" & "*Akash" Rudra* is the name of lord Shiva. Akash means "*Tear*". It is said that the planet of Rudraksha is originated from the tear drops of lord Shiva. As per the Vedic.

- Rudraksha can nullify the effects of malefic planets to a great extent. Shastras say rudraksha of nay mukhis can never do any harm to the wearer unlike navratnas. Which have to be carefully chosen. No other necklace or bead is auspicious & powerful as rudraksha
- Rudraksha came in different mukhis or the clefts or furrows on the surface. Shastras speak of 1 to 14 mukhis rudraksha are used for astrological benefits. Each bead has a different effect on you, depending on the number of mukhis it has. Each rudraksha is very individualistic & has to be carefully matched with one's horoscope for it to be beneficial
- Tantra, Yantra, Mantra has a very important place for rudraksha. Vedas have given special weightage to rudraksha. As it is belived that rudraksha has originated from the tears of lord Shiva. Rudraksha have tremendous energy & power. Rudraksha is best known for its biomedical properties & in controlling stress, hypertension & blood pressure.
- Rudraksha chain of 108 beads or 54 beads if worn or worshiped provides all types of benefits. Therefore, it is important that Rudraksha should be always respected & keeps pure. One should not touch with dirty hands & must be removed before entering the toilets. It is blessing to mankind.
- Rudraksha one who wear on their bodies it is believed that can not be affected by sins. Even if one wear Rudraksha on his body, without doing worship & saying the sacred mantra does not get near any sinful deed or thought
- Rudraksha are worn for their specific benefits. These are much more powerful and can help to achieve wonders, if energized & empowered the write way
- Rudraksha of different mukhis pleases the corresponding planets. It may be sufficient to go in for only those mukhis who ruling planets, cause malefic effects

Amazing function of rudraksha

- **Rudraksha takes the radiance from the atmosphere and converts it into oil:** If we chant '*Om Namaha Shivaya*' sitting under a rudraksha tree, fragrant oil will emanate from a rudraksha for 24 hours. This oil will spill out if we blow into the hollow of the rudraksha. The oil of rudraksha has a pleasant odour. This oil is extracted from its tree too. Once the rudraksha is made effective, it emits air instead of oil.
- **Transformation of sound waves and light waves:** The rudraksha transforms light waves of Deities in the universe into sound waves of the human body and vice versa. As a result, man can absorb waves of Deities and human thoughts can get converted into the language of the Deities.
- **Absorbtion of sama (Sattva) waves:** The rudraksha absorbs sama (Sattva) waves. Similarly, sama waves are emitted by its crests. A real rudraksha can be recognised by the vibrations felt upon holding it. At that time, the body absorbs the sama waves emitted by the rudraksha. If a rudraksha is held between the thumb and the ring finger, vibrations will be felt anywhere in the body. Even if kept nearby, the effect of a rudraksha is felt up to half an hour. Thus, during that period we are able to perceive vibrations even if any other object is held with the fingers. However, if the hands are washed with water, the vibrations cannot be perceived.

Different Types of Rudraksha Beads and their benefits

Rudraksha is comprised of two words Rudra, which is another name for Lord Shiva, and Aksha, which means teardrops. Hence, Rudraksha means tears of Lord Shiva. It is said to have originated from the eyes of Lord Shiva in the form of tears that landed on earth and formed the Rudraksha tree. The tree grows mostly in the Himalayan regions of India, Nepal, Sumatra, Java, Myanmar, and Indonesia. However, there are different types of Rudraksha beads that grow on the tree. They are based on the vertical lines seen running down on the surface. These lines are known as Mukhi, or in other words, "*the clefts or furrows on the surface*". (For instance, if there are two vertical lines on the surface, then it is known as 2 Mukhi Rudraksha.) Each Rudraksha bead contains 50.031% carbon, 0.95% nitrogen, 17.897% hydrogen, 30.53% oxygen, and each bead takes 15 to 16 years to mature. The Rudraksha comes with different "*Mukhis*" or "*Face*", ranging from 1 to 21 Faces. Among them, 1 to 14 Mukhis are commonly found. There are different types of Rudraksha with more than 22 vertical lines, but they are extremely rare, and their properties haven't been studied yet.

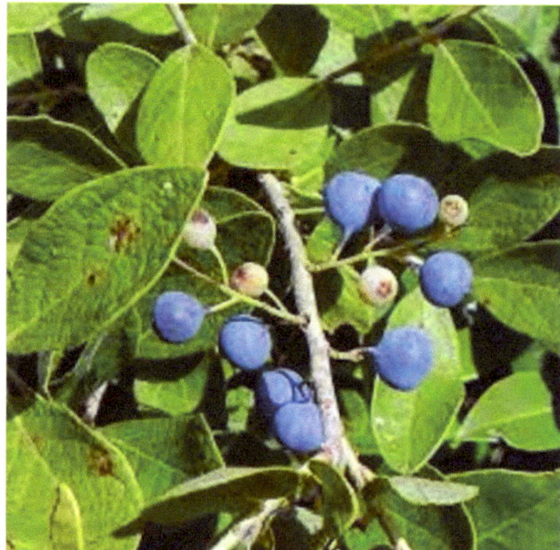

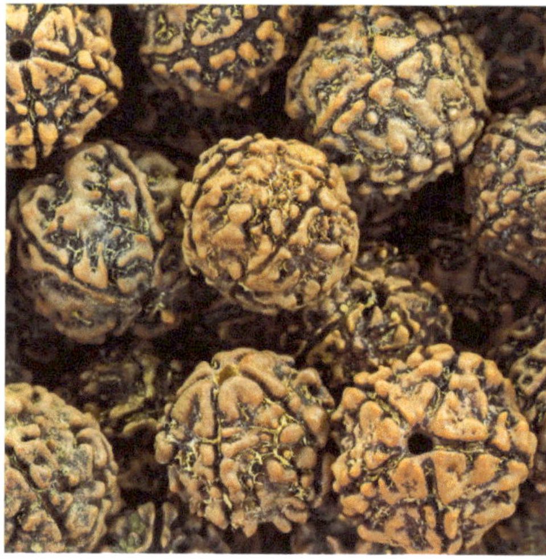

Fig. 38.6: *(top) showing Rudraksha tree (Elaeocarpus ganitrus) with leaves, ripened and unripened seeds containing typical dry Rudraksha (bottom)*

Elaeocarpus ganitrus is the scientific name of the Rudraksha tree which produces a typical seed called the "*rudraksha*". This particular tree species usually grows at a specific altitude in the mountains, especially along the Himalayan region. One can find these trees in Burma, Nepal, Thailand, India, Indonesia, etc. Many people use the different parts of the trees to make sleeper coaches for the railways. Hence, the trees are continually decreasing in number over the period. There are many varieties of Rudraksha available for different uses in the market. Many people use Rudraksha beads in the form of mala and bracelets. They use it to chant their religious hymns or use it for their varied benefits. Many online stores offer affordable elegant jewellery designs for the people who love to wear such Rudraksha mala in gold designs.

Although Rudraksha is very popular for its uses in the world, yet many people do not use it as they fail to understand the varied benefits of this fruit. Even if you do not believe in spiritual theories, you can refer to the scientific studies about Rudraksha. The scientific research shows that there are plenty of reasons as to why one should use Rudraksha for their daily life.

1 Mukhi Rudraksha

It represents the Hindu Lord Shiva, and many people consider this to be an auspicious gift of nature to humankind. The ruling planet of this Rudraksha is the Sun. This type of Rudraksha helps to increase the concentration and self-confidence in the man.

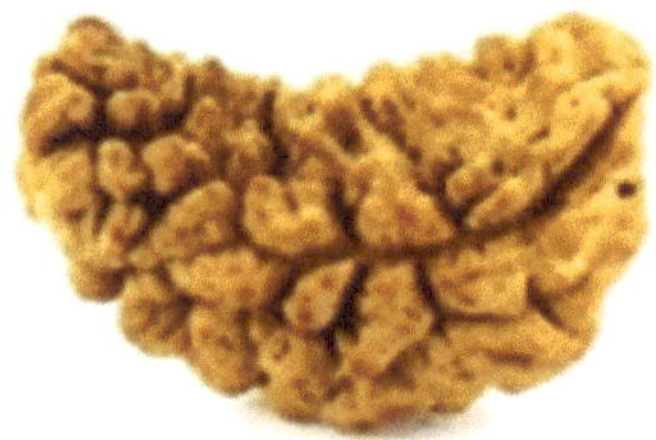

- **Ruling God:** Shiva
- **Ruling Planet:** All
- **Beeja Mantra:** || *Om Namah Shivaya* ||

Benefits of 1 Mukhi Rudraksha

- 1 *Mukhi Rudraksha* is ruled by Lord Shiva himself and is beneficial for attaining super consciousness.
- *Ek Mukhi Rudraksha* Has the capacity to destroy all sins and lead one to moksha
- Elevation of awareness towards the absolute consciousness of the divine
- Only a few selected ones who have been graced with Lord Shiva and divine karma gets to wear this rare 1 *Mukhi Rudraksha bead.*
- On a mental level, the mind shifts towards the supreme element known as *Partattva Dharana cha jayate Tatprakashnam.*
- On a physical level, 1 Mukhi Rudraksha helps to cure migraines and other mental diseases.

2 Mukhi Rudraksha

Original Rudraksha of this kind represents the union of the Hindu Gods Lord Shiva and Parvati. Two mukhi Rudraksha represents the Moon and helps the person to maintain a healthy balance between their family and professional life. In many people, this Rudraksha has been effective in curing eye diseases and other health issues.

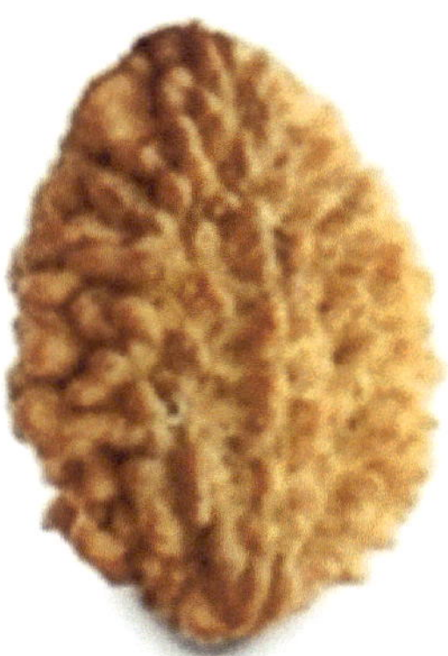

- **Ruling God:** Ardhanareshwar
- **Ruling Planet:** Moon
- **Beeja Mantra:** || Om Namah ||

Benefits of 2 Mukhi Rudraksha

- It represents two images of Shiva and Shakti. Thus, the wearer would be blessed with unity and harmony
- It symbolizes Guru-Shishya, parents-children, husband-wife relationship
- It maintains Oneness in the relationship
- On a spiritual level, it removes the negative elements of the planet moon.
- On a physical level, it cures emotional instability, releases fear, insecurity, and gives inner happiness and fulfillment.

3 Mukhi Rudraksha

The three mukhi Rudraksha symbolises the Fire God and the Trinity Gods, i.e. Lord Shiva, Lord Vishnu and Lord Brahma. The ancient history states that three mukhi Rudraksha provides relief to people suffering from stress and anxiety issues.

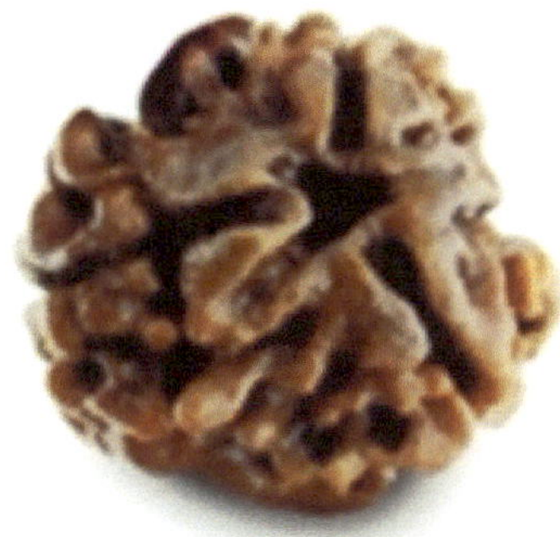

- **Ruling God:** Agni
- **Ruling Planet:** Sun
- **Beeja Mantra:** || Om Kleem Namah ||

Benefits of 3 Mukhi Rudraksha

- It symbolizes the fire god Agnidev.
- The three Mukhi Rudraksha helps a person to free himself from the bondage of past birth, the karmas related to his path and then pave the way for success based on the karma of his current life.
- The wearer of 3 Mukhi Rudraksha doesn't fall in the loop of the cycle of life; it means that he attains moksha after the current life.
- On a mental level, the wearer is uplifted from low self-esteem so that he can rise to the illuminated pure self.
- On a physical level, it heals stomach and liver ailments.

4 Mukhi Rudraksha

The four mukhi Rudraksha represents the Hindu Goddess Saraswati and and Lord Brahma. This Rudraksha helps to heal the overall body and increases the person's logical thinking.

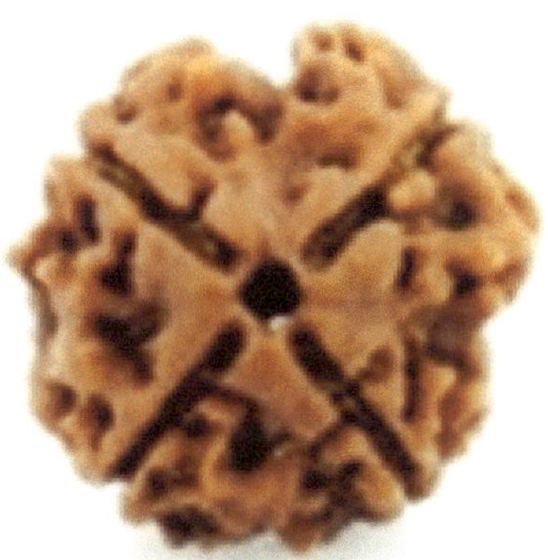

- **Ruling God:** Brihaspati
- **Ruling Planet:** Jupiter
- **Beeja Mantra:** || Om Hreem Namah ||

Benefits of 4 Mukhi Rudraksha

- 4 Mukhi Rudraksha is for those seeking the power of knowledge and creativity as wearing the rudraksha improves mental power, vocal power, wit, intelligence
- The wear of four Mukhi Rudraksha is also blessed with melodious speech.

5 Mukhi Rudraksha

This form of Rudraksha represents a unique form of Lord Shiva, Kalagni Rudra. The five mukhi Rudraksha signifies the five elements of the human body. Many people use this as a means to wash away their sins to lead a happy and pleasurable life.

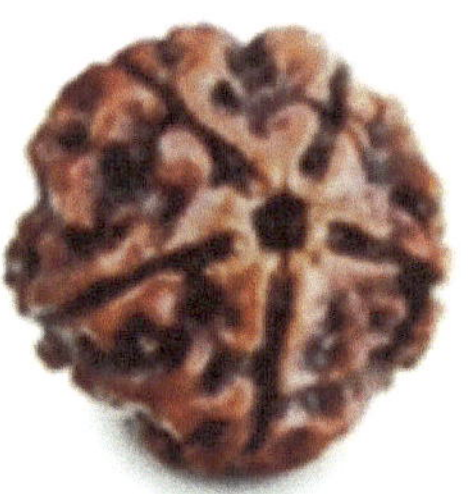

- **Ruling God:** Rudra Kalagni
- **Ruling Planet:** Jupiter
- **Beeja Mantra:** || Om Hreem Namah ||

Benefits of 5 Mukhi Rudraksha

- 5 Mukhi Rudraksha is beneficial for those seeking to find their own higher selves, UpaGuru
- Panch Mukhi Rudraksha enhances awareness, memory, word power and intellect.
- This type of Rudraksha is mostly used while chanting mantras as it helps them to connect with the grace of Shiva more easily.
- Pachmukhi Rudraksha removes the wearer from the negative energy of planet Jupiter.

6 Mukhi Rudraksha

The 6 mukhi rudraksha symbolizes the Hindu Lord Kartikeya and is also called Shatrunjaya Rudraksha. Lord Kartikeya is the son of the Hindu god Shiva according to Hindu Mythology. Many people use this Rudraksha to control their emotions like anxiety, anger, jealousy and mental excitement. This type of Rudraksha is quite beneficial in enhancing the vital aspects of the human body.

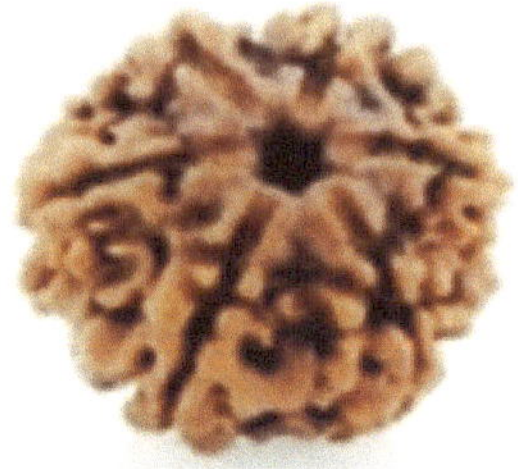

- **Ruling God:** Kartikeya
- **Ruling Planet:** Mars
- **Beeja Mantra:** || Om Hreem Hoom Namah ||

Benefits of 6 Mukhi Rudraksha

- It symbolizes stability and pacifies the planet Mars.
- The wearer is strengthened with willpower and focus as he gets free from mental lethargy, emotional instability.
- The wearer is also blessed with luck for properties and vehicles

7 Mukhi Rudraksha

According to Hindu mythology, the7 mukhi rudraksha represents the seven ages or the famous seven goddesses and “Saptrishis”. This Rudraksha is believed to protect its wearer from dangers and bestow fortune. Thereby, this particular type of Rudraksha helps to reduce the frequency of obstacles in one’s life.

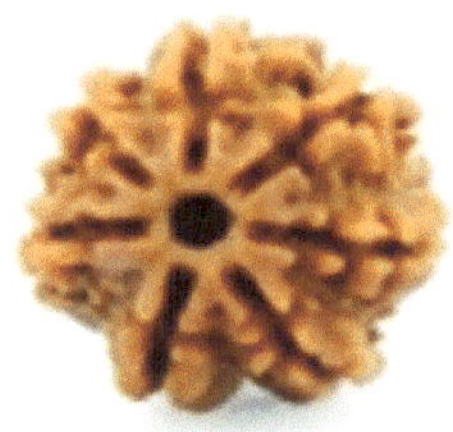

- **Ruling God:** Laxmi
- **Ruling Planets:** Venus
- **Beeja Mantra:** || Om Hoom Namah ||

Benefits of 7 Mukhi Rudraksha

- It symbolizes health, wealth, and new opportunities.
- For those suffering from financial and luck-related miseries, 7 Mukhi Rudraksha is suitable.
- The wearer progresses with name, fame, and abundance.

8 Mukhi Rudraksha

The eight mukhi Rudraksha signifies the Lord Ganesha and eight other Goddesses and hence called “ashtadeviya”. People who use this Rudraksh are able to overcome the difficulties related to spiritual, physical, or mental well-being.

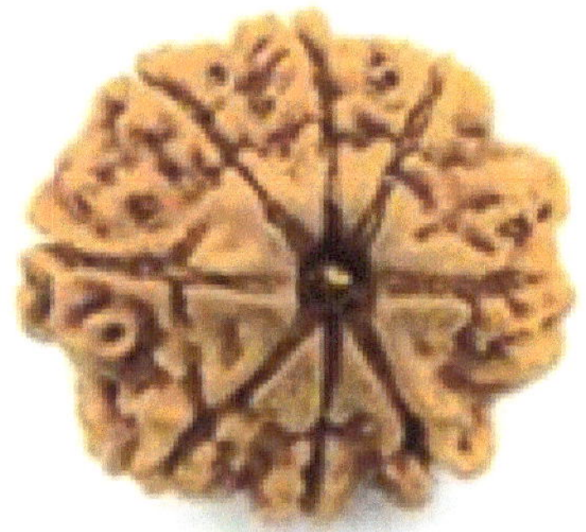

- **Ruling God:** Ganesh
- **Ruling Planets:** Ketu
- **Beeja Mantra:** || Om Hoom Namah||

Benefits of 8 Mukhi Rudraksha

- 8 Mukhi Rudraksha has the power to eliminate obstacles, evils in a person's path to success
- The person who wears it will be blessed with knowledge, wisdom, and wealth

9 Mukhi Rudraksha

The 9 mukhi Rudraksha symbolizes the nine forms of Goddess Durga which are also known as "Nau Shakti". Many people consider this Rudraksha to be another form of Bhairav. It is essential to wear this Rudraksha on Monday. This one helps people to control their sudden anger issues in many circumstances.

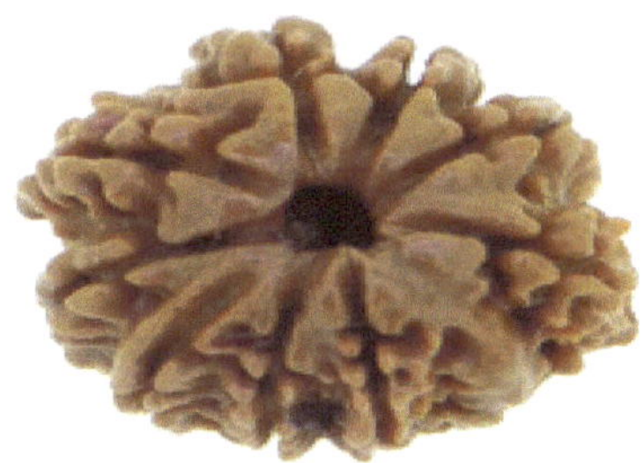

- **Ruling God:** Durga
- **Ruling Planets:** Rahu
- **Beeja Mantra:** || Om Hreem Hoom Namah ||

Benefits of 9 Mukhi Rudraksha

- 9 Mukhi Rudraksha symbolizes energy, power, dynamism, fearlessness.
- It gives two things : Bhogha – worldly comforts and desire fulfillment, and Moksha – liberation.

10 Mukhi Rudraksha

The ten mukhi Rudraksha represents the Hindu Lord Vishnu and brings peace and prosperity in one's life. People using this kind of Rudraksha can get relief from all types of fear in their lives. Also, in many cases, this Rudraksha helps to keep the troubles away.

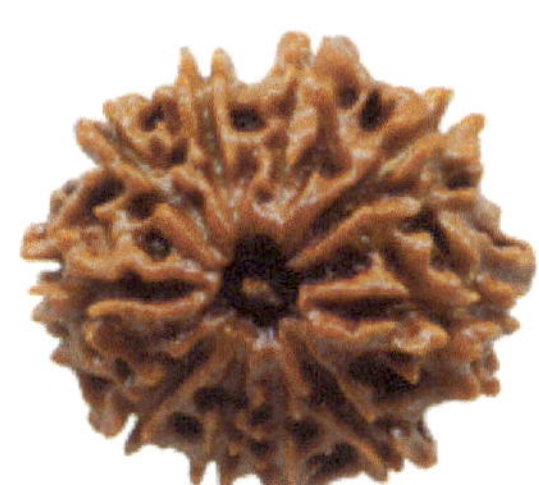

- **Ruling God:** Krishna
- **Ruling Planets:** All
- **Beeja Mantra:** || Om Hreem Namah Namah ||

Benefits of 10 Mukhi Rudraksha

- This Rudraksha symbolizes eternal peace.
- The wearer is protected from negative energies by the shield of Rudraksha.
- It is also worn for getting success in court cases, land deals, debts, and other losses.
- Texts say that it is one of the most powerful Rudrakshas that can pacify all the nine planets.

11 Mukhi Rudraksha

This type of Rudraksha represents Lord Shiva and the other eleven forms of Rudra. The eleven mukhi Rudraksha also symbolizes Lord Hanuman who is the eleventh incarnation of Lord Shiva. People who regularly wear this type of Rudraksha have blessed a successful life. This Rudraksha is also capable of producing incredible results in meditation and yogic practices.

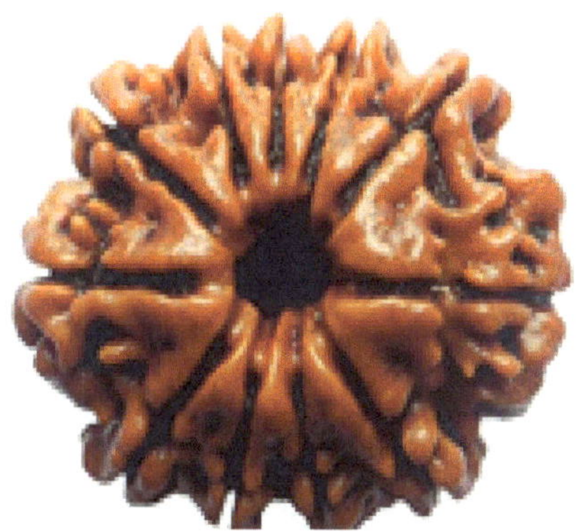

- **Ruling God:** 11 Rudras
- **Ruling Planets:** All
- **Beeja Mantra:** || Om Hreem Hoom Namah ||

Benefits of 11 Mukhi Rudraksha

- The power of wearing this bead is equivalent to performing 1000 Ashavamedh Yajna and 100 Vajpaye Yajna.
- It has the capacity to improve the high level of awareness, divine consciousness, wisdom, right judgment, control over senses, vocabulary, fearlessness, success, and adventure.
- It also pacifies all planets.

12 Mukhi Rudraksha

12 mukhi Rudraksha symbolizes the Hindu Lord Vishnu. As this Rudraksha offers the blessings of twelve Aditya Gods, hence it is commonly known as Aditya Rudraksha. Twelve faced Rudraksha helps to remove body pain and provides inner strength to the body.

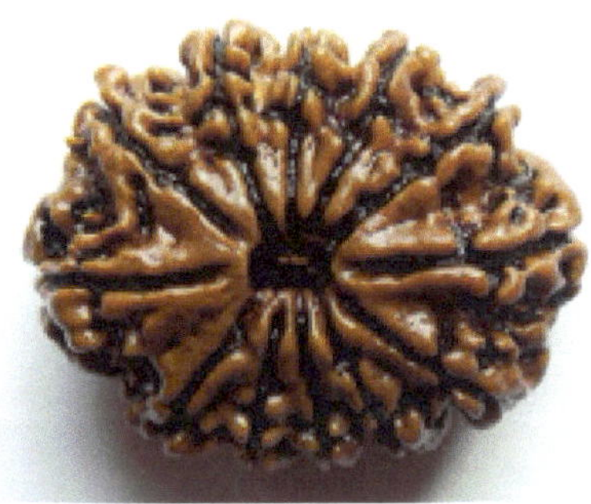

- **Ruling God:** Sun
- **Ruling Planets:** Sun
- **Beeja Mantra:** || Om Kraum Ksaum Raum Namah ||

Benefits of 12 Mukhi Rudraksha

- This is mostly for leaders as the wearer obtains the qualities of the sun : rule with brilliance, radiance, and power
- It also helps to release stress, anger, worries, suspicion, and low self-esteem
- The wearer is also blessed with self-motivation

13 Mukhi Rudraksha

The thirteen mukhi Rudraksha signifies the Hindu Lord Indra. This type of Rudraksha bestows wealth, good luck and prosperous health on its wearers.

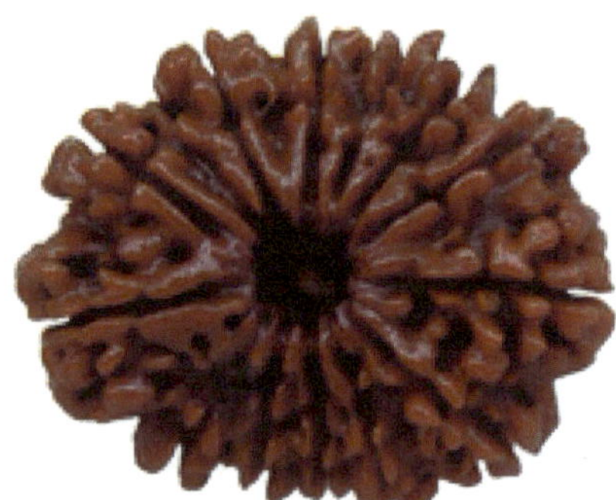

- **Ruling God:** Kamadeva
- **Ruling Planets:** Venus
- **Beeja Mantra:** || Om Hreem Namah ||

Benefits of 13 Mukhi Rudraksha

- It is for worldly desires
- It has the power of attraction with the hypnotic power of Vashikaran to the wearer
- It also raises *Kundalini energy* and awakens many Siddhis

14 Mukhi Rudraksha

The fourteen mukhi Rudraksha symbolises the Hindu Lord Hanuman. The benefits of Rudraksha beads include the development of immense courage and victory in the person. Along with these, the wearer of this Rudraksha also develops self-confidence and focus in his life.

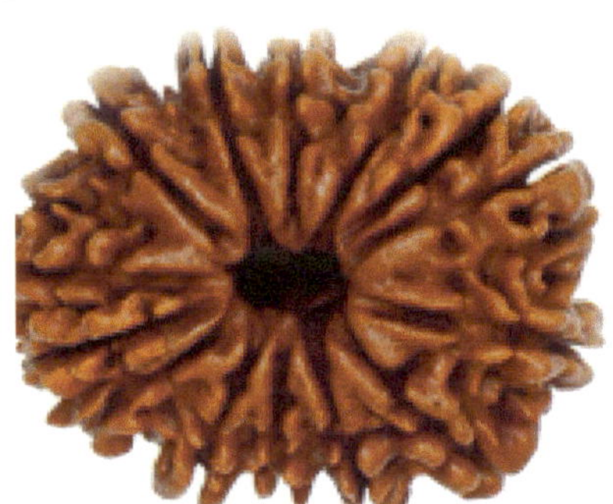

- **Ruling God:** Hanuman
- **Ruling Planets:** Mars
- **Beeja Mantra:** || Om Namah ||

Benefits of 14 Mukhi Rudraksha

- 14 Mukhi Rudraksha is known as the Deva mani or the most precious divine gem.
- 14 Mukhi Rudraksha symbolizes brevity, strong willpower, and courage, the qualities of Hanuman
- The wearer is invoked with the Hanuman inside, thus everything comes naturally after that
- *14 Mukhi Rudraksha* is the ultimate protector of the negative effects of Mars and is said to pacify "mangal dosha" in the chart.

15 Mukhi Rudraksha

People believe that this Rudraksha can destroy all the sins of the present life as it represents Pashupathinath. It is also known to be useful in controlling the effects of the planet Jupiter in one's life.

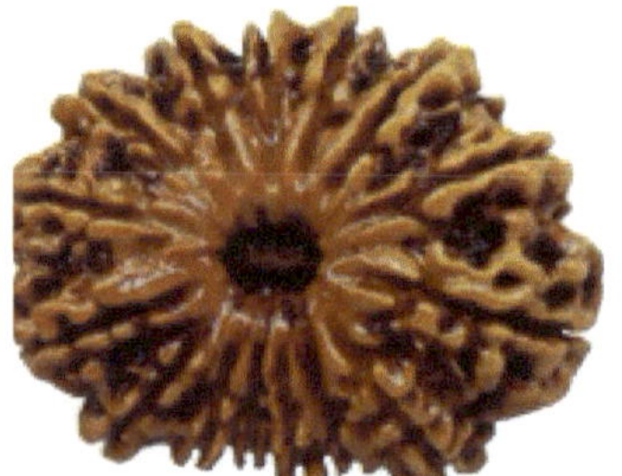

- **Ruling God:** Pashupatinath
- **Ruling Planet:** Mercury
- **Beeja Mantra:** || Om Hreem Namah ||

Benefits of 15 Mukhi Rudraksha

- It is known to heal the heart chakra
- The wearer is freed from grief, depression, loneliness, and other illness related to heart
- Wearing this would raise the person from worldly attachments and focus towards knowledge, creation, wealth generation

16 Mukhi Rudraksha

The sixteen mukhi Rudraksha symbolises the combination of Lord Vishnu and Shiva and hence represents victory. Prolonged use of this Rudraksha can help one to get rid of diseases and fears from life.

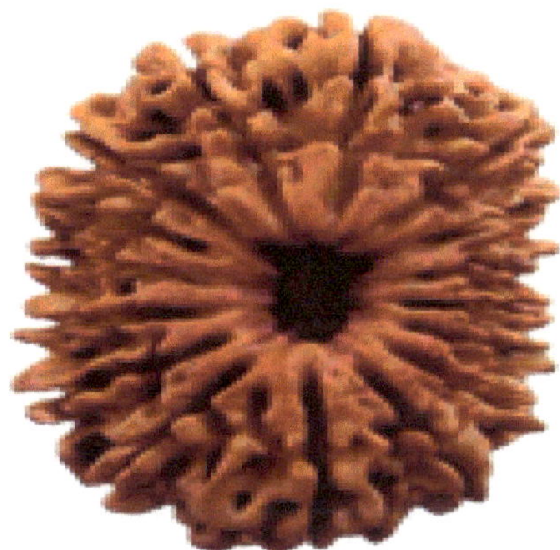

- **Ruling God:** Mahamrityunjaya Shiva
- **Ruling Planet:** Moon
- **Beeja Mantra:** || Om Hreem Hoom Namah ||

Benefits of 16 Mukhi Rudraksha

- On a physical level, it has the power to cure different diseases, release fear, and insecurities. It protects from illness.
- On a spiritual level, it liberates the person from fear of death
- On the energy level, it protects people from negative people and negative energies.
- It is for those who have fear of loss of a loved one, or fear of loss of name or fame, or loss of faith in oneself or God or death or nightmares.
- Wearing the 16 Mukhi Rudraksha is equivalent to chanting the Mahamritunjaya mantra 125,000 times every day.
- It is also said that even Lord Yama turns back from the wearer of 16 Mukhi Rudraksha

17 Mukhi Rudraksha

Seventeen mukhi Rudraksha marks the symbol of Lord Krishna. It also represents the builder of the world, Lord Vishwakarma in Hinduism. Many people use it with the belief of winning lotteries and fulfilling all their wishes.

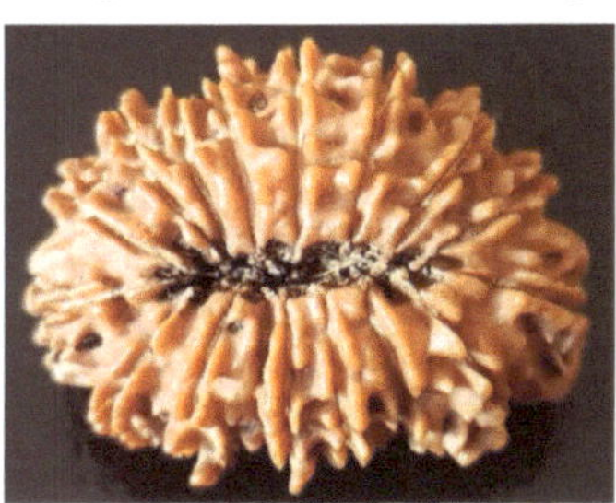

- **Ruling God:** Katyani Devi
- **Ruling Planet:** Saturn
- **Beeja Mantra:** || Om Hreem Hoom Hoom Namah ||

Benefits of 17 Mukhi Rudraksha

- The wearer of the 17 Mukhi Rudraksha is blessed with the fruits of Artha, Dharma, Kama, and Moksha.
- It is especially suited for project leaders, businessmen, political leaders with desiring growth in their career and luck
- It also frees oneself from losses, sadness, diseases, and other fears
- Other desires such as progeny, prosperity, getting a life partner is fulfilled by wearing this 17 Mukhi Rudraksha
- Katyani tantra says that the rudraksha is ruled by Mata Katyani, the sixth form of Goddess Durga, and thus, the wearer is blessed with fortune, wealth, and materialistic desires.

18 Mukhi Rudraksha

The eighteen mukhi Rudraksha symbolises the Lord Bahirav as well as Goddess Earth. The benefits of Rudraksha of this kind include the attainment of victory in all the affairs of one's life. It is quite beneficial in making people lead in a disciplined and healthy life.

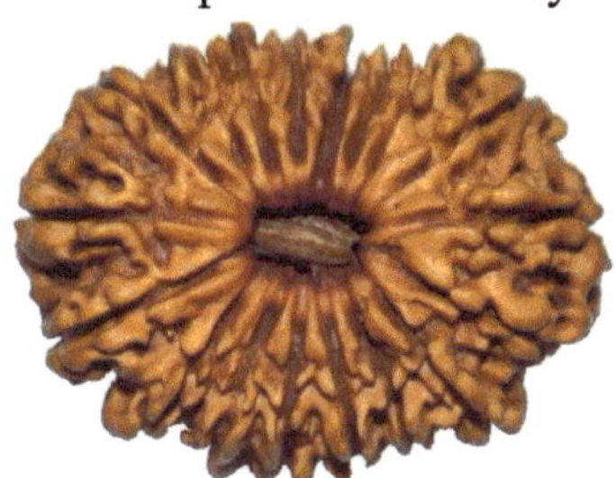

- **Ruling God:** Bhumi Devi
- **Ruling Planet:** Earth
- **Beeja Mantra:** || Om Hreem Shreem Vasudhaye Swaha ||

Benefits of 18 Mukhi Rudraksha

- It is blessed by the divine wife of Lord Vishnu, Bhumi Devi
- It is considered to be one of the most powerful Rudraksha designed for prosperity
- Katyani Tantra says that the wearer is blessed with health, intelligence, prosperity
- Bhumi represents the mother earth. Thus, the wearer of her rudraksha paves ways for success in business, wealth, land, and other transactions.

19 Mukhi Rudraksha

The nineteen mukhi Rudraksha symbolises Lord Shiva and the Goddess Parvati. It also represents the Lord Narayana, who provides happiness ad wealth. This kind of Rudraksha benefits in developing stamina, tolerance and patience in one's life.

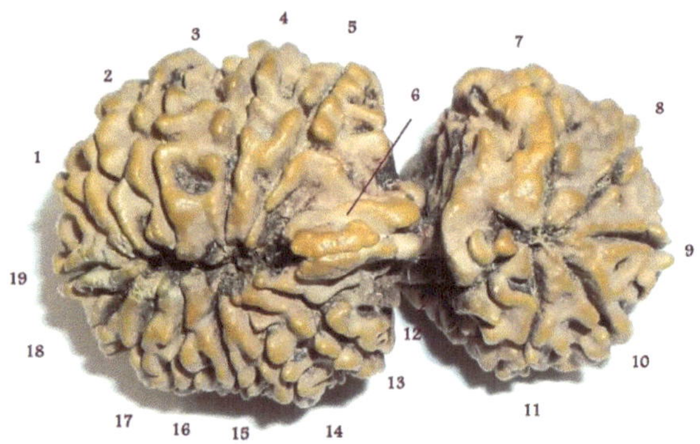

- **Ruling God:** Narayana
- **Ruling Planet:** Mercury
- **Beeja Mantra:** || Om Vam Vishnave Sheershayane Swaha ||

Benefits of 19 Mukhi Rudraksha

- The wearer will have everything fulfilled in life; there will not be lack of anything : be it wealth, success, health, abundance
- It is also meant for attracting a perfect life partner.

20 Mukhi Rudraksha

This Rudraksha is known for its ultimate benefit of attaining Moksha as it represents the power of Lord Brahma. This type of Rudraksha also represents Lord Janardhan.

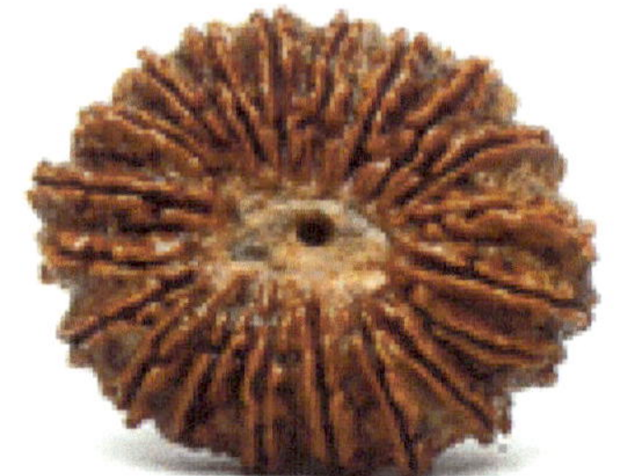

- **Ruling God:** Brahma
- **Ruling Planet:** Earth
- **Beeja Mantra:** || Rudrarupaye Kalpante Namastubhyam Trimurtaye ||

Benefits of 20 Mukhi Rudraksha

- It is meant for attaining divine knowledge in Creation, science, arts, and music.
- Wearing it would increase the creativity, knowledge, and intellect too
- It is most suitable for those with the desire to manifest projects for benefit of humanity

21 Mukhi Rudraksha

The final one symbolises Lord Kuber, who is also known as the God of wealth and prosperity. It is one of the rare kinds of Rudraksha, and people believe that the gods reside within this kind.

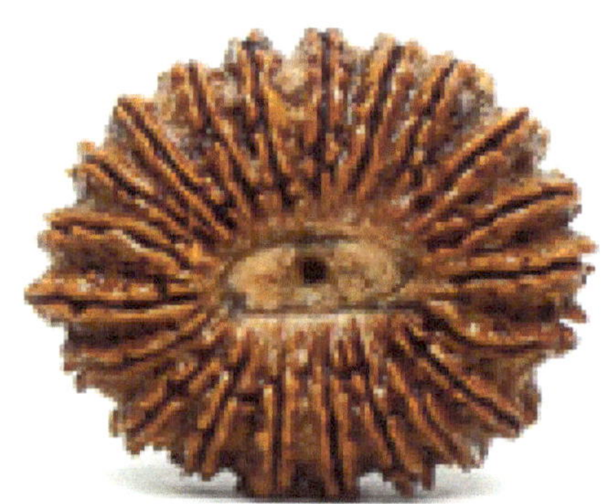

- **Ruling God:** Kubera
- **Ruling Planet:** Earth
- **Beeja Mantra:** || Om Yakshaya Kuberaya Vaishravanaya, Dhan Dhanyadhipataye, Dhan Dhanya Srimdhim mein Dapya Dapya Swaha ||

Benefits of 21 Mukhi Rudraksha

- It is one of the rarest among all the Rudrakshas and is ruled by Kubera, the lord of wealth. He also owns the title of "*king of the whole world*", "*King of Kings*" (Rajaraja), "*Giver of wealth*" (Dhanada), "*Lord of the riches*" and the "*Wealthiest Deva*"

- It removes all kinds of diseases.
- It has the power to increase wealth, even for the poor.
- The power also extends to protection from evil energies.
- The rudraksha is also suitable for travelers as Kubera is known to be the guardian of travelers

Ganesh Rudraksha

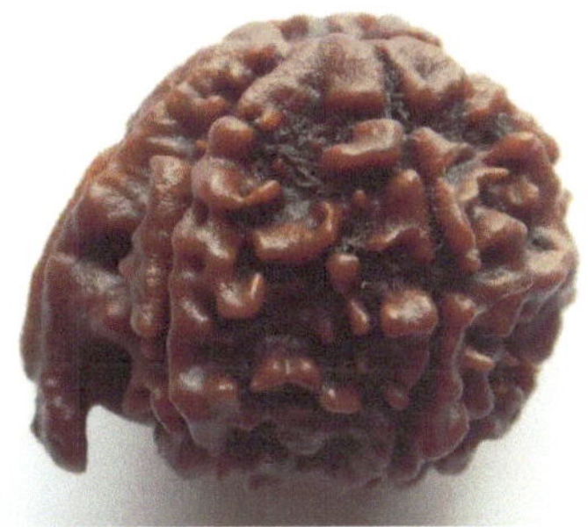

- **Ruling God:** Ganesh
- **Beeja Mantra:** || Om Hoom Namah ||

Benefits of Ganesh Rudraksha

- The trunk that's elevated looks like the face of Ganesh
- It provides perfection for worshipper in every aspect of life

Garbh Gauri Rudraksha

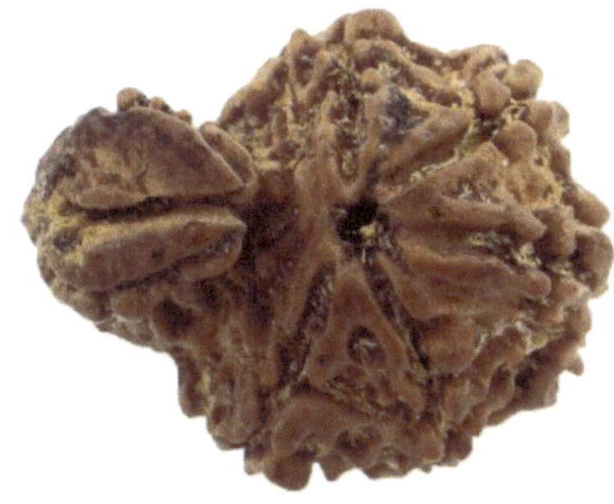

- **Ruling God:** Parvati and Ganesh
- **Ruling Planet:** Sun
- **Beeja Mantra:** || Om Trimurti Devaya Namah ||

Benefits of Garbh Gauri Rudraksha

- It is also one of the rarest Rudrakshas and is known as Trijuti
- It represents all three trinities : Brahma, Vishnu, and Shiva
- The wearer gets power for great achievement and is most suitable for leaders, project managers, and spiritual seekers

Gauri Shankar Rudraksha

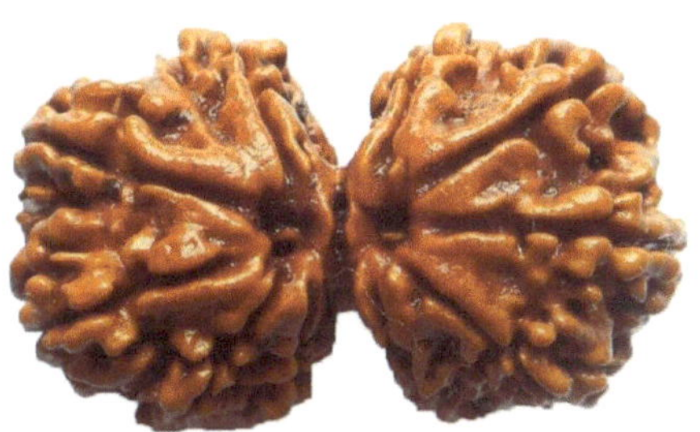

- **Ruling God:** Shiva and Parvati
- **Ruling Planet:** Sun
- **Beeja Mantra:** || Om Shree Gauri Shankaraya Namah ||

Benefits of Gauri Shankar Rudraksha

- It represents the united form of both Shiva and Parvati
- Gauri Shankar Rudraksha is known to open the Hrit Padma Chakra and aligns the inner soul to the Universal Love.
- It is also suitable for meditation, harmonizing relationships with partners while also attracting the suitable life partner with the grace of Shiva and Shakti

Apart from these types, another particular type Rudraksha available in the market is the Trijuti Rudraksha. It is a natural type of Rudraksha which has three unique Rudraksha attached on the tree itself. People believe that this kind of Rudraksha enhances creativity, along with the mind power of the person.Hence, Rudraksha holds a special place in Hindu mythology as it remains connected with the several Hindu Gods and Goddesses

Fake rudrakshas

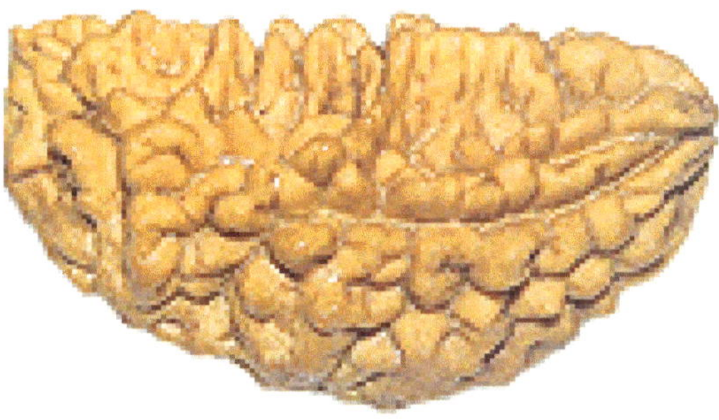

Its tree resembles a rudraksha tree; but its fruits and seeds are round. Its seeds, known as bhadrakshas, do not have openings, that is, they have no upper and lower ends. Use of bhadrakshas increases the unfavourable waves. Generally, bhadrakshas are sold as rudrakshas. Birds do not eat its fruits and if they do, they perish.

Vikrutaksha

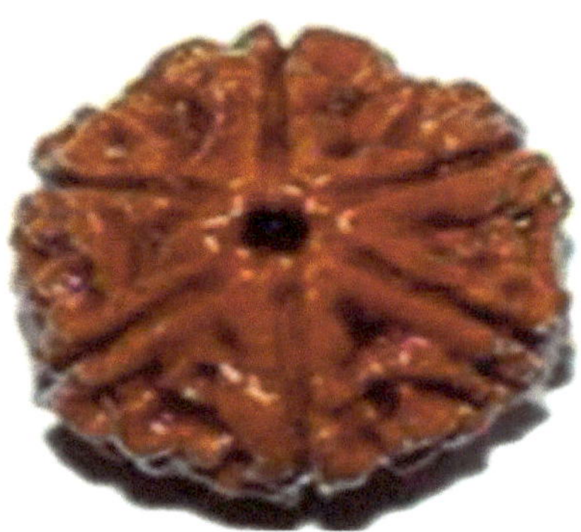

Nowadays, mostly a vikrutaksha is sold as a rudraksha. This is the seed of a type of wild berry. A gypsy tribe in Nepal known as the Gurangs first began using the vikrutaksha. An opening is made in the seed with a hot needle.

Similarly, figures like Om, swastik, a conch, a wheel etc. are carved on it with a hot needle. Immersing in water containing catechu dyes it. That is why its colour runs when it is dipped in water.

Artificial rudrakshas

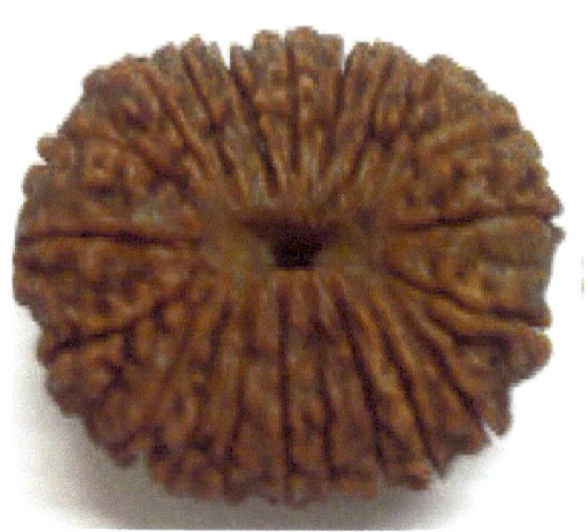

Table 38.2: *Difference between a real and a fake rudraksha*

	A real rudraksha	A fake rudraksha
1. Form	Flat like a fish	Round
2. Colour (reddish)	Permanent	Gets washed away with water
3. If put in water	Sinks immediately	Either floats or sinks gradually with wavy movements
4. Hollow from one end to the other	Present	Has to be made with a needle
5. Rotation about itself when hung in a copper vessel or in water	Takes place	Does not take place
6. Eaten away by termites after sometime	No	Yes
7. Cost of each (In theYear 2008)	₹4,000 – ₹40,000	₹20 – ₹200
8. Which waves does it absorb ?	Sama (Sattva)	–
9. Are the vibrations felt ?	Yes	No

An ideal rudraksha (Characteristics)

- Heavy and radiant
- With distinct openings
- One adorned with auspicious symbols such as an Om, Shivalinga, a swastik etc.
- The bigger the rudraksha and the smaller the shaligram, the more ideal it is. – Merutantra
- A rudraksha obtained from a rudraksha tree whose girth is more the span of the arms of a human, meaning, one obtained from a very old tree.
- A rudraksha obtained from a rudraksha tree situated at a great height above the sea level, and for the same tree, one obtained from the top of the tree : Rudrakshas at a greater height are more effective since they receive the Sattva component coming from above in greater proportion.
- A white colour rudraksha is the best. Rudrakshas of inferior quality in the ascending order are crimson, yellow or black. Generally, white and yellow rudrakshas are uncommon, while red and black ones are common.

Bibliography and Acknowledgement

- Dancing with Siva". www.himalayanacademy.com. Retrieved 2018-04-07.
- Jawla, Sunil; Rai, D. V. (2016-06-08). "QSAR Descriptors of Rudrakine Molecule of Rudraksha (Elaeocarpus ganitrus) Using Computation Servers". *German Journal of Pharmacy and Life Science* (GJPLS). 1 (1).
- Koul, M. K. (2001-05-13). "*Bond with the beads*". Spectrum. India: The Tribune.
- Laatsch, M. (2010). Rudraksha. Die Perlen der shivaitischen Gebetsschnur in altertümlichen und modernen Quellen.

Munich: Akademische Verlagsgemeinschaft München. ISBN 978-3-89975-411-7.

- Lee, D. W. (1991). "Ultrastructural Basis and Function of Iridescent Blue Color of Fruits in Elaeocarpus". *Nature*. 349 (6306): 260–262.
- Ruppel, A.M. (2017). The Cambridge Introduction to Sanskrit. Cambridge CB2 8BS, United Kingdom: Cambridge University Press. ISBN 978-1-107-45906-9.
- Seetha, K. N. (2008). Power of Rudraksha (4th ed.). Mumbai, India: Jaico Publishing House. ISBN 978-81-7992-844-8.
- Seetha, Kamal Narayan (2005). Power of rudraksha. India. pp. 15, 20 and 21.
- Seetha, Kamal Narayan (January 2009). Power of Rudraksha. ISBN 9788179929810. Retrieved 2009-01-01.
- Singh M Parashar (13 November 2019). Inner and Outer Meanings of Hinduism. Xlibris UK. pp. 229–. ISBN 978-1-984592-11-8.
- Singh, B; Chopra, A; Ishar, MP; Sharma, A; Raj, T (2010). "Pharmacognostic and antifungal investigations of Elaeocarpus ganitrus (Rudrakasha)". *Indian J Pharm Sci.* 72 (2): 261–5..
- Stutley, M. (1985). The Illustrated Dictionary of Hindu Iconography. New Delhi, India: Munshiram Manoharlal Publishers. ISBN 978-81-215-1087-5.
- Subramuniyaswami, Sivaya (1997). Dancing with Siva. USA. Search for "*Rudraksha*"in the page. ISBN 9780945497974.
- system, varna. "*varna system*". wikipedia. Retrieved 28 February 2021.
- The translation of rudrākṣa as "Rudra's Teardrops" and definition as berries of Elaeocarpus ganitrus see: Stutley, p. 119.
- What Significance Rudraksha holds in Hinduism?". NewsGram. 19 June 2017.

The Science of Vastu Shastra In Architectural Designing Brings Life Close To Nature And Health Wellness.

Historical Background

Vastu shastra is a traditional Indian system of architecture originating in India. Texts from the Indian subcontinent describe principles of design, layout, measurements, ground preparation, space arrangement, and spatial geometry. Vastu Shastras incorporate traditional Hindu and Buddhist beliefs.

The foundation of vastu is traditionally ascribed to the mythical sage Mamuni Mayan who is believed to be first author and the creator of vasthu shastra and expert in vastu constructions of ancient times.

According to Jessie Mercay, Chancellor and Professor (Volunteer) at American University of Mayonic Science and Technology, authentic vaastu science is based upon ancient principles discovered thousands of years ago by a rishi scientist/carpenter named Mamuni Mayan. Mayan is the one of the five sons of Vishwakarma. Mayan is mentioned throughout Indian literature. Most notably, he built the city of Dwarka for Krishna. Theories tracing links of the principles of composition in vastu shastra and the Indus Valley Civilization have been made, but scholar *Kapila Vatsyayan* is reluctant to speculate on such links given the Indus Valley script remains undeciphered. According to Chakrabarti, Vastu Vidya is as old the Vedic period and linked to the ritual architecture. According to Michael W. Meister, the Atharvaveda contains verses with mystic cosmogony which provide a paradigm for cosmic planning, but they did not represent architecture nor a developed practice.

Varahamihira's Brihat Samhita dated to the sixth century CE, states Meister, is the first known Indian text that describes "something like a vastupurusamandala to plan cities and buildings" The emergence of Vastu vidya as a specialised field of science is speculated to have occurred significantly before the 1st-century CE Vastu Shastra, the ancient Indian and medieval knack that deals with the subject of Vastu which means Environment. One may also regard Vastu Shastra as good practice of designing buildings and spaces that are free from metaphysical forces and conducts human life in harmony such that they will bring health, wealth and serenity to the inhabitants.

1. Vastu Shastra follows the *Vastu Purusha Mandal*. The mandala helps in deciding the whereabouts of various activities in a building.
2. Vastu Shastra has been a part of the Indian culture for thousands of years. Even today people consult Vastu experts before buying a new property. Vastu Shastra has its origin in Sthapatya Veda which is a part of Atharva Veda.
3. The early principles were drafted according to the sun rays and their differing positions at different times of the day. In ancient times, this science was only confined to the architects, known as Sthapathis, and was passed on either verbally or through hand-written monographs. The significance of Vastu Shastra is established by the fact that in earlier days, the architecture of temples and palaces was completely based on it.
4. Vastu Shastra has also been mentioned in our ancient scriptures like the Mahabharata and the Ramayana. The architecture of the city of Ayodhya bears a resemblance to the plans mentioned in the Indian architectural text Manasara. Setu bridge built by Lord Ram was based on Vastu principles. The excavations at Harappa and Mohenjo-daro also indicate that Vastu Shastra had an influence on the Indus Valley Civilization.

According to Indian mythology, Vastu is an Asur (Demon) who prayed to Bramhadev and got boons. This, in turn, spurred an insatiable hunger in him. His power grew to such an extent that he attacked the Devas (Gods) in an attempt to consume their energies. The Devas then asked Bramhadev to help them get rid of this peril. Bramhadev asked the Devas to wage a war with Vastu. During the fight, Vastu was pushed back to Earth and he fell flat on his back with this legs pointing towards Nirrtikon and his head to the Eshankon. Bramhadev then asked the Gods to jump and sit on each organ of Vastu as this will be the only way he can be killed. Bramhadev himself sat on the middle of Vastu, and defeated and killed Vastu.

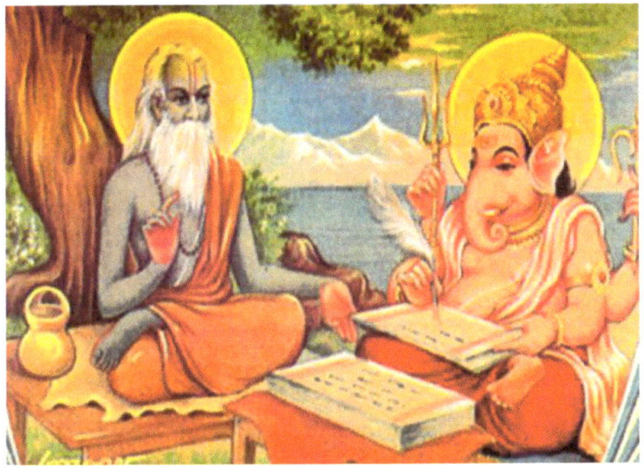

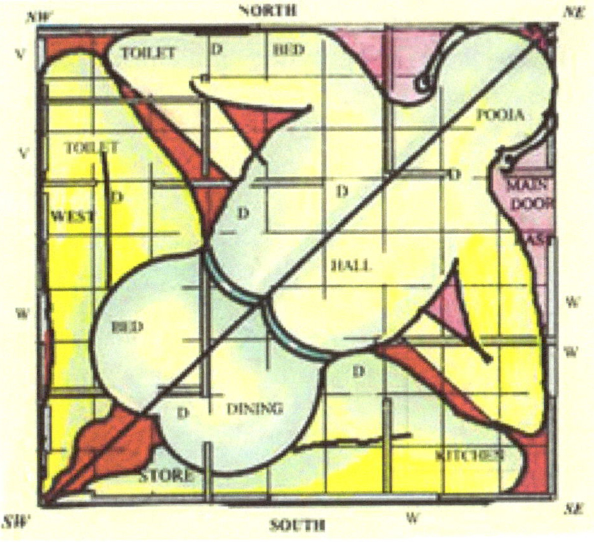

Fig. 39.1: *(Left) In the Mahabharata, a number of tall and majestic houses were built for the kings who were invited to the city Indraprastha for the Rajasuya Yagna of King Yuddhistira. The houses were free from obstructions, had compounds with high walls and their doors were of uniform height and inlaid with numerous metal ornaments. Again, Ramayana's site plan finds its similarity to the plan found in the great architectural text Manasara.(right) House design of Vastu purush mandala, the square grid (pada)*

It is said that '*The Vastupurusan*' still lies in the same position with his hands resting on his chest. The formation in which the Devas sat on Vastu was used to draft a grid diagram, which helps Vastu experts to decide favourable directions in a dwelling.

Even after thousands of years since its establishment, this science of direction remains to be very popular with people and many housing firms like Tata Housing adhere to it while designing their projects.

In Vastu purush mandala, the square grid (pada) are associated with certain deities

- North – Ruled by lord of wealth (Money)
- South – Ruled by lord of death (Death)
- East – Ruled by the solar deity- (Prosperity)
- West – Ruled by lord of water (Physical)
- North-East – Ruled by Shiva (Divine)
- South-East – Ruled by the fire deity (Energy)
- North-West -Ruled Lord of Air (Travelling)
- South-West – Ruled by Nairuti & ancestors (ancestors blessing)
- Center – Rules by the creator of the universe (balancing)

Vastu Direction According to Gods

North-West Vayvya		North		North-East Ishan
	Vayu Deity of air	Kuber Deity of wealth	Shiva God	
West	Varun Deity of water	Brahma	Surya Deity of Light	East
	Piter Ancestor	Yamraj Deity of death	Agnidev Deity of fire	
South-West Neshrtya		South © - AFE		South-East Aagneya

Fig. 39.2: *showing the directions and the angels in vasushatra*

- East – The direction of sunrise : Deity - Sun
- North – Towards the left side of East : Deity - Kuber
- West – Front of the East direction : Deity - Varun
- South – Front of the North direction : Deity - Yamraj
- Ishan Kon – East-North corner : Deity - Shiva
- Agni Kon – East-South corner : Deity - Agni or Fire
- Vayavya Kon – North-West corner : Deity-Vaau or Air
- Neshrty Kon – South-West corner : Deity - Pitar
- Center – Centre of all directions : Deity - Brahma

Vastu Principles for Different Parts of the House

1. Vastu Tips for Plot

The selection of plot is very important since it represents the form location and orientation of the house. These three factors further affect the radiation of positive as well as negative energies. So for the selection of a plot, these few factors must be considered-

- Regularly shaped plots such as rectangular or square are the most auspicious ones according to Vastu Shastra because these plot shapes help in financial growth, brings prosperity and happiness in the house.
- Shapes such as oval circular or semi-circular are not considered auspicious as this kind of plots tend to restrict the growth of an individual and also causes various health problems losses and lack of happiness in the house.
- Plot with either pathway on all four sides or plots with roads in north or east direction is considered the best options as they ensure good health, wealth and happiness for the residents.
- As per the Vastu Shastra, all the directions are considered good. The plot can face in any of the direction either on east west north or south. Each of the direction has its own advantages.

2. Vastu Tips for Main Entrance Gate

Entrance it the gateway from which all the energies constantly enter or exit the house. Hence the position of this gate must be decided with utmost care so as to abstain the house from further problems.

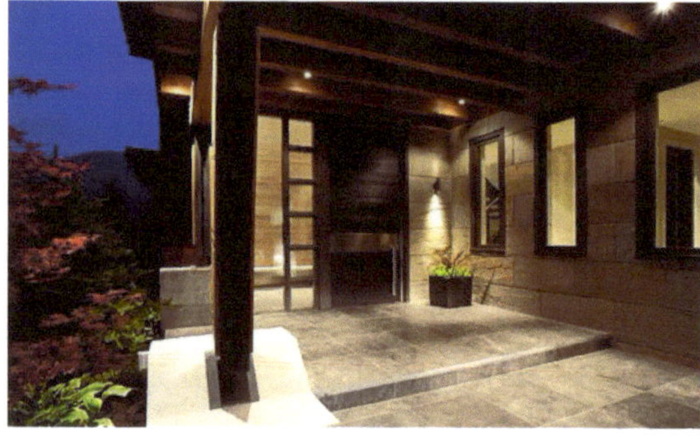

Fig. 39.3: *Photograph showing the best direction for the entrance gateway is north and east sides.*

- The best direction for the entrance gateway is north and east sides.
- Make sure that the entrance is free from any sort of trash or clutter to make the surrounding positive.
- Avoid placing any underwater or septic tank under the entrance gateway.
- The entrance should always be well lit as it invites positive energies.

3. Vastu Tips of Kitchen

Kitchen plays a vital role in maintaining the positive and negative energies in the house as it is the hub where all the energies prevail. So few things that must be considered are as follows:

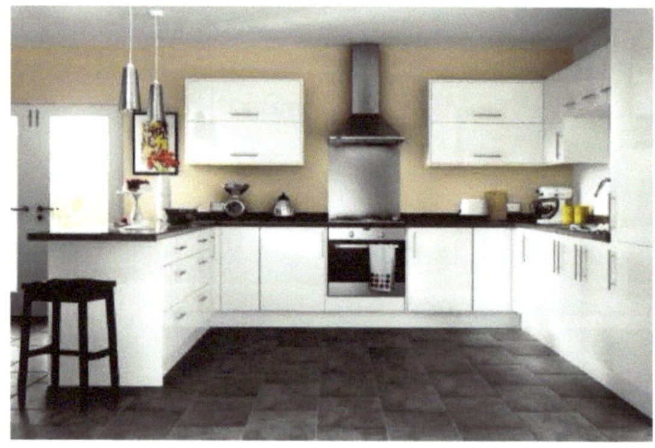

Fig. 39.4: *Photograph showing the best directions for the placement of kitchen are south-east or north-west*

- The best directions for the placement of kitchen are south-east or north-west.
- The south-east direction is governed by the fire lord hence it must the first priority.
- Water sink must be placed in the northeast direction.
- There should be no toilets adjoining or above the kitchen.
- The door of the kitchen should never face the toilet.

4. Vastu Tips for Living Room / Drawing Room

It is that part of the house where the members of the family spend most of their time and are also used to entertain guests as well as visitors. Hence this component of the house reveals whether the house bodes well with the family members or not. So to ensure that we need to take an account of the following considerations:

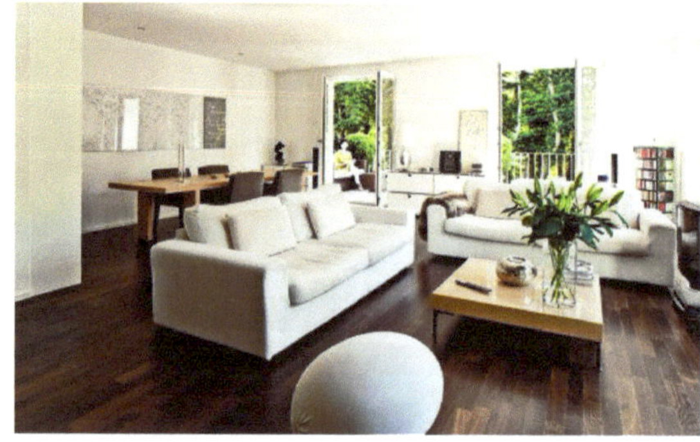

Fig. 39.5: *Photograph make sure that the northeast corner of the living room/drawing room is clutter free.*

- Colour walls with lighter shades as they promote calmness and affection.
- Make sure that the northeast corner of the living room/ drawing room is clutter free.
- Use of potted plants and paintings related to nature or scenery not only enhances the tranquillity of the room but also generates positive energy.
- Keeping artificial flowers or dried flowers are considered inauspicious and also attracts misfortune.

5. Best Sleeping direction for a better night's rest

Ayurveda's Triad of Health includes aahar (diet), vihar (balanced living), and nidra (sleep). So much importance is accorded to restful sleep, and so, of course, Ayurveda has a lot of recommendations about how to get better sleep.

Scientific Significance of the direction we sleep in?

The study of science is a quest for truth, proving a theorem and asserting that 'hence' is always pure joy. It would seem to me, as a scientist, that the direction of sleep is meant to avoid geomagnetic interference. The earth is a huge (albeit weak) magnet; but is its impact on human beings statistically significant?

The earth's magnetic positive pole is to the North, and the negative, to the South. A human's head is the positive side of a magnet, and feet, negative. Positive poles repel, so I'm assuming if we lay with our head to the North, the repelling forces will cause exhaustion.

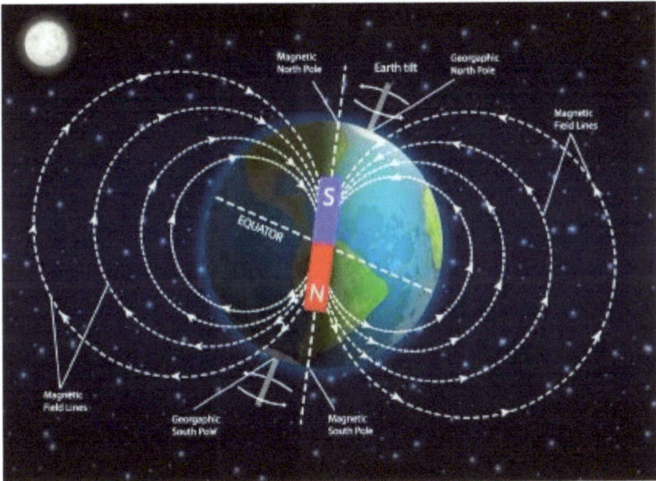

Fig. 39.6: *This diagram explains as to how magnetic field in our surroundings affect us in all the diections Hence we should avoid geomagnetic interference.during sleep. and choose the direction and position of sleep with its least harmful effect .*

Vastu, Ayurveda's sister science, deals with directions; it is the ancient science of architecture and environmental harmony and well-being. The objective of Vastu is to create a congenial setting to live and work within by using the Panchamahabhutas, (the five great elements of ether, air, fire, water and earth), directions, and energy fields for enhanced health, wealth, prosperity, and happiness.

When asked Michael Mastro, a leading North American Vastu expert, about sleep directions, and this was his advice : "We never sleep with our head to the North, because positive magnetic energy comes from the North Pole, and our body is a magnet with a positive polarity in our head, so this is like bringing two positive ends of magnets together (hence!); they repel each other and disturb blood flow, circulation, and digestion, which does not give restful sleep. If you have health issues, sleeping in the south direction is very beneficial (these recommendations don't change in the Southern Hemisphere)."

Ayurveda and Vastu concur on correct sleeping direction

1. South-North : Sleep with the head towards the South and feet towards the North.
2. East-West : East is a good direction too; sleep with the head towards the East and feet towards the West.
3. Avoid sleeping with the head towards the West.
4. Never sleep with the head towards the North.

North Direction

While finding our true North is spiritually and navigationally sound (the North Star has always been used for navigation), north-facing sleep is not recommended at all, as it can cause issues with blood circulation, increased stress, physical and psychiatric issues, and insomnia. Dr. Vasant Lad says, "Only dead people sleep facing North. Indeed, the Hindu custom is to arrange a corpse with the head pointing northwards till the body is cremated, because the belief is that that is the route for the soul to exit the body, as the legend of Lord Ganesha's head suggests.

East Direction: Head towards East

Sleeping with your head towards the East is supposed to be great for everyone, particularly students, because it enhances memory, improves concentration, and is good for overall health. The sun rises in the East, and it is considered a direction of positive waves and force of action. It makes a person feel rejuvenated and energized. It is also supposed to be good for meditation, and other spiritual pursuits. Vastu consultants often advise that a kid's bed should be placed with its head to the East and feet to the West. Sleeping in the East-West direction enhances creativity, is good for conception, and balances all three doshas (Vata, Pitta and Kapha constitutions). Studies have shown that people who sleep in this direction have shorter REM (Rapid Eye Movement) sleep cycles and eye movement (compared to sleeping in the North-South direction), implying fewer dreams and a more sound sleep.

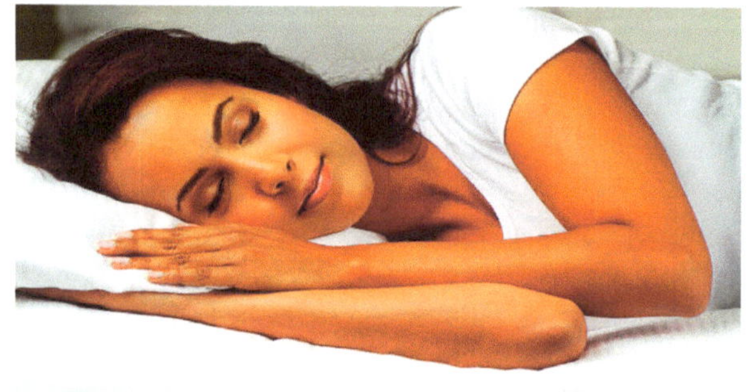

Fig. 39.7: *Photograph of a young lady is sleeping with your head towards the East which is supposed to be great for everyone, particularly students, because it enhances memory, improves concentration, and is good for overall health.*

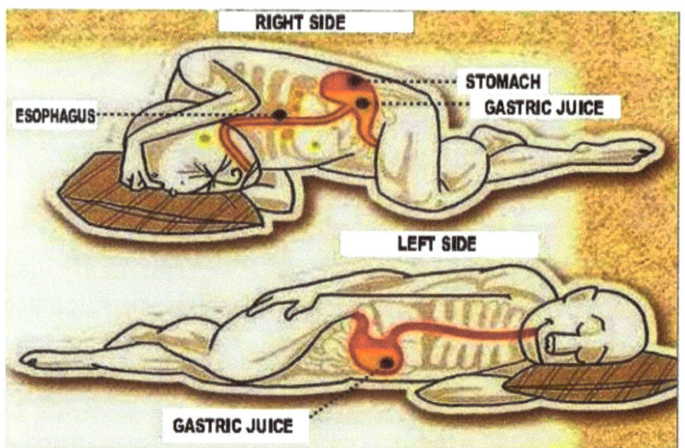

Fig.39.8:*Illustrations showing. the best sleeping position which is on your left side The Gastric juices can escape the stomach if you sleep on your right side. This acid can ruin you esophagus, some research say it can cause throat cancers, it can enter your lungs and also damage your teeth..*

West Direction

Sleeping West to East is not advised. There are some who suggest that it increases Rajas, or ambition and restlessness, but there are better ways to do that; some even consider it to be a neutral sleeping position. However, according to Vastu, sleeping with one's head to the West can lead to restless and disturbed sleep, nightmares, and a tendency towards violence.

South Direction

If one goes by the theory of magnets, a mutual attraction between the negative South and positive head creates harmony in sleep. According to mythology, South is the direction of Lord Yama, and promotes heavy, deep sleep, like the restorative sleep of death. Vastu practitioners consider this to be the best type of sleep for health, lowering blood pressure, and promoting positive energy, wealth, prosperity, and harmony.

For Vata people, who often have anxiety and cold hands, sleeping with the head towards the South or southeast is recommended. People with Pitta aggravation can sleep towards the northwest (for a limited time). Sleeping with the head facing West may bring a Kapha vikruti back to balance - again for a limited time.

Also consider *magnetic therapy*, which is an alternative medical practice that uses static (i.e. unmoving) magnets to alleviate pain and other health concerns; while science is expressing reservations until the benefits have been proven by allopathic testing, a 2015 estimate by BBC pegs the sale of global therapeutic magnets at US$ 1 billion, showing how popular this form of therapy is.

In 2009, a study in India in the Department of Physiology at Himalayan Institute of Medical Sciences was undertaken to observe whether sleeping with the head in a direction has any effect on heart rate, blood pressure, and serum cortisol during supine rest. It found that those instructed to sleep with their head in the South direction had the lowest SBP (systolic blood pressure), DBP (diastolic blood pressure), HR (heart rate), and SC (serum cortisol). These were statistically significant findings, though it was recommended that further studies were needed in different groups.

Can earth's weak geomagnetic field impact our neural signals?

Now here's the good news! A 2019 scientific study found evidence of humans having working magnetic sensors that send signals to the brain. Bees, turtles, fish, birds, and some mammals (whales, bats, cows) use their magnetic sense as homing devices and for navigation, in conjunction with cues like sight, smell, and hearing. These animals share the same ancestors we do. Thus far, science was looking for uniquely human behavioral responses to magnetic fields, but when the parameters of the study were changed to whether humans can sense the magnetic field, we obtained the evidence we were looking for : there is a sensory ability in our subconscious brain to detect magnetic signals. Indeed, humans can sense the earth's magnetic field. Scientifically, there is so much unexplored about the world, and I'm awed by the fact that we don't know what we don't know. Does sleep direction actually impact our quality of rest?

6. Vastu Tips for Bedroom

The bedroom is as important as the other parts of the room. It is that place where we relax and gather energy for the whole day. So, it is necessary to make sure that the room is in a favourable concord.

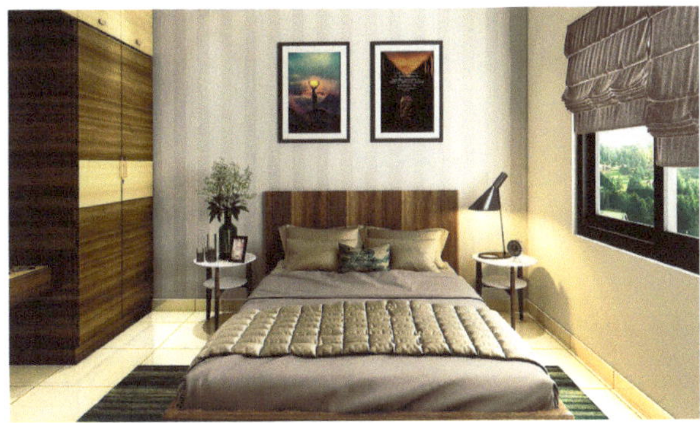

Fig. 39.9: *Photograph of a bed room. Make sure that the bed should be located such that your head is towards the south or east direction as these directions bring good sleep and ensure long life*

1. The bedroom should not be in the south-east direction.
2. Mirrors should not be located inside the bedroom as they lead to frequent quarrels amongst the members of the house.
3. The bed should be located such that your head is towards the south or east direction as these directions bring good sleep and ensure long life.
4. Ancient sages suggested that the place attached to the room which is towards the N.W. on the North is good to be used as a Bedroom. It is good to lie down on bed keeping one's head on the West side, because the sun rises in the East, the presiding deity of which is Indira, the Lord of devatas (Gods). After rising from bed in the morning, if one offers one's salutations, turning towards the East, it amounts to offering salutations to all the Gods. It is also recommended that one may sleep on one's bed putting the head towards the South and look towards the North. The presiding deity is Kubera, the Lord of Wealth. So it goes without saying that one is Worshipping *Kubera* by living on bed facing North. If one sleeps putting the head on the East and looking towards the West, one offers salutations to *Varuna*, the presiding deity of the West. The salutations benefit very much one's philosophical thinking, belief and practice. But, under any circumstances one should not sleep putting his head towards the North and looking towards the South, because the presiding deity of the South is*Yama*. Only the corpse of a person is laid on pyre, putting the head towards the North, facing the South. If one sleeps, for any unknown reason, putting the head towards the North and facing the South, one will have nightmares and sleepless nights. Today, Health Science reiterates that a man needs adequate sleep to keep himself fit and healthy. So one has to pay heed to the rules enumerated above.

7. Vastu Tips for Puja Room

- The *pooja room* must be situated in the northeast direction of the house.
- Ideally there should be no idols in the pooja room. But if one wants to keep then the height of the idol should be from 9 to 2 inches.
- The worship rooms should have doors or windows on either north or east side.
- The colour of the walls should be lighter in shade for e.g. white, cream, yellow, light blue.
- For the worshiping of fire lord the kund must be made in the southwest direction.
- A pooja room should not be made in a bedroom or a wall or adjacent to a bathroom wall.

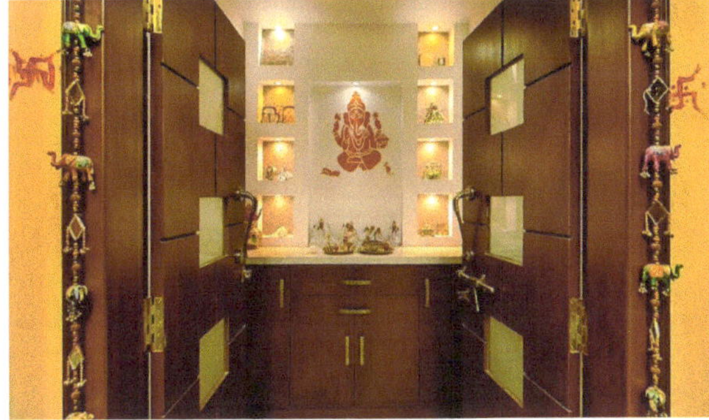

Fig.39.10: *Photograph of a puja room. This must be situated in the northeast direction of the house.*

8. Vastu Tips for Bathroom

- A *bathroom* must be placed in the eastern portion of the house.
- A toiled should be constructed to the west of the building.
- Shower taps must be attached on the northern wall.
- If the toilet is attached along with the bathroom then the WC should be placed on the north-west side of the space.
- Overhead tank must be placed in the south west portion.
- Ventilator should be placed in the east or north direction

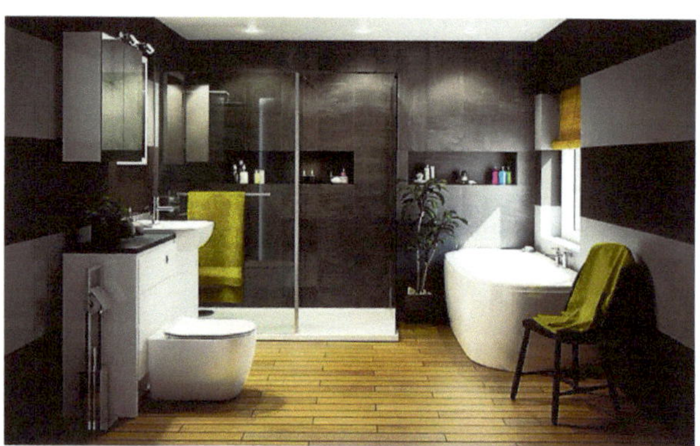

Fig.39.11: *Photograph of a bath room. This must be placed in the eastern portion of the house.*

9. Vastu Tips For Staircase

Most of the houses these days are multi storied so to bridge the gap between the two floors we need to build a staircase. So for that we need to first consider vastu shastra which would help us decide the shape size or direction of the stair.

- A *staircase* must be placed in the southern or western part of the house.
- External staircase can be placed in the southern direction facing the east direction of the house.
- A stair must not touch northern or eastern walls.
- The first stair must commence from north direction and end in the south direction.

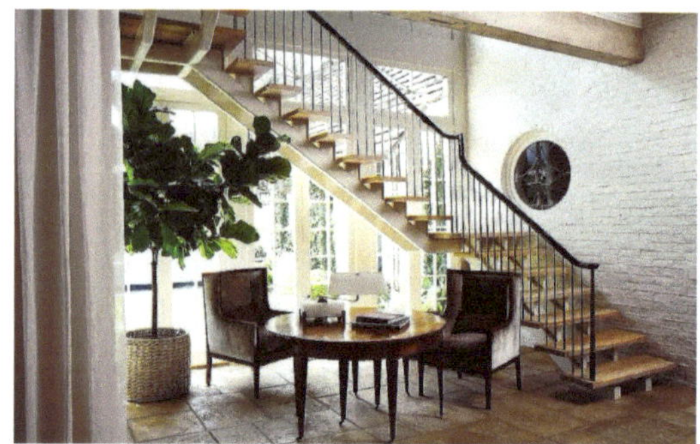

Fig. 39.12: *Photograph of a staircase .A staircase must be placed in the southern or western part of the house*

- The number of stair should always be in odd digits.
- Circular stairs are considered inauspicious according to vastu as they can cause bad health.
- The space below the staircase can be used for storage but rooms such as bathroom, kitchen, or pooja room should never be built.

10. Vastu tips for Choosing Colors for Your Home

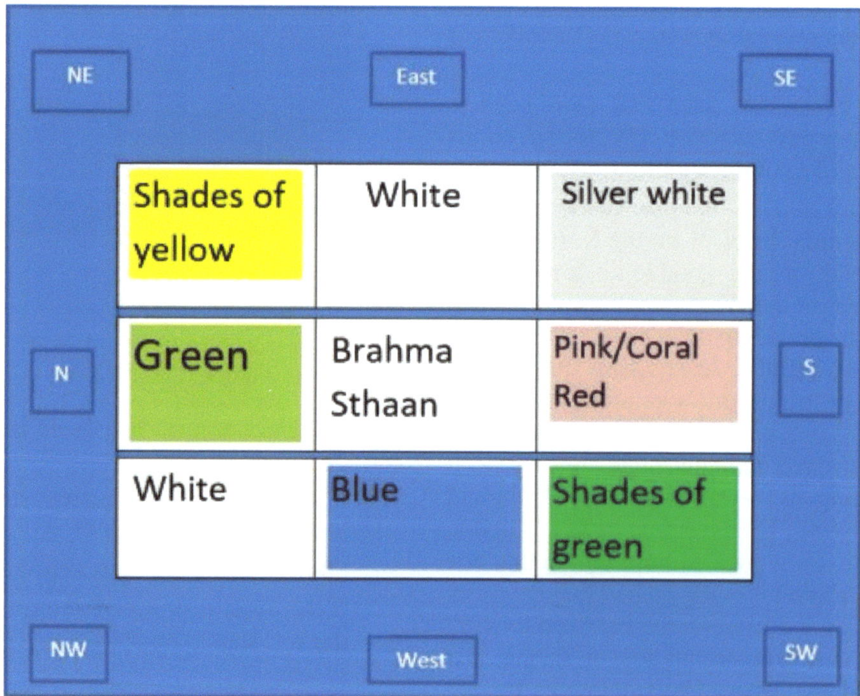

Fig. 39.13:*Color chart showing different colors which can be choosen to paint your interior wallsof different locations of your house.. Psychologists believe that the use of lighter colour can make us feel calm and relax whereas brighter colours can trigger our anger and sometimes one may even feel suffocated.*

The colours must be chosen aesthetically as they can either enhance your mood or doze you off. Psychologists believe that the use of lighter colour can make us feel calm and relax whereas brighter colours can trigger our anger and sometimes one may even feel suffocated. Colours like red orange and yellow are considered as bright colours which depicts boldness anger and warmth. Whereas blue, white, green, pastel and neutral colours are considered as light colours which depict coolness, calmness, peace and compromise.

11. Vastu tips for Basement

According to vastu any vacant space beneath the house or a building is considered as inauspicious but in case we want to have a basement then the following guidelines must be taken in account:

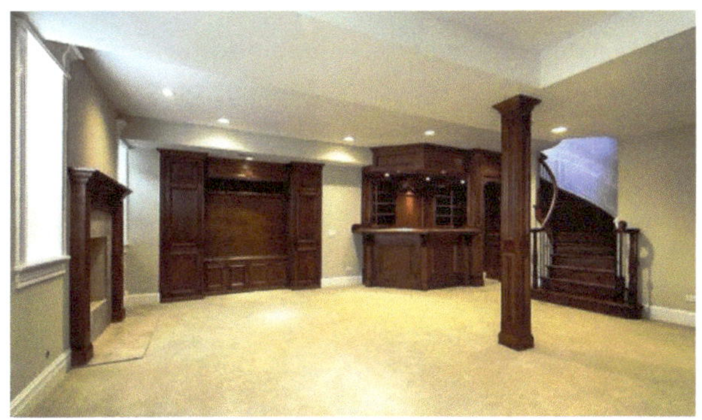

Fig. 39.14: *Photograph of a basement of the house It should be built in northern or eastern direction of the house.*

- A staircase must be placed in the southern or western part of the house
- Basement should be built in northern or eastern direction of the house.
- The purpose of basement can be for anything accept for living purpose.
- Basement must be of regular or geometrical shape. Irregular shaped basement can cause health problems to the members of the house.
- About ¼ area of the basement must be above the ground level. As it allows space for better ventilation.
- Minimum height of the basement should be at least 2.5 meters.
- Dark tints of colour must be avoided for basement as it can attract negative energy.

12. Vastu tips for Place to Keep Oils and Ghee

In olden days people used to have a grinding machine to squeeze oil in the South leaving the South East. By this, it was convenient for cooks to reach oil etc. easily. But now a days it is not necessary to have a grinding machine, as there are Mixes and grinding machines run by electric current. They may be put in the South.

13. Vastu tips for Lounge

This should be in the middle on the South side so that the members of a family may take rest after lunch. But sages did not recommend to sleep in lounge in nights.

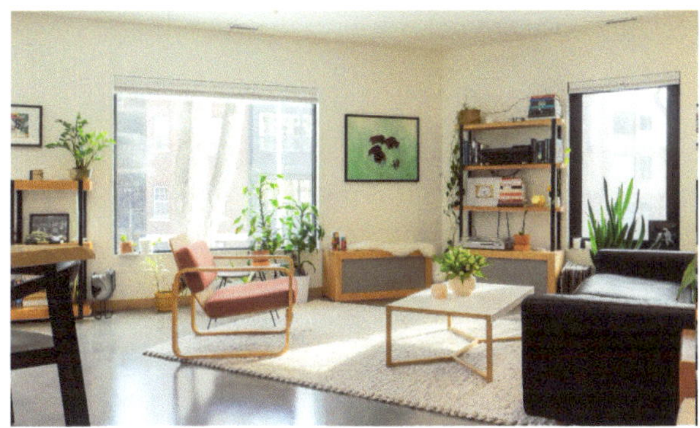

Fig. 39.15: *Photograph of a lounge of the house This should be in the middle on the South side*

14. Vastu tips for Study Room

In olden days it was considered good that the place on the West towards S.W. is the best one for studies. The reason is the planets mercury, Jupiter, the Moon and Venus influence the place as mentioned below.

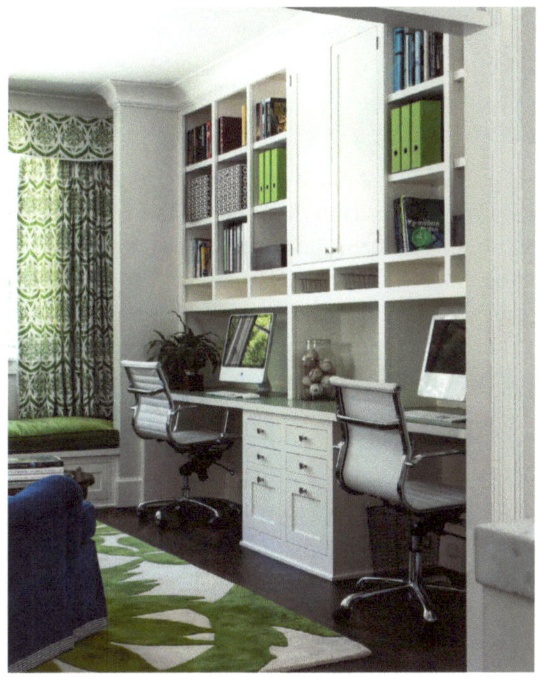

Fig. 39.16: *Photograph of a study room of the house. This should be in S.W. direction*

Jupiter: Accelerates desire to study and curiosity to learn.

Mercury: Develops intelligence.

The Moon: Lays strength on the nerves of the brain.

Venus: Functions like a coordinator and makes the man efficient. Therefore the study-room must be in the West and one should sit facing N.E., East or North. The "*Vaastu Shastra*" lays stress on the point that if one sits for studies as per the directions given above, one becomes quite an expert and enlightened.

15. Vastu tips for dining Hall

For taking food, the central part on the West is a useful one. Whatever one eats it is digested very easily.

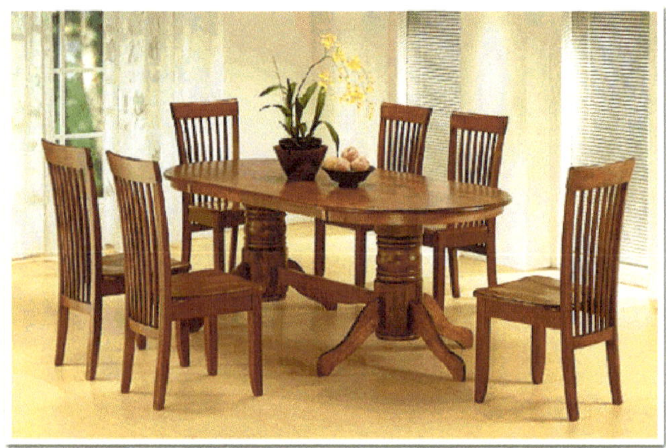

Fig. 39.17: *Photograph of a dining hall of the house. This should be in the central part on the West*

16. Vastu tips Room for Expressing Condolences and Sympathy

For this purpose best place is the Western portion attached to the N.W. The reason for this is the influence of the planets i.e. the Saturn, the Moon and Ketu. In addition to mourning that is the most suitable place to take a quick decision. When time is short and an immediate decision is to be taken, if one ponders here over any problem, he gets the solution in no time.

17. Vastu tips for place to Keep Tame Animals, Cattle and Birds

The N.W. of a plot is the best side to keep the above said living beings. Granary also must be on the same side. If the N. W. increases or decreases, it affects the health of cattle.

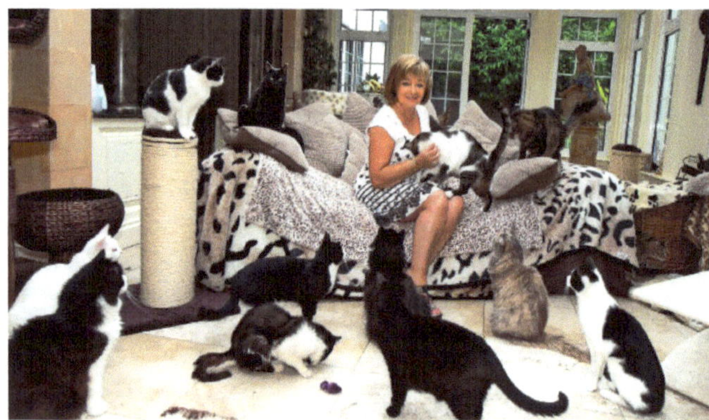

Fig. 39.18 *Photograph of a room of the house where pet animals can be kept safely. This should be in the N.W. of a plot is the best side to keep the above said living beings*

18. Vastu tips for Place for Keeping Valuable Things

The best place for keeping valuable things and property is the central portion on the North. The presiding deity of the North is Kubera. So the North is the best side to keep safely most valuable things and property.

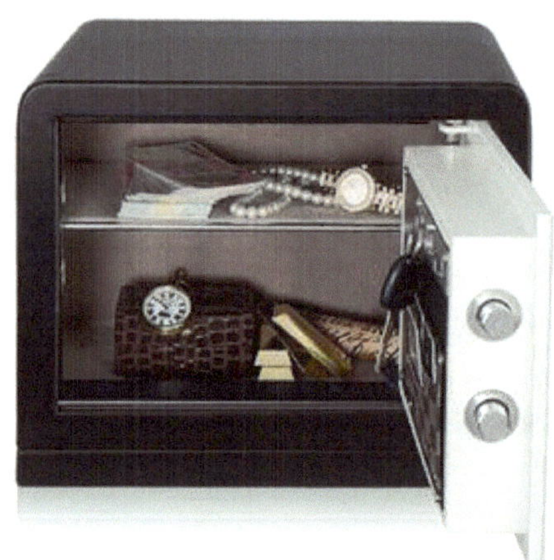

Fig. 39.19: *Photograph of a home safe locker. The valuable things and property should be kept in the central portion on the North*

19. Vastu tips for Place of Keeping Medicines

Our ancestors suggested that medicines should be kept in the N.E., because the sun – rays which have nourishing quality required for human health, fall at dawn, on the medicine and make them powerful to help human beings become hale and healthy. Today's Health – Science also agrees to this suggestion.

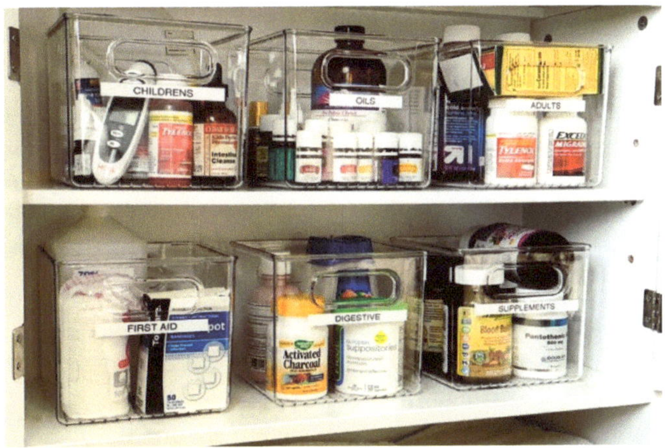

Fig. 39.20: *Photograph of a home medicine storage. These medicines should be kept in the N.E.*

20. Vastu Tips for Kids' Bedroom

Your child's room is the most special place in your house which consists of not just vibrant energy but is also a hub of creative energy and ideas. While parents make sure that they take good care of their child's health and provide them with proper nutrition, there are a few things that should be kept in mind when you design your kid's bedroom. No parent would want anything to act as a hurdle between their child's growth and his success. From the position of the kid's bed to the direction of his study table, everything should align properly in order to ensure your kids' progress. In fact, proper placement of things in stills positive thinking in children's mind to work harder and making them cheerful.

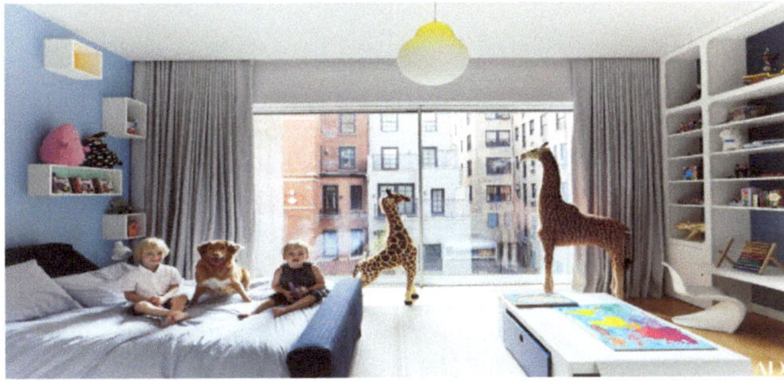

Fig. 39.21:*Photograph of a room for children. Keep the bed in South-west portion of room and let your child sleep with head towards South or East direction for peace of mind.*

Children room is a hub of recreation, fun and frolic; however some basic things should be taken care of to make your child an all-rounder. Vastu complaint room suggests placing every thing at its proper location according to corresponding direction such as study table, bed, bathroom, and clock, and window, door and so on. Proper placement of things instills positive thinking in children's mind to work harder and making then cheerful.

Every parent is keen to see their child's progress in every sphere of life while thereVastu Tips for Children Room are some negative things that every house has due to Vastu defects which affects children behaviour and mind. Improper placement of things transforms children into brat, stubborn and low in concentration pushing their parents to get on nerves. Converting your child's room with Vastu set of rules can perhaps give you positive results making your child obedient and progressive. These are as follows:

- *West direction* is ideal for children room and must be place there.
- Vastu for Drawing Room
- Keep the bed in South-west portion of room and let your child sleep with head towards South or East direction for peace of mind.
- Door of children room should not directly face the bed.
- South-west direction is best for placing furniture while avoid any kind of furnishing in middle or centre of the room which creates obstruction.
- Keep all the furnishing 3away from the wall.
- Cabinets and closets should be placed in South or West direction.
- Avoid recruiting TV, computer/laptop in children room as they effect child concentration. But seeing today's scenario and compulsion computers should be located in North and Television in South-east.
- Avoid any exposed mirror in children room and do not place any kind of mirror in front for bed.
- Study table should face East, North or North-east.
- Study area should be clutter free in order to boosts concentration and clutter free ambience is good for generating new ideas.
- Good lights should be placed in South-east direction while avoid sharp lamps on study table which begets strain.
- To add freshness in your child's mood brush up his room with Green or Blue hue.
- Doors in children room are best at East or North.
- Green color proves the best for kids' room, as it is associated with freshness and peace and increases brain power as well.

How do you relate the elements of nature with their directions?

For harmony and peace, the balance needs to be achieved between the elements and directions.

1. **Earth:** Earth is the most important element which influences our life in every aspect in every way.
2. **Water:** It is an element of the northeast and positioning of water bodies is made as such.
3. **Fire:** It is considered to be an element of the southeast, the sun rising from the east. So provisions are to be made for proper reception of sunlight in this direction.
4. **Air:** It is an element of the northeast and directions are important when you plan windows and doors so as to receive good healthy air.
5. **Space:** The sky or the universe is the centre of the whole system and that is the reason why the space in the centre of the house also called the 'Brahmasthan' is very important.

When you know about the five elements and their favoured direction, the need for positioning of objects and colours makes sense.

So now is the time to go into some aspects of Vastu and see how it can be incorporated into our daily lives. What are the things that need to be avoided, what are the things that you need to go for and what is the reason behind all these?

Five tips that can make your home vastu compliant and usher in peace and happiness:

1. Avoid Dark Colors

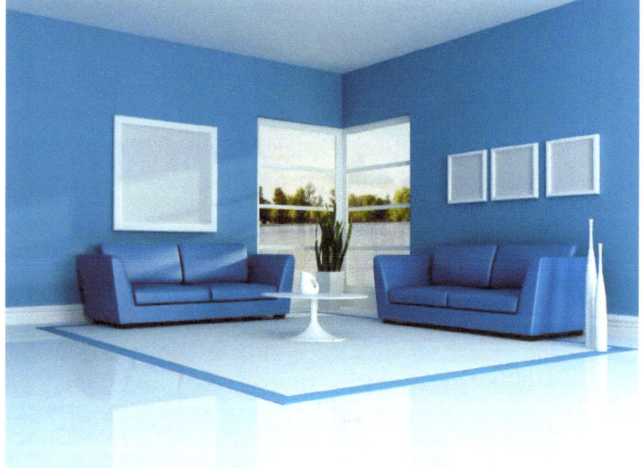

Fig. 39.22:*Photograph of a living room of the house This has been painted in blue color which indicates serenity, contentment and beauty*

Hues and its significance

Colours are mood indicators. Colours are the joys of life. Colours are the sadness in life. In short, colours have the power to affect our moods. Colours have the power to heal. Colours have the power to depress. When colours are everything in our life, we need to ensure that the right colour combinations are selected so that it brings out the best in everyone.

So what do colours signify?

- *Red* stands for power, aggressiveness, energy, passion and materialism.
- *Blue* stands for serenity, contentment and beauty.
- *White* stands for purity, truth, simplicity and luxury.
- *Orange* stands for health, warmth and determination.
- *Green* stands for abundance, fertility and prosperity.
- *Yellow* stands for happiness, optimism and intelligence.

Go in for colours accordingly. Like for example in a master bedroom go in for a combination of blue and pink. In your kids' room, go in for yellow and light green. Avoid using red here lest you face the wrath of your kids. In the kitchen you could use red combined with orange or white. According to Vaastu, the colours used in your home have significant effect on the mood and character of the inmates.

Colours to avoid: red, black and grey in the entrance

Colours to go for: blue, yellow, white and dark green

Also, if you are fond of the colour-break concept, then paint one wall on the east or south in a darker shade. Let your rooms breathe style and comfort.

2. Avoid Cactus and Thorny Plants

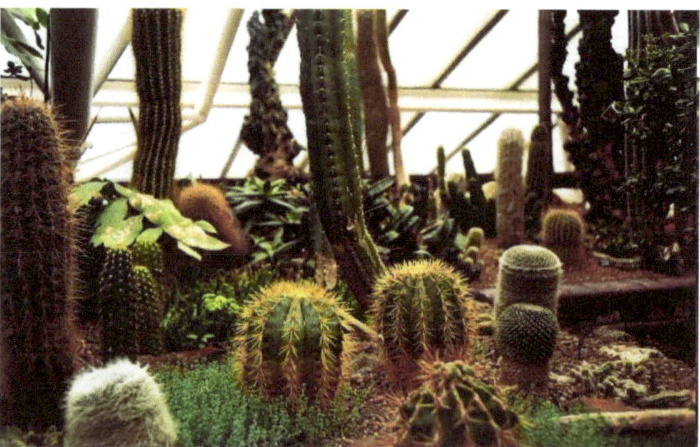

Fig. 39.23:*Showing cactus plants According to Vastu, cactus or related plants should never be kept in the house. Similarly, plants with red lowers and bonsai trees should not be kept inside the house.*

Plants bring in a lot of energy. Some plants are especially known for their medicinal value and benefits. Plants in general are known to purify the air around us. So it is not a hidden fact that good plants are always welcome at home both indoors and outdoors. Vastu supports the placing of plants according to directions and it tells us to avoid some plants.

According to Vastu, cactus or related plants should never be kept in the house. Similarly, plants with red flowers and bonsai trees should not be kept inside the house.

To Avoid – Plants in the northeast corner of the house and potted-plants along the north and east walls of the house.

To go for – Place auspicious plants like Tulsi (basil) or money plant for prosperity and happiness.

In addition, bamboo is considered very lucky both in Vastu and Feng-Shui. They are considered to bring good luck and protect the people of the house from evil powers. Money plant inside the house is considered to bring prosperity to the house. Basil is a very auspicious plant and its uses and benefits are widely known and used. It is to be placed in the north or east direction of the house.

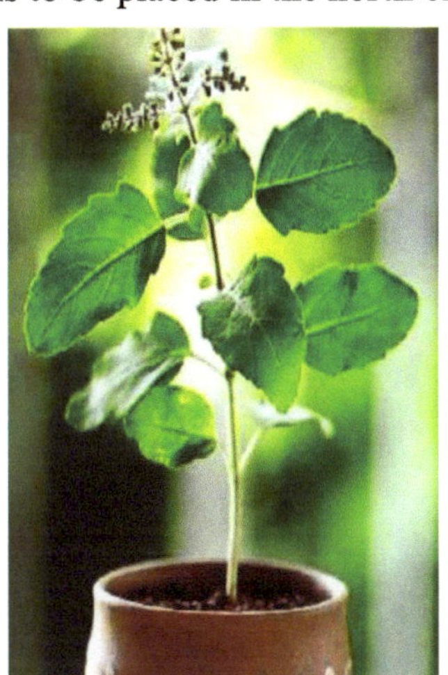
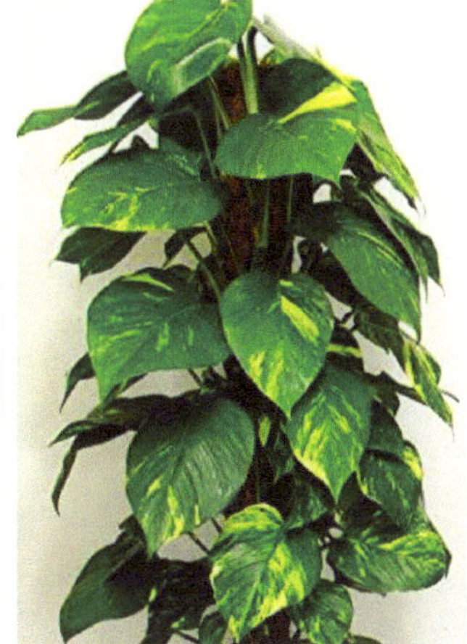

Fig. 39.24: *(Left) Placing a Tulasi/tulsi plant in the northeast or north or east sector of the house can transform any bad energy into positive and good energy. (Right) Showing typical color of leaves of money plant .*

Vastu Shastra plays an important role in deciding the location of your house as well as the items placed inside your house. Not only does it help in aligning good vibes with the directions of your furniture and doors but guides us the rules where few things should and shouldn't be kept at one's abode. People love decorating their homes with pictures and portraits of various things, plants like tulsi etc. However, is your positioning of keeping plants is wrong then this habit may not always result in your benefit. Acharya Indu Prakash talks about the directions which are considered auspicious to keep the *Tulsi plant.*

According to Vastu Shastra, the north, north-east or east direction should be selected for the basil plant in the house. This creates positive energy in the house and helps in destroying negative energy. However, it should be kept in mind that the basil plant should not be planted in the south direction of the house. Otherwise, you may have to face the loss. Therefore, on the basis of Vastu Shastra, you should try to keep the Tulsi plant only after choosing the right direction.

The Tulsi plant has a special significance in Hinduism. Planting a basil plant at home gives auspicious results. According to Vastu Shastra, if the Tulso plant is kept in the wrong direction then it can affect our life negatively. If you keep these things in mind then it will have a positive effect on you. According to Vastu Shastra, the north-east direction is considered to be the direction of Kuber, the god of wealth. So to increase the economic condition of the house, Tulsi should be planted in the north-east direction. Meanwhile, have a look at the video for more such tips:

If there is any flaw in Vastu Shastra of your house then there will always be some problem in your house. For this, you should then plant basil in south-east direction. If the basil plant dries then it should be put in a river or a nearby well. If you cannot do this, then the plant should be pressed into the pot of soil.

3. Choice of Paintings and Statues

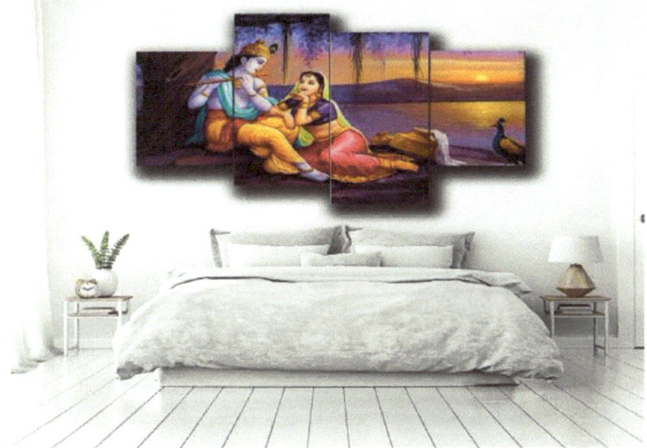

Fig.39.25: *Photograph of Radha-Krishana in bed room. This usher in good health and better living.*

Vaastu suggests paintings and statues placed in the house affect family members of the house too.

Painting or idol of Radha-Krishna together is best advised to be kept in the master bedroom as it symbolizes love between couples. Also the statue or painting of two white swans swimming together indicates the closeness and love of couples. It can be placed in the bedroom. It is advised that your place of worship be in the northeast direction. Also you can place an idol of Buddha in the northeast direction of your living room. This indicates spirituality and helps in seeking connection with oneself and God. Similarly wind chimes in the west direction signify your overall development both professionally and personally.

To avoid: paintings depicting scary marks, scenes of Ramayana or Mahabharata, nude portraits, aggressive and abstract paintings with conflicting colours. Also, heavy statues should not be placed in the northeast area of the room. Statues or figures of wild beasts and birds should be avoided.

To go for: Temples, paintings of nature scenes, prayer, and temples usher in good health and better living. Rangoli, Om and Swastika symbols can be safely used as they ward off evil spirits and influences.

4. Avoid Overhead Beams

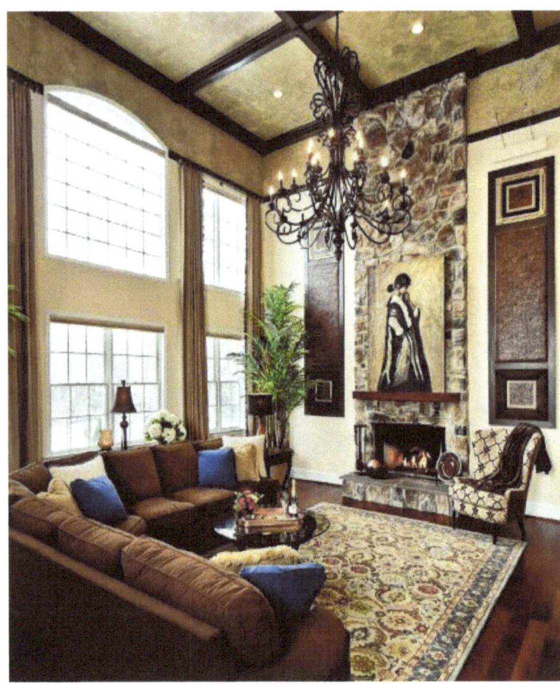

Fig. 39.26: *Photograph of a small living room. This is decorated with a chandelier on the beam to balance the energies.*

Beams and columns are the base for strong foundation of the house. The floors and walls and in total, your house is held together by the beam. Such is the strength of beam. So it is obvious that if a person sits or sleeps under an overhead beam for long hours, then the negative effects of beam are felt. Exposed beams in the living room are said to have depressing effects, which can lead to disagreements and argument in the family as per principles of Vastu. Also exposure to beam leads to reduced work efficiency and ill health. A point to be noted here is the height of the ceiling. If the ceiling is at a considerable height then the affect of beam is reduced. But if the ceiling is low then the beam causes lot of negative energy to flow. And also if the beam is a very structurally important one, then its side effects will be felt. So the effect of the beam is influenced by the height of ceiling, the type of beam and the time you spend under the beam.

To avoid: Sitting below the overhead beams for they will lead to you constantly worrying about something or the other.

To go for: Try masking the beams with a false ceiling or hang a lighting fixture or chandelier on the beam to balance the energies.

5. No Clutter in Bedrooms

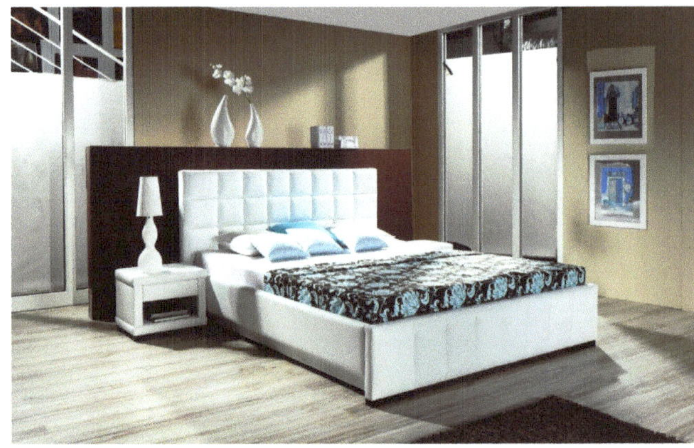

Fig. 39.27: *Photograph of a clean and neat modern bed room which is clutter free, giving us peaceful and calm atmosphere.*

Collecting and preserving things from the past is said to hinder your growth for the future. It makes you stuck in an endless circle of emotions. So it is advisable that you just keep a limited amount of things if at all it is to be stored as valuable memory treasures. Vastu believes that cluttering of objects leads to negative vibrations especially in the bedroom. In fact, bedroom is a room where you should be able to calm yourself totally and be at peace. That is the reason that things should be neatly organised be it your home or in cupboards or shelves. This leads to you being organised in life too. Clean all the shelves periodically.

This helps in disposing all the unwanted stuff and that is how you reduce the clutter at home.

To avoid: Things under the bed as they affect the subconscious mind and cause disruptions during your sleep, even footwear should not be placed under the bed.

To go for: Clean and neat bedroom area for a peaceful and calm atmosphere which helps you to live life optimally and in a well organized manner.

Clutter at home disturbs or cuts the passage of energy flow. When your home becomes free from clutter, it increases the productivity in you. It makes you less distractive and more productive.

Vastu Shastra is all about tapping the positive reserves of energy and utilizing it in a fruitful way. Follow the above tips to channelize and harness the positive energy. Let positive aura flow throughout your house and surroundings. Also let your home emit positive vibes while attracting positive energies. Vastu is not tough to incorporate or tough to heed. But the effects of Vastu are enormous enough to let you and your family live a happy and contented life. And this applies both to your personal as well as professional front.

Your home is where your heart is and hence you need to ensure it is rightly filled with the most suitable and essential things which bring in positive and peaceful vibrations.

Precautions as per Vastu for home

- Never keep a dustbin in the northeast corner of your house. This corner is the most auspicious sacred corner according to Vastu Shastra.
- Extension of the house other than north-east is a Vastu defect and needs a strong Vastu correction.
- The nonworking clocks or watches at home or office should be removed as they generate negative energy. Clocks should always be kept in ready to use condition.
- Vastu Shasta does not recommend a spiral staircase. It acts like a corkscrew creating negative energy.
- Avoid materials from an old building to build a new one. Otherwise, those old materials may repeat negative incidents that occurred in the old house.
- Avoid Vastu house adjacent to dilapidated buildings and cemeteries. They are without any life.
- According to Vastu, the shadow of the tree should not fall on your house between 9 am to 3 pm. Its called a "Chhaya Vedh" according to Vastu Shastra.

The energy of your house- Purifying your home for more positivity.

Purify your house by moping a floor with *Himalayan rock salt* once a week. It mobilizes fresh energy inside the house and also removes the negative one. Cobwebs symbolize being wrapped up and stuck physically & financially. Clear them away so you can move forward. Always keep the corners very bright. Corners in a Vastu are very potent energy sources. To protect your house from the pollutant energy, toilet lids should always be closed when not in "active use.

Bibliography and Acknowledgement

- Acharya P.K. (1933), Manasara (English translation), Online proofread edition including footnotes and glossary
- Acharya P.K. (1946), An Encyclopedia of Hindu Architecture, Oxford University Press - Terminology of Ancient Architecture
- Acharya P.K. (1946), An Encyclopedia of Hindu Architecture, Oxford University Press
- Acharya P.K. (1946), Bibliography of Ancient Sanskrit Treatises on Architecture and Arts, in An Encyclopedia of Hindu Architecture, Oxford University Press - pages 615-659
- Alice Boner and Sadāśiva Rath Śarmā (1966), Silpa Prakasa Medieval Orissan Sanskrit Text on Temple Architecture at Google Books, E.J. Brill (Netherlands)
- Arya, Rohit Vaastu: the Indian art of placement : design and decorate homes to reflect eternal spiritual principles Inner Traditions / Bear & Company, 2000, ISBN 0-89281-885-9.
- B. B. Puri, Applied vastu shastra vaibhavam in modern architecture, Vastu Gyan Publication, 1997, ISBN 978-81-900614-1-4.
- B.B. Dutt (1925), Town Planning in Ancient India at Google Books
- D. N. Shukla, Vastu-Sastra: Hindu Science of Architecture, Munshiram Manoharial Publishers, 1993, ISBN 978-81-215-0611-3.
- Dutt (1925), Town planning in Ancient India at Google Books, ISBN 978-81-8205-487-5; See critical review by LD Barnett, Bulletin of the School of Oriental and African Studies, Vol 4, Issue 2, June 1926, pp 391
- Gautum, Jagdish (2006). Latest Vastu Shastra (Some Secrets). Abhinav Publications. p. 17. ISBN 978-81-7017-449-3.
- GD Vasudev (2001), Vastu, Motilal Banarsidas, ISBN 81-208-1605-6, pp 74-92
- George Michell (1988), The Hindu Temple: An Introduction to Its Meaning and Forms, University of Chicago Press, ISBN 978-0226532301, pp 21-22
- Golden Principles of Vastu Shastra Vastukarta". www. vastukarta.com. Retrieved 8 May 2016.
- Gudrun Bühnemann (2003). Mandalas and Yantras in the Hindu Traditions. BRILL Academic. pp. 251–254. ISBN 90-4-12902-2.

- IVVRF (2000), *Journal of International Conference Vastu Panorama 2000*, Main Theme - The Study of Energetic Dimension of Man and Behavior of Environment
- IVVRF (2004), *Journal of International Conference Vastu Panorama* 2004
- IVVRF (2008), *Journal of International Conference Vastu Panorama* 2008, Main Theme - Save Mother earth and life- A Vastu Mission
- IVVRF (2012), *Journal of International Conference Vastu Panorama* 2012, Main Theme- Vastu Dynamics for Global Well Being
- Jack Hebner (2010), Architecture of the Vāstu Śastra - According to Sacred Science, in Science of the Sacred (Editor: David Osborn), ISBN 978-0557277247, pp. 85-92; N Lahiri (1996), Archaeological landscapes and textual images: a study of the sacred geography of late medieval Ballabgarh, World Archaeology, 28(2), pp 244-264
- K, George Varghese (2003). "Globalisation Traumas and New Social Imaginary: Visvakarma Community of Kerala". Economic and Political Weekly. 38 (45): 4794–4802. JSTOR 4414253 – via JSTOR.
- Kumar, Vijaya (2002). Vastushastra. New Dawn/Sterling. p. 5. ISBN 978-81-207-2199-9.
- LD Barnett, Bulletin of the School of Oriental and African Studies, Vol 4, Issue 2, June 1926, pp 391
- Meister, Michael W. (1983). "Geometry and Measure in Indian Temple Plans: Rectangular Temples". Artibus Asiae. 44 (4): 266–296. doi:10.2307/3249613. JSTOR 3249613.
- Milton Singer (1991). Semiotics of Cities, Selves, and Cultures: Explorations in Semiotic Anthropology. Walter de Gruyter. p. 117. ISBN 978-3-11-085775-7.
- Narlikar, Jayant V. (2009). "Astronomy, pseudoscience and rational thinking". In Percy, John; Pasachoff, Jay (eds.). Teaching and Learning Astronomy: Effective Strategies for Educators Worldwide. Cambridge University Press. p. 165. ISBN 9780521115391.
- Prabhu, Balagopal, T.S and Achyuthan, A, "A text Book of Vastuvidya", Vastuvidyapratisthanam, Kozhikode, New Edition, 2011.
- Prabhu, Balagopal, T.S and Achyuthan, A, "Design in Vastuvidya", Vastuvidyapratisthanam, Kozhiko
- Prabhu, Balagopal, T.S and Achyuthan, A, "Manusyalaya candrika- An Engineering Commentary", Vastuvidyapratisthanam, Kozhikode, New Edition, 2011.
- Prabhu, Balagopal, T.S, "Vastuvidyadarsanam", (Malayalam) Vastuvidyapratisthanam, Kozhikode.
- Quack, Johannes (2012). Disenchanting India: Organized Rationalism and Criticism of Religion in India. Oxford University Press. p. 119. ISBN 9780199812608. Retrieved 17 August 2015.
- R Arya, Vaastu: The Indian Art of Placement, ISBN 978-0892818853
- Sherri Silverman (2007), Vastu: Transcendental Home Design in Harmony with Nature, Gibbs Smith, Utah, ISBN 978-1423601326.
- Siddharth, Dr. Jayshree Om: The Ancient Science of Vastu, 2020, ISBN 978-93-90030-07-1
- Stella Kramrisch (1976), The Hindu Temple Volume 1 & 2, ISBN 81-208-0223-3
- Susan Lewandowski (1984), Buildings and Society: Essays on the Social Development of the Built Environment, edited by Anthony D. King, Routledge, ISBN 978-0710202345, Chapter 4
- V. Chakraborty, Indian Architectural Theory: Contemporary Uses of Vastu Vidya at Google Books
- Vastu: Transcendental Home Design in Harmony with Nature, Sherri Silverman
- Vastu-Silpa Kosha, Encyclopedia of Hindu Temple architecture and Vastu/S.K.Ramachandara Rao, Delhi, Devine Books, (Lala Murari Lal Chharia Oriental series) ISBN 978-93-81218-51-8 (Set)
- Vibhuti Chakrabarti (2013). Indian Architectural Theory and Practice: Contemporary Uses of Vastu Vidya. Routledge. pp. 1–2. ISBN 978-1-136-77882-7.
- Vibhuti Chakrabarti, Indian Architectural Theory: Contemporary Uses of Vastu Vidya Routledge, 1998, ISBN 978-0-7007-1113-0.
- Vibhuti Sachdev, Giles Tillotson (2004). Building Jaipur: The Making of an Indian City. pp. 155–160. ISBN 978-1861891372.
- Vibhuti Sachdev, Giles Tillotson (2004). Building Jaipur: The Making of an Indian City. p. 147. ISBN 978-1861891372.

Element of Water,Its Sources, Conservation,Desalination And Health Benefits - Overview

History of water on Earth

One factor in estimating when water appeared on Earth is that water is continually being lost to space. H_2O molecules in the atmosphere are broken up by photolysis, and the resulting free hydrogen atoms can sometimes escape Earth's gravitational pull (see : *Atmospheric escape*). When the Earth was younger and less massive, water would have been lost to space more easily. Lighter elements like hydrogen and helium are expected to leak from the atmosphere continually, but isotopic ratios of heavier noble gases in the modern atmosphere suggest that even the heavier elements in the early atmosphere were subject to significant losses.

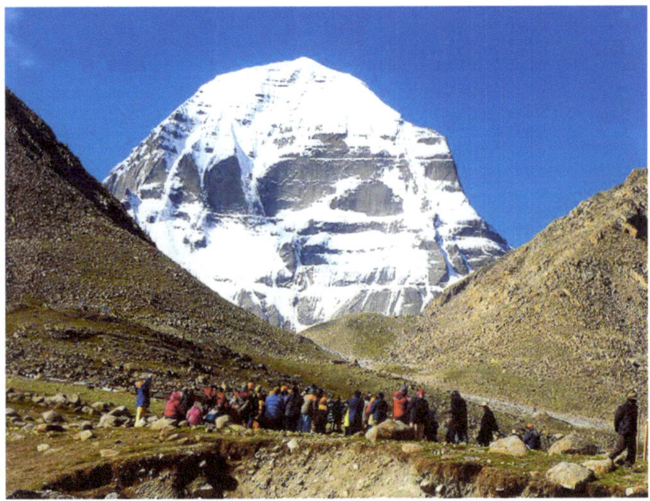

Fig. 40.1: *Mount Kailash is the most visited holy mountain in the world. A historical point in the world, with the origination of four of the most sacred rivers ensuring that Mount Kailash sits at a very high position of religious virtue. The four sacred streams which flow from M ount K ailash are – T he Indus River, Sutlej River, Brahmaputra River, and Karnali River.*

In particular, xenon is useful for calculations of water loss over time. Not only is it a noble gas (and therefore is not removed from the atmosphere through chemical reactions with other elements), but comparisons between abundances of its nine stable isotopes in the modern atmosphere reveal that the Earth lost at least one ocean of water early in its history, between the Hadean and Archean eras.

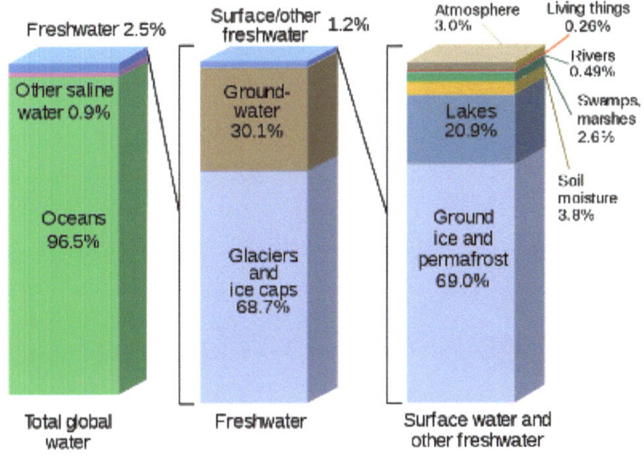

Fig. 40.2: *A graphical distribution of the locations of water on Earth. Only 3% of the Earth's water is fresh water. Most of it is in icecaps and glaciers (69%) and groundwater (30%), while all lakes, rivers and swamps combined only account for a small fraction (0.3%) of the Earth's total freshwater reserves.*

Any water on Earth during the later part of its accretion would have been disrupted by the Moon-forming impact (>4.5 billion years ago), which likely vaporized much of Earth's crust and upper mantle and created a rock-vapor atmosphere around the young planet. The rock vapor would have condensed within two thousand years, leaving behind hot volatiles which probably resulted in a majority carbon dioxide atmosphere with hydrogen and water vapor. Afterwards, liquid water oceans may have existed despite the surface temperature of 230 °C (446 °F) due to the increased atmospheric pressure of the CO_2 atmosphere. As cooling continued, most CO_2 was removed from the atmosphere by subduction and dissolution in ocean water, but levels oscillated wildly as new surface and mantle cycles appeared

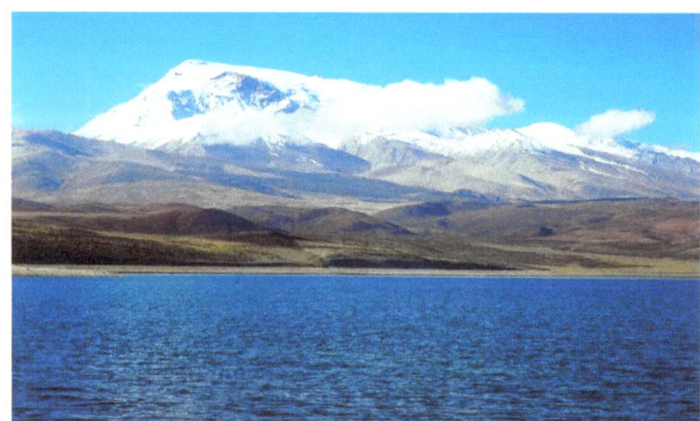

Fig. 40.3:*Photograph showing Kailash Mansarovar one of the four river emerging from Mount Kailash*

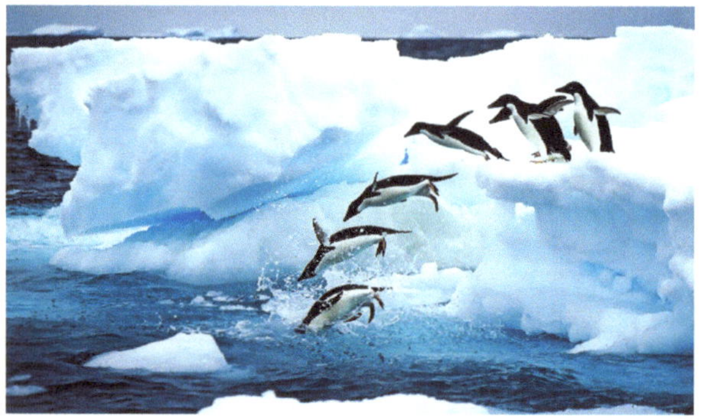

Fig.40.4:*Glaciers are the natural storage of water. Photograph of One of Antarctica's biggest glaciers Is eroding faster than thought*

Global Water Scarcity Scenario

Six hundred sixty three million people in the world do not have access to clean water and over 2.7 billion people face water shortages for at least one month out of the year. Fresh water sources account for less than 3 percent of the world's water supply, and the majority of earth's naturally occurring, fresh water is in *glaciers* — inaccessible to be used for consumption. Water usage has increased at twice the rate as that of the world's population growth. The agriculture industry is attributed to 70 percent of the world's water withdrawal. At the current rate, nearly two-thirds of the world could face water shortages by 2025. In much of the developing world, clean water is a commodity that requires funding, transportation and physical labor to obtain.

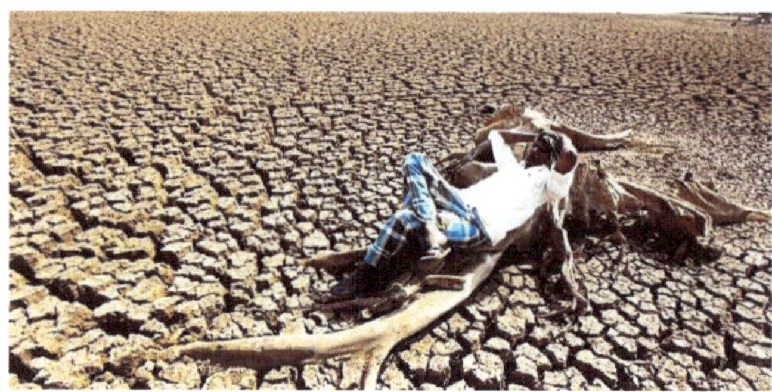

Fig, 40.5 *After Rajasthan, Karnataka has most drought-ravaged land in the country. Photograph of one of the agricultural land under severe drought in Karnataka, India*

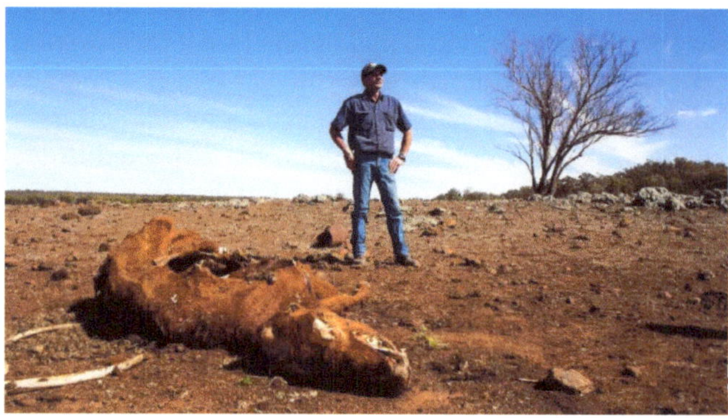

Fig, 40.6: *Greg Jerry, owner of a 3,300 hectare farm near the town of Coonabarabran in Australia, has lost 60 sheep and a dozen cows to the drought.*

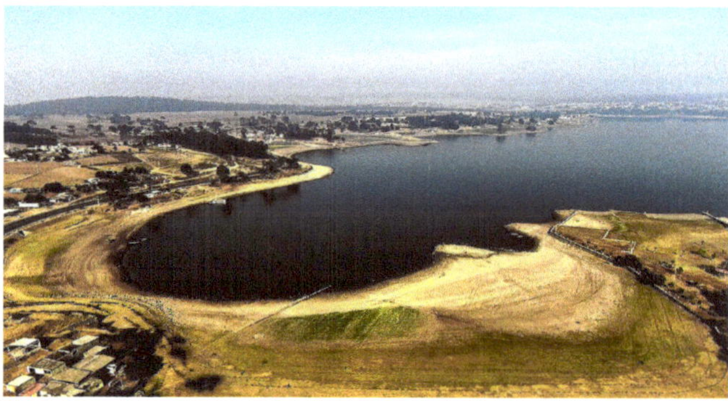

Fig. 40.7: *An aerial view of Villa Victoria Dam, the main water supply for Mexico City residents, on the outskirts of Toluca, Mexico Thursday, April 22, 2021. Drought conditions now cover 85% of Mexico, and in areas around Mexico City and Michoacán, the problem has gotten so bad that lakes and reservoirs are drying up. (AP Photo/Fernando Llano)*

Women around the world spend a total of 200 million hours a day traveling to collect water, taking time away from their economic activities and families. Fifty percent of those facing water scarcity live in India and China, and 500 million people live in regions where the water supply cannot keep up with the rate of water consumption. Though there is sufficient water on the planet to meet the needs of the world population, water distribution, usage, climate and pollution limit the amount of consumable water available from region to region, causing water stress or scarcity. Water scarcity may be caused by a lack of water supply altogether, or a lack of consumable supply due to contamination or salination. When there is insufficient water supply for irrigation, certain crops and products can become scarce, causing food shortages in already strained regions. Just 2.5 percent of the world's water is freshwater, and only 0.007 percent of all water is both fresh and available for use. An estimated 326,000,000,000,000,000,000 gallons — or 326 quintillions — of water are on the planet, and if just 0.007 percent of that volume is available and fresh, 2,282,000,000,000,000,000 gallons — over 2 quadrillions — of freshwater are readily accessible for human use.

Hypotheses for the origins of Earth s water

Extraplanetary sources

Water has a much lower condensation temperature than other materials that compose the terrestrial planets in the Solar System, such as iron and silicates. The region of the protoplanetary disk closest to the Sun was very hot early in the history of the Solar System, and it is not feasible that oceans of water condensed with the Earth as it formed. Further from the young Sun where temperatures were cooler, water could condense and form *icy planetesimals.* The boundary of the region where ice could form in the early Solar System is known as the frost line (or snow line), and is located in the modern asteroid belt, between about 2.7 and 3.1 astronomical units (AU) from the Sun. It is therefore necessary that objects forming beyond the frost line–such as comets, trans-Neptunian objects, and water-rich meteoroids (protoplanets)–delivered water to Earth. However, the timing of this delivery is still in question.

One hypothesis claims that Earth accreted (gradually grew by accumulation of) icy planetesimals about 4.5 billion years ago, when it was 60 to 90% of its current size. In this scenario, Earth was able to retain water in some form throughout accretion and major impact events. This hypothesis is supported by similarities in the abundance and the isotope ratios of water between the oldest known carbonaceous chondrite meteorites and meteorites from Vesta, both of which originate from the Solar System's asteroid belt. It is also supported by studies of osmium isotope ratios, which suggest that a sizeable quantity of water was contained in the material that *Earth* accreted early on. Measurements of the chemical composition of lunar samples collected by the Apollo 15 and 17 missions further support this, and indicate that water was already present on Earth before the Moon was formed.

One problem with this hypothesis is that the noble gas isotope ratios of Earth's atmosphere are different from those of its mantle, which suggests they were formed from different sources. To explain this observation, a so-called "*late veneer*" theory has been proposed in which water was delivered much later in Earth's history, after the Moon-forming impact.

However, the current understanding of Earth's formation allows for less than 1% of Earth's material accreting after the Moon formed, implying that the material accreted later must have been very water-rich. Models of early Solar System dynamics have shown that icy asteroids could have been delivered to the inner Solar System (including Earth) during this period if Jupiter migrated closer to the Sun.

Yet a third hypothesis, supported by evidence from molybdenum isotope ratios, suggests that the Earth gained most of its water from the same interplanetary collision that caused the formation of the Moon.

The various sources of Water

We all know how important water is to us. 3/4 of the earth's surface is covered with water. This water is distributed throughout the planet in various forms and shapes, called the various water bodies. These water bodies differ in size, right from huge ones like oceans and seas to the small ones like ponds. Thus the various water bodies we see on the earth's surface are in the form of oceans, seas, lakes, rivers, ponds, waterfalls etc.

Different Bodies of Water and their Characteristics

Let us travel the earth and learn about these various water bodies found only on our beautiful planet.

Oceans

The oceans are vast and deep bodies of water. Usually, it is these oceans that separate continents from one another. The oceans are bodies of salt water. We have five oceans in our world. They are the Pacific Ocean, the *Atlantic* Ocean, *Indian Ocean*, *Arctic Ocean,* the Southern Ocean or Antarctic Ocean. The largest and deepest ocean in the world is the *Pacific ocean*, covering one-third of the earth's surface.

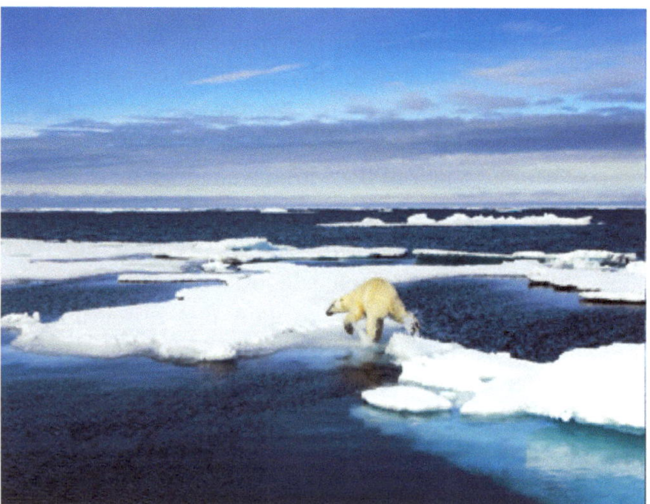

Fig. 40.8: *Arctic Ocean, is the smallest and shallowest of all other oceans. It is located near the North pole Polar bears hunt for seals through polar ice.*

This is followed by the Atlantic ocean and the Indian ocean in order of size. Oceans are home to a variety of plants and seaweed and thousands of sea creatures like the sea urchins,whales, sharks, octopus, a variety of fish, snakes, squids etc. In fact, oceans also contain millions of tiny dead animals called coral polyps which form the beautiful coral reefs, Australia being the largest coral reef in the world. Oceans are useful to us in many ways as they are a rich source of minerals, they provide energy and valuable fuels like petroleum. They work as an important channel of transportation.

Seas

Seas are also big water bodies but are definitely smaller than oceans. They are partly enclosed by a land mass and open into the ocean. We see many seas eventually connecting to the oceans. For example we have the Mediterranean Sea which is attached or joins the Atlantic Ocean. Some of the seas are the Red Sea, the Black Sea, the *Arabian Sea*, *Caribbean Sea* and the *Mediterranean Sea*. The Red and the Black Sea, have got their names because the Red Sea has millions of red tiny plants growing at the bottom and the *Black Sea* because of the thick black mud that lies at its bottom. Under the seas we find huge plains, high mountains and even deep valleys, interesting isn't it, that these various landforms are also present under the sea. The largest of the seas is the South China Sea which is supposed be holding hundreds of islands in its waters .

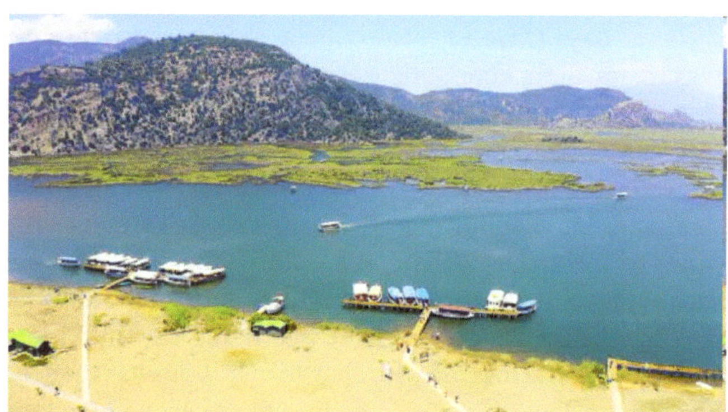

Fig. 40.9: *Aerial top view of a beach on the Mediterranean Sea*

The sea, like the oceans is useful to us in many ways.It is a rich source of food providing us with various kinds of sea food. It also works as a channel for transportation. Like oceans, seas are a source of food, and are also usually used extensively as transport lanes for ships.

Lakes

A lake is a water body surrounded by land on all sides. It is actually the opposite of an island, which is a piece of land surrounded by water on all sides. Lakes can be salty or fresh water lakes. Salty lakes are due to a lot of evaporation taking place. Some famous lakes are-Lake Superior, Caspian Sea, *Lake Victoria*, Lake Aral and the *Dal Lake*. In fact the Caspian Sea is the world's largest salt lake, it is so big that it is referred to as sea. Lake Superior is the biggest fresh water lake. The Dead Sea is a salt water lake. It is said that nothing can survive in the Dead Sea because it is very salty.

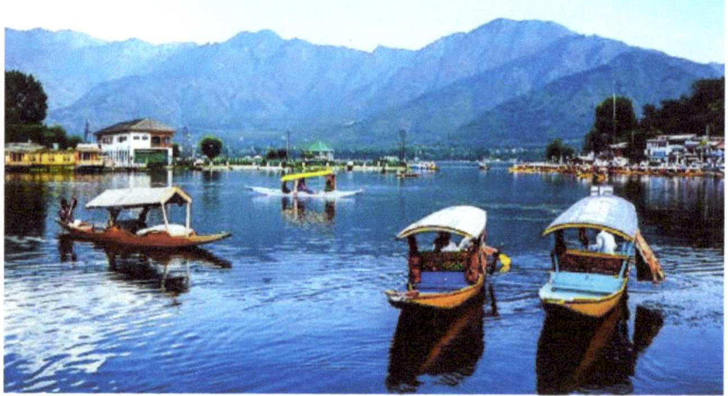

Fig.40.10: showing view of Dal Lake Srinagar with floating shikaras

Rivers

Rivers are large streams that flow over the land. They are hence large flowing water bodies, they usually end up in an ocean or sea. Rivers are fresh water bodies which generally originate in mountainous areas or elevated areas. We have basically two kinds of rivers which are, the Snow-fed rivers and the second is the Rain-fed rivers.

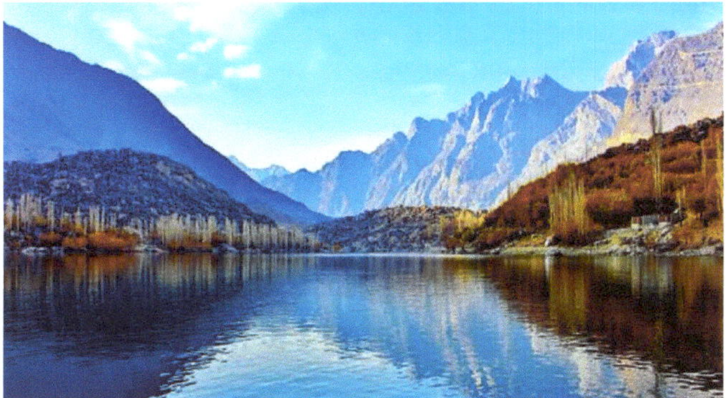

Fig.40.11: *The Indus civilisation flourished along a course abandoned by the major Himalayan river Sutlej, and did not develop around a flowing river as believed, scientists from India and the UK have found.*

Snow-fed rivers find their source in the snow capped mountains, where the snow melts, flowing down forming rivers, rain-fed rivers as the name suggests are formed in areas where it rains a lot giving rise to these rivers. The place where a river starts its journey, is called the source and the place where it ends its journey, is called the mouth of a river. Rivers again are very useful as we have seen in history,that most civilizations were formed near the banks of the rivers, like the Egyptian Civilization on the banks of the River Nile, the *Indus Valley Civilization* on the banks of the *River Indus*. This is because the rivers deposit a lot of fertile soil called silt which is excellent for the growing of crops.

Gulf

A gulf is a large area of an ocean or a sea that is partially enclosed by land. For Example the *Gulf of Mexico.*

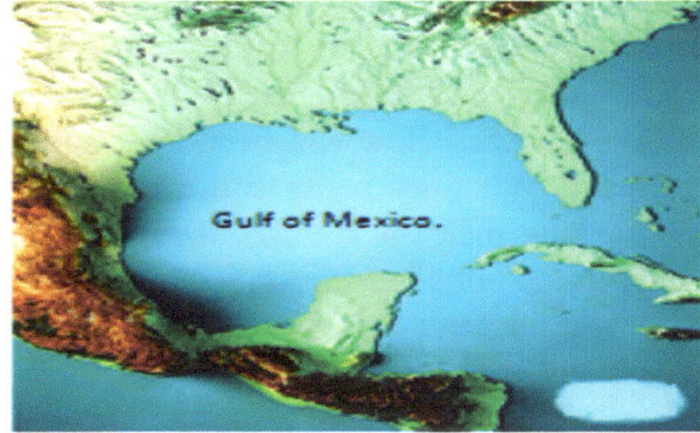

Fig. 40.12: *showing view of the Gulf of Mexico.*

Bay

A bay is a body of water, which is again partially enclosed by land. It is a wide mouth opening of land, where the water is surrounded by land on three sides and is joined to the sea on the fourth side.

For example the *Bay of Bengal*

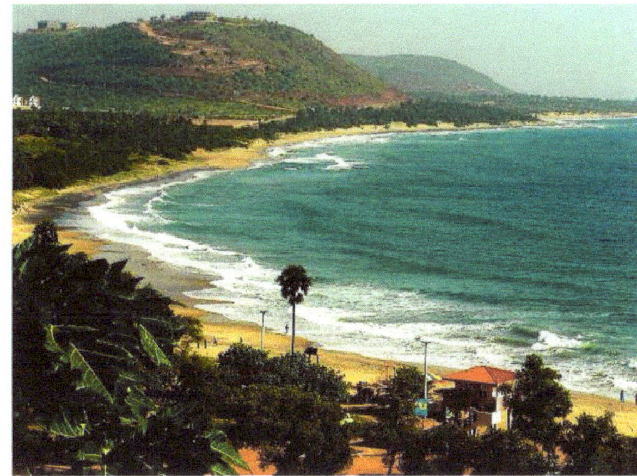

Fig. 40.13: *view of beach of Bay of Bengal*

Lagoon

A lagoon is a lake separated from the open sea by sand or rocks. *Lake Chilika* in Orissa, India is an example of a lagoon.

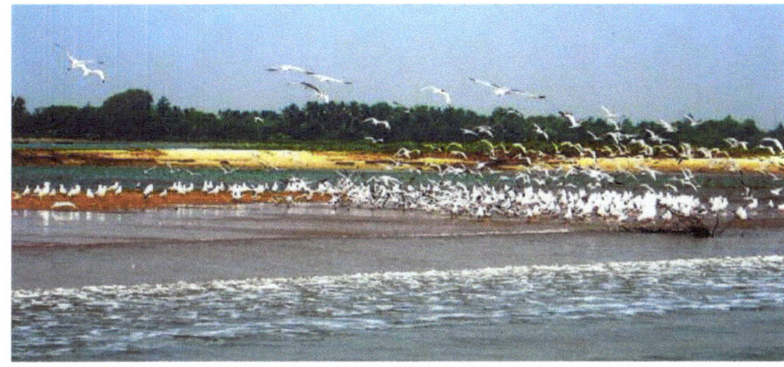

Fig.40.14: *view of Chilika lake which is the largest brackish water lagoon of Asian continent situated on East coast of India. It runs along the borders of three districts of Puri, Khurda and Ganjam and finally j oins t he B ay o f Bengal through a narrow mouth, forming an enormous lagoon of brackish water.*

Starait

A strait is a narrow stretch of water which joins two larger water bodies. For example : *Palk Strait* joining the Bay of Bengal and the Indian Ocean.

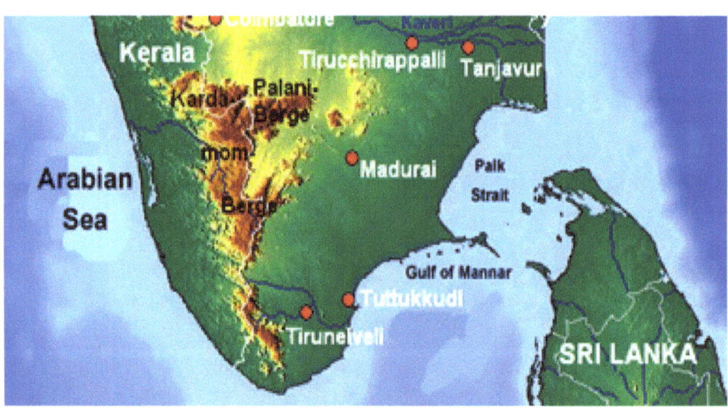

Fig. 40.15:*view of the Gulf of Mannar is a shallow bay, part of the Laccadive Sea in the Indian Ocean. A chain of low islands and reefs known as Adam's Bridge, also called Ramsethu, which includes Mannar Island, separates the Gulf of Mannar from Palk Strait, which lies to the north between India and Sri Lanka*

Waterfall

Water falling from a height is usually called a waterfall. A waterfall is formed when a river flows over an edge of hard rocks and falls from a great height. Waterfalls make beautiful tourist spots and are helpful in generating hydroelectric power. *The Angel falls* in South America are the world's highest waterfall.

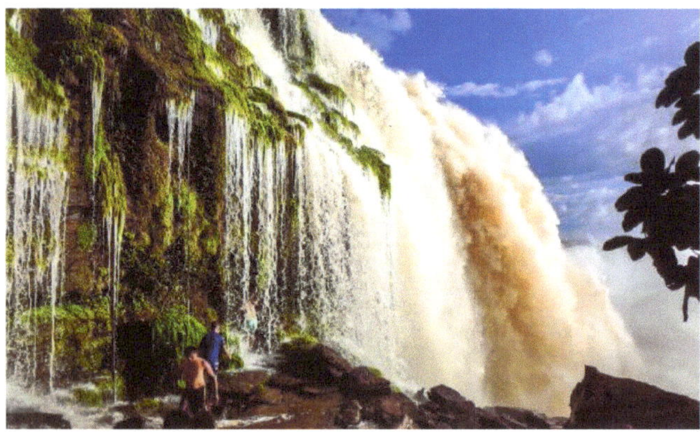

Fig 40.16: *Showing view of The Angel falls in South America. It is the world's highest waterfall, the main drop being 807.1 metres (2,648 ft.) with a total vertical drop of 979 metres (3,212 ft.). It drops over the edge of Auyán Tepuy, a table top mountain in the Canaima National Park*

Important questions frequently asked regarding the water

Where does water come from?

Water is made up of hydrogen and oxygen, and it exists in gaseous, liquid, and solid states. Water is one of the most plentiful and essential compounds, occurring as a liquid on Earth's surface under normal conditions, which makes it invaluable for human uses and as plant and animal habitat. Since water is readily changed to a vapour (gas), it can travel through the atmosphere from the oceans inland, where it condenses and nourishes life.

Why do cold water bottles and soft-drink bottles sweat?

A cold water bottle appears to sweat because it's a cooling source for the water vapour in the layer of air that surrounds the bottle. Air that is relatively warm can hold more water vapour than cooler air. When the cold water bottle is introduced, the warm air near the bottle cools and some of the water vapour condenses into liquid water, which is then deposited on the outside of the bottle.

When does water boil?

Boiling occurs when bubbles form within a liquid, marking a change from a substance's liquid or solid phase into a gas. The normal boiling point is the temperature at which the liquid's vapour pressure equals the standard sea level atmospheric pressure (760 mm [29.92 inches] of mercury). At sea level, atmospheric pressure is high, and water boils at 100 °C (212 °F); at higher altitudes it is lower, so water boils at a lower temperature.

Why is water blue?

Water appears blue for two important reasons. In small quantities water appears colourless, but water actually has an intrinsic blue colour caused by the slight absorption of light at red wavelengths. For larger bodies of water—ponds, rivers, lakes, and oceans—water appears blue on clear days because it mirrors the blueness of the sky. On overcast days, larger water bodies appear gray

When is water the most dense?

Water's density is greatest at about 4 °C (39.2 °F), in the liquid phase. Ice, water's solid phase, is more buoyant, so it forms at the surface of water bodies and freezes downward. Lakes and rivers rarely freeze completely, and the liquid water below can become a winter refuge for aquatic life. When ice melts in the spring, the slowly warming surface meltwater sinks, displacing the water below and mixing nutrients throughout the water column.

Extraterrestrial liquid water

Extraterrestrial liquid water (from the Latin words : extra ["outside of, beyond"] and terrestris ["of or belonging to Earth"]) is water in its liquid state that naturally occurs outside Earth. It is a subject of wide interest because it is recognized as one of the key prerequisites for life as we know it and thus surmised as essential for extraterrestrial life.

Though there are several *celestial bodies* in the Solar system to have a hydrosphere Earth still is the only celestial body known to have stable bodies of liquid water on its surface, with oceanic water covering 71% of its surface, and liquid water is essential to all known life forms on Earth. The presence of water on the surface of Earth is a product of its atmospheric pressure and a stable orbit in the Sun's circumstellar habitable zone, though the origin of Earth's water remains unknown.

The main methods currently used for confirmation are absorption spectroscopy and geochemistry. These techniques have proven effective for atmospheric water vapour and ice. However, using current methods of astronomical spectroscopy it is substantially more difficult to detect liquid water on terrestrial planets, especially in the case of subsurface water. Due to this, astronomers, astrobiologists and planetary scientists use habitable zone, gravitational and tidal theory, models of planetary differentiation and radiometry to determine potential for liquid water. Water observed in volcanic activity can provide more compelling indirect evidence, as can fluvial features and the presence of antifreeze agents, such as salts or ammonia.

Using such methods, many scientists infer that liquid water once covered large areas of Mars and Venus. Water is thought to exist as liquid beneath the surface of some planetary bodies, similar to *groundwater* on Earth. Water vapour is sometimes considered conclusive evidence for the presence of liquid water, although atmospheric water vapour may be found to exist in many places where liquid water does not. Similar indirect evidence, however, supports the existence of liquids below the surface of several moons and dwarf planets elsewhere in the Solar System. Some are speculated to be large extraterrestrial "oceans". Liquid water is thought to be common in other planetary systems, despite the lack of conclusive evidence, and there is a growing list of extrasolar candidates for liquid water. In June 2020, NASA scientists reported that it is likely that exoplanets with oceans may be common in the Milky Way galaxy, based on mathematical modeling studie

Liquid water in the Solar System

As of December 2015, the confirmed liquid water in the Solar System outside Earth is 25–50 times the volume of Earth's water (1.3 billion cubic kilometers).

Mars

The Mars ocean hypothesis suggests that nearly a third of the surface of *Mars* was once covered by water, though the water on Mars is no longer oceanic (much of it residing in the ice caps).

A cross-section of Mars underground ice is exposed at the steep slope that appears bright blue in this enhanced-color view from the MRO. The scene is about 500 meters wide. The scarp drops about 128 meters from the level ground in the upper third of the image

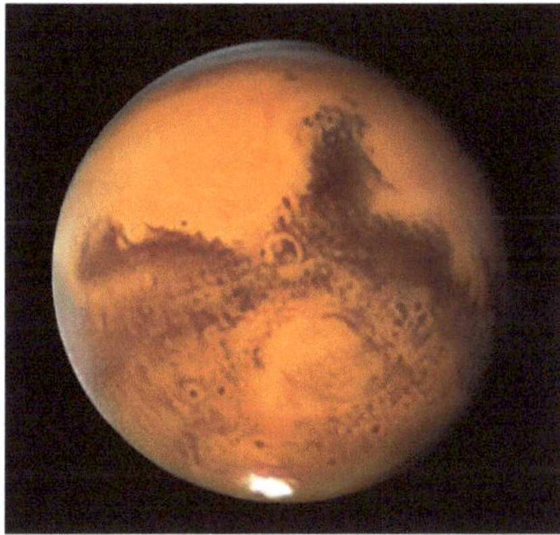

Fig. 40.17: *showing view of Mars which is at its biggest and brightest right now as the Red Planet lines up with Earth on the same side of the Sun. Every 26 months, the pair take up this arrangement, moving close together, before then diverging again on their separate orbits around our star.*

Water on Mars exists today almost exclusively as ice, with a small amount present in the atmosphere as vapour. Some liquid water may occur transiently on the Martian surface today but only under certain conditions.. No large standing bodies of liquid water exist because the atmospheric pressure at the surface averages just 600 pascals (0.087 psi)—about 0.6% of Earth's mean sea level pressure—and because the global average temperature is far too low (210 K (−63 °C)), leading to either rapid evaporation or freezing. Features called recurring slope lineae are thought to be caused by flows of brine — hydrated salts.

In July 2018, scientists from the Italian Space Agency reported the detection of a *subglacial lake on Mar*s, 1.5 kilometres (0.93 mi) below the southern polar ice cap, and spanning 20 kilometres (12 mi) horizontally, the first evidence for a stable body of liquid water on the planet. Because the temperature at the base of the polar cap is estimated at 205 K (−68 °C; −91 °F), scientists assume that the water may remain liquid by the antifreeze effect of magnesium and calcium perchlorates. The 1.5-kilometre (0.93 mi) ice layer covering the lake is composed of water ice with 10 to 20% admixed dust, and seasonally covered by a 1-metre (3 ft 3 in)-thick layer of CO_2 ice..

Europa (Moon of Jupiter)

Scientists' consensus is that a layer of liquid water exists beneath *Europa's (moon of Jupiter)* surface, and that heat from tidal flexing allows the subsurface ocean to remain liquid.It is estimated that the outer crust of solid ice is approximately 10–30 km (6–19 mi) thick, including a ductile "warm ice" layer, which could mean that the liquid ocean underneath may be about 100 km (60 mi) deep. This leads to a volume of Europa's oceans of 3 × 1018 m3, slightly more than two times the volume of Earth's oceans.

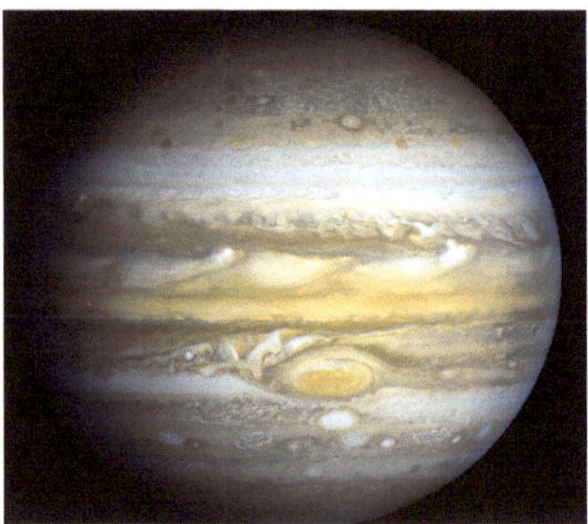

Fig. 40.18:*showing high-resolution global view of Europa (moon of Jupiter) Jupiter from Voyager 1 A 14-frame mosaic of Jupiter from Voyager 1.*

Enceladus (Moon of Saturn)

Enceladus, a moon of Saturn, has shown geysers of water, confirmed by the Cassini spacecraft in 2005 and analyzed more deeply in 2008. Gravimetric data in 2010–2011 confirmed a subsurface ocean.

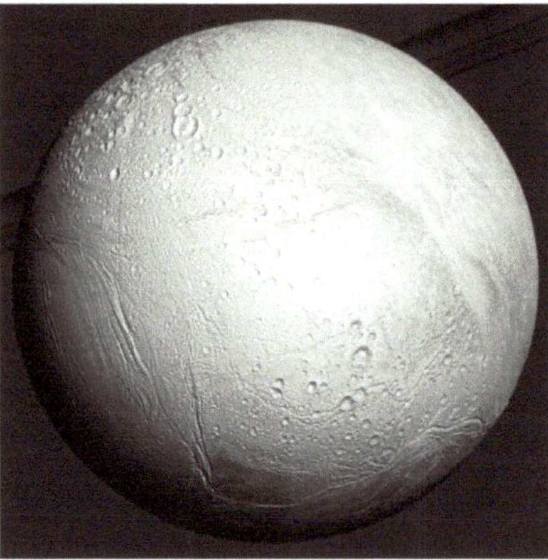

Fig. 40.19: *showing the grayscale image of Enceladus (moon of Saturn) is from NASA/JPL/Space Science Institute.*

"Saturn's moon Enceladus reflects sunlight brightly while the planet and its rings fill the background of this Cassini view. Enceladus is one of the most reflective bodies in the solar system because it is constantly coated by fresh, white ice particles.

While previously believed to be localized, most likely in a portion of the southern hemisphere, evidence revealed in 2015 now suggests the subsurface ocean is global in nature. In addition to water, these geysers from vents near the south pole contained small amounts of salt, nitrogen, carbon dioxide, and volatile hydrocarbons. The melting of the ocean water and the geysers appear to be driven by tidal flux from Saturn.

Ganymede (Satellite of Jupiter)

A subsurface saline ocean is theorized to exist on *Ganymede*, a moon of Jupiter, following observation by the Hubble Space Telescope in 2015. Patterns in auroral belts and rocking of the magnetic field suggest the presence of an ocean. It is estimated to be 100 km deep with the surface lying below a crust of 150 km of ice.

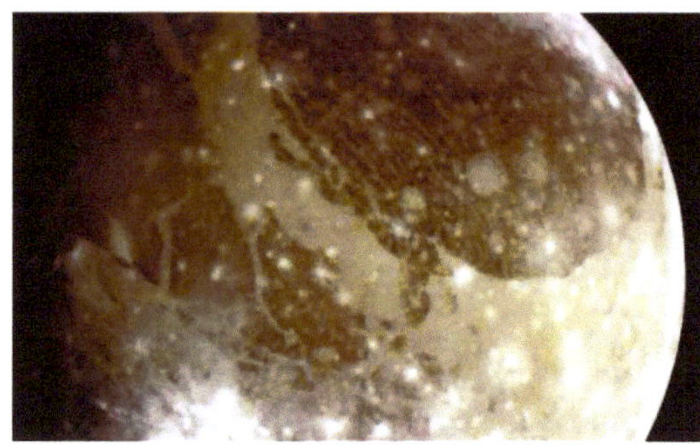

Fig. 40.20: *Showing view of Ganymede. Unlike Callisto, Ganymede, an equally icy satellite, reveals distinct patches of dark and light terrain.Ganymede's auroras change when interacting with Jupiter's magnetic field reveal t he likely existence of a subsurface ocean about 100 km (60 miles) thick. The trace components identified i n Ganymede's icy surface include a smaller amount of the same claylike dust found on Callisto and the same traces of solid carbon dioxide, hydrogen peroxide, and sulfur compounds, plus evidence for molecular oxygen and ozone trapped in the ice.*

Ceres

Ceres appears to be differentiated into a rocky core and icy mantle, and may have a remnant internal ocean of liquid water under the layer of ice. The surface is probably a mixture of water ice and various hydrated minerals such as carbonates and clay. In January 2014, emissions of water vapor were detected from several regions of Ceres. This was unexpected, because large bodies in the asteroid belt do not typically emit vapor, a hallmark of comets. Ceres also features a mountain called Ahuna Mons that is thought to be a cryovolcanic dome that facilitates the movement of high viscosity cryovolcanic magma consisting of water ice softened by its content of salts.

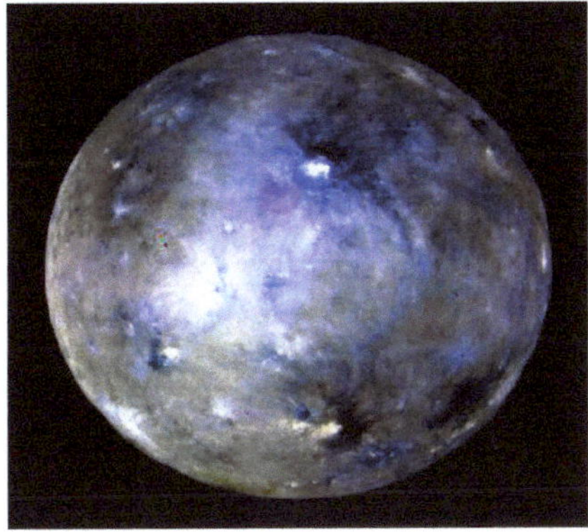

Fig.40.21:*Showing view of Ceres. This enhanced color image of Ceres' surface was made from data obtained on April 29, 2017, when NASA's Dawn spacecraft was exactly between the sun and Ceres. The brightest region on Ceres, called Cerealia Facula, is highlighted in Occator Crater in the center of this image. Vinalia Faculae, the set of secondary bright spots in the same crater, are located to the right of Cerealia Facula. The blueish color is generally found in association with young craters. Scientists believe the color relates to processes that occur when an impact ejects and redistributes material on the surface. The continuous bombardment of Ceres' surface by micrometeorites alters the texture of the exposed material, leading to its reddening.*

Ice giants (planets Uranus and Neptune)

The *"ice giant"* (sometimes known as "water giant") planets *Uranus* and *Neptune* are thought to have a supercritical water ocean beneath their clouds, which accounts for about two-thirds of their total mass, most likely surrounding small rocky cores, although a 2006 study by Wiktorowicz and Ingersall ruled out the possibility of such a water *"ocean"* existing on Neptune. This kind of planet is thought to be common in extrasolar planetary systems.

Outer Atmosphere, the upper cloud layer
Atmosphere (hydrogen, helium, methane gases)
Mantle (water, ammonia, methane ices)
Core (silicate/Fe-Ni rock)
A
B
C

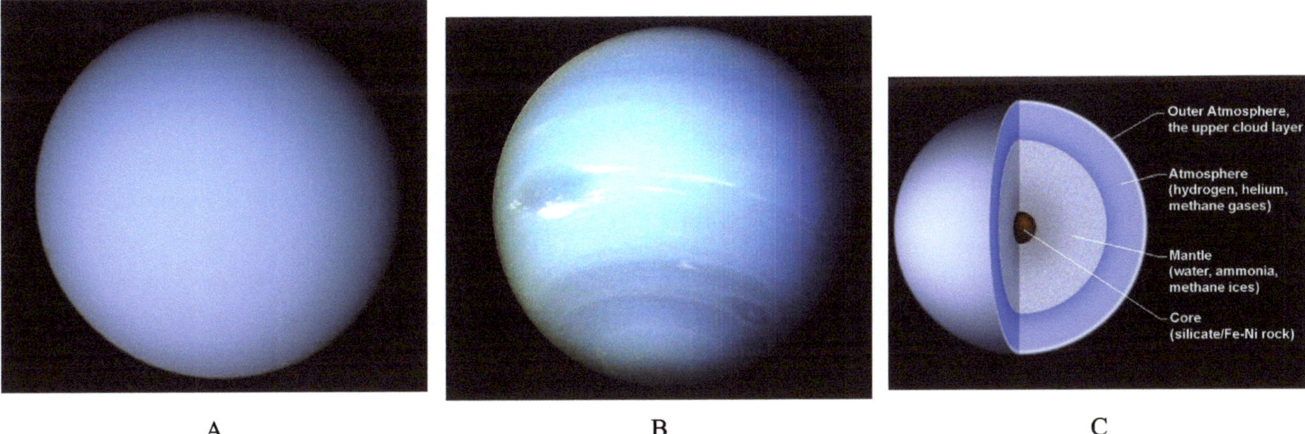

Fig. 40.22: *Within our solar system there are two ice giants that take the form of Uranus and Neptune and are named ice giants due to the ice compounds that have been incorporated in to the planets during their formation A. Showing features of Uranus B. Features of Neptune.C. The ice within the ice giants?takes the form of heavier volatile substances that are referred to as 'ices', although no there is very little ice left in the structure of the planets. With their main constituents being made up of substances heavier than hydrogen and helium, in the form of oxygen, carbon, nitrogen, and sulfur.*

Pluto

In June 2020, astronomers reported evidence that the dwarf planet *Pluto* may have had a subsurface ocean, and consequently may have been habitable, when it was first formed. Both Arrokoth (recently visited by NASA's New Horizons mission) and Pluto are in the Kuiper Belt – a donut-shaped region of icy bodies beyond the orbit of Neptune. There may be millions of these icy objects, collectively referred to as Kuiper Belt objects (KBOs) or trans-Neptunian objects (TNOs), in this distant region of our solar system. Till recently, similar to the asteroid belt, the *Kuiper Belt* is a region of leftovers from the solar system's early history. Like the asteroid belt, it has also been shaped by a giant planet, although it's more of a thick disk (like a donut) than a thin belt. The Kuiper

Belt shouldn't be confused with the Oort Cloud, which is a much more distant region of icy, comet-like bodies that surrounds the solar system, including the Kuiper Belt. Both the Oort Cloud and the Kuiper Belt are thought to be sources of comets. The Kuiper Belt is truly a frontier in space – it's a place we're still just beginning to explore and our understanding is still evolving.

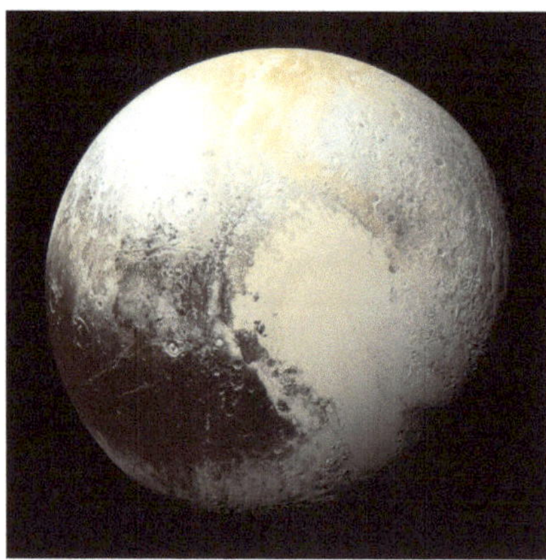

Fig. 40.23: *Showing view of planet Pluto. This is the most accurate natural color images of Pluto taken by NASA's New Horizons spacecraft in 2015.*

Water rich circumstellar disks

Long before the discovery of water on asteroids on comets and dwarf planets beyond Neptune, the Solar System's circumstellar disks, beyond the snow line, including the asteroid belt and the Kuiper Belt were thought to contain large amounts of water and these were believed to be the Origin of water on Earth. Given that many types of stars are thought to blow volatiles from the system through the photoevaporation effect, water content in *circumstellar disks* and rocky material in other planetary systems are very good indicators of a planetary system's potential for liquid water and a potential for organic chemistry, especially if detected within the planet forming regions or the habitable zone. Techniques such as interferometry can be used for this. In 2007, such a disk was found in the habitable zone of MWC 480. In 2008, such a disk was found around the star AA Tauri. In 2009, a similar disk was discovered around the young star HD 142527.

In 2013, a water-rich debris disk around GD 61 accompanied by a confirmed rocky object consisting of magnesium, silicon, iron, and oxygen. The same year, another water rich disk was spotted around HD 100546 has ices close to the star.

There is, of course, no guarantee that the other conditions will be found that allow liquid water to be present on a planetary surface.

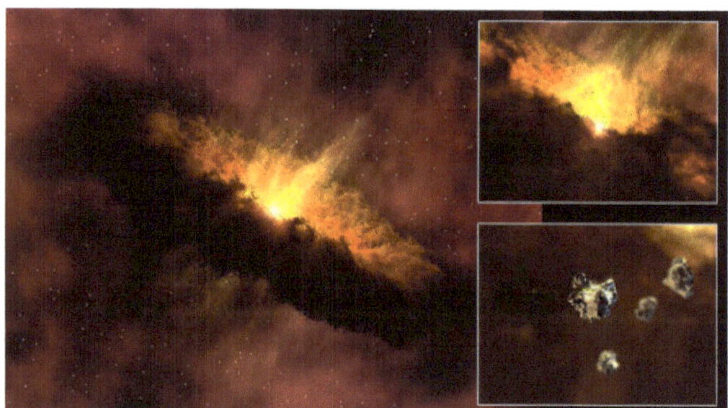

Fig 40.24: *Showing the Solar System's circumstellar disks, beyond the snow line, including the asteroid belt and the Kuiper Belt were thought to contain large amounts of water and these were believed to be the Origin of water on Earth. Using the Spitzer Space Telescope, astronomers are probing the chemistry of circumstellar disks, the dusty disks that surround stars, to understand the first moments in planetary life. Spitzer has turned its ultra-sensitive infrared spectrograph instrument toward five young stars in the constellation Taurus. These stars are still surrounded by thick, dusty disks – relics of the gravitational collapse that formed them only a few million years ago. The five disks have similar chemistry, indicating dusty material rich in silicates and organic compounds, as well as both water and carbon dioxide ices. Despite their similarities, there are also intriguing differences between the disks that may hold important clues about the evolution of stars and their young planetary systems.*

Should planetary mass objects be present, a single, gas giant planet, with or without planetary mass moons, orbiting close to the circumstellar habitable zone, could prevent the necessary conditions from occurring in the system. However, it would mean that planetary mass objects, such as the icy bodies of the solar system, could have abundant quantities of liquid within them.

Ancient water on Venus

NASA's Goddard Institute for Space Studies and others have postulated that *Venus* may have had a shallow ocean in the past for up to 2 billion years, with as much water as Earth. Depending on the parameters used in their theoretical model, the last liquid water could have evaporated as recently as 715 million years agoCurrently, the only known water on Venus is in the form of a tiny amount of atmospheric vapor (20 ppm). Hydrogen, a component of water, is still being lost to space nowadays as detected by ESA's Venus Express spacecraft.

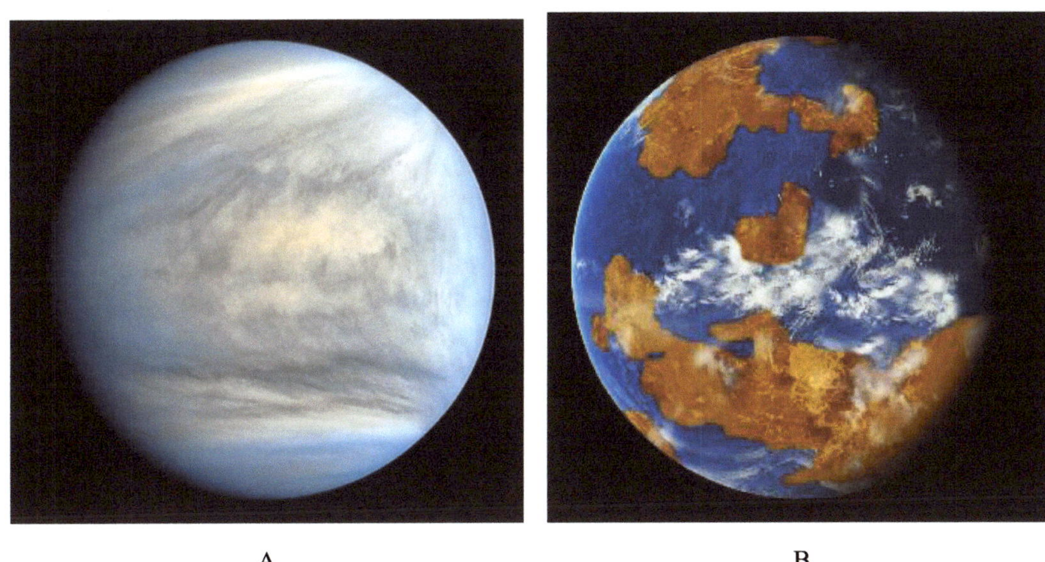

Fig 40.25: *(A) Showing view of planet venus. Photographed in ultraviolet light and rendered in false color, this view reveals the complexities of the clouds that coat Venus. The ochre hues correspond to sulfur dioxide. image credit : JAXA Way and his team of researchers created five simulations assuming different levels of water coverage and found that Venus was able to maintain stable temperatures between a maximum of about 50 degrees Celsius and a minimum of about 20 degrees Celsius for around three billion years. This could've been the temperature of Venus even now but a series of unfortunate events changed its course of evolution around 700-750 million years ago.(B) An artist illustration of how Venus would've looked like 2 billion years ago. image credit : NASA*

Evidence of past surface water

Assuming that the giant-impact hypothesis is correct, there were never real seas or oceans on the Moon, only perhaps a little moisture (liquid or ice) in some places, when the Moon had a thin atmosphere created by degassing of volcanoes or impacts of icy bodies. The Dawn space probe found possible evidence of past water flow on the *asteroid Vesta*, leading to speculation of underground reservoirs of water-ice. Astronomers speculate that Venus had liquid water and perhaps oceans in its very early history. Given that Venus has been completely resurfaced by its own active geology, the idea of a primeval ocean is hard to test. Rock samples may one day give the answer.

It was once thought that Mars might have dried up from something more Earth-like. The initial discovery of a cratered surface made this seem unlikely, but further evidence has changed this view. Liquid water may have existed on the surface of Mars in the distant past, and several basins on Mars have been proposed as dry sea beds. The largest is Vastitas Borealis; others include Hellas Planitia and Argyre Planitia.

There is currently much debate over whether Mars once had an ocean of water in its northern hemisphere, and over what happened to it if it did. Recent findings by the Mars

Exploration Rover mission indicate it had some long-term standing water in at least one location, but its extent is not known. The Opportunity Mars rover photographed bright veins of a mineral leading to conclusive confirmation of deposition by liquid water.

On 9 December 2013, NASA reported that the planet Mars had a large freshwater lake (which could have been a hospitable environment for microbial life) based on evidence from the Curiosity rover studying Aeolis Palus near Mount Sharp in Gale Crater.

Liquid water on comets and asteroids

Comets contain large proportions of water ice, but are generally thought to be completely frozen due to their small size and large distance from the Sun. However, studies on dust collected from comet Wild-2 show evidence for liquid water inside the comet at some point in the past. It is yet unclear what source of heat may have caused melting of some of the comet's water ice.

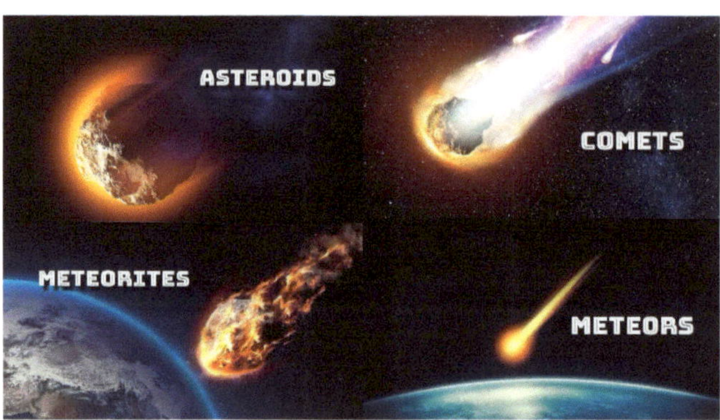

Fig.40.26: *showing photos of Comets and Asteroids. Asteroids and comets are debris left over from the formation of the moon and planets. Comets are located in the outermost regions of the solar system, while, asteroids are located in a belt between Jupiter and Mars. Occasionally, comets and asteroids change their orbital path due to gravitational disturbances, sometimes bringing them close to a planet. Craters on the moon and planets are evidence of the history of impacts with comets and asteroids.*

Nevertheless, on 10 December 2014, scientists reported that the composition of water vapor from *comet Churyumov–Gerasimenko*, as determined by the Rosetta spacecraft, is substantially different from that found on Earth. That is, the ratio of deuterium to hydrogen in the water from the comet was determined to be three times that found for terrestrial water. This makes it very unlikely that water found on Earth came from comets such as comet Churyumov–Gerasimenko according to the scientists. The asteroid 24 Themis was the first found to have water, including liquid pressurised by non-atmospheric means, dissolved into mineral through ionising radiation. Water has also been found to flow on the large asteroid 4 Vesta heated through periodic impacts.

Extrasolar habitable zone candidates for water

Most known extrasolar planetary systems appear to have very different compositions to the Solar System, though there is probably sample bias arising from the detection methods. The goal of current searches is to find Earth-sized planets in the habitable zone of their planetary systems (also sometimes called the Goldilocks zone). Planets with oceans could include Earth-sized moons of giant planets, though it remains speculative whether such 'moons' really exist. The Kepler telescope might be sensitive enough to detect them. There is speculation that rocky planets hosting water may be common place throughout the *Milky Way*.

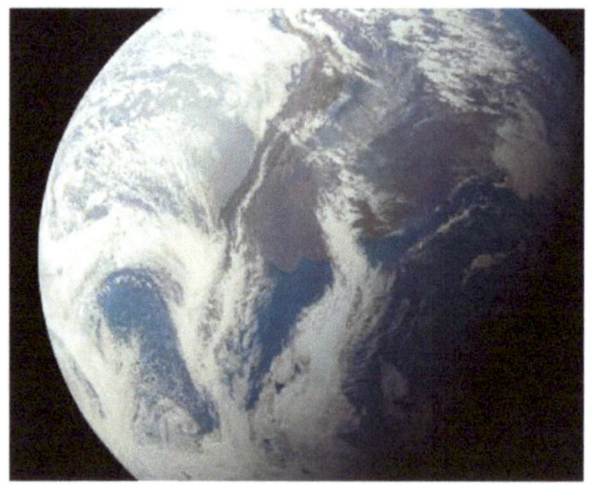

A

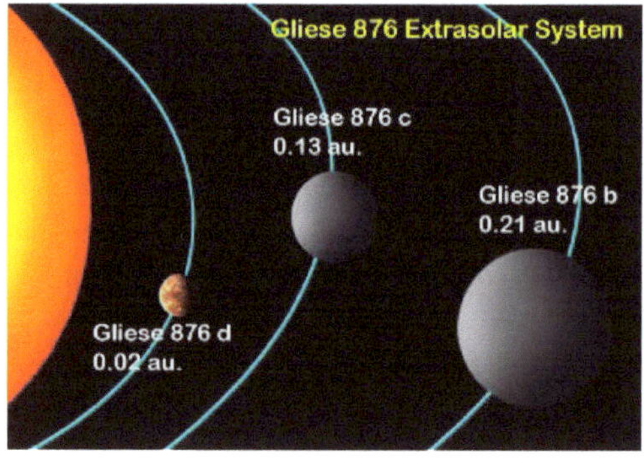

B

Fig. 40.27: *(A&B) Earth-sized planets in the habitable zone of their planetary systems (also sometimes called the Goldilocks zone). Planets with oceans could include Earth-sized moons of giant planets*

The Importance of Water

Water is one of the most important resources on the planet. Without water, life cannot exist. But what makes water so important? Water has several unique characteristics that make it an extremely valuable resource. Some such properties of water are listed below.

- Water is a very good solvent – it has the ability to dissolve many substances.
- The boiling point and freezing point of water make it easily available in all three states (solid, liquid, and gaseous).
- The specific heat of water is quite high. This enables water to absorb and release heat slowly, thereby regulating the temperature of its environment.
- Owing to its transparency, water can allow light to reach the life forms that are submerged in it. This is crucial for the survival of plant life in the oceans, lakes, and rivers.

- Water is neither acidic nor basic in nature. It has a pH of 7, making it a neutral substance.

These unique qualities of water, along with its abundance on the planet (approximately 71% of the Earth's surface is made up of water), make it a crucial resource for plants, animals, and human beings.

A. Importance of Water in Living Organisms

- Water is the medium through which all essential vitamins and minerals are transported in the bodies of living organisms (owing to its ability to dissolve a wide range of substances).
- Water also plays a vital role in facilitating the work of enzymes in living organisms. For example, the sodium bicarbonate secreted by the pancreas is broken down into ions by water, making the medium sufficiently alkaline for the enzymes to work.
- Water helps maintain body temperatures in plants and animals. In order to decrease the temperature in their bodies, animals lose water via perspiration (sweating) and plants lose water via transpiration.
- Since water can rise in capillary tubes without any external help, it can be transported from the roots of trees to every other part of the tree.
- Water is an integral part of *photosynthesis*. Without it, autotrophic plants would not be able to produce their own food.
- Water serves as a habitat for more than 50% of all life on Earth.

B. Importance of Water in Human Beings

- Insufficient water content in the human body results in severe dehydration, which is often accompanied by kidney failure, seizures, and swelling in the brain.
- Water helps improve the circulation of oxygen throughout the body.
- It also plays a crucial role in the digestion of food.
- Water is a very important component of saliva, which helps break down food.
- The excretion of waste in the human body requires water. Insufficient water levels in the body may increase the strain on the kidneys, resulting in the formation of kidney stones.

C. Other Important Uses of Water

- If not for the high specific heat of water, the temperature of the Earth's surface would be much lower. This would make it difficult for life to survive.
- The water in the Earth's oceans absorb heat from the sun during the day and help maintain the temperature during the night.
- Water is necessary for the irrigation of crops and is, therefore, an integral part of agriculture.
- It is widely used in cooking activities since it boils at a temperature of 100°
- Humans make use of water for a wide range of domestic activities such as washing and cleaning.
- Water also serves as a medium for the transportation of cargo. Many goods are transported between the Earth's continents via ships.

D. Industrial Uses of Water

- Many industries require large quantities of water for processing, cooling, and diluting products. Examples of industries that consume large quantities of water include the paper industry, the food industry, and the chemical industry.
- Water is also used as an industrial solvent for the production of several commercially important products. Almost all power plants that generate electricity employ water to spin turbines.
- Heavy water, an important form of water, is widely used in nuclear reactors as a neutron moderator.

Health Benefits of Water Backed by Scientific Research

your body weight is about 60 percent water, according to the U.S. Geological Survey. Your body uses water in all its cells, organs, and tissues to help regulate temperature and maintain other bodily functions. Because your body loses water through breathing, sweating, and digestion, it's important to rehydrate by drinking fluids and eating foods that contain water. The amount of water you need depends on a variety of factors, according to the Mayo Clinic : The climate you live in, how physically active you are, and whether you're experiencing an illness or have any other health problems all affect recommended intake.

Here are the reasons why water is such a powerful element when it comes to your health.

1. Water Protects Your Tissues, Spinal Cord, and Joints

Water does more than just quench your thirst and regulate your body's temperature; it keeps the tissues in your body moist, according to the Mayo Clinic Health System. You know how it feels when your eyes, nose, or mouth gets dry? Keeping your body hydrated helps it retain optimum levels of moisture in these sensitive areas, as well as in the blood, bones, and brain. In addition, water helps protect the spinal cord, and it acts as a lubricant and cushion for your joints.

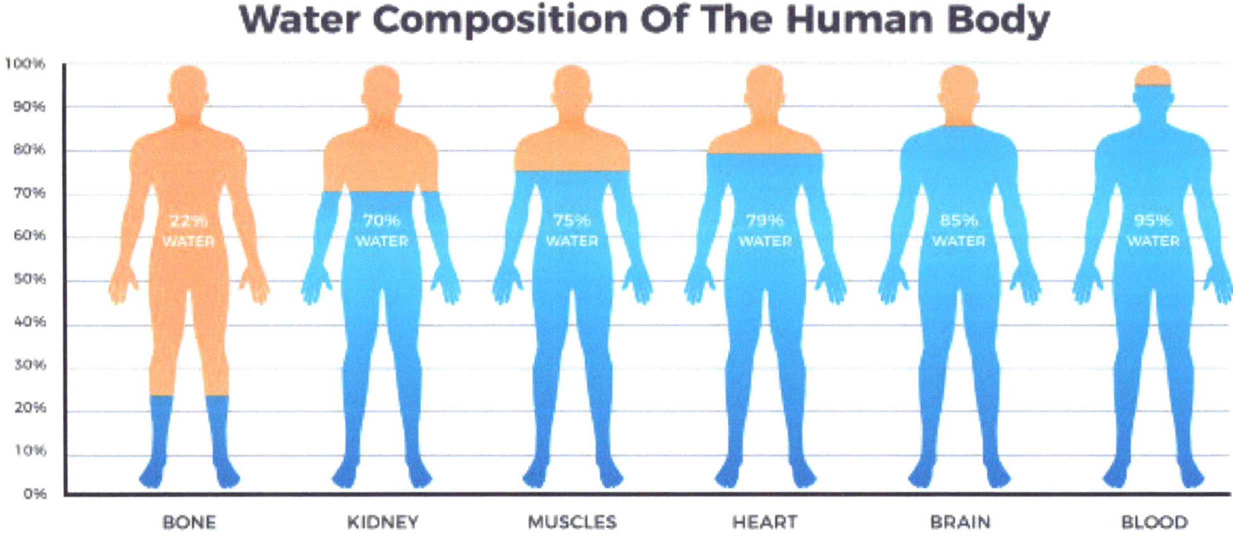

Fig.40.28: *Diagram showing water composition of the human body*

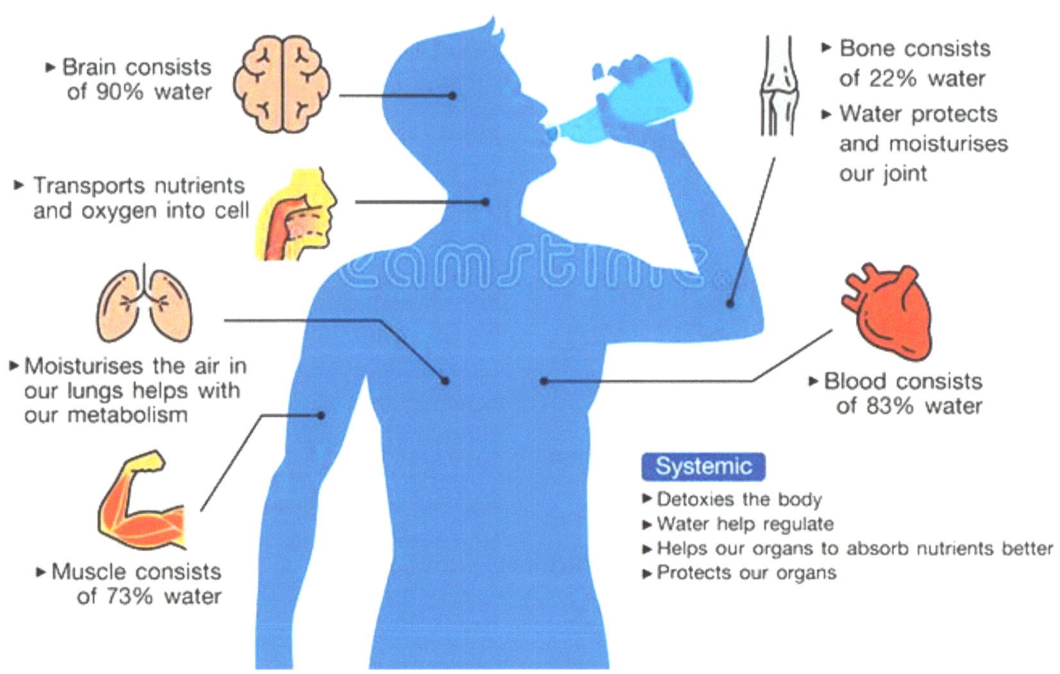

Fig.40.29: *Diagram showing function of water in the human body*

2. Water Helps Your Body Remove Waste

Adequate water intake enables your body to excrete waste through perspiration, urination, and defecation. Water helps your kidneys remove waste from your blood and keep the blood vessels that run to your kidneys open and

filter Water is also important for helping prevent constipation, points out the University of Rochester Medical Center. However, as research notes, there is no evidence to prove that increasing your fluid intake will cure constipation.

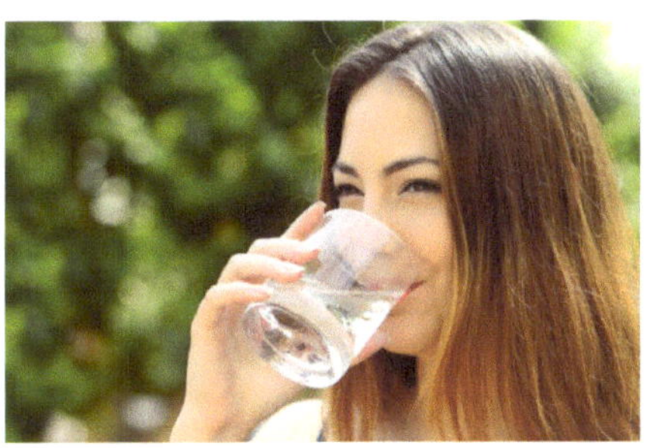

Fig.40.30: *A young lady is quenching her thrust by drinking a clean and fresh water*

3. Water Aids in Digestion

Water is important for healthy digestion. As the Mayo Clinic explains, water helps break down the food you eat, allowing its nutrients to be absorbed by your body. After you drink, both your small and large intestines absorb water, which moves into your bloodstream and is also used to break down nutrients. As your large intestine absorbs water, stool changes from liquid to solid, according to the National Institute for Diabetes and Digestive and Kidney Diseases. Water is also necessary to help you digest soluble fiber, per MedlinePlus. With the help of water, this fiber turns to gel and slows digestion.

4. Water Prevents You From Becoming Dehydrated

Your body loses fluids when you engage in vigorous exercise, sweat in high heat, or come down with a fever or contract an illness that causes vomiting or diarrhea, according to the Centers for Disease Control and Prevention. If you're losing fluids for any of these reasons, it's important to increase your fluid intake so that you can restore your body's natural hydration level. Your doctor may also recommend that you drink more fluids to help treat other health conditions, like bladder infections and urinary tract stones. If you're pregnant or nursing, you may want to consult with your physician about your fluid intake because your body will be using more fluids than usual, especially if you're breastfeeding.

5. Water Helps Your Brain Function Optimally

Ever feel foggy headed? Take a sip of water. Research shows that dehydration is a drag to memory, attention, and energy, per a small study on adult men from China published in June 2019 in the International Journal of Environmental Research and Public Health. It's no wonder, considering H_2O makes up 75 percent of the brain, the authors point out. One reason for that foggy-headed feeling? "Adequate electrolyte balance is vital to keeping your body functioning optimally. Low electrolytes can cause issues including muscle weakness, fatigue, and confusion," says Gabrielle Lyon, DO, a functional medicine physician in New York City.

6. Water Keeps Your Cardiovascular System Healthy

Water is a huge part of your blood. (For instance, plasma — the pale yellow liquid portion of your blood — is about 90 percent water, notes Britannica.) If you become dehydrated, your blood becomes more concentrated, which can lead to an imbalance of the electrolyte minerals it contains (sodium and potassium, for example), says Susan Blum, MD, founder of the Blum Center for Health in Rye Brook, New York. These electrolytes are necessary for proper muscle and heart function. "Dehydration can also lead to lower blood volume, and thus blood pressure, so you may feel light-headed or woozy standing up," she says.

7. Water Can Help You Eat Healthier

It may be plain, but it's powerful. In a study of more than 18,300 American adults, people who drank just 1 percent more water a day ate fewer calories and less saturated fat, sugar, sodium, and cholesterol, according to a study published in February 2016 in the Journal of Human Nutrition and Dietetics. Water may help fill you up, especially if you drink it before eating a meal, a notion that was backed up in a small study of 15 young, healthy participants that was published in October 2018 in Clinical Nutrition Research.

Biological Roles of Water: Why is water necessary for life?

Water makes up 60-75% of human body weight. A loss of just 4% of total body water leads to dehydration, and a loss of 15% can be fatal. Likewise, a person could survive a month without food but wouldn't survive 3 days without water. This crucial dependence on water broadly governs all life forms. Clearly water is vital for survival, but what makes it so necessary?

The Molecular Make-up of Water

Many of water's roles in supporting life are due to its molecular structure and a few special properties. Water is a simple molecule composed of two small, positively charged hydrogen atoms and one large negatively charged oxygen atom. When the hydrogens bind to the oxygen, it creates an asymmetrical molecule with positive charge on one side and negative charge on the other side.. This charge differential is called polarity and dictates how water interacts with other molecules.

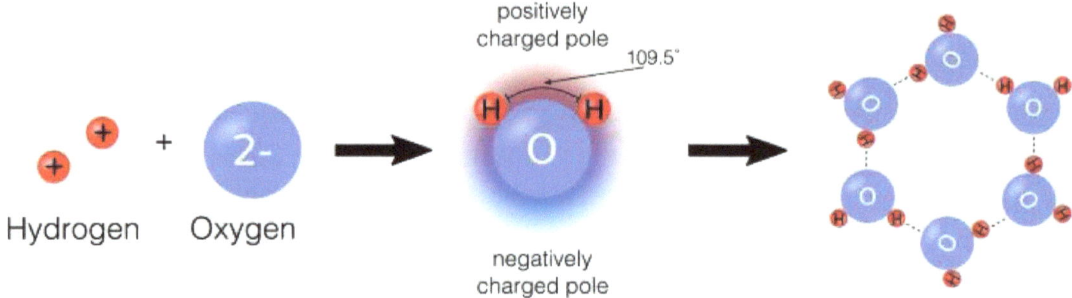

Fig. 40.31: *Water Chemistry. Water molecules are made of two hydrogens and one oxygen. These atoms are of different sizes and charges, which creates the asymmetry in the molecular structure and leads to strong bonds between water and other polar molecules, including water itself.*

Water is the "Universal Solvent"

As a *polar molecule*, water interacts best with other polar molecules, such as itself. This is because of the phenomenon wherein opposite charges attract one another : because each individual water molecule has both a negative portion and a positive portion, each side is attracted to molecules of the opposite charge. This attraction allows water to form relatively strong connections, called bonds, with other polar molecules around it, including other water molecules. In this case, the positive hydrogen of one water molecule will bond with the negative oxygen of the adjacent molecule, whose own hydrogens are attracted to the next oxygen, and so on. Importantly, this bonding makes water molecules stick together in a property called cohesion. The cohesion of water molecules helps plants take up water at their roots. Cohesion also contributes to water's high boiling point, which helps animals regulate body temperature.

Furthermore, since most biological molecules have some electrical asymmetry, they too are polar and water molecules can form bonds with and surround both their positive and negative regions. In the act of surrounding the polar molecules of another substance, water wriggles its way into all the nooks and crannies between molecules, effectively breaking it apart are dissolving it. This is what happens when you put sugar crystals into water : both water and sugar are polar, allowing individual water molecules to surround individual sugar molecules, breaking apart the sugar and dissolving it. Similar to polarity, some molecules are made of ions, or oppositely charged particles. Water breaks apart these ionic molecules as well by interacting with both the positively and negatively charged particles. This is what happens when you put salt in water, because salt is composed of sodium and chloride ions. Water's extensive capability to dissolve a variety of molecules has earned it the designation of "universal solvent," and it is this ability that makes water such an invaluable life-sustaining force. On a biological level, water's role as a solvent helps cells transport and use substances like oxygen or nutrients. Water-based solutions like blood help carry molecules to the necessary locations. Thus, water's role as a solvent facilitates the transport of molecules like oxygen for respiration and has a major impact on the ability of drugs to reach their targets in the body.

Water Supports Cellular Structure

Water also has an important structural role in biology. Visually, water fills cells to help maintain shape and structure. The water inside many cells (including those that make up the human body) creates pressure that opposes external forces, similar to putting air in a balloon. However, even some plants, which can maintain their cell structure without water, still require water to survive. Water allows everything inside cells to have the right shape at the molecular level. As shape is critical for biochemical processes, this is also one of water's most important roles.

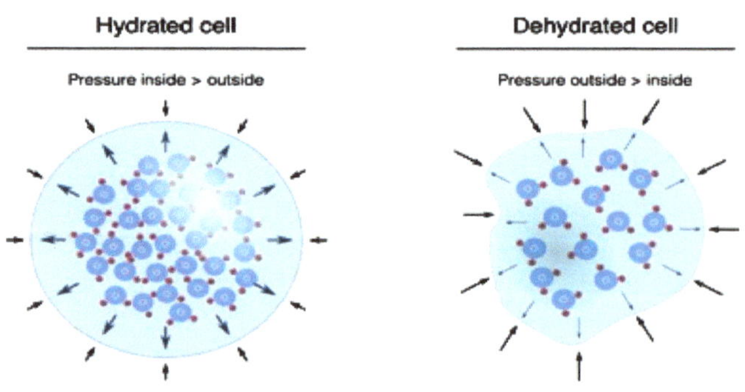

Fig.40.32: *Water impacts cell shape. Water creates pressure inside the cell that helps it maintain shape. In the hydrated*

cell (left), the water pushes outward and the cell maintains a round shape. In the dehydrated cell, there is less water pushing outward so the cell becomes wrinkled. Water also contributes to the formation of membranes surrounding cells. Every cell on Earth is surrounded by a membrane, most of which are formed by two layers of molecules called phospholipidis. The phospholipids, like water, have two distinct components : a polar "head" and a nonpolar "tail." Due to this, the polar heads interact with water, while the nonpolar tails try to avoid water and interact with each other instead. Seeking these favorable interactions, phospholipids spontaneously form bilayers with the heads facing outward towards the surrounding water and the tails facing inward, excluding water. The bilayer surrounds cells and selectively allows substances like salts and nutrients to enter and exit the cell. The interactions involved in forming the membrane are strong enough that the membranes form spontaneously and aren't easily disrupted. Without water, cell membranes would lack structure, and without proper membrane structure, cells would be unable to keep important molecules inside the cell and harmful molecules outside the cell.

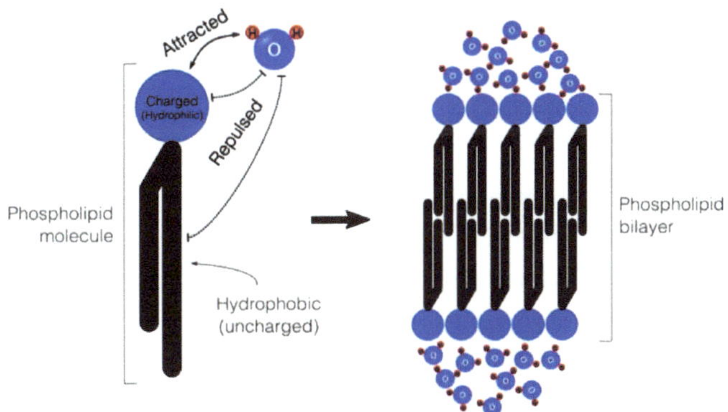

Fig.40.33: *Phospholipid bilayers. Phospholipids form bilayers surrounded by water. The polar heads face outward to interact with water and the hydrophobic tails face inward to avoid interacting with water.*

In addition to influencing the overall shape of cells, water also impacts some fundamental components of every cell : DNA and proteins. Proteins are produced as a long chain of building blocks called amino acids and need to fold into a specific shape to function correctly. Water drives the folding of amino acid chains as different types of amino acids seek and avoid interacting with water. Proteins provide structure, receive signals, and catalyze chemical reactions in the cell. In this way, proteins are the workhorses of cells. Ultimately proteins drive contraction of muscles, communication, digestion of nutrients, and many other vital functions. Without the proper shape, proteins would be unable to perform these functions and a cell (let alone an entire human) could not survive. Similarly, DNA needs to be in a specific shape for its instructions to be properly decoded. Proteins that read or copy DNA can only bind DNA that has a particular shape. Water molecules surround DNA in an ordered fashion to support its characteristic double-helix conformation. Without this shape, cells would be unable to follow the careful instructions encoded by DNA or to pass the instructions onto future cells, making human growth, reproduction, and, ultimately, survival infeasible.

Chemical Reactions of Water

Water is directly involved in many chemical reactions to build and break down important components of the cell. *Photosynthesis*, the process in plants that creates sugars for all life forms, requires water. Water also participates in building larger molecules in cells. Molecules like DNA and proteins are made of repetitive units of smaller molecules. Putting these small molecules together occurs through a reaction that produces water. Conversely, water is required for the reverse reaction that breaks down these molecules, allowing cells to obtain nutrients or repurpose pieces of big molecules.

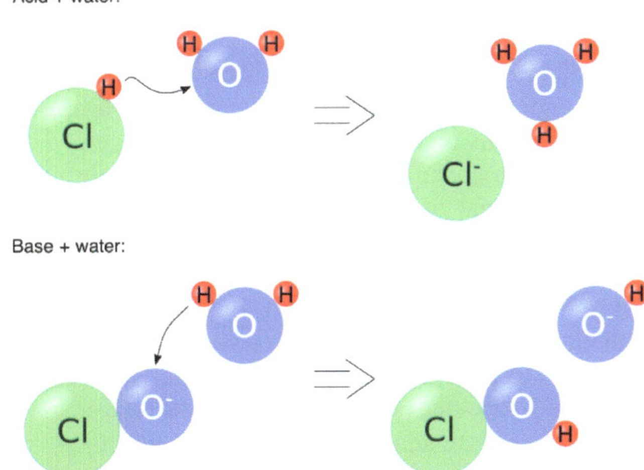

Fig. 40.34: *Water acts as a buffer by releasing or accepting hydrogen atoms.*

Additionally, water buffers cells from the dangerous effects of acids and bases. Highly acidic or basic substances, like bleach or hydrochloric acid, are corrosive to even the most durable materials. This is because acids and bases release excess *hydrogens* or take up excess hydrogens, respectively, from the surrounding materials. Losing or gaining positively-charged hydrogens disrupts the structure of molecules. As we've learned, proteins require a specific structure to function properly, so it's important to protect them from acids and bases. Water does this by acting as both an acid and a base. Although the chemical bonds within a water molecule are very stable, it's possible for a water molecule to give up a hydrogen and become OH–, thus acting as a base, or accept another hydrogen and become H_3O+, thus acting as an acid. This adaptability allows water to combat drastic changes of pH due to acidic or basic substances in the body in a process called buffering. Ultimately, this protects proteins and other molecules in the cell.

In conclusion, water is vital for all life. Its versatility and adaptability help perform important chemical reactions. Its simple molecular structure helps maintain important shapes for cells' inner components and outer membrane. No other molecule matches water when it comes to unique properties that support life. Excitingly, researchers continue to establish new properties of water such as additional effects of its asymmetrical structure. Scientists have yet to determine the physiological impacts of these properties. It's amazing how a simple molecule is universally important for organisms with diverse needs.

Amazing Benefits of Drinking Water and How it Makes Kids Smarter

Benefits of Drinking Water

This infographic helps you to understand how important water is for all your child's bodily functions. Notice the different organs of the body and the percentage of how much water is contained within each organ. Water is the main component of every organ in the body. Water is essential. And everyone, including your children, needs to drink plenty of this life-giving substance every day. Did you know that people can go for up to three weeks without food? Water is a different story. Survival rates connected to water? Only a few days. Water is necessary for life! Seventy-five percent of your child's body is made up of water. As an adult, it's 70%. And interestingly, our earth is also 70% water. Your children lose water every day through sweat and urine and need to replenish what is lost. And fever, vomiting or diarrhea will also cause your child to lose water. Even if your child doesn't feel thirsty, it doesn't mean his/her body doesn't need water. Check out the water recommendations below. And notice on this infographic how much water is contained in all of our vital organs.

A. How Much Daily Water Intake?

There are recommendations for water intake according to age. But these are only recommendations. Other factors should be considered—are your kids involved in sports? Is the weather hot, dry or humid? If so, your child (and you) will need more water. Don't wait until your child is thirsty—by that time his body is already dehydrated.

As the Mayo Clinic notes, the National Academies of Sciences, Engineering, and Medicine recommends that men consume 3.7 liters (15.5 cups) and women get 2.7 liters (11.5 cups) of fluids per day, which can come from water, beverages in general, and food (such as fruits and vegetables). You can also try the Urine Color Test, courtesy of the U.S. Army Public Health Command, to evaluate how you're doing on drinking up. After going to the bathroom, look at the color of your urine. If it is very pale yellow to light yellow, you're well hydrated. Darker yellow is a sign of dehydration. Brown or cola-colored urine is a medical emergency, and you should seek medical attention.

Recommended for daily water intake

- **Children Ages 5-8:** Five (8oz/ea.) glasses of water each day or 40 ounces
- **Ages 9-12:** Seven (8oz/ea.) glasses of water daily or at least 56 ounces
- **Ages 13+** : Eight to ten (8 oz./ea.) glasses of water or at least 80 ounces

Reasons Kids Need to Drink Water

Here are 10 important reasons for you and your kids to drink plenty of water every single day:

- Water Eliminates Dehydration
- Water helps kids stay hydrated–which is important for their brains to work and for them to stay healthy! Dehydration means that your body doesn't have enough water to function properly. Seventy-five percent of people (including children) are chronically dehydrated. Even mild dehydration will
- slow down your child's metabolism as much as 3% and cause fatigue
- cause your child to feel grumpy or tired
- give your child headaches
- The human body has no stored water to draw on during dehydration so it's vitally important that your child drinks water throughout the day.

Suggestion

- Dehydration can happen very quickly—keep water with you in the car for thirsty kids. If they play sports or are involved in strenuous extra-curricular activities, send them with plenty of water in their backpacks or sports packs.

- If your children come home from school grumpy or tired—give them a glass of water. I personally prefer room-temperature water for younger kids. Sometimes a very cold glass of water can trigger a headache particularly when they are already tired or experiencing mild dehydration.

B. Water Helps Kids Suffering from Asthma and Allergies

Your children need water for their cells to grow. As they grow, 75% of the cell volume must be filled with water. This is one reason why children develop asthma and allergies during the growth stage of their physical development– they don't have enough water for their body systems to function. Some research indicates that asthma can be caused by chronic dehydration and by increasing water and adding a bit of salt to the tongue, asthma coughing disappears. Kids are also susceptible to allergies if they increase their food intake but not their water intake.

Suggestion

If you have a child who suffers from asthma or allergies, water obviously will help. Kids with allergies should drink a glass of water Before eating food. And kids with asthma need to drink more water. They also need to stop drinking sodas containing caffeine and reduce their orange juice consumption which can trigger an allergic reaction in some children.

C. Water Lessens Hunger Pains

In a University of Washington study, it was discovered that dieters who drink one glass of water before bed will shut down late-night hunger pains by almost 100%! Drinking water helps separate the feelings of thirst and hunger. Thirty-seven percent of Americans suffer from a very weak thirst mechanism. In fact, it is so weak that it is often mistaken for hunger. Many kids and parents who feel hungry are really in need of water.

Suggestion

Does your child get up at night complaining of hunger or thirst? If so, either give him/her a glass of water an hour before bedtime or even 30 minutes before bed. If they get up feeling hungry or thirsty—give them another glass of water. You're probably thinking, "they are going to be up all night going to the bathroom." Possibly, but if your child's body is in need of water, the water they drink will be used to replenish their organs and cells. If you want your child's brain to operate at peak performance– they need to drink water. It helps with energy, thinking, concentrating and focusing. It helps with energy, thinking, concentrating and focusing.

D. Water Reduces Fatigue and Helps Kids Learn

When your kids are thirsty, they get tired very easily. In fact, studies show that not replenishing the body with water is the #1 trigger of daytime fatigue. According to F. Batmanghelidj, MD, water is the main source of energy and is called the "cash flow" of the body. Recently one of my friends on Facebook was complaining about the principal at her children's school. The kids were not being allowed to drink any water until lunch time and after that, they had to wait until they were ready to go home to have more water. This rule was probably given to eliminate kids from leaving class and going to the bathroom.

Kids in school need water to help:

- Keep their brains alive and working
- Water gives a child electrical energy for brain functions, particularly thinking.
- It is needed for sustained focus energy
- Water can also help prevent attention deficit disorder in children (and adults). In fact, kids who drink plenty of water, their attention spans actually increase.
- Water integrates mind and body functions. It helps kids and teens with the desire to make goals and have a purpose. Hard to believe that water can do this–but research indicates it can and does.

Suggestion

Send bottled water with your children to school. Let their teachers know exactly why you are doing this. If they don't understand, encourage them to read the research connecting water to learning.

Children at school need to have water throughout the day to keep their minds clear to learn

E. Drink Water to Ease Growing Pains & Back and Joint Pains

Back, joint and muscle pain are not relegated to the aging. It can also happen to your kids. Growing pains are common among children. Preliminary research indicates that 8-10 glasses of water a day can significantly ease back, joint and muscle pain for up to 80% of sufferers.

Suggestion

If your kids are experiencing growing pains, give them plenty of water throughout the day and a glass of water about one hour prior to them going to bed (so they can empty their bladder before they nod off). It should help.

F. Drinking Water Helps With Short-term Memory

Did you know that a mere 2% drop in body water can trigger fuzzy short-term memory? It can also cause kids to have problems understanding basic math, and have difficulty focusing on a computer screen or printed page in a book. Drinking water every day can help prevent memory loss well into old age.

Suggestion

Before starting their homework, make certain your kids have had a big glass of water to drink. And as I said above, send them to school with a bottle of water or thermos of water. It's necessary for their memories and learning. Even a 2% drop in water in the body will cause fuzzy thinking. Are you or your kids tired? grumpy? Grab a glass of thirst-quenching and brain-boosting water!

G. Water Decreases the Risk of Certain Cancers

Drinking water can help ward off certain cancers. For instance:

- Drinking 5 glasses of water daily help to decrease the risk of colon cancer by 45%
- Drinking 5 glasses of water each day can slash the risk of breast cancer by 79%
- When a person drinks at least 5 glasses of water a day, they are 50% less likely to develop bladder cancer
- Water also helps to normalize the blood-manufacturing system in the bone marrow which helps prevent childhood leukemia and lymphoma.

Suggestion

Although some of these forms of cancer are not cancers common in children, it's a good idea to get your kids in the habit of drinking plenty of water every day. It just may help prevent certain cancers when they are adults because water keeps the immune system working at peak performance and can fight infections and cancer cells where they are formed.

H. Sip or Guzzle?

If your child sips water throughout the day, they will keep their systems hydrated and their abilities to learn and function will substantially increase. If they guzzle water (drinking it very rapidly) they will cleanse their systems. Both are helpful for their bodies and minds.

Suggestion

Either sipping or guzzling water is good for your child's health. I would suggest that they sip water throughout the day to keep their minds in tip-top shape. If they need to cleanse their system—guzzle it.

Drinking sodas, juices, or even milk does not count toward your daily intact of water. Soda dehydrates the body not to mention the high sugar content in both sodas and juices. When in doubt–grab a glass of water!

I. Drinking Soda, Juice or Milk Doesn't Count Toward Water Intake

Many parents think that as long as their child is getting some form of liquid (milk, juice, soda) in their systems, they will be hydrated. This is partially correct. However, sodas and juices are loaded with sugar and sugar drains water from the colon and can cause constipation and/or diarrhea. Plus, the sodium in sodas increases dehydration. Kids don't need excess salt or sugar in their diets. It impedes their ability to learn. They need water.

Suggestion

Make water your family's #1 beverage choice. You'll be glad you did. You will notice your children having sustained, focused energy; their brains will work better and more efficiently which all translates into a healthier more positive learning experience.

J. Drinking Water Helps Clear Teen Skin

When your kids get to be teens, they will be concerned about their skin. Having healthy, acne-free skin is important for teens and their self-esteem. There are many reasons for teen acne, but several things that can help is drinking plenty of water, giving up sodas and eating plenty of fruits and veggies. Fruits and veggies are loaded with water and will help clean out the cells. Drinking water every day will help improve your teen's skin by:

- Eliminating toxins from the body
- Flushing out the system
- Hydrating the skin
- Making the skin smoother
- Decreasing the effects of aging

Suggestion

Encourage your teen to drink plenty of water every day. It definitely helps teens with problem skin. I know from my own personal experience and with my teen sons. The more water we drank, the more healthy and blemish-free skin we had. Last, here are some of my favorite books about water for your family. When I was studying towards my three nutrition certifications, one of the required reading books was–You're Not Sick You're Thirsty. It's an excellent book filled with documented research on the importance of drinking water. Become further enlightened by this amazing life-giving substance.

Box 40.1: *Importance of Water Consumption in Children*

Age	Males	Females
9 – 13	1.6L/day = 6 glasses	1.4L/day = 5 to 6 glasses
14 – 18	1.9L/day = 7 glasses	1.6L/day = 6 glasses
Adults	2.6L/day = 10 glasses	2.1L/day = 8 glasses

Water conservation at various levels

1. Conserve Water At Home

With the increase of population and more areas struggling with drought & conservation efforts, making a conscious decision to cut back on water usage means a lower utility bill, a better environment, & a continued effort to keep water drinkable and affordable for all humans & animals on our Earth.

We've gathered some ways to help conserve water at home. Deciding on just a few small challenges can make an impact on water usage, reducing hundreds of gallons of water each year.

1. Switch to a low-flow shower head:- Switching your shower head to a low-flow can save you around 15 gallons of water during a ten minute shower. An 8 minute shower with a low-flow shower head uses about 12 gallons of water; 1.5 gallons per minute, versus 24-64 gallons with other shower heads.

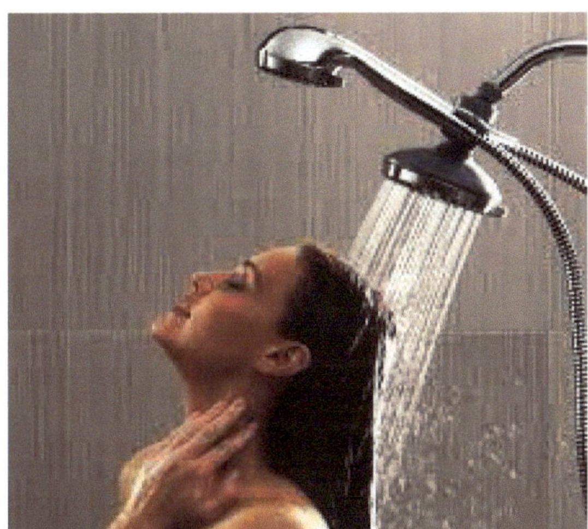

Fig.40.35: *A young lady taking bath under –low flow shower head*

2. Turn off the faucet when you are brushing your teeth or shaving:- Running a faucet flows about 2.2 gallons of water per minute. Turn off your *faucet* after you wet your toothbrush or razor, and leave it off until it's time for your rinse.

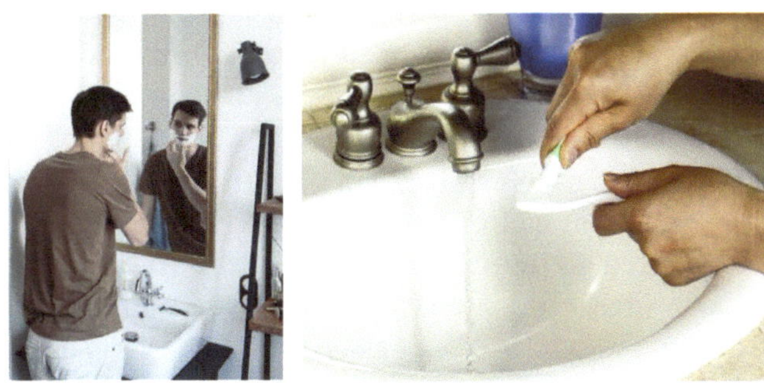

Fig.40.36: *Person is taking all precaution to save water during dental cleaning and shaving*

3. Turn off the faucet while you're washing your hands:- Use a squirt of soap, lather, and turn on the faucet to rinse. If you wash your hands for 15 seconds, 7 times a day, you're using about 7.7 gallons of water. Use water only after you're done with your lather and ready for your rinse!

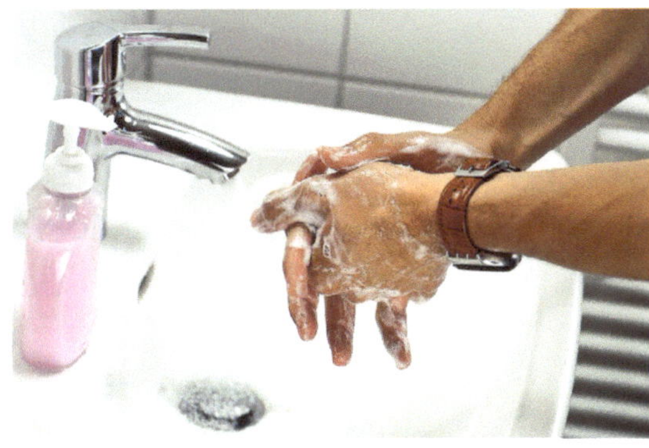

Fig.40.37: *Photograph of a man washing his hands with liquid soap and closing the faucet during this period.*

4. Upgrade to water conserving models of dishwashers and washing machines:- There are energy & *water conservation machines* available that help to conserve water while they're cleaning for you! This might be a bit pricey at first, but your utility bills go down, and you will be helping the planet big time!

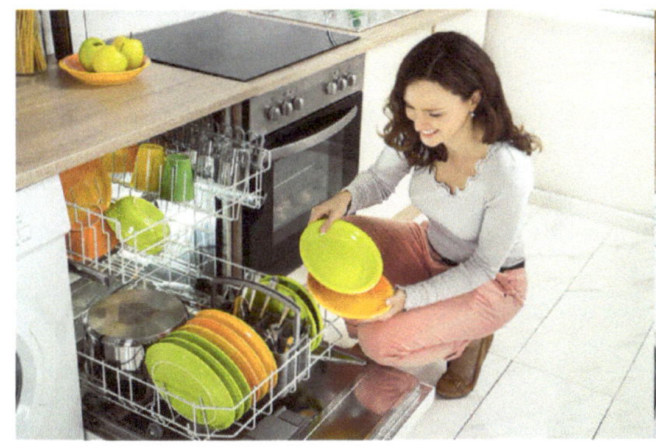

Fig.40.38: *A young house wife in cleaning dishes in a upgraded machine*

5. Run the dishwasher or washing machine only when it's full:- Doing half loads, or small laundry loads add up to gallons of wasted water. Adjust washer machine setting if you must do a small load.

6. Don't have a dishwasher? Fill your sink up with warm soapy water instead of letting the faucet run the whole time that you are scrubbing. Scrap foods in your compost bin to decrease the amount of times you may need to change the water.

7. Create a rain catcher:- Harvesting rain water is a fantastic way to keep your plants hydrated without using your hose or sprinklers.

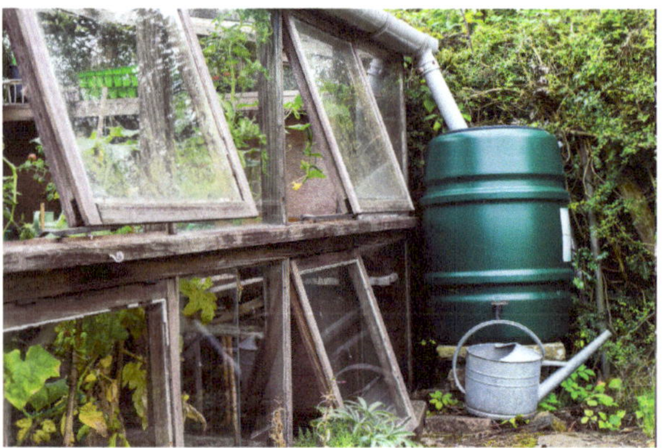

Fig.40.39: *Harvesting rain water at home.*

8. Water plants early in the morning:- It's cooler in the mornings, which translates to using less water. The cooler the temperature, the less the water will evaporate.

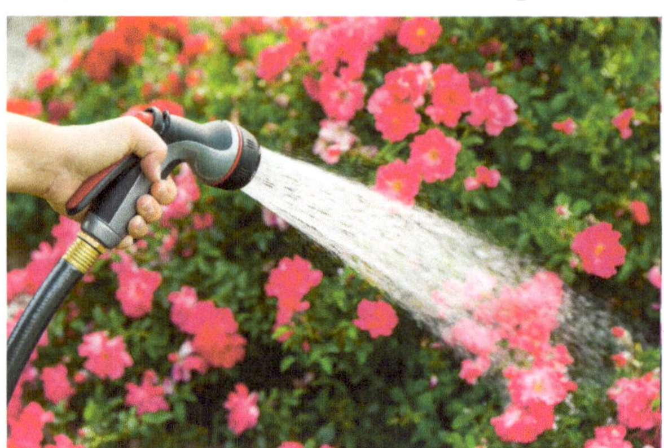

Fig.40.40: *A person is watering his plants in the early hours of morning.*

9. Fix your leaks! Fixing leaky faucets or running toilets can save gallons and gallons of water and hundreds of dollars per year.

10. Frugal Flusher:- Be a *frugal flusher* – if it's yellow, let it mellow. Flushing your toilet just 5 times a day with a conventional toilet uses about 3.5-5 gallons per flush; if flushed 5 times a day, this equates to 17.5-25 gallons used! If you install a high-efficiency toilet, 5 flushes equates to only 6.4 gallons used.

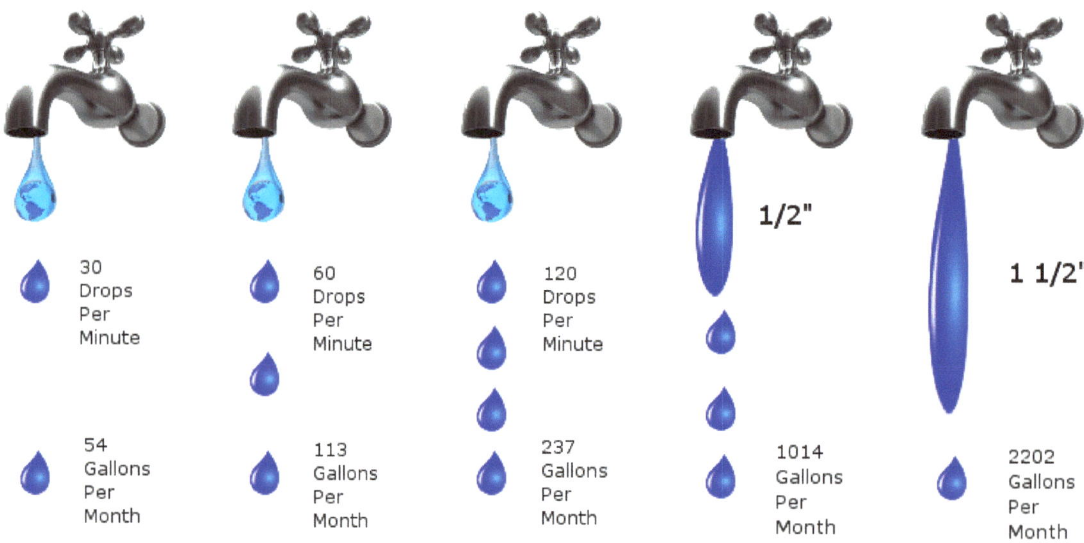

Fig.40.41: *Water Loss Chart Average Loss Of Water From Leaking Faucets Over A Period Of One Month*

11. Take shorter showers:- An easy way to cut down on water is to turn off the shower while soaping up and turning it back on to rinse. An 8 minute shower usesanywhere between 12-64 gallons of water depending on what type of shower head you are using.

12. Plant drought-resistant lawns & plants:- They have *drought-resistant grasses*, as well as artificial grasses that are a great option for decreases your utility bill and the amount of water you use. Plant succulents and native plants to your area. It's also smart to group plants together according to their watering needs – that way, you do not over water.

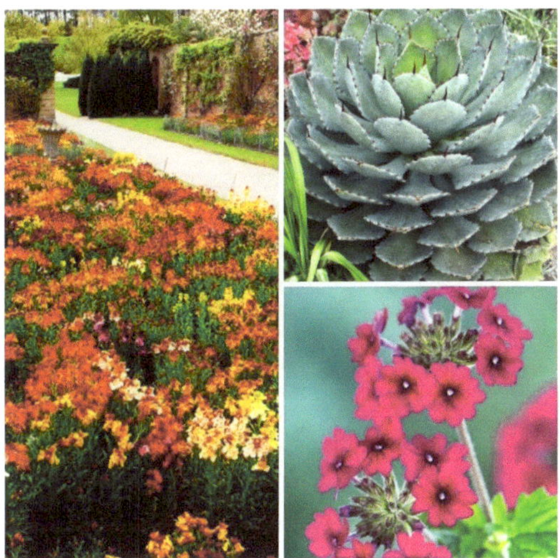

Fig.40.42: *showing drought –resistant flowers and plants for house lawn*

13. Position your sprinklers:- Position your sprinklers to water the things that need water. It's smart to check this positioning often, as sometimes external factors such as children or animals can move these out of place.

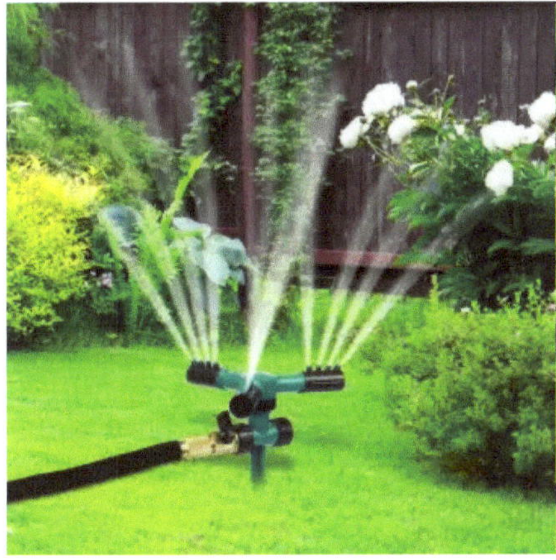

Fig.40.43: *showing automatic 360° rotating garden water sprinklers lawn irrigation*

14. Check for leaks:- Checking leaks both inside and outside can dramatically save a lot of water, as well as money. If you've experienced a huge spike in your water bill, call a plumber and have them check your water lines for you.

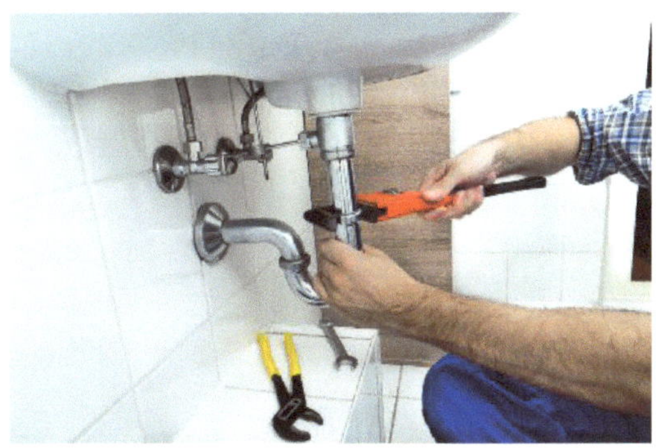

Fig.40.44: *Photograph showing Plumber checking the leaks and fixing these appropriately*

15. Use a shower bucket:- While waiting for your hot water, plentiful water gets drained from the shower. Get a bucket or pail and stick it under the faucet until it's your preferred temperature. You can use this water for watering plants, flushing the toilet, in your tea kettle, etc.

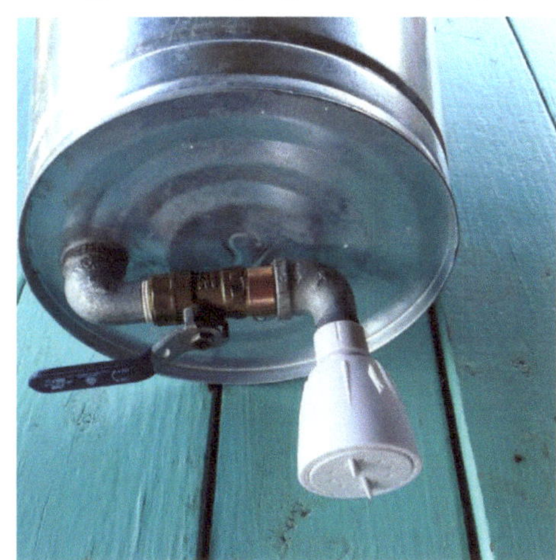

Fig.40.45: *Photograph showing the American Homestead shower bucket!*

16. Use a car wash that recycles water:- If you wash your car at home, don't leave the hose on; use buckets instead or install a hose nozzle

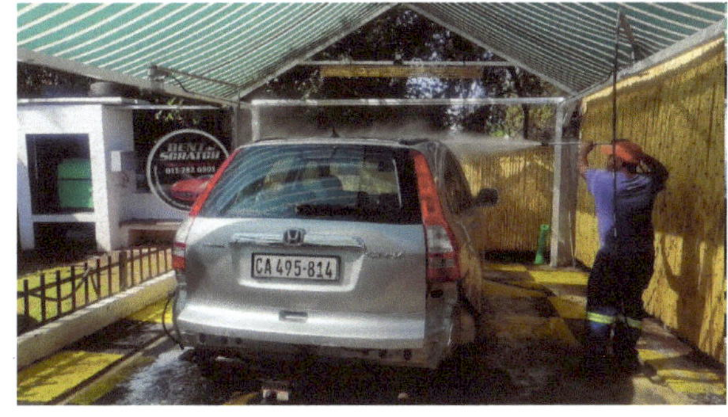

Fig. 40.46: *showing car washing with recycling the water.*

17. Washing fruits & vegetables:- It should be done in a pan or pot of water instead of letting the water run from the faucet.

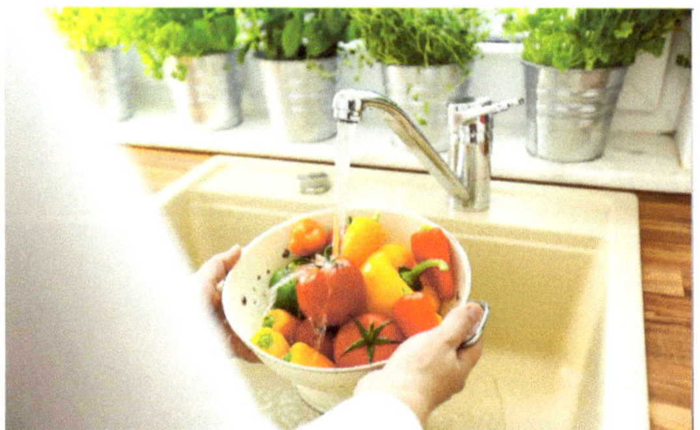

Fig. 40.47: *showing best way to wash your veggies and fruit in a pan to save water.*

18. Install gutters and downspouts:- You can re-direct rain water runoff to trees & plants essentially addressing two water issues at once!; Watering your plants, and upcycling rain water!

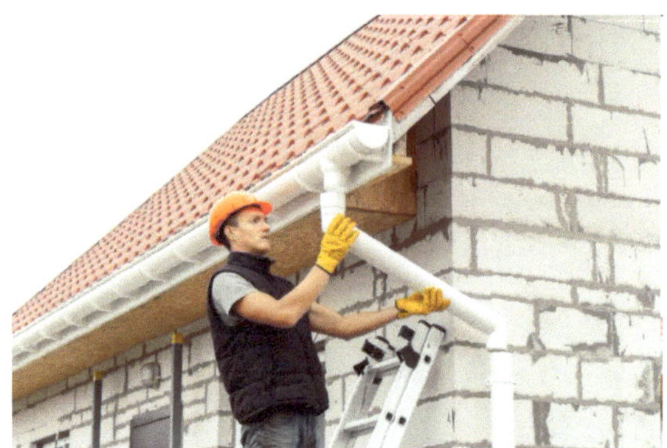

Fig.40.48: *A plumber is Instaling gutters and downspouts to re-direct rain water runoff to trees & plants*

19. Use the garbage disposal sparingly:- Garbage disposals use a lot of water. Compost vegetable food waste instead, and save gallons of water while reducing food waste.

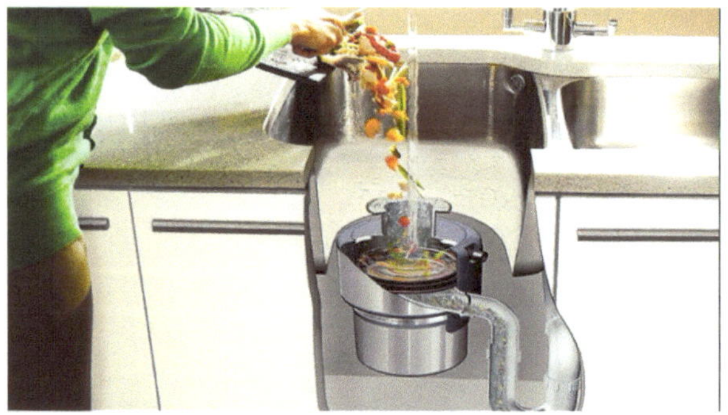

Fig.40.49: *showing the garbage disposal system to save water.*

20. Keep a pitcher or water bottle of drinking water in the fridge:- While waiting for the tap water to get cold for a fresh drink of water, collect the water in a pitcher or water bottle so it's not running down the drain instead, this way, you have fresh cold drinking water while helping reduce water waste!

21. Throw left -over ice cubes or ice chunks on a plant that needs watering.

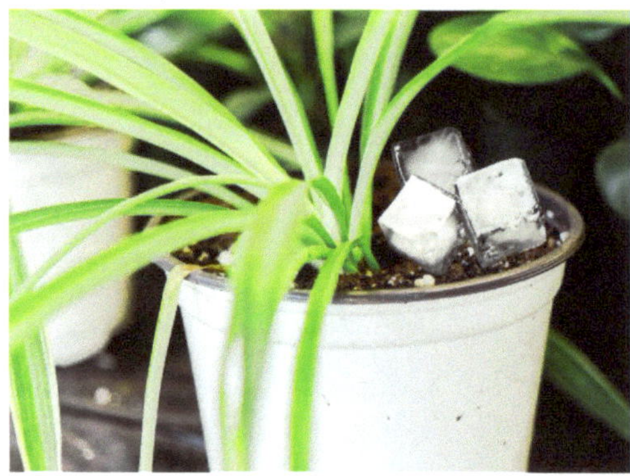

Fig.40.50: *showing plants are being watered with left over icechunks*

22. Soak pots & pans:- Soak pots and pans with water instead of scraping and cleaning the food off while the water is running.

Quick cleaning tip: Soak with water, add a few drops of *dish soap*, and put onto the stove with low heat; this will help clean stuck on food and debris easier with less water waste.

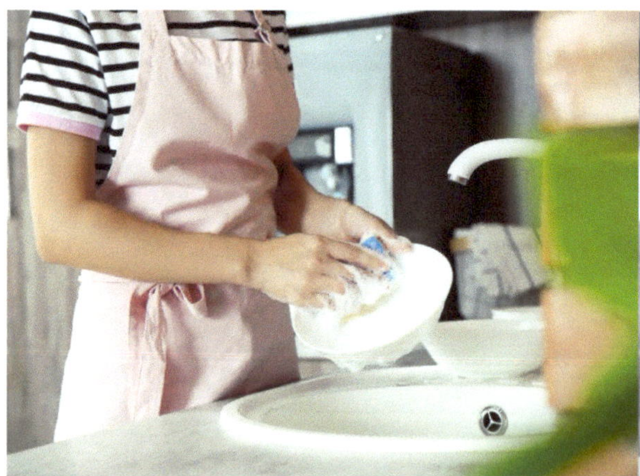

Fig.40.51: *How to clean stuck on food and debris. Soak with water, add a few drops of dish soap, and put onto the stove with low heat; this will help clean stuck on food and debris easier with less water waste.*

23. Don't use running water to de-thaw frozen foods! For both food safety and water conservation, defrost food in the refrigerator.

24. Ever have Throw leftover ice cubes or ice chunks on a plant that needs watering:- Instead of throwing this water down the drain, pour in a tea kettle to boil and make tea or use it to water plants.

25. Reuse your towels:- When at home, or at a hotel, reuse your bath towels. Let them dry properly. Wash after every 4th or 5th use. Towels don't need to be washed every time they're used, you're already clean when you come out of the shower!

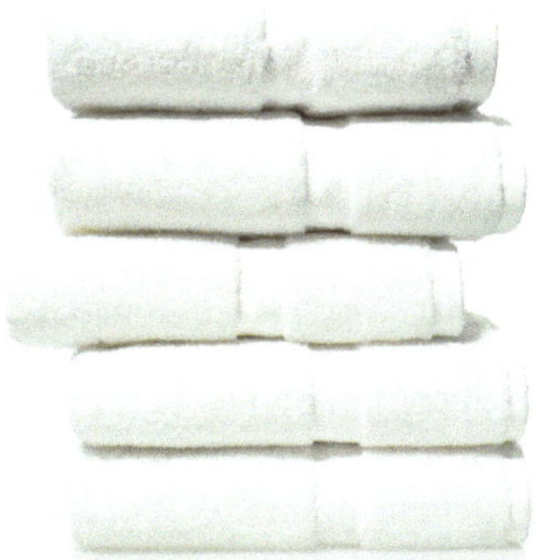

Fig.40.52: *One can reuse your bath towels at home or at hotel.*

2. Agricultural Water Conservation

While many farmers globally are relying on groundwater and other pumped resources to properly water their crops, the environmental effects of water waste are a big problem in agriculture. Water waste can lead to soil erosion, overwatered crops, and unnecessary spend. By better optimizing your water usage, you are not only doing your part to conserve one of nature's most precious resources, but you can also produce healthier crops, all with less water. Here are some tips for water conservation in agriculture.

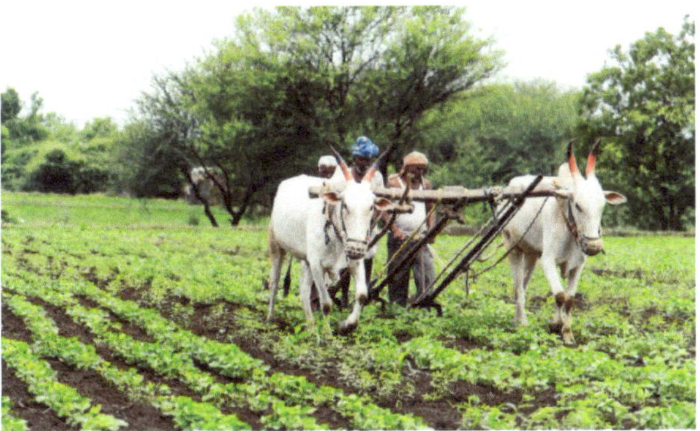

Fig.40.53: *Many Indian farmers are relying on groundwater and other pumped resources to properly water their crops, the environmental effects of water waste are a big problem in agriculture.*

Indian economy is dependent on agriculture, and the farmer's livelihood is dependent on the monsoon. Drastic climatic conditions like floods, drought, a shift in plant growing zones have resulted in the decline in crop productivity. In this scenario, it is imperative that effective provisions for saving water are made.

Go Organic

A 30-year trial found that organically-grown corn actually produced 30 percent more than non-organic fields, when drought was taken into consideration. *Organic methods of farming* help retain soil moisture, add more *groundwater*, and prevent pesticides from going into streams and other bodies of water.

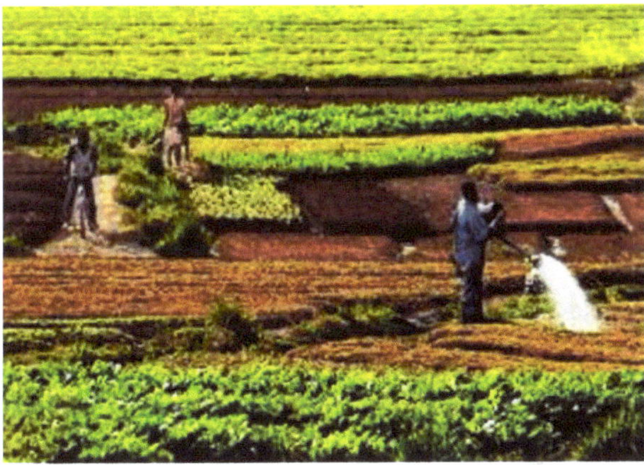

Fig 40.54: *showing Organic method of farming to retain soil moisture, add more groundwater,*

Install Better Watering Systems

Watering with drip irrigation instead of the traditional overhead spray method can decrease evaporation and save up to 80 percent more water. It also ensure that the water gets to the plants' roots, which can lead to better growth.

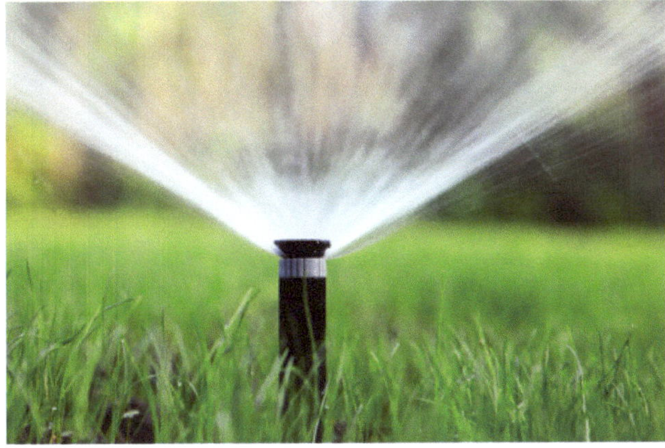

Fig.40.55: *showing watering plants with drip irrigation system*

Choose More Drought-Tolerant Crops

All crops you grow need to be ideal for your climate. If plants are native to your region, they will be more likely to succeed in natural weather conditions, such as periods of drought. In addition, if your region usually experiences periods of drought, consider planting crops that are acclimated to periods without enough water. This can help cut down on watering.

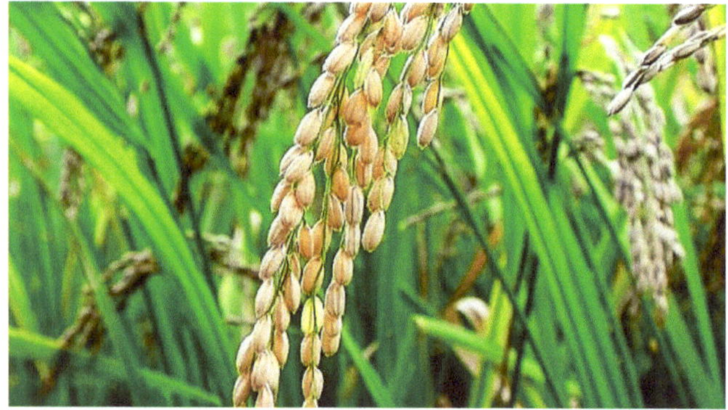

Fig. 40.56: *showing drought resistant rice variety in India*

Store Rain Water

Alternatively, in periods of regular rainstorms, consider building rain barrels to store precipitation. When rainy season turns into drought, you are able to use that natural rainwater for crop irrigation

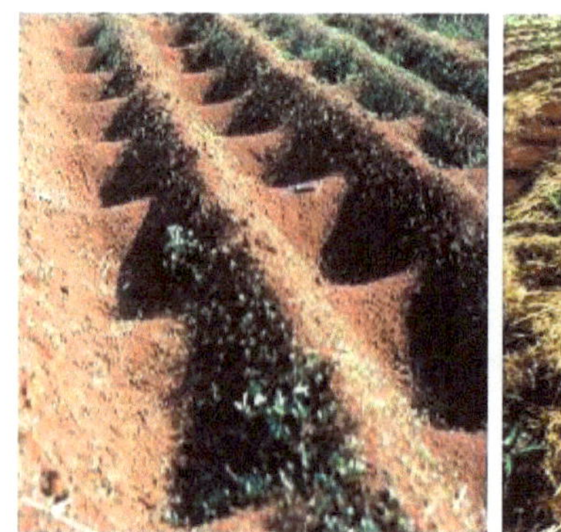

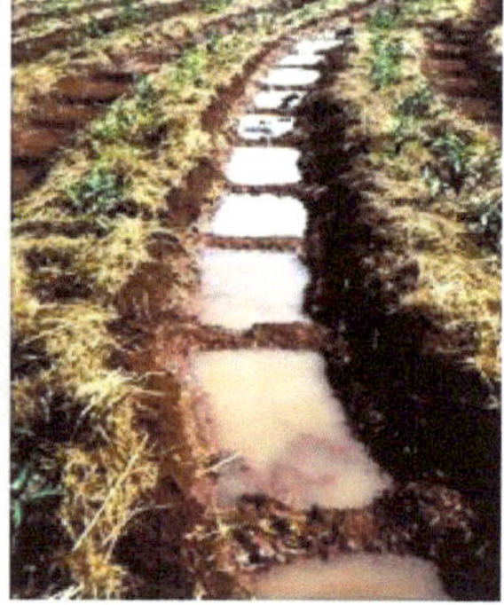

Fig.40.57: *showing one of the methods in harvesting rain water in a field*

Better Optimize Watering Times

It is essential to know enough information about your land and crops. Low cost and long-battery life connected sensors running on *Sigfox network* are able to tell farmers crucial data about their crops and soil, including soil moisture levels and soil temperature so it's easier to determine if and when to water.

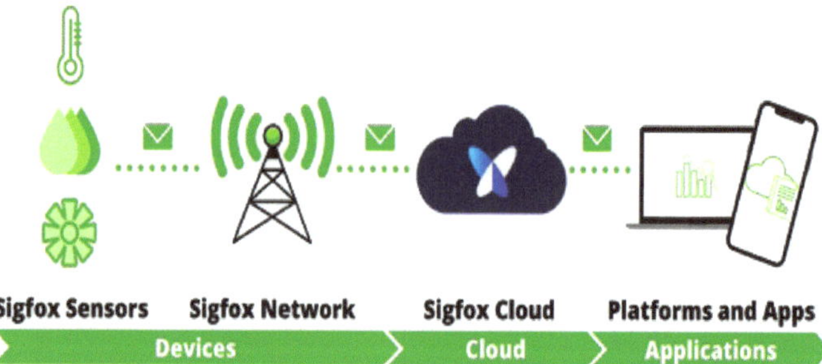

Fig.40.58: *Example of a Sigfox network from sensors to platforms. Sigfox offers a straightforward communications solution, where all network and computing complexity is managed in the Cloud, rather than on a device*

Follow Best Practices for Better Soil Quality

By focusing on better soil quality, your soil can better hold moisture and oxygen for plants to thrive. This will cut down on the amount of water needed on a regular basis. Good soil management practices include fertilizing with manure, adding compost, and reducing tillage frequency.

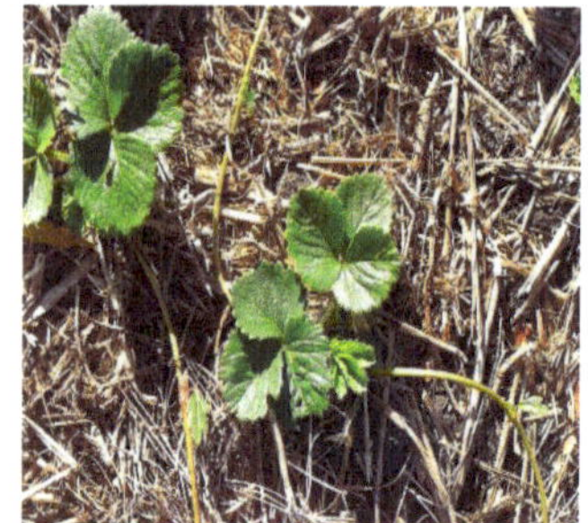

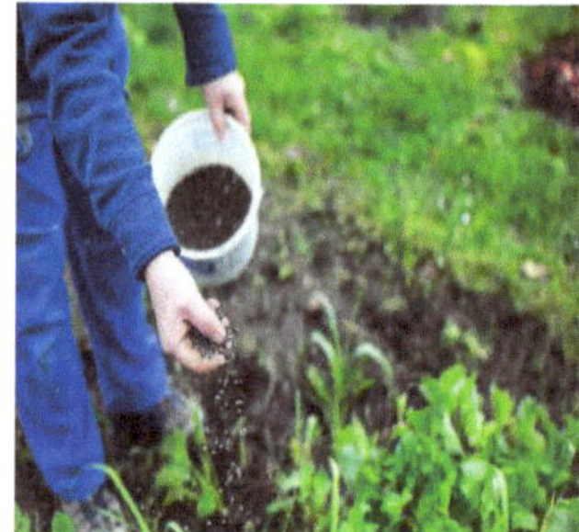

Fig.40.59: *(left) Plants nestled in mulch receive many benefits – p lus, i t greatly improves s oil microbiome health nearby. (right) Plants need nitrogen, and fertilizer is a way to grow better.*

Rotate Crops

Many farmers rotate the types of crops they plant by season or year, thus providing enough variety for the soil and plants to thrive. Different crops need different soil nutrients and water amounts. By constantly rotating the types of crops, there's usually a higher crop yield. Agricultural water conservation does take some effort, but the results are worth the effort. By better conserving water, you're not only saving a precious natural resource, you're also helping your crops thrive. Optimize your watering systems with better soil moisture monitoring. Sigfox-enabled sensors allow you to instantly collect soil moisture levels for your land and view it instantly on your phone, tablet, or computer.

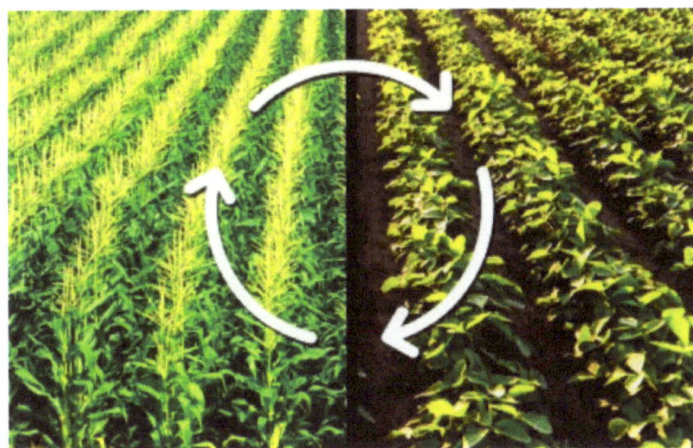

Fig.40.60: *showing farmers rotate the types of crops they plant by season or year with help of Sigfox-enabled sensors.*

Black Plastic and Organic Mulches:

Did you know that organic and *black plastic mulches* can save 25 percent in water requirements? Black Plastic or synthetic mulch not only reduces the water evaporation but also helps in controlling weeds and warms the soil, for an earlier crop. Organic mulches post decomposition provide nutrients to the soil and conserve moisture. Cover crops and Green Mulches can be used too.

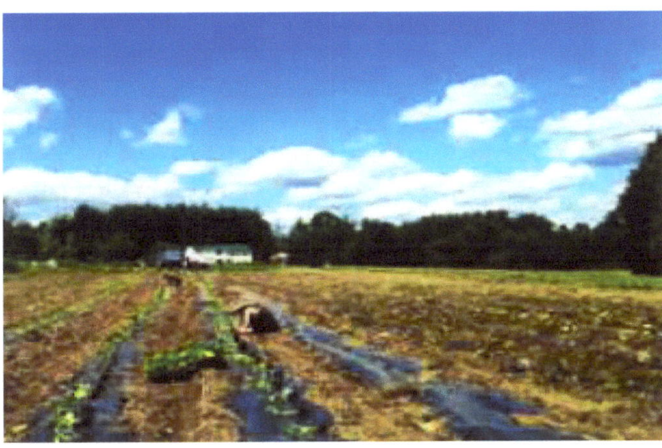

Fig.40.61: *Showing use of organic and black plastic mulches in farming technique*

Laser Leveling

Unevenness of the soil surface impacts germination, stand and yield of crops. Farmers spend considerable time and resources in leveling their fields properly. However, traditional methods of leveling land are cumbersome, time-consuming as well as expensive. *Laser land leveling* can be defined as leveling the area within a certain degree of the desired slope using a guided laser beam throughout the field.

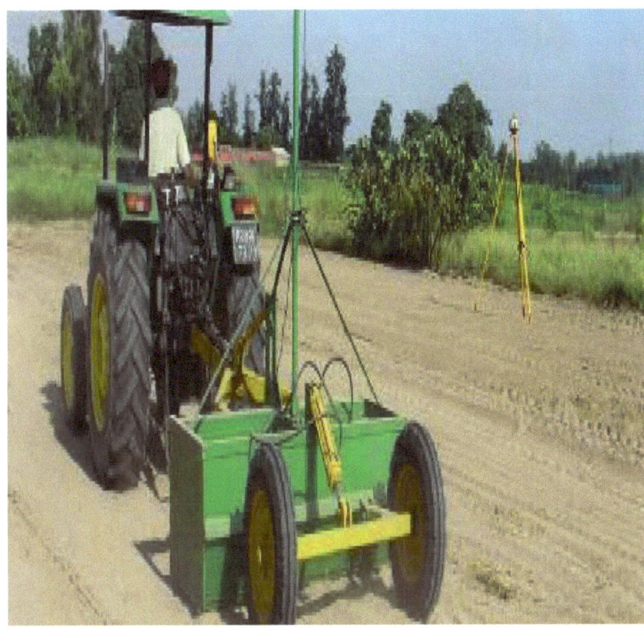

Fig 40.62: *Laser land levelling, a simple operation to prepare the land before sowing, can reap massive returns such as increasing yields, saving water and reducing greenhouse gas emissions.*

The benefits of Laser Land Levelling are:

- Accurate distribution of water
- Saving water
- Conservation of soil nutrients
- Precision Farming
- Higher crop productivity
- Fewer weed problems
- Saving time, energy and resources

Agroforestry

Agroforestry is a concept in which trees are used as a part of the landscape. This idea benefits the soil, animals and plants alike.

Advantages of Agroforestry are:

- Less evaporation rate due to which the soil and water run-off is prevented.
- Shade tolerant crops can be grown.
- Animals benefit from the shade.
- The leaves and fruits from trees can form an organic mulch.
- Multi-variety crops can be planted.
- By mixing trees, shrubs and seasonal crops the damage caused due to insects, diseases, drought, and the wind is prevented.

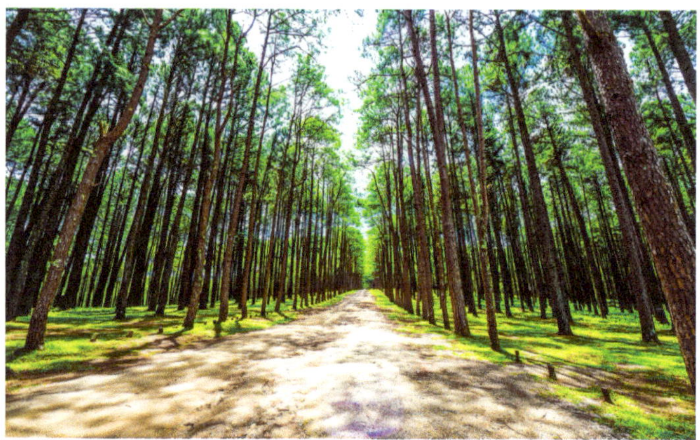

Fig. 40.63:*showing plantation of trees are used as a part of the landscape.in agroforestry which in turn lead Less evaporation rate due to which the soil and water run-off is prevented.*

Chinampas or Floating Gardens

This farming system was practiced by the Aztecs of Mexico's lake country for more than thousand years. *Chinampas* or floating gardens are long and narrow patches of ground, bordered by canals on both sides. Approximately 30 meters by 2.5 meters, they are built during canal excavation through stacking alternate layers of canal muck and rotting vegetation.

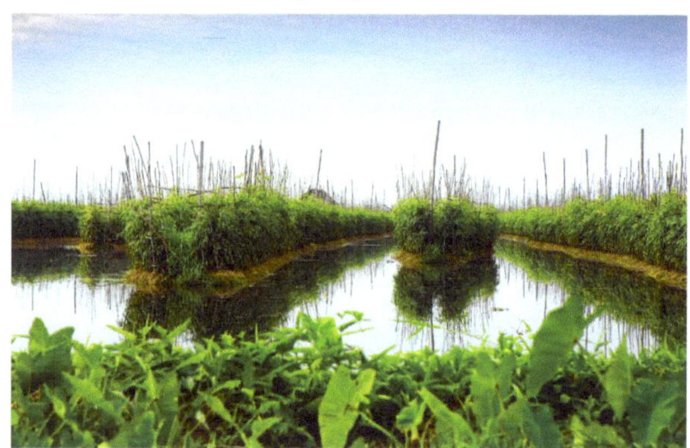

Fig 40.64: *showing use of Chinampas or f oating gardens with long and narrow patches of ground, bordered by canals on both sides as practiced by the Aztecs of Mexico's lake country .*

Sub-surface irrigation

This type of irrigation is suitable for hot, arid and windy regions. Its advantages are:

- Saving water
- High Yield
- Minimal evaporation
- Negligible soil and nutrient run-off
- Nutrients reach the root level
- Less disease infestation
- Fewer weeds problems
- Less labor
- Root zone is uniformly moist
- Less energy required for pumping

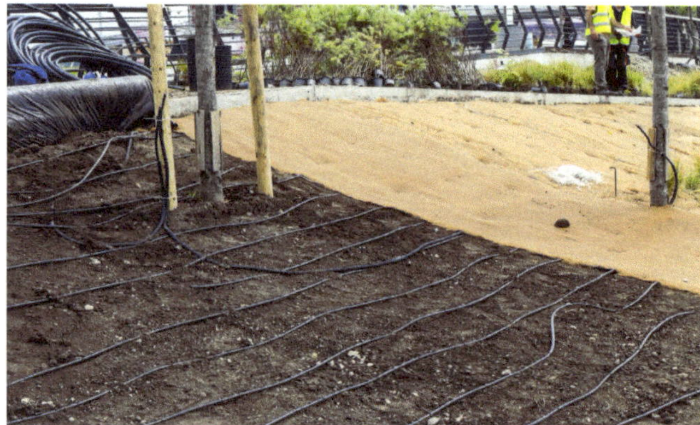

Fig.40.65 *showing use of Sub-surface irrigation technique. This type of irrigation is suitable for hot, arid and windy regions to save water and Negligible soil and nutrient run-off.*

Plastic buckets for starting trees

The waste baskets lying at the construction sites can be put to great use by starting young trees in them. All you need to do is, take a 5-gallon bucket, drill drainage holes at the bottom, place it next to a small tree and let gravity do the rest. You can also attach a small pipe to the holes and leave it close to the tree. This method helps in irrigating the crops slowly and gradually.

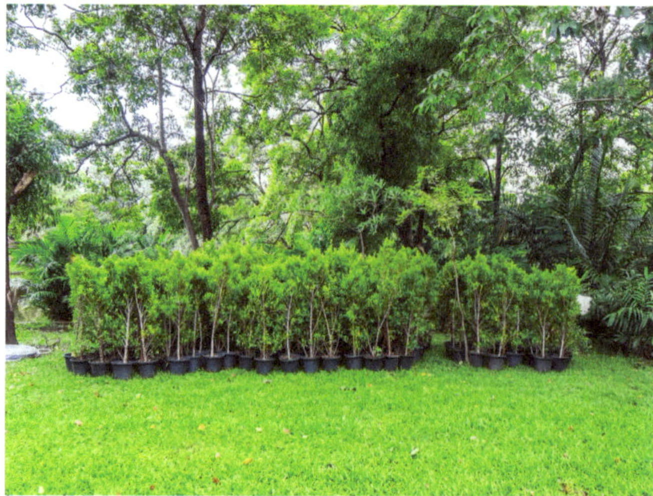

Fig.40.66: *showing use of Plastic buckets for starting trees. This method helpful in irrigating the crops slowly and gradually.*

Sand dams

Developed by the Romans in 400 BC, Sand Dams has been used in India, Africa, and South America for more than fifty years, but remains underutilized. It is a simple concept and can provide enough clean drinking water for gardening and farming in large quantity and an extensive period. *Sand Dams* are built by digging a deep trench and filling it with concrete. This drench is filled overtime with rains. The dams are usually located across small rivers which stop flowing in the dry season, the sand becomes about 40% saturated with water and can hold 2 to 10 million liters.

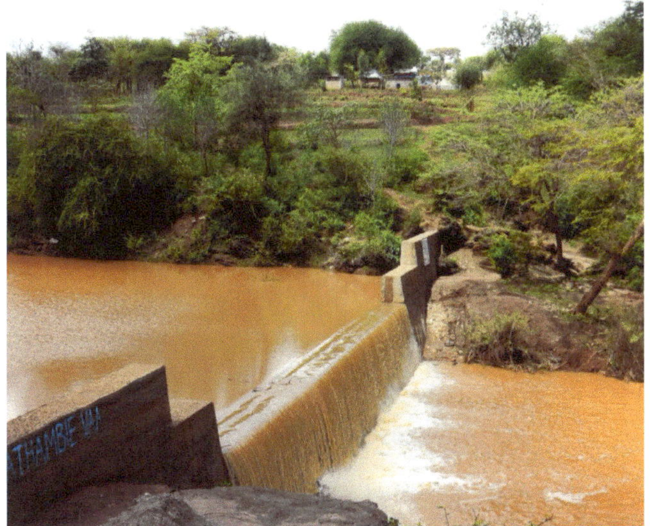

Fig.40.67: *showing use of sand dams as one of the techniques in farming. It is a simple concept and can provide enough clean drinking water for gardening and farming in large quantity and an extensive period*

3. Future Methods of Conserving Water in Agriculture

IoT Water Sensors

Many homeowners have embraced IoT (Internet of Things) technology to improve water and energy conservation in the home. From smart lights to smart refrigerators, it's easy to monitor and adjust energy consumption from a centralized dashboard. While some farmers are reluctant to share their well use data with regulators, using IoT technology is an efficient way to demonstrate compliance and avoid overpumping. Not only that, but smart water sensors can be used to monitor other variables as well, including pH level, salinity, and additional factors that impact crop health.

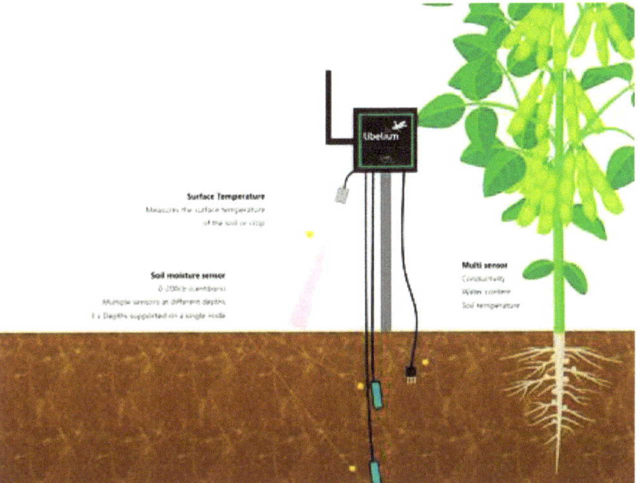

Fig 40.68: *Smart Agriculture Node – monitoring moisture, conductivity, surface temperature and soil temperature*

Remote Sensing Technology

IoT-connected well meters aren't the only way to monitor groundwater resources. Radio waves, electric currents, and even satellites have all been used to determine how much groundwater is available in a given region. One approach, called the *Metric technique,* uses "*evapo -transpiration*" to "retroactively determine water use from historical images."

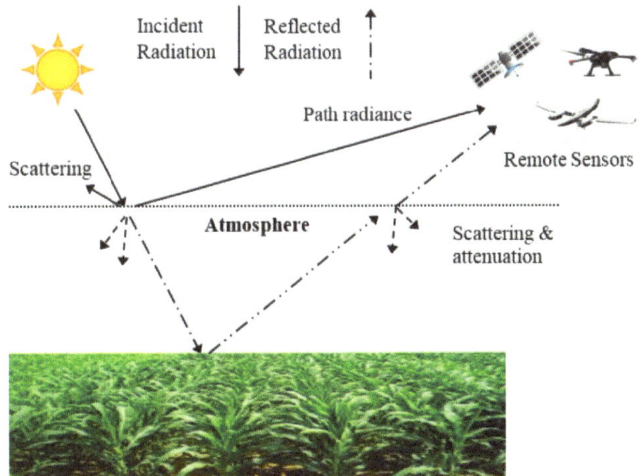

Fig.40.69: *showing remote sensing technique in acquiring data for farmers to conserve and replenish scarce ground-water resources.*

In another project, "a pair of twin satellites launched by NASA were able to estimate that Central Valley aquifers had (just between 2003 and 2010) lost 25 million acre-feet of groundwater." These approaches can help measure something that groundwater meters don't cover :

recharge, or the amount of water that returns to an aquifer after pumping. With better data, regulators can uphold pumping restrictions while also working with farmers to conserve and replenish scarce groundwater resources.

4. Better Methods of Conserving Water in Agriculture

New technologies and farming practices can help improve water use efficiency for its own sake. From more efficient irrigation to indoor farming, here are just a few ways that *water conservation* in agriculture is going to change in the future:

Improved Irrigation

Traditional farming practices rely on manual measurement of key metrics, such as soil humidity, soil temperature, and more. Not only is this a time-consuming process, but it can lead to overwatering or underwatering if the measurements are off. New IoT technologies can track all of these variables in real-time for more accurate – and actionable – data. According to IBM, these systems can help reduce waste and improve crop output by making use of both soil and environmental sensors. They can even take weather forecasts into account so farmers can "build advanced irrigation systems to save water and prevent pesticide waste by predicting rain."

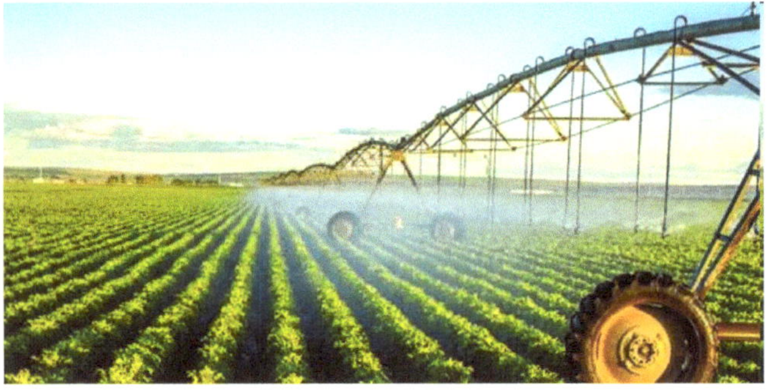

Fig. 40.70: *showing Improved irrigation method to save water and prevent pesticide waste.*

Reduced Evaporation

Another key driver of water waste is evaporation, especially when fields are left fallow for long periods : "Soils fallowed for a 21-month period (from harvest to spring of crop year) can be expected to lose three-fourths of the precipitation received." In California, SGMA is expected to lead to the retirement of as many as 1 million acres of land in the San Joaquin Valley alone, while in Arizona, a drought could lead farmers to leave up to 40% of their lands fallow for extended periods. Maintenance practices, such as covering fields in light-colored soil to reflect sunlight or using wheat-grass strips to prevent wind, can help reduce water loss. Other techniques include reducing tillage and maintaining crop residue on the surface of the soil. The world "to-till" originates from Proto-Germanic with the basic meaning "to cultivate", "to plow". The primary goals of *no-till agriculture* are to avoid cultivation with soil improvement in mind. No-till agriculture reduces soil erosion. Tillage breaks the earth's surface and turns it over, moving the cover layer inside. As a result, the bare soil is subject to erosion because of the loosened structure. Deprived of cover matter, it is subject to quick erosion due to water flows, especially in slope and steep areas, and winds. The rainsplash erosion is another issue to consider as flexible particles are easily removed when hit with heavy rains. Correspondingly, the absence of soil disturbance in no-till farming eliminates the issues.

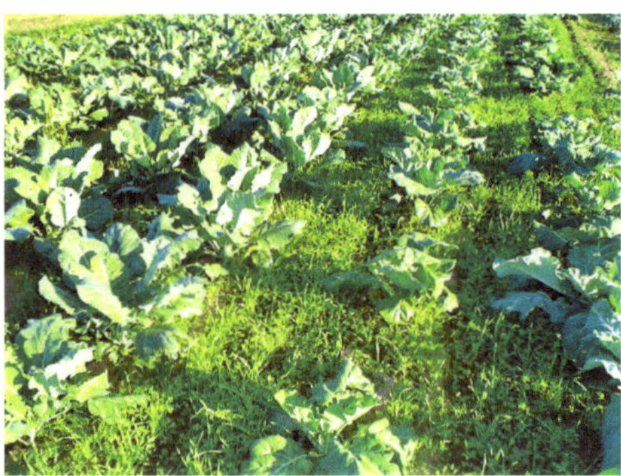

Fig.40.71: *showing A field of cover crops : in between the collards in this field is a cover crop mix of rye, hairy vetch and crimson clover, which provides a lush cover protecting the soil from harsh winds and eroding/compacting rains. Source : TILLER (2012)*

Benefits of No-Till

Maintaining soil health is just one of the advantages of no-till farming. It competes with alternative practices flaunting other merits as well. The major benefits of no-till farming include, among others:

- Savings on tillage equipment needed to plow the entire field. Modern machines allow sowing directly on the residue-covered strips instead. Furthermore, plants can get nutrients from the decomposed matter this way.
- Limited fossil fuel inputs for field operations (6 to 2 gallons of diesel fuel per acre, according to the U.S. Department of Agriculture).
- Shorted operation time. Sophisticated seeders do the job faster and complete it in one-field pass.
- Avoided human labor for tilling operations and maintaining tillage machines.

- Conserved moisture and decreased water spend due to slowed evaporation and low cracking.
- Eliminated herbicide leakage due to less frequent irrigation.

Weighing no-till farming pros and cons, more and more farmers convert to the new method year by year, encouraged with the USDA conservation programs and economic standpoints. The agriculture approach implementations vary across crops and regions. An ERS research gives the adoption data for 2002-2017 regarding separate crops.

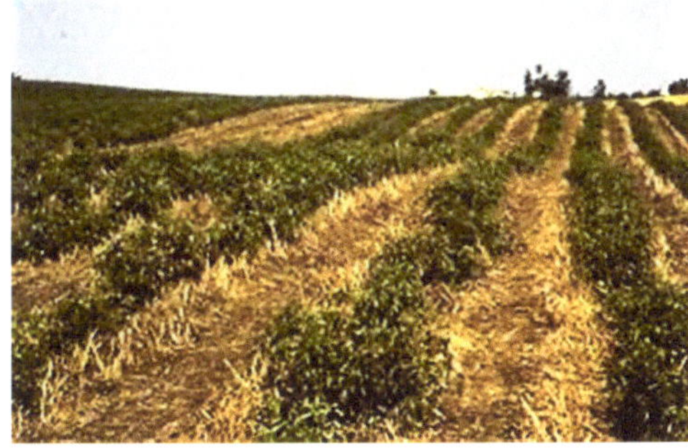

Fig. 40.72: *Even a small amount of crop residue can provide a benefit to a growing crop under extremely dry conditions. The residue moderates soil temperatures and help to reduce evaporation of soil water. Source : OMAFRA (2011)*

Indoor Farming

While *indoor farming* is well-established in some parts of the world, especially in Japan and the Netherlands, it's still an underdeveloped market in the U.S.

Many indoor farms rely on vertical farming to maximize the available growing space; controlled-environment agriculture (CEA) to create year-round growing conditions, and soil-free hydroponics to reduce evaporation and improve nutrient transfer. Some examples of indoor farms in the U.S. include:

- *Aero Farms*, which grows microgreens in New Jersey under LED lights and uses "95% less water than conventional agriculture on just one percent of the land required.
- *Bowery Farming*, which produces leafy greens and herbs in New Jersey and Maryland. It uses BoweryOS, its proprietary farm operating system that relies on "computer vision, automation, and machine learning to monitor our crops and all the variables that drive their growth," and allowing them to track the entire process "from seed to store."
- *Square Roots* creates indoor farms in shipping containers that it claims can replicate any climate based on historical data. Because of their small size and portability, these farms are primarily intended for use in crowded urban environments.

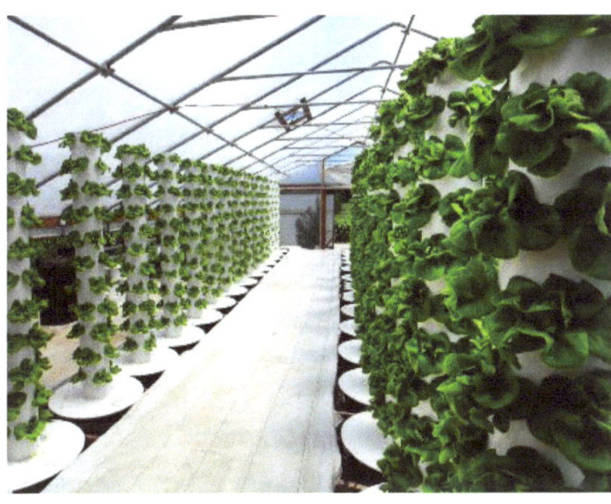

A

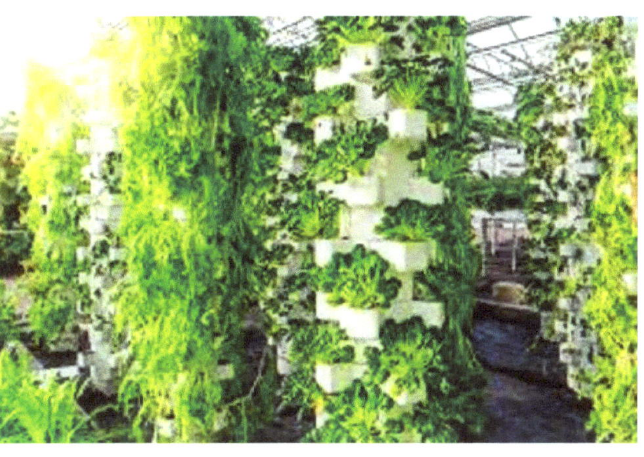

b

Fig.40.73: *Photographs A. Showing indoor farming. B. Vertical farming*

Smart Tractors and Drones

You don't have to farm indoors in order to make use of the latest agricultural technology. John Deere has been rolling out smart tractors as part of their precision agriculture line that can help people improve tillage, seed placement, irrigation, and more. These include touch-screen displays,satellite receivers that can pinpoint location to within an inch, and AutoTrac hands-free guidance systems. In Australia, scientists are developing smart drones that will allow farmers to "plan and deliver precise water and nutrients to their crops on a need-by-need basis."

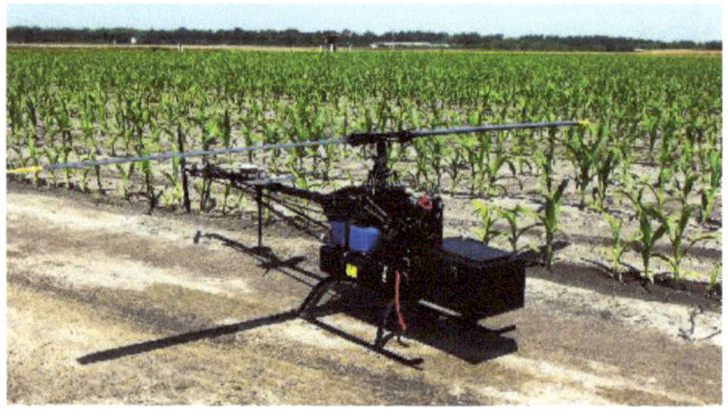

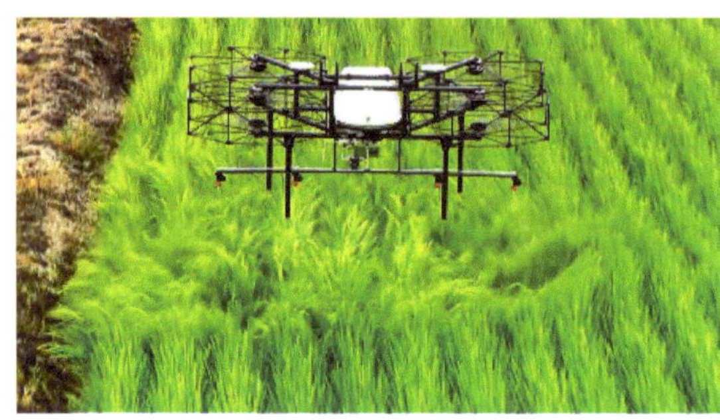

A b

Fig. 40.74:*Photographs showing (left) smart tracter and (right) drone that will allow farmers to "plan and deliver precise water and nutrients to their crops on a need-by-need basis.*

Other techniques that can be used by Indian farmers to save water are:

- Use a Water Flow Meter to Measure Water Usage
- Tailwater Return Systems
- Bottle Irrigation and Pitcher or Olla Irrigation
- Zai Pits
- System of Crop Intensification (SCI) or System of Root Intensification (SRI)
- Ripper-Furrower Planting System
- Acequias
- Organic Farm Soils
- Drought Tolerant Livestock Breeds
- Recycle Wastewater
- Half Moons, Bunds, and Terraces
- Mycorrhizal Fungus
- Soil Moisture Sensors
- Good Drainage

How much should you drink?

Being attentive to the amount of water you drink each day is important for optimal health. Most people drink when they're thirsty, which helps regulate daily water intake. According to the National Academies of Sciences, Engineering, and Medicine, general water intake (from all beverages and foods) that meet most people's needs are : about 15.5 cups of water (125 ounces) each day for menabout 11.5 cups (91 ounces) daily for women .People get about 20 percent of their daily water intake from food. The rest is dependent on drinking water and water-based beverages. So, ideally men would consume about 100 ounces (3.0 liters) of water from beverages, and women, about 73 ounces (2.12 liters) from beverages. You'll have to increase your water intake if you're exercising or living in a hotter region to avoid dehydration. Other ways to assess hydration include your thirst and the color of your urine. Feeling thirsty indicates your body is not receiving adequate hydration. Urine that is dark or colored indicates dehydration. Pale or non-colored urine typically indicates proper hydration.

Water-Based Therapies Used in Traditional and Alternative Medicine

Types and Benefits of Hydrotherapy

Hydrotherapy is the use of water, both internally and externally and at varying temperatures, for health purposes. Also known as water therapy or "water cures", hydrotherapy includes such therapeutic treatments as saunas, steam baths, foot baths, contrast therapy, sitz baths, and colonic cleansing.

Although some forms of hydrotherapy are commonly used in traditional medical practices, there are some hydrotherapy procedures that are not supported by science and border on pseudoscience.

History of Hydrotherapy

From Roman baths to hot mineral springs, cultures around the world have used water for centuries to treat a variety of health concerns. During the same period, Vincent Preissnitz founded the first hydrotherapy clinic in Gräfenberg, Germany as part of a larger naturalism movement, which involved eating only coarse foods and copious amounts of water. Soon after, hydrotherapy and the naturalism craze spread to the United States, where John Harvey Kellogg of Kellogg's cereal fame aimed to scientifically prove its benefits at Battle Creek Sanitarium in Michigan. Kellogg had a special fascination with colonic cleansing.

Hydrotherapy is popular in Europe, Asia, and parts of the United States (including Saratoga Springs in New York where Franklin Delana Roosevelt often frequented), where people regularly "take the waters" at hot mineral springs.

Principles

According to proponents of hydrotherapy, hot and cold water induce physiologic changes that are beneficial to human health. Among them:

- Hot water causes superficial blood vessels to dilate, activating sweat glands, loosening joints, and removing toxic wastes from tissues.
- Cold water causes superficial blood vessels to constrict, moving blood flow away from an affected area to relieve inflammation

There are different appliances used to deliver hydrotherapy, including full-body immersion tanks, body-specific tubs, whirlpool baths, and cold and hot water wraps (compresses).

Types

Hydrotherapy is often performed at health centers, spas, and physical therapy clinics and even at home. Common types of hydrotherapy include:

Aquatic exercises: Exercising in a pool of warm or cool water allows you to exercise with less resistance and pressure on joints. It can be helpful for people back pain, arthritis, obesity, advanced age, or physical disability.

Balneotherapy: Soaking in mineral-rich waters or natural mineral hot springs are thought to have curative benefits. Known as balneotherapy, the practice is said to treat arthritis, low back pain, immune dysfunction, and fibromyalgia, among others.

Colonic hydrotherapy: Also known as colonic cleansing or irrigation, the practice involves rinsing feces from the colon, which proponents claim can help clear toxins and improve health.

Compresses: This form of hydrotherapy involves wrapping towels soaked in warm or cool water on a body part to increase circulation or reduce inflammation. Aromatics are often added to the wraps for various therapeutic purposes.

Contrast hydrotherapy: Also known as water circuit therapy, it involves alternating immersion in hot and cold water to treat chronic pain or promote lymphatic drainage (thereby removing toxins from the immune system).

Floatation tanks: Also known as isolation tanks or immersion tanks, the practice involves floating atop a shallow pool of saltwater in a sealed, darkened tank. Doing so is said to relieve stress and anxiety, improve sleep, and relax muscles.

Foot baths: Soaking your feet can reduce swelling and pain after a long day on one's feet. But, it can also be used to soften tissues before a spa foot treatment. Some people even claim that food baths can balance circulation and decrease congestion in the head, lungs, and pelvic organs.

Hot fomentation: The application of warm compresses or hot water bottles to the chest is said to relieve acute symptoms of a cold or bronchitis.

Ice bath: Popular among athletes, ice baths involve soaking in a tub of water between 45 F and 65 F to speed recovery from an injury or extreme exercise. Also known as cold water immersion, ice baths have increasingly been replaced by cryotherapy, which exposes the body to short bursts of air as cold as -280 F.

Sauna: A sauna is a form of hydrotherapy in which dry, warm air induces sweating to release toxins, burn calories, relax muscles, and improve skin quality.

Sitz bath: A sitz bath involves sitting a tub of water to treat conditions affecting the anal, rectal, or genital areas. Sitz baths are commonly used for hemorrhoids, premenstrual syndrome (PMS), and anal fissures.

Steam baths: Steam baths involve rooms filled with warm, humid aid that proponents claim can amplify the benefits of a sauna. Turkish baths are a form of steam bathing that employs higher humidity and lower temperatures.

Therapeutic baths: Therapeutic baths involve soaking in a tub of warm water to treat skin conditions, joint problems, or emotional stress. Additives are commonly used, including Epsom salt, aromatherapy oils, dead sea salts, and herbs. Mud baths are a form of therapeutic bathing.

Watsu: This is an alternative massage technique (coined from words "*water*" and "*shiatsu*") in which a therapist performs massage while you float comfortably in a pool of warm water.

Whirlpool hydrotherapy: Rather than immersing a limb or body in still water, a whirlpool is said to offer additional benefits, including increased circulation and improved tissue repair after a burn, ulcer, or other skin injuries

Clinical Evidence

Although many of the health claims of hydrotherapy are unsupported (and several are far-fetched), other forms of are supported by a larger body of research. This is particularly true with respect to conditions like arthritis and the use of hydrotherapy among sports therapists.

1. Osteoarthritis

In a study published in *Clinical Rehabilitation* in 2018, researchers compared the effectiveness of twice-weekly aquatic exercise sessions to once-weekly group education in people with knee osteoarthritis. After eight weeks, people who engaged in aquatic exercises had reduced pain and improve joint function compared to those who managed their condition but didn't engage in hydrotherapy

2. Rheumatoid Arthritis

In people with rheumatoid arthritis, hydrotherapy may improve outcomes when used in combination with prescribed medications, according to a 2017 study in the International Journal of Rheumatic Diseases. For this study, half of the participants received hydrotherapy with rheumatoid arthritis medications, while the other half were treated with medications alone. After 12 weeks, the group receiving hydrotherapy had increases antioxidant levels and decreased oxidative stress, suggesting that the progression of the disease had been slowed.

3. Sports Recovery

Cold water immersion and contrast water therapy may improve recovery following sports and extreme physical activity, suggests a 2017 review of studies in the *Journal of Strength and Conditioning Research.*

According to the research, cold water immersion improves recovery in athletes after 24 hours as measured by sprint times and jump performance. Similarly, athletes who underwent contrast water therapy experienced better recovery after 48 hours compared to those who didn't. However, neither form of hydrotherapy improved the *perception* of recovery among athletes, meaning that the symptoms reported were more or less the same

Precautions

Hydrotherapy may not be appropriate for everyone. Exposure to sudden cold or prolonged heat can have adverse effects on the cardiovascular system. Prolonged soaking can lead to skin maceration and infection. Similarly, colonic cleansing can disrupt the normal bacterial flora in the lower intestine as well as the balance of electrolytes in the body if overused. Hydrotherapy may need to be avoided or used with caution in people with the following health conditions:

- Cardiovascular disease
- High blood pressure
- Colds, flu, or other respiratory infections
- High fever
- Incontinence
- Kidney disease
- Thrombosis
- Skin infections
- Cancer
- Pregnancy

Cardiac Functions with Hydrotherapy: (i.e., exercise in warm water) had been considered potentially dangerous in heart failure patientsdue to the increased venous return caused by the hydrostatic pressure. However, it is now known that cardiac function actually improves during water immersion due to theincrease in early diastolic filling and decrease in heart rate, resulting in improvements in stroke volume and ejection fraction. Studies with sauna therapy (i.e., warming) have demonstrated important improvements in neuro -hormonal attenuation and exercise status in heart failure patients. These data suggest that hydrotherapy is a good potential treatment for heart failure patients. However, few studies are available, and none have compared conventional rehabilitation to hydrotherapy

Will Turning Seawater Into Drinking Water Help Water Shortages?

With severe droughts affecting over 36 countries could the solution lie in the ocean? The ocean makes up 70 percent of the earth's surface and accounts for 96 percent of the water on the planet. The problem is, this water can't be consumed. It's oversaturated with salt. Desalination is the process of turning salty ocean water into drinking water. So with 783 million people lacking access to clean water and more areas facing severe droughts, could desalination be the silver bullet? The Middle East has been a leader in desalination so far. Saudi Arabia, United Arab Emirates, Kuwait, and Israel rely heavily on desalination as a source for clean water. Israel gets 40 percent of domestic water from desalination. These countries also have hardly any groundwater or fresh water sources so desalination is a case of innovation by necessity. These countries make up the one percent of the world currently relying on desalination to meet water needs. But the UN predicts that by 2025 14 percent of the world will rely on desalination to meet water needs

How does desalination work?

Desalination is the process of purifying saline water into a potable fresh water. Basically–turning ocean water into drinkable fresh water. Sounds pretty cool!

There are several ways to remove salt from water. Reverse osmosis and distillation are the most common ways to desalinate water. Reverse osmosis water treatment pushes water through small filters leaving salt behind. Distillation on a large scale involves boiling water and collecting water vapor during the process. Both require a lot of energy, infrastructure and are costly.

Is cost the reason why desalination isn't used?

The energy requirements are so high that the cost for a lot of countries is too much. That's why it's mainly used in regions lacking freshwater, ships, and military vessels. There are environmental concerns too. Desalination plants take in salt water straight from the ocean and can kill or harm fish and other small ocean life as water travels from the source to the plant. Lastly, salinity levels in oceans are predicted to rise, which would make filtering water more expensive. The more salt there is to filter out, the more energy required. That's why plants often convert brackish water (think lightly salted potato chips vs. regular) to clean water. But brackish water is not as prevalent as ocean water.

Can it work?

It's still very expensive compared to using freshwater sources. But companies are working on it. Israel invested in a large desalination plant in 2005 and will be producing enough water to supply half the country by the end of 2015. The building desalination plants is very costly but it is a safety net for places where drought conditions persist and freshwater is limited or lacking entirely. California, you know what I'm talking about. California is building seventeen new desalination plants after years of severe drought. And it's still controversial. Desalination is being used as a last resort in California. Cities in California have tried investing in infrastructure for desalination previously. Santa Barbara built a desalination plant years ago and is just now restarting it after initial costs were too high to run the plant previously. It will cost 55 million USD to restart and maintain. Water obtained from desalination costs twice the amount of water from freshwater sources. But now, parts of California don't have many other options.

The only way desalination can be a good option to solving the water crisis is if renewable energy is used, costs are lowered, and environmental protections are put in place for marine life too.

Companies and countries and trying to lower the amount of energy needed to desalinate water and look into using cleaner energy sources. For example, Saudi Arabia has pushed to use solar energy to power desalination plants.

In California, the California Coastkeepers Alliance is working with desalination plants on a plan to make sure marine life is minimally harmed by using techniques sub-surface water intake as opposed to sucking in water from the surface where marine life is more prevalent.

Desalination does allow for severely water-stressed areas to have their own water source, but it still comes at a high cost. But with climate change and severe drought affecting more and more areas, it's a process worth investing in to lower cost and cut carbon footprints of production. Combining renewable energy with improved technology could make desalination a more viable option. But it's still not going to be a first choice for most countries.

Desalination breakthrough could lead to cheaper water filtration

Producing clean water at a lower cost could be on the horizon after researchers from The University of Texas at Austin and Penn State solved a complex problem that has baffled scientists for decades, until now. *Desalination membranes* remove salt and other chemicals from water, a process critical to the health of society, cleaning billions of gallons of water for agriculture, energy production and drinking. The idea seems simple – push salty water through and clean water comes out the other side – but it contains complex intricacies that scientists are still trying to understand.

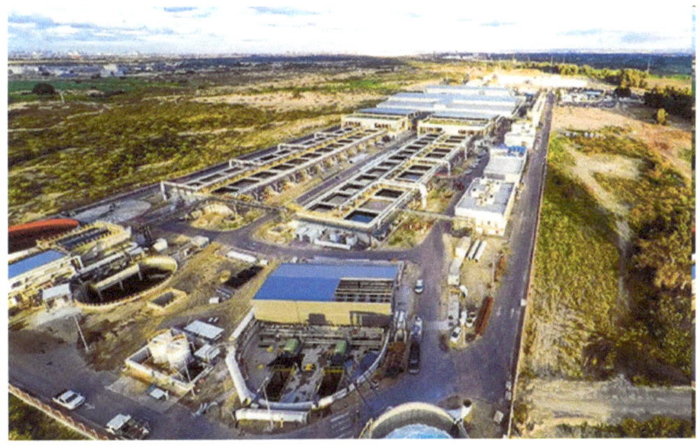

Fig.40.75: *Sorek Desalination Plant. Ten miles south of Tel Aviv, two concrete reservoirs the size of football fields and watch water pour into them from a massive pipe emerging from the sand. Mediterranean seawater pumped from an intake a mile offshore Credit : Photo courtesy of IDE Technologies.*

The research team, in partnership with DuPont Water Solutions, solved an important aspect of this mystery, opening the door to reduce costs of clean water production. The researchers determined desalination membranes are inconsistent in density and mass distribution, which can hold back their performance. Uniform density at the nanoscale is the key to increasing how much clean water these membranes can create.

"*Reverse osmosis membranes* are widely used for cleaning water, but there's still a lot we don't know about them," said Manish Kumar, an associate professor in the Department of Civil, Architectural and Environmental Engineering at UT Austin, who co-led the research. "We couldn't really say how water moves through them, so all the improvements over the past 40 years have essentially been done in the dark." The findings were published today in Science. The paper documents an increase in efficiency in the membranes tested by 30%-40%, meaning they can clean more water while using significantly less energy. That could lead to increased access to clean water and lower water bills for individual homes and large users alike.

Reverse osmosis membranes work by applying pressure to the salty feed solution on one side. The minerals stay there while the water passes through. Although more efficient than non-membrane desalination processes, it still takes a large amount of energy, the researchers said, and improving the efficiency of the membranes could reduce that burden.

"Fresh water management is becoming a crucial challenge throughout the world," said Enrique Gomez, a professor of chemical engineering at Penn State who co-led the research. "Shortages, droughts -- with increasing severe weather patterns, it is expected this problem will become even more significant. It's critically important to have clean water availability, especially in low-resource areas."

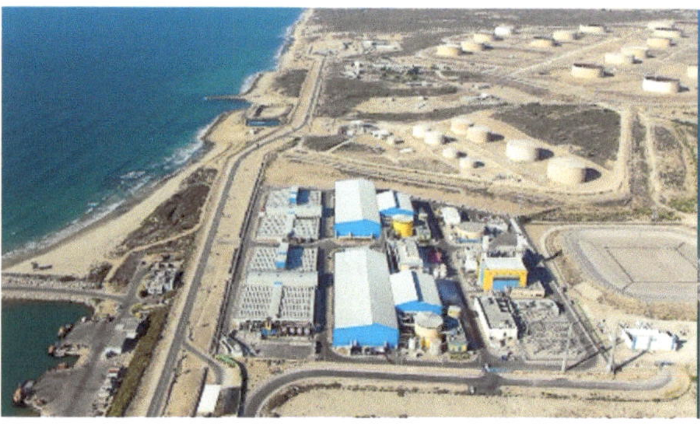

Fig.40.76: *IDE's Israel seawater RO desalination plant. IDE Technologies announced that its seawater reverse osmosis desalination plant in the coastal city of Ashkelon, Israel, has reached a world record with its delivery process*

The National Science Foundation and DuPont, which makes numerous desalination products, funded the research. The seeds were planted when DuPont researchers found that thicker membranes were actually proving to be more permeable. This came as a surprise because the conventional knowledge was that thickness reduces how much water could flow through the membranes.

The team connected with Dow Water Solutions, which is now a part of DuPont, in 2015 at a "water summit" Kumar organized, and they were eager to solve this mystery. The research team, which also includes researchers from Iowa State University, developed 3D reconstructions of the nanoscale membrane structure using state-of-the-art electron microscopes at the Materials Characterization Lab of Penn State. They modeled the path water takes through these membranes to predict how efficiently water could be cleaned based on structure. Greg Foss of the Texas Advanced Computing Center helped visualize these simulations, and most of the calculations were performed on Stampede2, TACC's supercomputer.

Seawater turns into freshwater through solar energy: A new low-cost technology

According to FAO estimates, by 2025 nearly 2 billion people may not have enough drinking water to satisfy their daily needs. One of the possible solutions to this problem is desalination, namely treating seawater to make it drinkable. However, removing salt from seawater requires 10 to 1000 times more energy than traditional methods of freshwater supply, namely pumping water from rivers or wells.

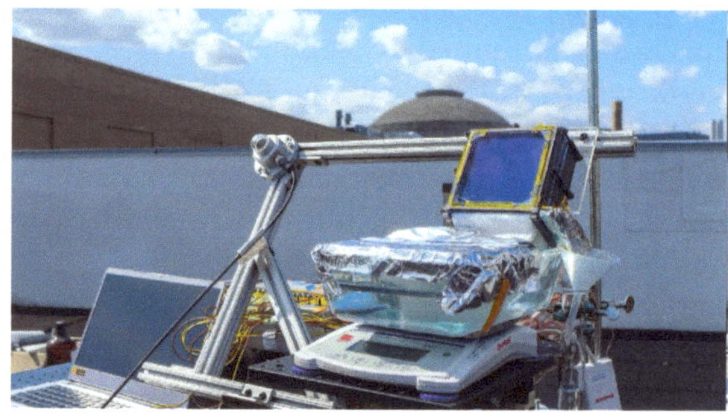

Fig.40.77: *Tests on an MIT building rooftop showed that a simple proof-of-concept desalination device could produce clean, drinkable water at a rate equivalent to more than 1.5 gallons per hour for each square meter of solar collecting area. Images courtesy of the researchers*

Motivated by this problem, a team of engineers from the Department of Energy of Politecnico di Torino has devised a new prototype to desalinate seawater in a sustainable and low-cost way, using *solar energy* more efficiently. Compared to previous solutions, the developed technology is in fact able to double the amount of water produced at given solar energy, and it may be subject to further efficiency improvement in the near future. The group of young researchers who recently published these results in the journal Nature Sustainability is composed of Eliodoro Chiavazzo, Matteo Morciano, Francesca Viglino, Matteo Fasano and Pietro Asinari (Multi-Scale Modeling Lab).

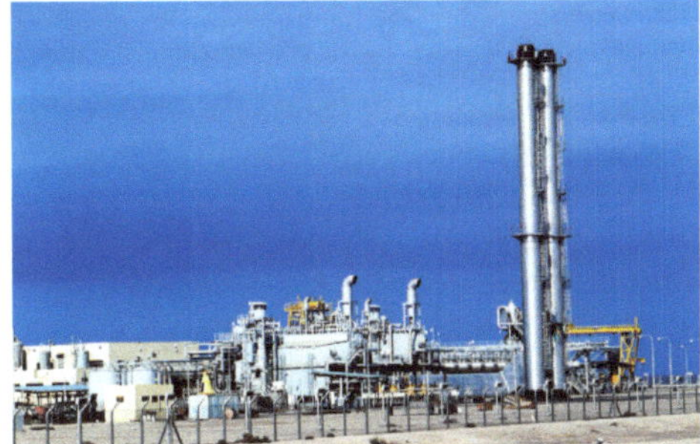

Fig. 40.78: *Saudi Arabia Pushes to Use Solar Power for Desalination Plants. A desalination plant in Al Khafji, Saudi Ar abia, is powered by fossil fuels. A new, solar-powered desalination plant is now being built in the city.*

The working principle of the proposed technology is very simple : "Inspired by plants, which transport water from roots to leaves by capillarity and transpiration, our *floating device* is able t o collect s eawater using a l ow-cost porous material, thus avoiding the use of expensive and cumbersome pumps. The collected seawater is then heated up by solar energy, which sustains the separation of salt from the evaporating water. This process can be facilitated by membranes inserted between contaminated and drinking water to avoid their mixing, similarly to some plants able to survive in marine environments (for example the mangroves)," explain Matteo Fasano and Matteo Morciano.

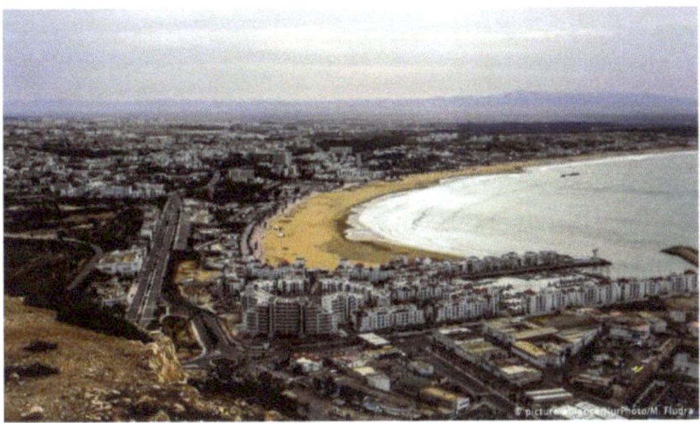

Fig.40.79: *Agadir, Morocco. Abengoa's new desalination plant will serve the people of this city - and irrigate 13,600 hectares of nearby farmland, too*

While conventional 'active' desalination technologies need costly mechanical or electrical components (such as pumps and/or control systems) and require specialized technicians for installation and maintenance, the desalination approach proposed by the team at Politecnico di Torino is based on spontaneous processes occurring without the aid of ancillary machinery and can, therefore, be referred to as 'passive' technology. All this makes the device inherently inexpensive and simple to install and repair. The latter features are particularly attractive in coastal regions that are suffering from a chronic shortage of drinking water and are not yet reached by centralized infrastructures and investments.

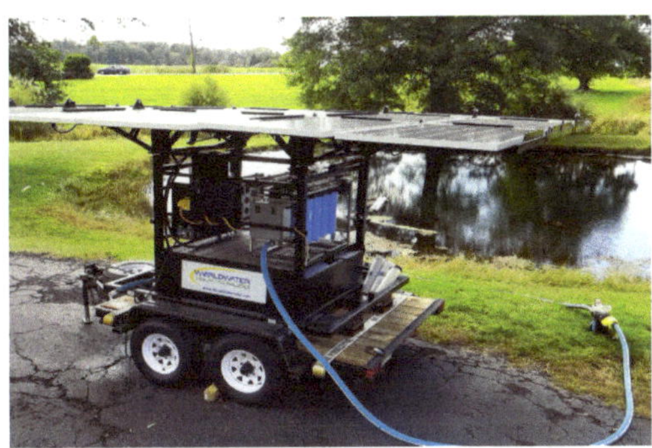

Fig. 40.80:*A solar-powered MaxPure system turns pond water into clean drinking water*

Up to now, a well-known disadvantage of *'passive' technologies* for desalination has been the low energy efficiency as compared to 'active' ones. Researchers at Politecnico di Torino have faced this obstacle with creativity : "While previous studies focused on how to maximize the solar energy absorption, we have shifted the attention to a more efficient management of the absorbed solar thermal energy. In this way, we have been able to reach record values of productivity up to 20 litres per day of drinking water per square meter exposed to the Sun. The reason behind the performance increase is the 'recycling' of solar heat in several cascade evaporation processes, in line with the philosophy of 'doing more, with less'. Technologies based on this process are typically called 'multi-effect', and here we provide the first evidence that this strategy can be very effective for 'passive' desalination technologies as well."

After developing the prototype for more than two years and testing it directly in the Ligurian sea (Varazze, Italy), the Politecnico's engineers claim that this technology could have an impact in isolated coastal locations with little drinking water but abundant solar energy, especially in developing countries. Furthermore, the technology is particularly suitable for providing safe and low-cost drinking water in emergency conditions, for example in areas hit by floods or tsunamis and left isolated for days or weeks from electricity grid and aqueduct. A further application envisioned for this technology are floating gardens for food production, an interesting option especially in overpopulated areas. The researchers, who continue to work on this issue within the Clean Water Center at Politecnico di Torino, are now looking for possible industrial partners to make the prototype more durable, scalable and versatile. For example, engineered versions of the device could be employed in coastal areas where over-exploitation of groundwater causes the intrusion of saline water into freshwater aquifers (a particularly serious problem in some areas of Southern Italy), or could treat waters polluted by industrial or mining plants.

Bibliography and Acknowledgement

- Abbott, George Knapp (2007). Elements of Hydrotherapy for Nurses. Brushton, New York: Teach Services. ISBN 978-1-57258-521-8.
- Acharya, Keya (2012-08-01). "How India's cities came to drown in sewage and waste". Guardian Environment Network.
- Ahmadi, Esmaeil; McLellan, Benjamin; Ogata, Seiichi; Mohammadi-Ivatloo, Behnam; Tezuka, Tetsuo (2020). "An Integrated Planning Framework for Sustainable Water and Energy Supply". Sustainability. 12 (10): 4295.
- Albuquerque Bernalillo County Water Utility Authority (2009). "Xeriscape Rebates". Albuquerque, NM. Retrieved 2010.
- Alhaj, Mohamed; Mabrouk, Abdelnasser; Al-Ghamdi, Sami G. (2018). "Energy efficient multi-effect distillation powered by a solar linear Fresnel collector". Energy Conversion and Management. 171: 576–586..
- Ali, Muhammad Tauha; Fath, Hassan E.S.; Armstrong, Peter R. (October 2011). "A comprehensive techno-economical review of indirect solar desalination". Renewable and Sustainable Energy Reviews. 15 (8): 4187–4199.
- Attari, S. Z. (8 April 2014). "Perceptions of water use". Proceedings of the National Academy of Sciences. 111 (14): 5129–5134.
- Attia, Ahmed A.A. (September 2012). "Thermal analysis for system uses solar energy as a pressure source for reverse osmosis (RO) water desalination". Solar Energy. 86 (9): 2486–2493.
- Banat, Fawzi; Jwaied, Nesreen (March 2008). "Economic evaluation of desalination by small-scale autonomous solar-powered membrane distillation units". Desalination. 220 (1–3): 566–573..
- Banat, Fawzi; Jwaied, Nesreen; Rommel, Matthias; Koschikowski, Joachim; Wieghaus, Marcel (November 2007). "Performance evaluation of the "large SMADES" autonomous desalination solar-driven membrane distillation plant in Aqaba, Jordan". Desalination. 217 (1–3): 17–28.
- Basic Information about Nonpoint Source Pollution". Washington, DC: US Environmental Protection Agency (EPA). 2020-10-07.
- Bell, David R.; Rossman, George R. (1992). "Water in Earth's Mantle: The Role of Nominally Anhydrous Minerals". Science. 255: 1391–1397.
- C. J. Vörösmarty, P. Green, J. Salisbury, R. B. Lammers, Global water resources: Vulnerability from climate change and population growth. Science 289, 284–288 (2000)
- Dail, Clarence; Thomas, Charles (1989). Hydrotherapy: Simple Treatments for Common Ailments. Brushton, New York: Teach Services. ISBN 0-945383-08-8.
- Delgado, J. A.; Groffman, P. M.; Nearing, M. A.; Goddard, T.; Reicosky, D.; Lal, R.; Kitchen, N. R.; Rice, C. W.; Towery, D.; Salon, P. (1 July 2011). "Conservation practices to mitigate and adapt to climate change". Journal of Soil and Water Conservation. 66 (4): 118A–129A..
- Delyannis, E. (2003). Historic background of desalination and renewable energies, Solar Energy, 75(5), 357-366.
- Deniz, Emrah (2015-10-28). "Solar-Powered Desalination". Desalination Updates. Archived copy". Archived from the original on 2015-11-01. Retrieved 2015-10-29.
- DeOreo, William B. (2016). Residential End Uses of Water, Version 2. Water Research Foundation. ISBN 978-1-60573-235-0. [page needed]
- Desalination" (definition), The American Heritage Science Dictionary, via dictionary.com. Retrieved August 19, 2007.
- Description of the Hydrologic Cycle". nwrfc.noaa.gov/rfc/. NOAA River Forecast Center.
- Dziegielewski, B. J.; Kiefer, C. (January 22, 2010). "Water Conservation Measurement Metrics: Guidance Report" (PDF). American Water Works Association. Great Lakes – U.S. EPA". Epa.gov. 2006-06-28. Retrieved 2011-02-19.
- Eakins, B.W. and G.F. Sharman, Volumes of the World's Oceans from ETOPO1, NOAA National Geophysical Data Center, Boulder, CO, 2010.
- Earth's water distribution". United States Geological Survey. Retrieved 2009-05-13.
- Ebrahimi, Atieh; Najafpour, Ghasem D; Yousefi Kebria, Daryoush (2019). "Performance of microbial desalination cell for salt removal and energy generation using different catholyte solutions". Desalination. 432: 1. doi:10.1016/j. desal.2018.01.002.
- Elimelech, M.; Phillip, W. A. (5 August 2011). "The Future of Seawater Desalination: Energy, Technology, and the Environment". Science. 333 (6043): 712–717. Bibcode:2011Sci. 333.712E..
- Ercin, A. Ertug; Hoekstra, Arjen Y. (2014). "Water footprint scenarios for 2050: A global analysis". Environment International. 64: 71–82.
- FAO Hot issues: Water scarcity Archived 25 October 2012 at the Wayback Machine. Fao.org. Retrieved on 27 August 2013.
- FAO Water Unit | Water News: water scarcity". Fao.org. Retrieved 2009-03-12.
- Fatta-Kassinos, Despo; Dionysiou, Dionysios D.; Kümmerer, Klaus (2016). Wastewater Reuse and Current Challenges -Springer. The Handbook of Environmental Chemistry. 44.
- Fawcett, William; Hughes, Martin; Krieg, Hannes; Albrecht, Stefan; Vennström, Anders (2012). "Flexible strategies for long-term sustainability under uncertainty". Building Research. 40 (5): 545–557.
- Filley, S. "How much does a cow need ?" (PDF). Archived from the original (PDF) on 12 May 2012. Retrieved 17 March 2012.
- Fischetti, Mark (September 2007). "Fresh from the Sea". Scientific American. 297 (3): 118–119. Bibcode:2007 SciAm.297c.118F..
- García-Rodríguez, Lourdes; Palmero-Marrero, Ana I.; Gómez-Camacho, Carlos (2002). "Comparison of solar thermal technologies for applications in seawater desalination". Desalination. 142 (2): 135–42.
- Grüber, C; Riesberg, A; et al. (March 2003). "The effect of hydrotherapy on the incidence of common cold episodes in children: A randomised clinical trial". European Journal of Pediatrics. 162 (3): 168–76.

• H. H. G. Savenije, Water scarcity indicators; the deception of the numbers. Physics and Chemistry of the Earth B 25, 199–204 (2000).

• Han, Songlee; Rhee, Young-Woo; Kang, Seong-Pil (February 2017). "Investigation of salt removal using cyclopentane hydrate formation and washing treatment for seawater desalination". Desalination. 404: 132–137.Report Water Waste". Cal Water. 2015. Retrieved 2017-07-11.

• Hermoso, Virgilio; Abell, Robin; Linke, Simon; Boon, Philip (June 2016). "The role of protected areas for freshwater biodiversity conservation: challenges and opportunities in a rapidly changing world: Freshwater protected areas". Aquatic Conservation. 26: 3–11. doi:10.1002/aqc.2681.

• Hirschmann, Marc; Kohlstedt, David (2012-03-01). "Water in Earth's mantle". Physics Today. 65 (3): 40.

• J H Lienhard, G P Thiel, D M Warsinger, L D Banchik (2016). "Low Carbon Desalination: Status and Research, Development, and Demonstration Needs". Report of a Workshop Conducted at the Massachusetts Institute of Technology in Association with the Global Clean Water Desalination Alliance, MIT Abdul Latif Jameel World Water and Food Security Lab, Cambridge, Massachusetts.

• Kalogirou, S. (2009). Solar energy engineering: Processes and systems. Burlington, MA: Elsevier/Academic Press.

• Kameri-Mbote, Patricia (January 2007). "Water, Conflict, and Cooperation: Lessons from the nile river Basin" (PDF). Navigating Peace. Woodrow Wilson International Center for Scholars (4). Archived from the original (PDF) on 2010-07-06.

• Kohlstedt, D. L.; Keppler, H.; Rubie, D. C. (1996). "Solubility of water in the α, β and γ phases of (Mg,Fe) 2 SiO 4". Contributions to Mineralogy and Petrology. 123 (4): 345–357.

• Kumar Kurunthachalam, Senthil (2014). "Water Conservation and Sustainability: An Utmost Importance". Hydrol Current Res. LUHNA Chapter 6: Historical Landcover Changes in the Great Lakes Region". Biology.usgs.gov. 2003-11-20. Archived from the original on 2012-01-11. Retrieved 2011-02-19.

• Li,Chennan; Goswami, Yogi; Stefanakos, Elias (2013-03-01). "Solar assisted sea water desalination: A review". Renewable and Sustainable Energy Reviews. 19: 136–163..

• Mayer, Peter W.; DeOreo, William B. (1999). Residential End Uses of Water (PDF). AWWA Research Foundation and American Water Works Association. ISBN 978-1-58321-016-1.

• Molden, D. (Ed.) (2007) Water for food, Water for life: A Comprehensive Assessment of Water Management in Agriculture. Earthscan/IWMI. National Archives, https://www.archives.gov/research/guide-fed-records/groups/380.html

• National Water Commission (2010). Australian environmental water management report. NWC, Canberra Natural Resource Management and Environmental Dept. "Crops Need Water". Archived from the original on 16 January 2012. Retrieved 17 March 2012.

• Pearson, D. G.; Brenker, F. E.; Nestola, F.; McNeill, J.; Nasdala, L.; Hutchison, M. T.; Matveev, S.; Mather, K.; Silversmit, G.; Schmitz, S.; Vekemans, B. (March 2014). "Hydrous mantle transition zone indicated by ringwoodite included within diamond". Nature. 507 (7491): 221–224..

• Pulitzer Center on Crisis Reporting Archived July 23, 2009, at the Wayback Machine Qiblawey, Hazim Mohameed; Banat, Fawzi (2008). "Solar thermal desalination technologies". Desalination. 220 (1–3): 633–44.

• S. L. Postel, G. C. Daily, P. R. Ehrlich, Human appropriation of renewable fresh water. Science 271, 785–788 (1996). SAWS Report Water Waste - What is Water Waste?". Saws.org. Retrieved 2017-07-11.

• Sarwar, J.; Mansoor, B. (2016-07-15). "Characterization of thermophysical properties of phase change materials for non-membrane based indirect solar desalination application". Energy Conversion and Management. 120: 247–256. Statistics and Facts | WaterSense | US EPA". Epa.gov. 2017-01- 23.Retrieved 2017-07-11.

• Sinclair, Marybetts (2008). Modern Hydrotherapy for the Massage Therapist. Philadelphia: Wolters Kluwer/Lippincott Williams & Wilkins. ISBN 978-0-7817-9209-7.

• Thrash, Agatha; Thrash, Calvin (1981). Home Remedies: Hydrotherapy, Massage, Charcoal and Other Simple Treatments. Seale, Alabama: Thrash Publications. ISBN 0-942658-02-7.

• Tulloch, James (August 26, 2009). "Water Conflicts: Fight or Flight?".Allianz. Archived from the original on 2008-08-29. Retrieved 14 January 2010. EPA (2010-01-13). "How to Conserve Water and Use It Effectively". Washington, DC. Retrieved 2010-02-03.

• Tyler E. Culp et al. Nanoscale control of internal inhomogeneity enhances water transport in desalination membranes. Science, Jan 1st, 2021 DOI: 10.1126/science.abb8518

• Utrik RO unit a big success "Marshall Islands Journal Jan 17th 2014 Water Conflict Chronology". Pacific Institute. Retrieved April 14, 2014.

• Vickers, Amy (2002). Water Use and Conservation. Amherst, MA: water plow Press. p. 434. ISBN 978-1-931579-07-0.

• Water – Use It Wisely." U.S. multi-city public outreach program. Park & Co., Phoenix, AZ. Accessed 2010-02-02.

• Water & Drought Update - Palo Alto Water Use Guidelines". Retrieved 2017-08-06.

• Water and Climate Change: Understanding the Risks and Making Climate-Smart Investment Decisions". World Bank. 2009. Archived from the original on 7 April 2012. Retrieved 2011-10-24.

•Watts, Jonathan (2005-06-07). "100 Chinese cities face water crisis, says minister". The Guardian.Time for universal water metering?" Innovations Report. May 2006.

•Wheeler, N., Evans, W., (1870) Improvements in Evaporating and Distilling by Solar Heat. http://www.google.com/patents/US102633

•Winpenny, James (March 2003). Financing Water for All (PDF). World Water Council. ISBN 92-95017-01-3. Archived from the original (PDF) on 2009-03-19.

•Zaragoza, G.; Andrés-Mañas, J. A; Ruiz-Aguirre, A. (2018- 10-30). "Commercial scale membrane distillation for solar desalination". NPJ Clean Water. 1 (1 Ohtani, Eiji (2020). "Hydration and Dehydration in Earth's Interior". Annual Review of Earth and Planetary Sciences.

•Zhang, S.X.; V. Babovic (2012). "A real options approach to the design and architecture of water supply systems using innovative water technologies under uncertainty". Journal of Hydroinformatics. 14 (1): 13–29..

Health Implications of Human Body Earthing ToThe Earth's Surface Electrons

Environmental medicine focuses on interactions between human health and the environment, including factors such as compromised air and water and toxic chemicals, and how they cause or mediate disease. Omnipresent throughout the environment is a surprisingly beneficial, yet overlooked global resource for health maintenance, disease prevention, and clinical therapy: the surface of the Earth itself. It is an established, though not widely appreciated fact, that the Earth's surface possesses a limitless and continuously renewed supply of free or mobile electrons. The surface of the planet is electrically conductive (except in limited ultradry areas such as deserts), and its negative potential is maintained (i.e., its electron supply replenished) by the global atmospheric electrical circuit Mounting evidence suggests that the Earth's negative potential can create a stable internal bioelectrical environment for the normal functioning of all body systems. Moreover, oscillations of the intensity of the Earth's potential may be important for setting the biological clocks regulating diurnal body rhythms, such as cortisol secretion It is also well established that electrons from antioxidant molecules neutralize reactive oxygen species (ROS, or in popular terms, free radicals) involved in the body's immune and inflammatory responses. The National Library of Medicine's online resource PubMed lists 7021 studies and 522 review articles from a search of "antioxidant + electron + free radical" . It is assumed that the influx of free electrons absorbed into the body through direct contact with the Earth likely neutralize ROS and thereby reduce acute and chronic inflammation

Throughout history, humans mostly walked barefoot or with footwear made of animal skins. They slept on the ground or on skins. Through direct contact or through perspiration-moistened animal skins used as footwear or sleeping mats, the ground's abundant free electrons were able to enter the body, which is electrically conductive. Through this mechanism, every part of the body could equilibrate with the electrical potential of the Earth, thereby stabilizing the electrical environment of all organs, tissues, and cells. Modern lifestyle has increasingly separated humans from the primordial flow of Earth's electrons. For example, since the 1960s, we have increasingly worn insulating rubber or plastic soled shoes, instead of the traditional leather fashioned from hides. Rossi has lamented that the use of insulating materials in post-World War II shoes has separated us from the Earth's energy field . Obviously, we no longer sleep on the ground as we did in times past. During recent decades, chronic illness, immune disorders, and inflammatory diseases have increased dramatically, and some researchers have cited environmental factors as the cause . However, the possibility of modern disconnection with the Earth's surface as a cause has not been considered. Much of the research reviewed in this paper points in that direction. In the late 19th century, a back-to-nature movement in Germany claimed many health benefits from being barefoot outdoors, even in cold weather .

In the 1920s, White, a medical doctor, investigated the practice of sleeping grounded after being informed by some individuals that they could not sleep properly "unless they were on the ground or connected to the ground in some way," such as with copper wires attached to grounded-to-Earth water, gas, or radiator pipes. He reported improved sleeping using these techniques . However, these ideas never caught on in mainstream society.

At the end of the last century, experiments initiated independently by Ober in the USA and K. Sokal and P. Sokal in Poland revealed distinct physiological and health benefits with the use of conductive bed pads, mats, EKG- and TENS-type electrode patches, and plates connected indoors to the Earth outside. Ober, a retired cable television executive, found a similarity between the human body (a bioelectrical, signal-transmitting organism) and the cable used to transmit cable television signals. When cables are "grounded" to the Earth, interference is virtually eliminated from the signal. Furthermore, all electrical systems are stabilized by grounding them to the Earth. K. Sokal and P. Sokal, meanwhile, discovered that grounding the human body represents a "universal regulating factor in Nature" that strongly influences bioelectrical, bioenergetic, and biochemical processes and appears to offer a significant modulating effect on chronic illnesses encountered daily in their clinical practices. Earthing (also known as grounding) refers to contact with the Earth's surface electrons by walking barefoot outside or sitting, working, or sleeping indoors connected to conductive systems, some of them patented, that transfer the energy from the ground into the body. Emerging scientific research supports the concept that the Earth's electrons induce multiple physiological changes of clinical significance, including reduced pain, better sleep, a shift from sympathetic to parasympathetic tone in the autonomic nervous system (ANS), and a blood-thinning effect.

Review of Earthing Papers

The studies summarized below involve indoor-testing methods under controlled conditions that simulate being barefootoutdoors

1. Sleep and Chronic Pain

In a blinded pilot study, Ober recruited 60 subjects (22 males and 28 females) who suffered from self-described sleep disturbances and chronic muscle and joint pain for at least six months . Subjects were randomly divided for the month-long study in which both groups slept on conductive carbon fiber mattress pads provided by Ober. Half the pads were connected to a dedicated Earth ground outside each subject's bedroom window, while the other half were "sham" grounded—not connected to the Earth. Most grounded subjects described symptomatic improvement while most in the control group did not. Some subjects reported significant relief from asthmatic and respiratory conditions, rheumatoid arthritis, PMS, sleep apnea, and hypertension while sleeping grounded. These results indicated that the effects of earthing go beyond reduction of pain and improvements in sleep.

2. Sleep, Stress, Pain, and Cortisol

A pilot study evaluated diurnal rhythms in cortisol correlated with changes in sleep, pain, and stress (anxiety, depression, and irritability), as monitored by subjective reporting.Twelve subjects with complaints of sleep dysfunction, pain, and stress were grounded to Earth during sleep in their own beds using a conductive mattress pad for 8 weeks.

In order to obtain a baseline measurement of cortisol, subjects chewed Dacron salvettes for 2 minutes and then placed them in time-labeled sampling tubes that were stored in a refrigerator. Self-administered sample collections began at 8 AM and were repeated every 4 hours. After 6 weeks of being grounded, subjects repeated this 24-hour saliva test. The samples were processed using a standard radioimmunoassay. A composite of the results is shown in Figure 1.

Subjective symptoms of sleep dysfunction, pain, and stress were reported daily throughout the 8-week test period. The majority of subjects with high- to out-of-range nighttime secretion levels experienced improvements by sleeping grounded. This is demonstrated by the restoration of normal day-night cortisol secretion profiles

Eleven of 12 participants reported falling asleep more quickly, and all 12 reported waking up fewer times at night. Grounding the body at night during sleep also appears to positively affect morning fatigue levels, daytime energy, and nighttime pain levels.

About 30 percent of the general American adult population complain of sleep disruption, while approximately 10 percent have associated symptoms of daytime functional impairment consistent with the diagnosis of insomnia. Insomnia often correlates with major depression, generalized anxiety, substance abuse, dementia, and a variety of pain and physical problems. The direct and indirect costs of chronic insomnia have been estimated at tens of billions of dollars annually in the USA alone [14]. In view of the burdens of personal discomfort and health care costs, grounding the body during sleep seems to have much to offer.

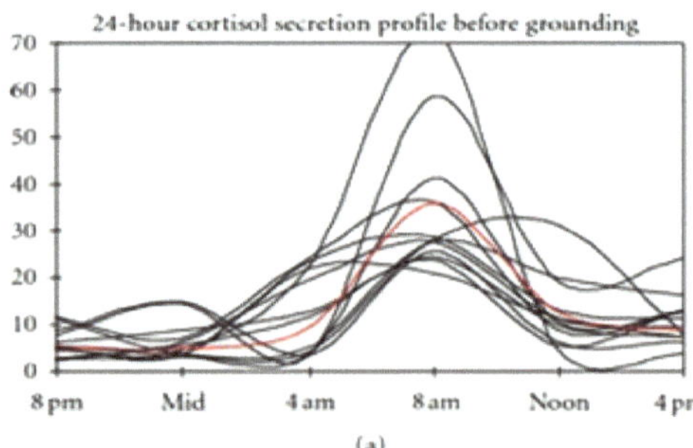

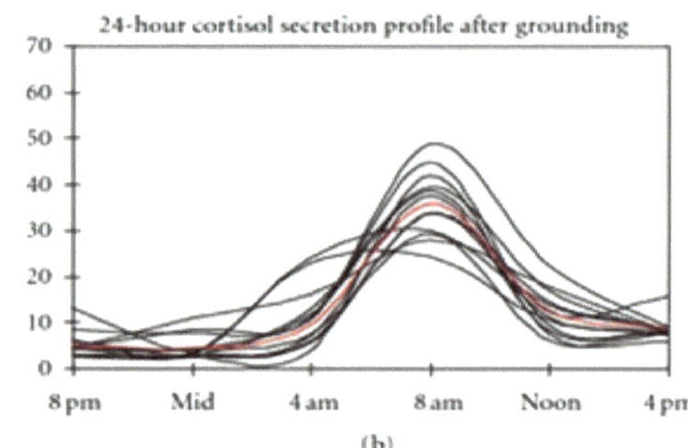

Fig.41.1 *Cortisol levels before and after grounding. In unstressed individuals, the normal 24-hour cortisol secretion profile follows a predictable pattern: lowest around midnight and highest around 8 a.m. Graph (a) illustrates the wide variation of patterns among study participants prior to grounding, while (b) shows a realignment and normalization trend of patterns after six weeks of sleeping grounded.*

3. Earthing Reduces Electric Fields Induced on the Body

Voltage induced on a human body from the electrical environment was measured using a high-impedance measurement head. Apple white, an electrical engineer and expert in the design of electrostatic discharge systems in the electronic industry, was both subject and author of the study . Measurements were taken while ungrounded and then grounded using a conductive patch and conductive bed pad. The author measured the induced fields at three positions: left breast, abdomen, and left thigh.

Each method (patch and sheet) immediately reduced the common alternating current (AC) 60 Hz ambient voltage induced on the body by a highly significant factor of about 70 on average. Figure 2 shows this effect.

The study showed that when the body is grounded, its electrical potential becomes equalized with the Earth's electrical potential through a transfer of electrons from the Earth to the body. This, in turn, prevents the 60 Hz mode from producing an AC electric potential at the surface of the body and from producing perturbations of the electric charges of the molecules inside the body. The study confirms the "umbrella" effect of earthing the body explained by Nobel Prize winner Richard Feynman in his lectures on electromagnetism . Feynman said that when the body potential is the same as the Earth's electric potential (and thus grounded), it becomes an extension of the Earth's gigantic electric system. The Earth's potential thus becomes the "working agent that cancels, reduces, or pushes away electric fields from the body."

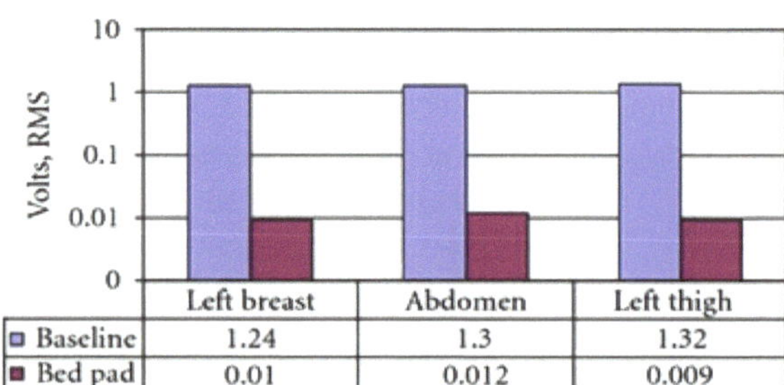

Fig.41.2 *Effect of bed pad grounding on 60 Hz mode.*

Apple white was able to document changes in the ambient voltage induced on the body by monitoring the voltage drop across a resistor. This effect clearly showed the "umbrella effect" described above. The body of the grounded person is not subject to the perturbation of electrons and electrical systems. Jamieson asks whether the failure to appropriately ground humans is a factor contributing to the potential consequences of electropollution in office settings.Considerable debate exists on whether electromagnetic fields in our environment cause a risk to health , but there is no question that the body reacts to the presence of environmental electric fields. This study demonstrates that grounding essentially eliminates the ambient voltage induced on the body from common electricity power sources.

4. Physiological and Electrophysiological Effects Reductions in Overall Stress Levels and Tension and Shift in ANS Balance

Fifty-eight healthy adult subjects (including 30 controls) participated in a randomized double-blind pilot study investigating earthing effects on human physiology .Earthing was accomplished with a conductive adhesive patch placed on the sole of each foot.Abio feed back system recorded electrophysiological and physiological parameters. Experimental subjects were exposed to 28 minutes in the unearthed condition followed by 28 minutes with the earthing wire connected. Controls were unearthed for 56 minutes

Upon earthing, about half the subjects showed an abrupt, almost instantaneous change in root mean square (rms) values of electroencephalograms (EEGs) from the left hemisphere (but not the right hemisphere) at all frequencies analyzed by the biofeedback system (beta, alpha, theta, and delta). All grounded subjects presented an abrupt change in rms values of surface electromyograms (SEMGs) from right and left upper trapezius muscles. Earthing decreased blood volume pulse (BVP) in 19 of 22 experimental subjects (statistically significant) and in 8 of 30 controls (not significant). Earthing the human body showed significant effects on electrophysiological properties of the brain and musculature, on the BVP, and on the noise and stability of electrophysiological recordings. Taken together, the changes in EEG, EMG, and BVP suggest reductions in overall stress levels and tensions and a shift in ANS balance upon earthing. The results extend the conclusions of previous studies.

Confirming Shift from Sympathetic to Parasympathetic Activation

A multiparameter double-blind study was designed to reproduce and expand on previous electrophysiological and physiological parameters measured immediately after grounding with an improved methodology and state-of-the-art equipment . Fourteen men and 14 women, in good health, ages 18–80, were tested while seated in a comfortable recliner during 2-hour grounding sessions, leaving time for signals to stabilize before, during, and after grounding (40 minutes for each period). Sham 2-hour grounding sessions were also recorded with the same subjects as controls. For each session, statistical analyses were performed on four 10-minute segments: before and after grounding (sham grounding for control sessions) and before and after ungrounding (sham ungrounding for control sessions). The following results were documented: 1. an immediate decrease (within a few seconds) in skin conductance (SC) at grounding and an immediate increase at ungrounding. No change was seen for the control (sham grounding) sessions.

2. respiratory rate (RR) increased during grounding, an effect that lasted after ungrounding. RR variance increased immediately after grounding and then decreased;

3. blood oxygenation (BO) variance decreased during grounding, followed by a dramatic increase after ungrounding;

4. pulse rate (PR) and perfusion index (PI) variances increased toward the end of the grounding period, and this change persisted after ungrounding.

The immediate decrease in SC indicates a rapid activation of the parasympathetic nervous system and corresponding deactivation of the sympathetic nervous system. The immediate increase in SC at cessation of grounding indicates an opposite effect. Increased RR, stabilization of BO, and slight rise in heart rate suggest the start of a metabolic healing response necessitating an increase in oxygen consumption.

Immune Cell and Pain Responses with Delayed-Onset Muscle Soreness Induction

Pain reduction from sleeping grounded has been documented in previous studies . This pilot study looked for blood markers that might differentiate between grounded and ungrounded subjects who completed a single session of intense, eccentric exercise resulting in delayed-onset muscle soreness (DOMS) of the gastrocnemius . If markers were able to differentiate these groups, future studies could be done in greater detail with a larger subject base. DOMS is a common complaint in the fitness and athletic world following excessive physical activity and involves acute inflammation in overtaxed muscles. It develops in 14 to 48 hours and persists for more than 96 hours . No known treatment reduces the recovery period, but apparently massage and hydrotherapyand acupuncture can reduce pain.

Eight healthy men ages 20–23 were put through a similar routine of toe raises while carrying on their shoulders a barbell equal to one-third of their body weight. Each participant was exercised individually on a Monday morning and then monitored for the rest of the week while following a similar eating, sleeping, and living schedule in a hotel. The group was randomly divided in half and either grounded or sham grounded with the use of a conductive patch placed at the sole of each foot during active hours and a conductive sheet at night.

Complete blood counts, blood chemistry, enzyme chemistry, serum and saliva cortisol, magnetic resonance imaging and spectroscopy, and pain levels (a total of 48 parameters) were taken at the same time of day before the eccentric exercise and at 24, 48, and 72 hours afterwards. Parameters consistently differing by 10 percent or more, normalized to baseline, were considered worthy of further study. Parameters that differed by these criteria included white blood cell counts, bilirubin, creatine kinase, phosphocreatine/inorganic phosphate ratios, glycerolphosphorylcholine, phosphorylcholine, the visual analogue pain scale, and pressure measurements on the right gastrocnemius. The results showed that grounding the body to the Earth alters measures of immune system activity and pain. Among the ungrounded men, for instance, there was an expected, sharp increase in white blood cells at the stage when DOMS is known to reach its peak and greater perception of pain This effect demonstrates a typical inflammatory response. In comparison, the grounded men had only a slight decrease in white blood cells, indicating scant inflammation, and, for the first time ever observed, a shorter recovery time. Brown later commented that there were "significant differences" in the pain these men reported . The rapid change in skin conductance reported in an earlier study led to the hypothesis that grounding may also improve heart rate variability (HRV), a measurement of the heart's response to ANS regulation. A double-blind study was designed with 27 participants [27]. Subjects sat in a comfortable reclining chair. Four transcutaneous electrical nerve stimulation (TENS) type adhesive electrode patches were placed on the sole of each foot and on each palm.

Participants served as their own controls. Each participant's data from a 2-hour session (40 minutes of which was grounded) were compared with another 2-hour sham-grounded session. The sequence of grounding versus sham-grounding sessions was assigned randomly. During the grounded sessions, participants had statistically significant improvements in HRV that went way beyond basic relaxation results (which were shown by the nongrounded sessions). Since improved HRV is a significant positive indicator on cardiovascular status, , it is suggested that simple grounding techniques be utilized as a basic integrative strategy in supporting the cardiovascular system, especially under situations of heightened autonomic tone when the sympathetic nervous system is more activated than the parasympathetic nervous system.

Reduction of Primary Indicators of Osteoporosis, Improvement of Glucose Regulation, and Immune Response

K. Sokal and P. Sokal, cardiologist and neurosurgeon father and son on the medical staff of a military clinic in Poland, conducted a series of experiments to determine whether contact with the Earth via a copper conductor can affect physiological processes . Their investigations were prompted by the question as to whether the natural electric charge on the surface of the Earth influences the regulation of human physiological processes.

Double-blind experiments were conducted on groups ranging from 12 to 84 subjects who followed similar physical activity, diet, and fluid intake during the trial periods. Grounding was achieved with a copper plate (30 mm × 80 mm) placed on the lower part of the leg, attached with a strip so that it would not come off during the night. The plate was connected by a conductive wire to a larger plate (60 mm × 250 mm) placed in contact with the Earth outside. In one experiment with nonmedicated subjects, grounding during a single night of sleep resulted in statistically significant changes in concentrations of minerals and electrolytes in the blood serum: iron, ionized calcium, inorganic phosphorus, sodium, potassium, and magnesium. Renal excretion of both calcium and phosphorus was reduced significantly. The observed reductions in blood and urinary calcium and phosphorus directly relate to osteoporosis. The results suggest that Earthing for a single night reduces primary indicators of osteoporosis

Earthing continually during rest and physical activity over a 72-hour period decreased fasting glucose among patients with non-insulin-dependent diabetes mellitus. Patients had been well controlled with glibenclamide, an antidiabetic drug, for about 6 months, but at the time of study had unsatisfactory glycemic control despite dietary and exercise advice and glibenclamide doses of 10 mg/day.K. Sokal and P. Sokal drew blood samples from 6 male and 6 female adults with no history of thyroid disease. A single night of grounding produced a significant decrease of free tri-iodothyronine and an increase of free thyroxin and thyroid-stimulating hormone. The meaning of these results is unclear but suggests an earthing influence on hepatic, hypothalamus, and pituitary relationships with thyroid function. Ober et al. have observed that many individuals on thyroid medication reported symptoms of hyperthyroid, such as heart palpitations, after starting grounding. Such symptoms typically vanish after medication is adjusted downward under medical supervision.

Through a series of feedback regulations, thyroid hormones affect almost every physiological process in the body, including growth and development, metabolism, body temperature, and heart rate. Clearly, further study of earthing effects on thyroid function is needed. In another experiment, the effect of grounding on the classic immune response following vaccination was examined. Earthing accelerated the immune response, as demonstrated by increases in gamma globulin concentration. This result confirms an association between earthing and the immune response, as was suggested in the DOMS study. K. Sokal and P. Sokal conclude that earthing the human body influences human physiological processes, including increasing the activity of catabolic processes and may be "the primary factor regulating endocrine and nervous systems."

Altered Blood Electrodynamics

Since grounding produces changes in many electrical properties of the body , a next logical step was to evaluate the electrical property of the blood. A suitable measure is the zeta potential of red blood cells (RBCs) and RBC aggregation. Zeta potential is a parameter closely related to the number of negative charges on the surface of an RBC. The higher the number, the greater the ability of the RBC to repel other RBCs. Thus, the greater the zeta potential the less coagulable is the blood.Ten relatively healthy subjects participated in the study . They were seated comfortably in a reclining chair and were grounded for two hours with electrode patches placed on their feet and hands, as in previous studies. Blood samples were taken before and after. Grounding the body to the earth substantially increases the zeta potential and decreases RBC aggregation, thereby reducing blood viscosity. Subjects in pain reported reduction to the point that it was almost unnoticeable. The results strongly suggest that earthing is a natural solution for patients with excessive blood viscosity, an option of great interest not just for cardiologists, but also for any physician concerned about the relationship of blood viscosity, clotting, and inflammation. In 2008, Adak and colleagues reported the presence of both hypercoagulable blood and poor RBC zeta potential among diabetics. Zeta potential was particularly poor among diabetics with cardiovascular disease

Until now, the physiological significance and possible health effects of stabilizing the internal bioelectrical environment of an organism have not been a significant topic of research. Some aspects of this, however, are relatively obvious. In the absence of Earth contact, internal charge distribution will not be uniform, but instead will be subject to a variety of electrical perturbations in the environment.

It is well known that many important regulations and physiological processes involve events taking place on cell and tissue surfaces. In the absence of a common reference point, or "ground," electrical gradients, due to uneven charge distribution, can build up along tissue surfaces and cell membranes.

We can predict that such charge differentials will influence biochemical and physiological processes. First, the structure and functioning of many enzymes are sensitive to local environmental conditions. Each enzyme has an optimal pH that favors maximal activity. A change in the electrical environment can alter the pH of biological fluids and the charge distribution on molecules and thereby affect reaction rates. The pH effect results because of critical charged amino acids at the active site of the enzyme that participate in substrate binding and catalysis. In addition, the ability of a substrate or enzyme to donate or accept hydrogen ions is influenced by pH. Another example is provided by voltage-gated ion channels, which play critical biophysical roles in excitable cells such as neurons. Local alterations in the charge profiles around these channels can lead to electrical instability of the cell membrane and to the inappropriate spontaneous activity observed during certain pathological states

Earthing research offers insights into the clinical potential of barefoot contact with the Earth, or simulated barefoot contact indoors via simple conductive systems, on the stability of internal bioelectrical function and human physiology. Initial experiments resulted in subjective reports of improved sleep and reduced pain . Subsequent research showed that improved sleep was correlated with a normalization of the cortisol day-night profile . The results are significant in light of the extensive research showing that lack of sleep stresses the body and contributes to many detrimental health consequences. Lack of sleep is often the result of pain. Hence, reduction of pain might be one reason for the benefits just described.Pain reduction from sleeping grounded has been confirmed in a controlled study on DOMS. Earthing is the first intervention known to speed recovery from DOMS . Painful conditions are often the result of various kinds of acute or chronic inflammation conditions caused in part by ROS generated by normal metabolism and also by the immune system as part of the response to injury or trauma. Inflammation can cause pain and loss of range of motion in joints. Inflammatory swelling can put pressure on pain receptors (nocireceptors) and can compromise the microcirculation, leading to ischemic pain. Inflammation can cause the release of toxic molecules that also activate pain receptors.

Modern biomedical research has also documented a close relationship between chronic inflammation and virtually all chronic diseases, including the diseases of aging, and the aging process itself. The steep rise in inflammatory diseases, in fact, has been recently called "inflamm-aging" to describe a progressive inflammatory status and a loss of stress-coping ability as major components of the aging process.Reduction in inflammation as a result of earthing has been documented with infrared medical imaging and with measurements of blood chemistry and white blood cell counts.

The logical explanation for the anti-inflammatory effects is that grounding the body allows negatively charged antioxidant electrons from the Earth to enter the body and neutralize positively charged free radicals at sites of inflammation Flow of electrons from the Earth to the body has been documented . A pilot study on the electrodynamics of red blood cells (zeta potential) has revealed that earthing significantly reduces blood viscosity, an important but neglected parameter in cardiovascular diseases and diabetes [29], and circulation in general. Thus, thinning the blood may allow for more oxygen delivery to tissues and further support the reduction of inflammation. Stress reduction has been confirmed with various measures showing rapid shifts in the ANS from sympathetic to parasympathetic dominance, improvement in heart rate variability, and normalization of muscle tension . Not reported here are many observations over more than two decades by Ober et al. and K. Sokal and P. Sokal indicating that regular earthing may improve blood pressure, cardiovascular arrhythmias, and autoimmune conditions such as lupus, multiple sclerosis, and rheumatoid arthritis. Some effects of earthing on medication are described by Ober et al. As an example, the combination of earthing and coumadin has the potential to exert a compounded blood thinning effect and must be supervised by a physician. Multiple anecdotes of elevated INR have been reported. INR (international normalized ratio) is a widely used measurement of coagulation. The influence of earthing on thyroid function and medication has been described earlier.From a practical standpoint, clinicians could recommend outdoor "barefoot sessions" to patients, weather, and conditions permitting. Ober et al. have observed that going barefoot as little as 30 or 40 minutes daily can significantly reduce pain and stress, and the studies summarized here explain why this is the case. Obviously, there is no cost for barefoot grounding. However, the use of conductive systems while sleeping, approach working, or relaxing indoors offer a more convenient and routine-friendly approach.

"Earthing" or "Grounding"
Direct physical contact of the human body with the surface of the earth
reduces blood viscosity
improves cardiovascular health
better sleep
reduces pain
feeling of well-being

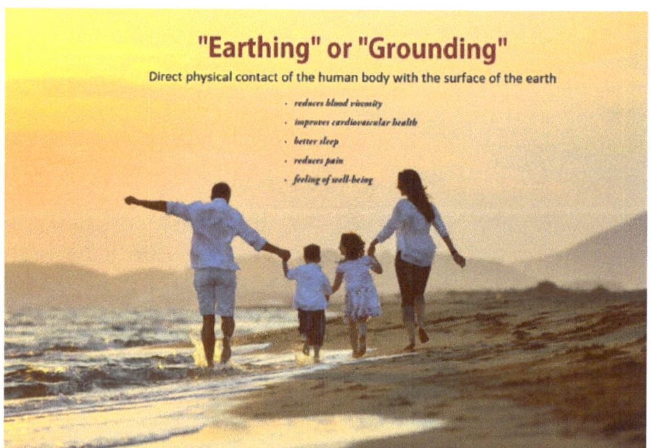

Fig.41.3 *Direct physical contactof the human body with the surface of the earth*

What Is Earthing?

The terms "earthing" and "grounding" are interchangeable. It is simply the act of placing your bare feet on the earth, or walking barefoot. When you do, free electrons are transferred from the earth into your body, and this grounding effect is one of the most potent antioxidants we know of. Unfortunately, few people ever walk barefoot anymore to experience it. Hopefully, as more and more people become aware of the importance of being grounded, this will change, or at the very least spawn a much needed change in the way most footwear is made. Synthetic rubber soles disconnect you from the earth. Leather soles do not. So you can still find shoes that allow you to remain grounded without going barefoot. Grounding has numerous benefits, aside from creating a general feeling of well-being. For example, walking barefoot can help ameliorate the constant assault of electromagnetic fields and other types of radiation from cell phones, computers and Wi-Fi. By getting outside, barefoot, touching the earth, and allowing the excess charge in your body to discharge into the earth, you can alleviate some of the stress put on your system. That is the grounding effect. I have personally prioritized grounding myself to the earth as much as possible for over 5 years.

Inflammation — The Root of Most Disease

One of the primary health benefits of grounding is its antioxidant effect. It helps alleviate inflammation throughout your body. Dr. Sinatra goes on to tell the inspiring story of a contractor he met about 23 years ago, who at one point worked with a group of Scandinavian carpenters who really understood the benefits of grounding and supported each other in maintaining this healthy habit:

According to Dr. Sinatra, inflammation thrives when your blood is thick and you have a lot of free radical stress, and a lot of positive charges in your body. Grounding effectively alleviates inflammation because it thins your blood and infuses you with negatively charged ions through the soles of your feet. But beware; not all surfaces allow you to ground.

What Surfaces Will Allow You to Properly Ground?

Good grounding surfaces include:

- Sand (beach)
- Grass (preferably moist)
- Bare soil
- Concrete and brick (as long as it's not painted or sealed)
- Ceramictile

The following surfaces will NOT ground you:

- Asphalt
- Wood
- Rubber and plastic
- Vinyl
- Tarortarmac

An interesting tidbit offered by Dr. Sinatra is how to ground while flying. I typically bring a grounding pad with me when I fly, but Dr. Sinatra claims that simply taking your shoes off and putting your feet (bare or with socks) on the steel struts will do the trick.

The Earth Is a Rich Source of Healthful Electrons

The earth is struck by lightning thousands of time each minute, primarily around the equator. Subsequently, the earth carries an enormous negative charge. It's always electron-rich and can serve as a powerful and abundant supply of antioxidant free radical-busting electrons.

The human body appears to be finely tuned to "work" with the earth in the sense that there's a constant flow of energy between our bodies and the earth. When you put your feet on the ground, you absorb large amounts of negative electrons through the soles of your feet. In today's world, this is more important than ever, yet fewer people than ever actually connect with the earth in this way anymore. Free radical stress from exposure to mercury pollution, cigarettes, insecticides, pesticides, trans fats, and radiation, just to name a few, continually deplete your body of electrons.

Recharge Your 'Batteries' with Grounding

Dr. Sinatra, like myself, is a proponent for CoQ10, as it is a major electron donor and helps turn over ATP, which is the energy generated within each of your body's cells.

Amazingly, grounding can also enhance ATP, via another mechanism. How do dietary-derived, oral antioxidants compare to the electrons transferred from the earth through your skin? According to Dr. Sinatra:

Walking Barefoot Is a Valuable Aspect of a Healthy Lifestyle

Exercising barefoot outdoors is one of the most wonderful, inexpensive and powerful ways of incorporating Earthing into your daily life and will also help speed up tissue repair, as well as easing the muscle pain you sometimes get from strenuous exercise. A review of the available research, published January 2012 in the Journal of Environmental and Public Health, agrees with the concept of reaping health benefits when connecting to the Earth. According to the authors:

"Mounting evidence suggests that the Earth's negative potential can create a stable internal bioelectrical environment for the normal functioning of all body systems. Moreover, oscillations of the intensity of the Earth's potential may be important for setting the biological clocks regulating diurnal body rhythms, such as cortisol secretion.

It is also well established that electrons from antioxidant molecules neutralize reactive oxygen species (ROS, or in popular terms, free radicals) involved in the body's immune and inflammatory responses. The National Library of Medicine's online resource PubMed lists 7021 studies and 522 review articles from a search of 'antioxidant + electron + free radical.' It is assumed that the influx of free electrons absorbed into the body through direct contact with the Earth likely neutralize ROS and thereby reduce acute and chronic inflammation.

Throughout history, humans mostly walked barefoot or with footwear made of animal skins. They slept on the ground or on skins. Through direct contact or through perspiration-moistened animal skins used as footwear or sleeping mats, the ground's abundant free electrons were able to enter the body, which is electrically conductive. Through this mechanism, every part of the body could equilibrate with the electrical potential of the Earth, thereby stabilizing the electrical environment of all organs, tissues, and cells.

Modern lifestyle has increasingly separated humans from the primordial flow of Earth's electrons. For example, since the 1960s, we have increasingly worn insulating rubber or plastic soled shoes, instead of the traditional leather fashioned from hides. Rossi has lamented that the use of insulating materials in post-World War II shoes has separated us from the Earth's energy field. Obviously, we no longer sleep on the ground as we did in times past.

During recent decades, chronic illness, immune disorders, and inflammatory diseases have increased dramatically, and some researchers have cited

environmental factors as the cause. However, the possibility of modern disconnection with the Earth's surface as a cause has not been considered. Much of the research reviewed in this paper points in that direction.

How Grounding Changes Your Blood

Grounding helps thin your blood by improving its zeta potential, which means it improves the energy between your red blood cells. Research has demonstrated it takes about 80 minutes for the free electrons from the earth to reach your blood stream and transform your blood

Do you know what a high-sugar diet, smoking, radio frequencies and other toxic electromagnetic forces, emotional stress, anxiety, high cholesterol, and high uric acid levels do to your blood?All of these make your blood hypercoagulable, meaning it makes it thick and slow-moving, which increases your risk of having a blood clot or stroke. Hypercoagulable blood is the essence of inflammation, because when your blood does not flow well, oxygen can't get to your tissues. In fact, grounding's effect on blood thinning is so profound if you are taking blood thinners you must work with your health care provider to lower your dose otherwise you may overdose on the medication. Zeta potential is the electrical potential of solids and liquids, also referred to as electrokinetic potential. Your red blood cells repel each other and function at the speed of light, traveling through your body at an astounding 186,000 miles per second. Grounding actually increases zeta potential by an average of 280 percent. According to Dr. Sinatra

"This is the most incredible discovery, because if you can increase the thinning of your blood naturally by grounding, you can fight off disease. Not only heart disease and stroke, but I'm thinking cancer, Alzheimer's, multiple sclerosis, or any illness that requires good oxygenation to the tissues."

Similarly, anything that lowers zeta potential of your blood will promote disease. For example, early (and some current) birth control pills were notorious for causing heart attacks in women. One of the mechanisms that causes this increased risk is that synthetic estrogens and progesterones increase blood viscosity, i.e., they decrease the zeta potential of your blood. There are currently studies being performed at the University of Arizona which will objectively document grounding effect on the zeta potential. They are anticipated to be completed this year.

Other Beneficial Changes Caused By Grounding

Animal experiments have also shown that ungrounded rats had higher blood sugar compared to their grounded counterparts, despite being fed identical diets. If disconnecting from the earth disrupts human sugar metabolism, we may have identified yet another contributing cause for the dramatic rise of diabetes in children. Experiments in Poland, the U.S. and Canada, using both animal and human models, show that grounding improves the human physiology. Other biochemical alterations caused by grounding include changes in:

- Phosphorus
- Calcium metabolism
- Fibroid metabolism
- White blood cells

Grounding also calms your sympathetic nervous system, which supports your heart rate variability. And, when you support heart rate variability, this promotes homeostatis, or balance, in your autonomic nervous system. In essence, anytime you improve heart rate variability, you're improving the entire organism — in this case, your entire body and all its functions.

Contraindications and Other Warnings

While walking barefoot is clearly one of the most natural things you can possibly do to improve your health, there are still some contraindications and situations in which you may want to use caution. *"I don't like people to ground when they're taking Coumadin," Dr. Sinatra warns. "It's a relative contraindication because we have had people ground, taking Coumadin at the same time, and their blood became like water. It was like red wine and then it got really thin. That could be dangerous. If you have high blood pressure, [or]... if you had a stroke and you have thin blood, it's a disaster. We basically tell people that if you're on Coumadin, you must work with your doctor, because your doctor's going to have to reduce the Coumadin."*

Depending on your health status and toxic load, your health may also get worse before it gets better when you start grounding on a regular basis. This is a classic detox reaction, which you may also experience with other detox methods

"Some patients with polyneuropathy would get worsening of their limb pain on grounding, and some would get better. I want to make that clear that grounding is not a panacea," Dr. Sinatra says. "But what I've learned with grounding is that the sicker you are, the more you need to ground."

The traditionally core components of alternative, lifestyle, and preventive medicine include nutrition, exercise, stress management, and relationships. One key component that is missing from this overall formula is the practice of Earthing, which is commonly referred to as grounding.

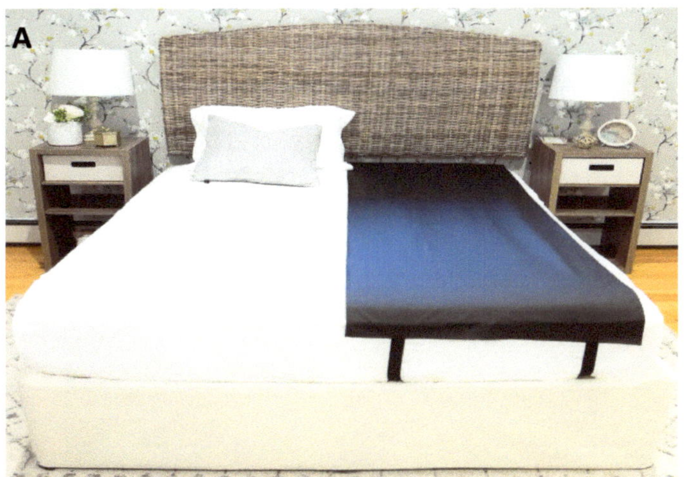

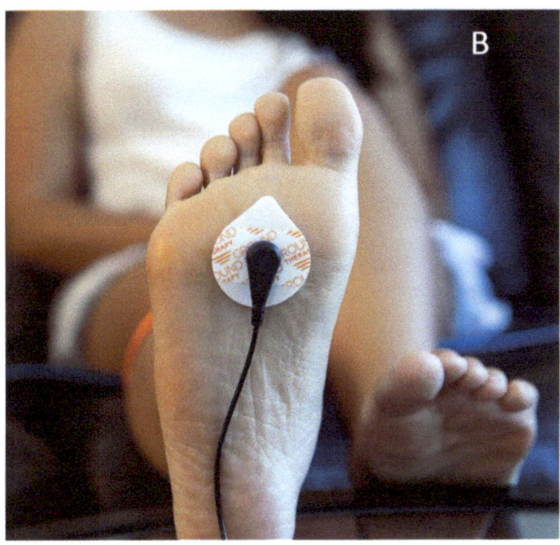

Fig.41.4 *Grounded sleep system. Notes: Grounded sleep system consists of a cotton sheet with conductive carbon or silver threads woven into it. The threads connect to a wire that leads out the bedroom window or through the wall to a metal rod inserted into the Earth near a healthy plant. Alternatively, it can be connected to the ground terminal of an electrical outlet. Sleeping on this system connects the body to the Earth. A frequent report from people using this system is that sleeping grounded improves the quality of sleep and reduces aches and pains from a variety of causes. B. Attachment of foot patch in body earthing.*

Grounding and the Cardiovascular System

In 1977, Steve Sinatra, MD became a board-certified cardiologist. After writing dozens of peer review articles, books, and chapters in medical text books over the past 40 years, I thought about my greatest discoveries as a physician. Indeed, it was the utilization of coenzyme Q10 in my patients as well as the cardiovascular implications of grounding, also known as Earthing the body. This chapter is a testimony to the incredible discovery of grounding to the natural electric charge of the planet

It was almost 15 years ago at an American College of Cardiology conference that I met Clint Ober in San Diego. He introduced to me the theory of grounding, and it made a lot of sense to me. I was excited about the entire concept, as well as trying to take it to a higher level. However, like anything else in medicine, the theory behind grounding needed intensive research. Ever since that encounter with Clint, more than 20 peer reviewed articles on the benefits of grounding have become available to mainstream medicine.

Over the past 4 decades, I have treated hundreds of patients with acute coronary syndrome and unstable angina, as well as acute myocardial infarction. Although the utilization of thrombolytic therapies, percutaneous transluminal coronary angioplasty, stents, and statin medications are crucial in the care of these patients, the grounding phenomena also needed to be recognized.

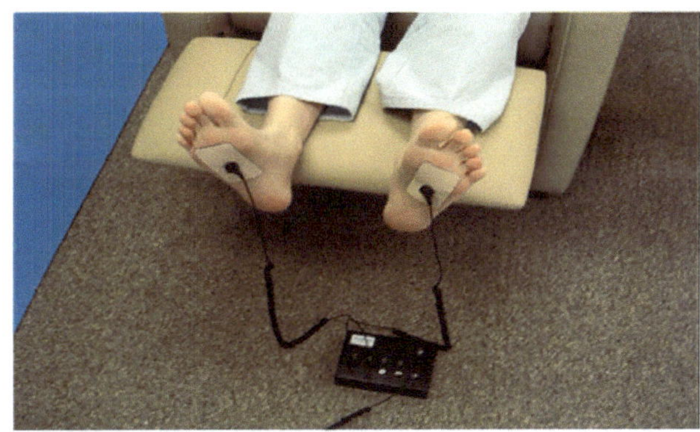

Fig 41.5 ***Grounding system showing patches, wires, and box connecting to a ground rod planted outside through a switch (not shown) and a fuse (not shown). Similar patches and wires from the hands were also connected to the box to ground the hands.***

Simply stated, when one grounds to the electron-enriched earth, an improved balance of the ANS occurs. Improvements in HRV can support patients with emotional stress, anxiety, fear, and any other symptoms of autonomic dystonia.A 2017 study performed at the Pennsylvania State University Children's Hospital Neonatal Intensive Care Unit in Hershey revealed that grounding premature infants produced immediate and significant improvements in measurements of the ANS. Grounding improves vagal tone and may support resilience to stress, which could lower the risk of neonatal mortality in preterm infants

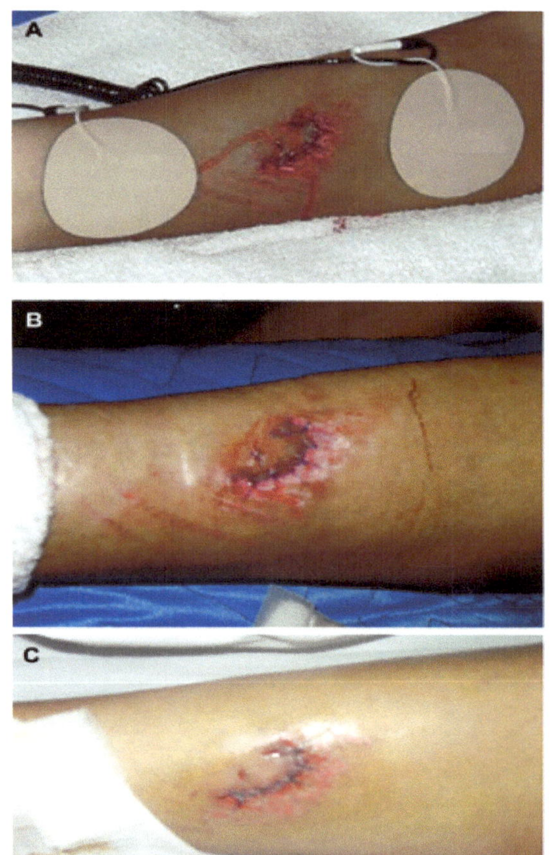

Fig. 41.6 *Rapid recovery from a serious wound with minimal swelling and redness expected for such a serious injury. Notes: Cyclist was injured in Tour de France competition – chain wheel gouged his leg. (A) Grounding patches were placed above and below wound as soon as possible after injury. Photo courtesy of Dr Jeff Spencer. (B) Day 1 after injury. (C) Day 2 after injury. There was minimal redness, pain, and swelling, and cyclist was able to continue the race on the day following the injury. (B and C) Copyright © 2014. Reprinted with permission from Basic Health Publications, Inc. Ober CA, Sinatra ST, Zucker M. Earthing: The Most Important Health Discovery Ever? 2nd ed. Laguna Beach: Basic Health Publications; 2014.*

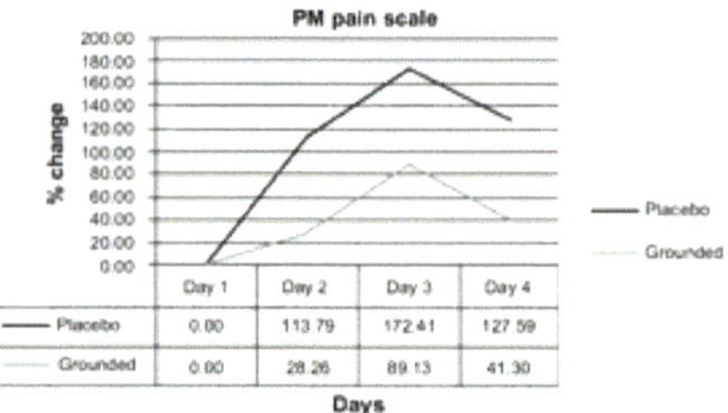

	Day 1	Day 2	Day 3	Day 4
Placebo	0.00	113.79	172.41	127.59
Grounded	0.00	28.26	89.13	41.30

Fig. 41.7 *Changes in afternoon (PM) visual analog pain scale was completely pain-free reports.*

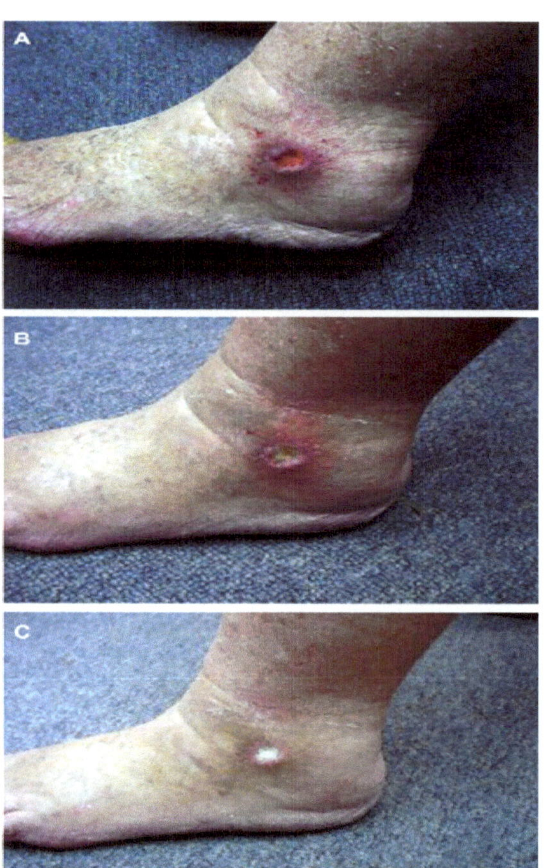

Fig.41.8 *Photographicimages documenting accelerated improvement of an 8-monthold, non-healing open wound suffered by an 84-year-old diabetic woman. Notes: (A) Shows the open wound and a pale-gray hue to the skin. (B) Taken after one week of grounding or earthing treatments, shows a marked level of healing and improvement in circulation, as indicated by the skin color. (C) Taken after 2 weeks of earthing treatment, shows the wound healed over and the skin color looking dramatically healthier. Treatment consisted of a daily 30-minute grounding session with an electrode patch while patient was seated comfortably. The cause of the wound adjacent to the left ankle was a poorly fitted boot. A few hours after wearing the boot, a blister formed, and then developed into a resistant open wound. The patient had undergone various treatments at a specialized wound center with no improvement. Vascular imaging of her lower extremities revealed poor circulation. When first seen, she had a mild limp and was in pain. After an initial 30 minutes of exposure to grounding, the patient reported a noticeable decrease in pain. After 1 week of daily grounding, she said her pain level was about 80% less. At that time, she showed no evidence of a limp. At the end of 2 weeks, she said she*

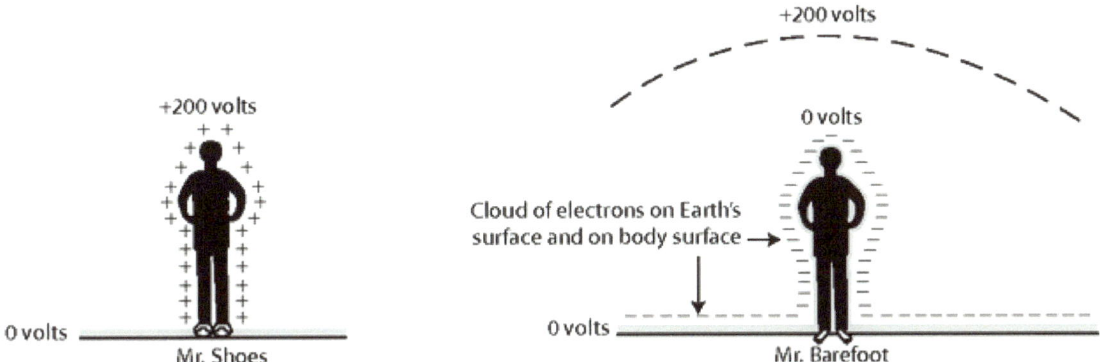

Fig.41.9 *The object is essentially residing within the protective "umbrella" of earth's natural electric field. This protective phenomenon also occurs inside your house or office if you are connected to the earth with an earthing device, such as a grounding wrist pad or a foot pad. Adapted from Richard Feynman's famous Berkeley Lectures on Physics. (From Ober C, Sinatra ST, Zucker M. Earthing: The Most Important Health Discovery Ever? Laguna Beach, CA: Basic Health Publications; Second Edition, 2014, p. 76.)*

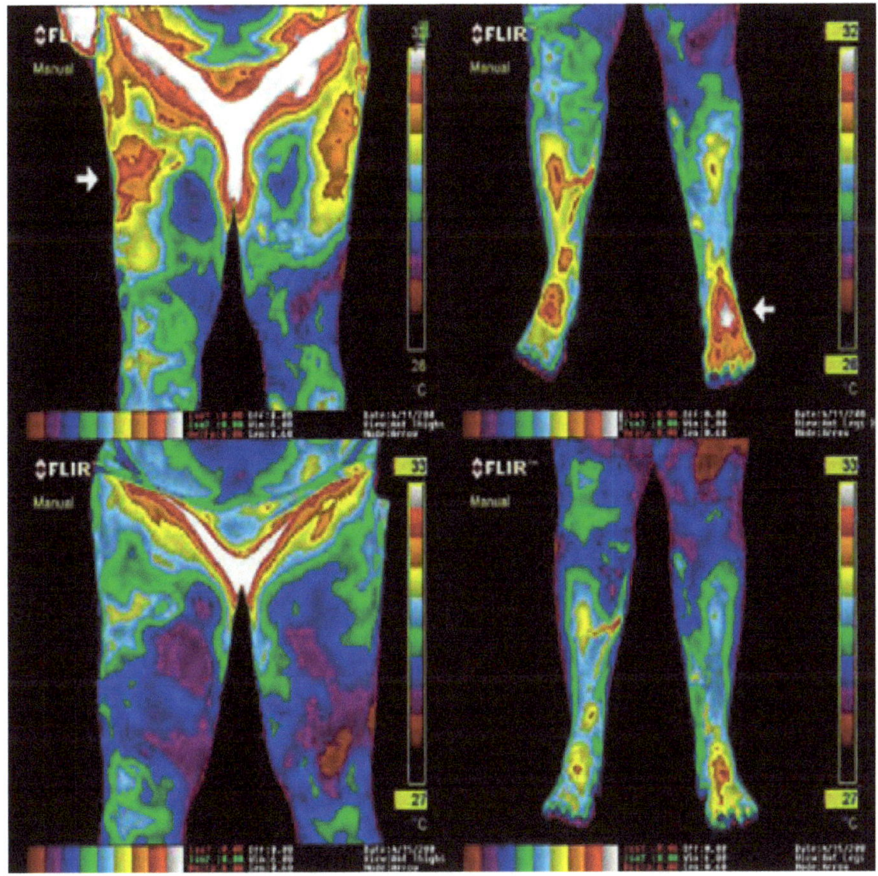

Fig.41.10 *Reduction in inflammation and pain after sleeping grounded for four nights. Medical infrared imaging shows warm and painful areas (arrows). Sleeping grounded for four nights resolved the pain and the hot areas cooled. (From Amalu W. Medical Thermography case studies. Clinical earthing application in 20 case studies.*

The traditionally core components of alternative, lifestyle, and preventive medicine include nutrition, exercise, stress management, and relationships. One key component that is missing from this overall formula is the practice of Earthing, which is commonly referred to as grounding. The simplicity and the multitude of benefits provided by Earthing are not understood by many people.

Before we proceed any further, let's examine exactly what Earthing means.

Earthing simply means reconnecting the conductive human body to the Earth's natural and subtle surface electric charge, an effortless lifestyle activity that systematically influences the basic bioelectrical function of the body Implementation of this simple lifestyle change surprisingly stabilizes the physiology, reduces inflammation, pain, and stress, enhances sleep, blood flow, and lymphatic/venous return to the heart, and produces greater well-being. People report very positive effects from a regular schedule of Earthing. They report that they feel and look healthier and younger. Those suffering from pain state that they feel less pain and their mood improves. Earthing is quite simple to implement and often achieves rapid results, particularly for individuals with chronicc health disorders

Our Lost Connection To The Earth

The Earth has long been recognized and utilized by the electrical industry as an essential source of stability and safety. All modern electrical systems, from large grids and power stations to homes, buildings, and factories, and the machinery and appliances powered by electricity, are all connected to the Earth for stability and safety. Essentially, electrical systems are "healthier" precisely because of their connection to the Earth

It is now time for the medical world to start recognizing that a body connected to the ground – a grounded body – is similarly more stable and healthier. It functions more naturally, a state lost over time because humans have become largely disconnected from the Earth

We obviously no longer sleep on the ground, rarely walk barefoot outdoors, and, for more than a half century, almost exclusively wear insulating synthetic soled shoes instead of traditional and conductive leather footwear. We live and work, and spend much or most of our time disconnected, often far above ground in high rises. This disconnection with the Earth may contribute to electrical imbalances, a build-up of disruptive static electricity (positive charges), and an unknown electron deficiency in the body, and with it, susceptibility to dysfunction, disorder, and disease .The electrical charge provided by Earth and its limitless supply of electrons and their diurnal frequencies, provides a form of "electric nutrition" so to speak Research supports the hypothesis that Earthing facilitates a significant transfer of free electrons into the body, a transfer resulting in rapid, sometimes instant, physiological changes Earthing restores and maintains a natural internal electrical environment. Research indicates that Earthing the human body represents a "universal regulating factor in Nature" strongly influencing bioelectrical, bioenergetics, and biochemical processes and appears to offer a significant modulating effect on chronic illnesses and dysfunction.

Earth ,the Original Anti-inflammatory

One of the most prevailing effects of Earthing, as documented over nearly 20 years of research, along with feedback from thousands of individuals around the world, is reduction and even elimination of chronic inflammation, a common cause or aggravating factor for chronic and aging-related diseases, as well as pain.

This finding suggests that the planet we live on is the original painkiller, the original anti-inflammatory: nature's way to counteract inflammation. Briefly, the hypothesis for this effect is as follows: Free radicals (also known as reactive oxygen species, ROS) are positively charged molecules produced normally, that strip electrons from healthy tissue, resulting in damage. Every cell produces billions of free radicals every day. Earthing allows huge numbers of free electrons to enter the body where they are believed to neutralize free radicals. The active mechanisms of electron transportation to a site of inflammation may encompass the nervous, meridian, and circulatory systems. It is indicated that the influx of free electrons absorbed into the body serves as a powerful anti-inflammatory reinforcement for the immune system.

Earthing typically reverses both acute and chronic inflammation, and does so rapidly. Interestingly, three studies based on a sports medicine research model called delayed onset muscular soreness (DOMS) documented clear evidence of pain relief and reduced inflammation from Earthing.. DOMS refers to the pain, tenderness, and stiffness felt in muscles several hours to days after unaccustomed or strenuous exercise.

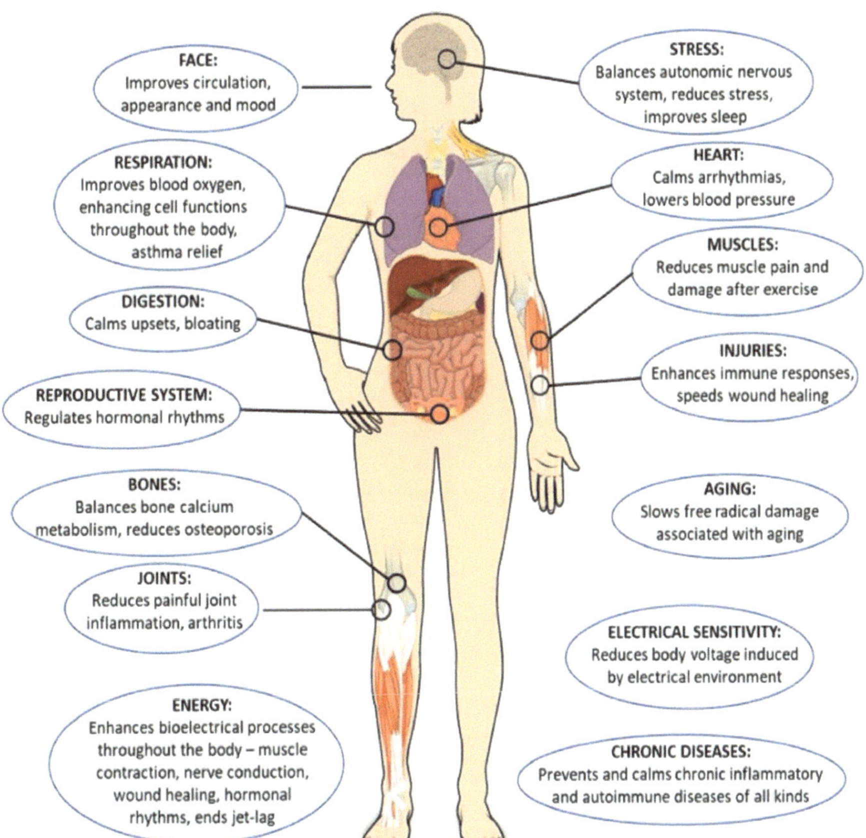

Fig.41.11 *Effects of earthing on our body system .*

Copper Plate Earthings

3E solutions supply the complete range of Copper Earthing Plates that are also used as a conventional earthing solution. We install Copper earthing plate installation as per IS:3043 in a 3 Feet Long x 3 Feet Wide x10 Deep earth hole with alternate layers of Salt and Charcoal. The salt helps to reduce the earthing resistance by creating an electrolytic environment surrounding earthing plate but over the time leach out deeper in the earth and need salt and water at more frequent intervals. Since salt also corrode the earthing plate and terminal strip that connect the copper plate with equipment and reduce the dependability, generally, chemical earthings are preferred. Earthing Copper Plate Size: As per Copper earthing Plate Design, Plates are available in 600mm x 600m (2 Feet x 2 Feet) and 300mm x 300mm (1 Feet x 1 Feet) dimensions with 3mm thickness or as per requirements. Earthing Plate is fixed with copper strip and GI Pipe. After digging 3 feet x 3 feet 10 feet hole, the earthing plate is inserted in and salt and charcoal added in alternate layers upto the level of the plate. Funnel / Wire mesh is used to avoid soil in water pipe.

The natural soil or 3E make backfill compound mixed with good quality (pref black cotton soil) to backfill till the top and a chamber is installed to measure the earthing resistance values once a year. After testing the earthing, the earthing is connected to the equipment through a test link. The test link is used to disconnect earthing with interconnection to equipotential bonding while testing of the earthings.

Table 41.1 *Following Items are used in installation as per Copper Plate Earthings Design*

1.Copper Earthing Plate
2.Copper Strip connected to GI Pipe at the bottom
3 GI Pipe for watering
4 Salt
5 Charcoal
6 Cast Iron Cover Brass Nut Bolts Washer

Conclusion

De Flora et al. wrote the following: "Since the late 20th century, chronic degenerative diseases have overcome infectious disease as the major causes of death in the 21st century, so an increase in human longevity will depend on finding an intervention that inhibits the development of these diseases and slows their progress".Could such an intervention be located right beneath our feet? Earthing research, observations, and related theories raise an intriguing possibility about the Earth's surface electrons as an untapped health resource—the Earth as a "global treatment table." Emerging evidence shows that contact with the Earth—whether being outside barefoot or indoors connected to grounded conductive systems—may be a simple, natural, and yet profoundly effective environmental strategy against chronic stress, ANS dysfunction, inflammation, pain, poor sleep, disturbed HRV, hypercoagulable blood, and many common health disorders, including cardiovascular disease. The research done to date supports the concept that grounding or earthing the human body may be an essential element in the health equation along with sunshine, clean air and water, nutritious food, and physical activity.

Summary

Environmental medicine generally addresses environmental factors with a negative impact on human health. However, emerging scientific research has revealed a surprisingly positive and overlooked environmental factor on health: direct physical contact with the vast supply of electrons on the surface of the Earth.

Modern lifestyle separates humans from such contact. The research suggests that this disconnect may be a major contributor to physiological dysfunction and unwellness. Reconnection with the Earth's electrons has been found to promote intriguing physiological changes and subjective reports of well-being. Earthing (or grounding) refers to the discovery of benefits—including better sleep and reduced pain—from walking barefoot outside or sitting, working, or sleeping indoors connected to conductive systems that transfer the Earth's electrons from the ground into the body. This paper reviews the earthing research and the potential of earthing as a simple and easily accessed global modality of significant clinical importance.

Bibliography ans Acknowledgement

Adak S, Chowdhury S, Bhattacharyya M. Dynamic and electrokinetic behavior of erythrocyte membrane in diabetes mellitus and diabetic cardiovascular disease. Biochimica et Biophysica Acta. 2008;1780(2):108–115. [PubMed] [Google Scholar]

Anisimov S, Mareev E, Bakastov S. On the generation and evolution of aeroelectric structures in the surface layer. Journal of Geophysical Research D. 1999;104(12):14359–14367. [Google Scholar]

Applewhite R. The effectiveness of a conductive patch and a conductive bed pad in reducing induced human body voltage via the application of earth ground. European Biology and Bioelectromagnetics. 2005;1:23–40. [Google Scholar]

Bobbert MF, Hollander AP, Huijing PA. Factors in delayed onset muscular soreness of man. Medicine and Science in Sports and Exercise. 1986;18(1):75–81. [PubMed]

Brown R, Chevalier G, Hill M. Pilot study on the effect of grounding on delayed-onset muscle soreness. Journal of Alternative and Complementary Medicine. 2010;16(3):265–273. [PMC free article] [PubMed] [Google Scholar]

Chahine M, Chatelier A, Babich O, Krupp JJ. Voltage-gated sodium channels in neurological disorders. CNS and Neurological Disorders—Drug Targets. 2008;7(2):144–158. [PubMed] [Google Scholar]

Chevalier G, Mori K, Oschman JL. The effect of Earthing (grounding) on human physiology. European Biology and Bioelectromagnetics. 2006;2(1):600–621. [Google Scholar]

Chevalier G, Sinatra S. Emotional stress, heart rate variability, grounding, and improved autonomic tone: clinical applications. Integrative Medicine: A Clinician's Journal. 2011;10(3) [Google Scholar]

Chevalier G, Sinatra ST, Oschman JL, Delany RM. Grounding the human body reduces blood viscosity—a major factor in cardiovascular disease. Journal of Alternative and Complementary Medicine. In press. [PMC free article] [PubMed] [Google Scholar]

Chevalier G. Changes in pulse rate, respiratory rate, blood oxygenation, perfusion index, skin conductance, and their variability induced during and after grounding human subjects for 40 minutes. Journal of Alternative and Complementary Medicine. 2010;16(1):1–7. [PubMed] [Google Scholar]

de Flora S, Quaglia A, Bennicelli C, Vercelli M. The epidemiological revolution of the 20th century. FASEB Journal. 2005;19(8):892–897. [PubMed] [Google Scholar]

Feynman R, Leighton R, Sands M. The Feynman Lectures on Physics. II. Boston, Mass, USA: Addison-Wesley; 1963. [Google Scholar]

Franceschi C, Bonaf M, Valensin S, et al. Inflamm-aging: an evolutionary perspective on immunosenescence. Annals of the New York Academy of Sciences. 2000;908:244–254. [PubMed] [Google Scholar]

Genuis SJ. Fielding a current idea: exploring the public health impact of electromagnetic radiation. Public Health. 2008;122(2):113–124. [PubMed] [Google Scholar]

Ghaly M, Teplitz D. The biologic effects of grounding the human body during sleep as measured by cortisol levels and subjective reporting of sleep, pain, and stress. Journal of Alternative and Complementary Medicine. 2004;10(5):767–776. [PubMed] [Google Scholar]

Holiday D, Resnick R, Walker J. Fundamentals of Physics, Fourth Edition. New York, NY, USA: John Wiley & Sons; 1993. [Google Scholar]

H bscher M, Vogt L, Bernh rster M, Rosenhagen A, Banzer W. Effects of acupuncture on symptoms and muscle function in delayed-onset muscle soreness. Journal of Alternative and Complementary Medicine. 2008;14(8):1011–1016.

Jamieson KS, ApSimon HM, Jamieson SS, Bell JNB, Yost MG. The effects of electric fields on charged molecules and particles in individual microenvironments. Atmospheric Environment. 2007;41(25):5224–5235. [Google Scholar]

Just A. Return to Nature: The True Natural Method of Healing and Living and The True Salvation of the Soul. New York, NY, USA: B. Lust; 1903. [Google Scholar]

NIH State-of-the-Science Conference on Manifestations and Management of Chronic Insomnia in Adults. http://consensus.nih.gov/2005/insomniastatement.htm, June 13-15, 2005.

Ober C, Sinatra ST, Zucker M. Earthing: The Most Important Health Discovery Ever? Laguna Beach, Calif, USA: Basic Health Publications; 2010. [Google Scholar]

Ober C. Grounding the human body to neutralize bioelectrical stress from static electricity and EMFs. ESD Journal, http://www.esdjournal.com/articles/cober/ground.htm, January 2000.

Oschman JL. Can electrons act as antioxidants? A review and commentary. Journal of Alternative and Complementary Medicine. 2007;13(9):955–967. [PubMed] [Google Scholar]

Oschman JL. Charge transfer in the living matrix. Journal of Bodywork and Movement Therapies. 2009;13(3):215–228.

Oschman JL. Perspective: assume a spherical cow: the role of free or mobile electrons in bodywork, energetic and movement therapies. Journal of Bodywork and Movement Therapies. 2008;12(1):40–57. [PubMed] [Google Scholar]

Rossi W. The Sex Life of the Foot and Shoe. Vol. 61. Hertfordshire, UK: Wordsworth Editions; 1989. [Google Scholar]

Sokal K, Sokal P. Earthing the human body influences physiologic processes. Journal of Alternative and Complementary Medicine. 2011;17(4):301–308. [PMC free article] [PubMed] [Google Scholar]

Stein R. Is Modern Life Ravaging Our Immune Systems? Washington Post; 2008. [Google Scholar]

Tartibian B, Maleki B, Abbasi A. The effects of ingestion of Omega-3 fatty acids on perceived pain and external symptoms of delayed onset muscle soreness in untrained men. Clinical Journal of Sport Medicine. 2009;19(2):115–119. [PubMed] [Google Scholar]

Vaile J, Halson S, Gill N, Dawson B. Effect of hydrotherapy on the signs and symptoms of delayed onset muscle soreness. European Journal of Applied Physiology. 2008;102(4):447–455. [PubMed] [Google Scholar]

White G. The Finer Forces of Nature in Diagnosis and Therapy. Los Angeles, Calif, USA: Phillips Printing Company; 1929. [Google Scholar]

Williams E, Heckman S. The local diurnal variation of cloud electrification and the global diurnal variation of negative charge on the Earth. Journal of Geophysical Research. 1993;98(3):5221–5234. [Google Scholar]

Zainuddin Z, Newton M, Sacco P, Nosaka K. Effects of massage on delayed-onset muscle soreness, swelling, and recovery of muscle function. Journal of Athletic Training. 2005;40(3):174–180. [PMC free article] [PubMed] [Google Scholar]

Artificial Intelligence-Based Smart Comrade Robot for Elders Healthcare.

Technology is a trend that affects human existence in every part of the world. Robots are an exciting example of what the future of technology holds. Robotics has enhanced human life and industry significantly, thanks to the technology . Adults with autism are already a regular thing in many industries, including healthcare, military service, and domestic assistance. The global population is growing, therefore making the requirements of this demographic an increasingly significant issue for health providers, government officials, caretakers, and families. Due to these reasons, buddy robots (which serve as aids to elderly people) are often seen as having an authoritarian function in helping individuals do their caring duties without assistance. An increased old population is often brought up as a method of dealing with the rising number of senior persons. Actually, robots are becoming more prevalent in the senior care sector. We should have been aware of certain ethical issues that have recently been brought to light as a result of these advances. Artificial intelligence approaches are applicable for various fields of utility. Digital smart systems, medical data analysis, healthcare system, and other applications are possible with AI model. Specifically, disease diagnosis with deep learning, radiology model with ML, automatic systems, and so forth are the most utilized healthcare systems of AI.

A rising need for new technology has emerged for older adults because of the greying of our current generation. The primary reasons in favour of this are that there are too few hospital workers and many individuals want to live as independently as possible rather than be placed in an institution . Additionally, we will need an adequate supply of healthcare professionals together with the use of cutting-edge technology. Robotics is playing a significant role in helping older people these days. A household use robot that is particularly intended for use at home may be regarded as a level of service robot. The business of making robots specifically for the house is expanding from scientific and commercial standpoints. In order for Comrade robot to be the most effective in the house, it should be able to carry out several activities such as home monitoring, gadget management, personal assistance, and entertaining.

When more and more robots are developed to engage with a human being to give the sort of care that is often provided by a licensed therapist, the lack of healthcare and the standard of living for the elderly will both improve . Designing a providing assurance "robotic arm" to supervise the old person is the method being used. The overall aim is to create a low rental Comradeship robot to assist an elderly person with daily home automation.

In the end, the house robot could traverse the usual home settings without any human assistance, carrying out duties such as senior citizens monitoring devices, home gadget management, and security and stability sensing, as well as in the case of an attack. This document has two distinct sections. One is a Comrade robot, while the other is a health monitoring band. A Comrade robot does so in the form of "making itself helpful"; that is, it is capable of assisting people in a household setting. The old person is constantly being kept under constant supervision by the Comrade robot . With the sensors incorporated in the design, the leaving comments industrial vehicle ensures both safe and secure environment in the family environment. Trespassers, gas leaks, and fire are all on the list. In the creative and emotional realm, Comrade robots and emotional synthetic avatars have now been created for graduate training. It may be difficult to extract a ministry of planning from both materials; therefore, teams that want to build Comrade robots must create their own website from scratch. Of course, there are many representations of structure for Comrade robot, but it is also tough to locate how the actual ones operate. Most articles concern themselves with how well an overall behavior performs, with little emphasis on the detailed architecture needed for replication.

The RoboCare program is dedicated to creating distributed applications where programming and autonomous agents all work together to accomplish an overall objective, which is to provide a supply of services that are ready for use in settings where people may need help and direction.

While we are also interested in supporting endangered elderly individuals to enjoy an inclusive environment in their own homes, our primary focus is on bringing the concept to market. According to recent data, Europe and Japan are gradually growing older. In order to increase public attention to this matter of "independence" and "ageing at home," new ways of supporting the seniors and persons with disabilities have been created.

This is why when it comes to RoboCare, most of the study deals with two potential situations, which are referred to as the RoboCare Household Atmosphere and the Quality of Life Institution setting . Robotic frameworks, wearable devices, activity monitoring in complicated settings, and human relationships are the main components of strong reliance for the future of robotic care. Here we will give the reader a short summary of the key findings that we have discovered so far and many lessons we have learnt from those efforts to custom-tailor AI for assisted living. Remote sensing data-based applications, image processing, video and audio recognition system, security system, and so forth are the applications of this research field. The major objective is to improve the performance state of medical data analysis and the robot model construction with efficient analysis is designed. This research contributes to improving the robot technology and availability of AI in medical healthcare system. Comrade robot model with AI utility helps to obtain a better performance result.

Why Robotic Help Would Be Required In Future?

Lifespans across the globe are rising, and therefore the percentage of the people in retirement ages is growing (Moyle et al. As visual acuity in older adults diminishes, this necessitates the provision of more services and has a larger impact on budgets for healthcare provision. The older population needs more research to help them retain emotional human fellow. Robotic technology may be used to assist both rehabilitative and sociable robots in relieving strain on social care facilities. Large data processing, overlapping issue, and feature set analysis difficulties are the major problem of conventional work.You may also look into Comradeship robotics, which are little robots that are made to look and behave like animals (Pu et al]). They aid creatures during rodent therapy by decreasing the dangers for the mammals individually. In general, Schr dinger, the mechanical seal, is a famous example. The advantages of getting to know Paro, a simulated nursing care Comrade for elderly people, include decreased irritation as well as depressive disorder in cognitive impairment, better immune responses, less burden on care providers, and enhanced affect and information exchange among both elderly people and their day care providers.. Furthermore, paracetamol may help to minimize the need for hallucinogenic and analgesia medications and may help to lower cholesterol levels.

The authors in and others examine the main methodologies, including designation as well as learning algorithms, which are essential in the development of developing quantum computing, as well as designation and learning algorithms, and computational efficiency that are applicable in the field of growing artificial intelligence and intricate their use .Research methods employed in data security, personal computing, and cloud services provide better findings, as diverse assessment criteria are taken into consideration.

The impact of robot animals upon autonomous older adults was examined in a clinical trial (Abubshait et al.) and also the researchers reported that robotic dogs may offer social enjoyment and relationships. While practical assistance was very attractive, the fact that the robot looked and felt more like a human created a conflict. People preferred soft fur and recommended play elements, such as plush toys, as potential improvements for the Comrade robots that are presently available. When new, brightly colored, child-oriented dogs were used, this restricted the kind of impressions respondents might create. Note that although older persons and individuals with memory are incorporated throughout Comrade robot creation, they are seldom, if ever, offered the opportunity to be engaged. Interaction typically happens in the project design whenever healthcare services are engaged.

It was recommended that the construction of something like an everyone around collapse detection technique be undertaken (Celis et al.). Utilizing just one aeration rate, an innovative wearable gadget for the detection of falls was created. Ubiquitous computing Remote Monitoring for the Old capable of detecting an individual's fall as maintaining the health of the patients. An Intelligent Home Security System based on GSM and ARM Architectural design: Industrial robots have lately been created utilizing a range of technologies, including the Web, wireless communications, wirelessly, and speech recognition.

Robotic Over Review In General

The word robot was originally derived from the Czech word robot, which means forced labor. Karel Capek, the Czech writer, introduced the term robot in his play "R.U.R." Capek used the term robotic in a series called "Rossum's Universal Robots" that premiered in Prague in 1921. The robots in R.U.R were built by man, and they were supposed to work for humanity. Thus, from generations to generations, human people have made use of robots to do various jobs. However, there is just no generally accepted definition for robots Despite this disagreement, the University of the Robot Society still sees a robot as a multipurpose fully programmable tool that is used to transfer credible commitments, tools, or optical disks in various ways using preprogrammed movements. This concept differentiates robots from other automated machines, because they are programmable. A robot may be described as an upgradeable, complex nervous, sentient, and transportable machine that uses energy to do work. Regardless of its form and size, a robot has seven major elements. This collaboration serves a particular goal. Figure 1 depicts the parts of a robot.

1. Controller

The commander is in charge of coordinating the robot's movements. The operational environment refers to the area within which a robot may operate . The microcontroller is also in charge of collecting input first from surrounding environment via the use of its sensing.

2. Power Conversion Unit

The fusion reactor supplies the robot's controls. Electricity, combustible materials, and battery storage are all commonplace power stations in robots . Most of the electricity that is provided to a building comes from the grid, and, in order to power the building, the system uses an AC/DC electrical power converter to change the AC electricity into DC electricity.

• Sensors

Robots may now have the sensor take a specific measurements of the surroundings, with the sensing' data helping to shape the robot's behaviors. To guarantee the robot's security, this is often done. Devices utilize a robot to respond to environmental variations.

• Actuator

In most of the robots, the actuators are often known as the muscles of the robot. The conversion takes place by using the energy that drives your robot's mobility.

• Control and Task Program

A collection of commands from the manufacturers of the robot's controller are known as the management plan, while a sequence of questions typically supplied by the user are called the task programme . To accomplish a particular job, the manipulator must carry out the movements task programmed by the task programme.

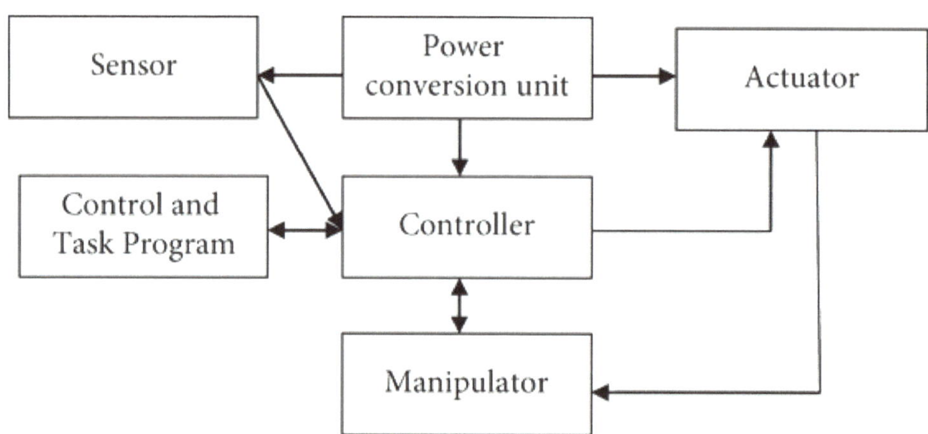

Fig. 42.1 *Components of a robot.*

3. Manipulator

The robotics have had the capacity to pick up, alter, and blow things up. The robot's manipulation imitates outstretched arm of something like a human individual. Manipulators typically refer to the joints connecting the arms with the upper arms, elbows, and wrists. Joints tend to be either rotational or sliding . Reaction kinetics refer to the way wherein the joints are arranged to define the potential stepper motor.

4. End Effector

The final part of the system, which connects to the input device, is known as the manipulation link. The instrument handle's link is known as an actuation. It imitates the mechanical arm, mimicking the results obtained.

Development Of Comrade Robot Structure

To develop up with a proper Comrade robot structure, we also must research the many needs that Comrade robots may have. Just one "perfect" Comrade robot might fulfill all these criteria. Meanwhile, theoretically speaking, the need of a Comrade robot does not quite apply; in reality, one is still required . The specifications for a given robot rely on a variety of different variables, including the kind of intended application and also the particular hardware components that are required.Here we provide a comprehensive list of all potential criteria an engineer should consider while designing a generic structure. The main task of the Comrade robot is to sense the environment around it, including hearing, seeing, and touching. Intercultural competence calls for synchronizing data; thus, various kinds of data need attention

In addition, inputs processing may be programmed to target specific sensor data, in response to predictions from a mixing process. Significance must be verified on every piece of data received, and all information collected must also be classified before it can be kept.

The Comrade robot was able to have a classroom discussion with the user. What this implies is not just to create effective sentences and also to take fundamental principles of communicating into consideration . A Comrade robot should constantly be likely to preserve the dialogue flowing in order to sustain a strong connection. The usage of live interaction also incorporates elements like this; for instance, in order to prevent boring or misunderstanding the user, lengthy pauses should not be present in a discussion. It should be able to communicate across all modalities and should do so in a logical and reasonable manner. Speech would overlap with proper lip motions, which have been prioritized about the present face animations and the robot dealing with the lips both of it. We illustrate the construction of a Comrade robot and address the specifications outlined above. However, observe that perhaps the design is abstracted from the specifics of various kinds of friend robotics, allowing its application to diverse kinds of robot Comrades. We are emphasizing again here that it was for a Comrade robot that also has an "overall" personality; nevertheless, you may build various parts without putting any content into them. Initial set of data processing uses dialogue engine and reasoning engine. Depending on the goals, rules, memory unit, and emotion recognitions are taken with heuristics approach. After that, the input and output processing states are determined with facial recognition with animation approach. Dataset uses source from camera, sound, and so forth and the speech recognition and facial recognition data are synchronized. With the low-level behavior, the animation controls are processed. Here this conflict scheduler, the performance of output state is determined.

AI and Robotic Technology in Elder Healthcare

By building a framework that incorporates current state-of-the-art AI technologies from an off way, RoboCare aims to help service providers fully appreciate the kind of assistance resources available . The difficult part is to find out whether the methods listed above might help create educational software parts that can be purchased off market. Robotic systems now provide us the ability to create robotic system with very accurate survival skills. We have effectively implemented these systems in both the home and hospital facility settings thanks to a variety of methods.

The professional diagnosis and management Comrade robot is able to provide guidance on prevention and prognosis by collecting data like clinical findings, a client's medical records, and previous medical instances. The robot was created by the robotics and artificial intelligence, that is, related to clinical texts, two million clinical data, and many individual instances The hospital is conducting a pilot programme in which people participate to evaluate the robot. When interacting with a client all through physical diagnosis, the robot "pays attention" to the dialogue and takes the sensor readings along with source information to help the clinician diagnose and prescribe medication . The clinician then collects information to interact with the clinician. It is anticipated that the robot would assist doctors to come to a conclusion about the cause of the patient's symptoms quicker and cut down on mistakes.

The Health System Mechanism, is made up of several AI industrial robots.

To arrive at a prognosis, the speech based EHR system and image natural antibiotic are both utilized. Comrade proposes a diagnosis and therapy in which all relevant information is collected.

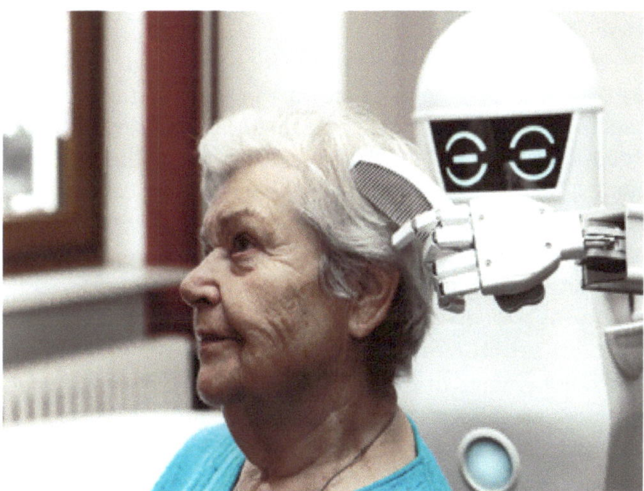

Fig.42.2 *AI chatbots can help fill the void by providing some companionship*

Thanks to advancements in technology, it is now possible to provide ambient independent living solutions to help seniors in their dwellings . The multidisciplinary approach that is required for robotics technology problems includes knowledge from fields like building, fashion, psychological, law, and ethics, as well as technology, computer programming, science, and medicine. In order to benefit everyone, robots and information and communication technology (ICT) must be made accessible across the populace at school, in hospitals, in home languages, and in smart neighborhoods. A high degree of acceptance and usefulness for the users may be achieved by integrating these approaches in the development of the surroundings.

Some basic suggestions for social order, together with technological and legal troubles, may be discovered through the applying load with actual customers in some kind of a contemporary context

Society Centered Design

Robotic technologies should be planned, manufactured, and

deployed to assist people in the day-to-day tasks in a societal architecture.The intelligent machines must be able to go from a user-centered design process to a social system design process, at which development process is properly considered and is further integrated with the society's requirements . Many of the ideas shown in the previous sections included users throughout the whole development process, starting with the study of end-users' requirements and leading all the way through the assessment of the prototype system for valuable suggestions..

Stakeholder Readiness

It is also essential to consider the speed to market in evaluating integrated services. That level of readiness indicates how soon the individuals and organizations are prepared to take and spread the technologies. The gap among study and implementation is the only problem with this topic.

Low Cost

Considering that personalized robotics are meant to be used by the individual, the price must be in line with their financial capability, in place to encourage for broad service usage. Robotic alternatives incur a reduced cost for the sake of a costing system , they are costly owing to the increased components they employ, but then on the other hand they are less costly for the public health system. Cloud automation solution models may enable a new breed of personalized robots for businesses.

Customizability, Flexibility, and Modularity

The requirements of the users will fluctuate. Having provided component services, it is essential to offer one that can respond to customer requirements and competences that vary.

Robustness, Dependability, Safety, and Security

Because the test equipment is expected to engage with those who are vulnerable and aged, it must have been secure and dependable.

Autonomy

Robotics institutions are expected to move independently and make choices based on the needs of consumers. They ought to be capable of identifying errors that users have made or they have made and make corrections on their own when required.

Social Informatics of Knowledge Embodiment

Our study has significance that are present in the system; it is applied to other comparable systems. Nonetheless, in order to validate our results, further research with healthcare practitioners in the field is required. In our research of AI-infused autonomous vehicles, we disregarded electronic archives, too. The usage of other things, like computers, may be affected by AI industrial robotics; however, in our research paper, we have not seen this. The possibility of further study includes research that compares cognitive manifestation in various entities in order to learn about how they support or replace one another.Lastly, we have not investigated the nature of senior executives' interest in, or usage of, AI machines. Understanding the four forms of information embodiment as a generative framework for finding motivators may be the most useful. Mechanistic explanation of cognitive immersion should rely on knowing the motive. From a social bioinformatics viewpoint, AI technology is relevant in the context.

It is vital to understand the sociospatial relationships AI has with people in order to fully comprehend its true worth. STIN analytic approach is particularly helpful, since it offers a paradigm for incorporating various social actors' perspectives while considering technologies. An excellent illustration of our findings is that, in contrast to the robots that were intended to make people's job and emphasizing, the AI humanoid systems that operate as rivals and magisters encounter greater opposition from economic systems than those that work as collaboration and guild mates.

This STIN study also showed that the automation technologies supplier has a minimal but nonetheless significant impact on the market. Requiring timely deployment of AI mobile robots for skilled employees, the supplier highlighted the technologies' complimentary and nonconfrontational character to help people gain confidence. This research confirms that our awareness of the use of AI industrial robotics in intellectual work requires a social information systems viewpoint.

By using powerful computers like AI robotic systems, researchers are showing that they can behave as an independent social actor in addition to just being a tool for humans. When humans and robots interact more naturally and intuitively, the difference between the humanity and the machine may become obsolete. Further refinement of the notion of interconnections in social bioinformatics as interpersonal relations and living organism connection converge may be required in order to help more people have social networks.

A manifestation of information changes understanding labor, and the introduction of new privacy practices is probable. Since making scientific have yet to comprehend the consequences of artificial intelligence, it is possible that the necessary training activities may need new methods of collecting, analyzing, and displaying data at employment. Social and community customers frequently need to work with machines, as well. Because of the resulting shift in the organization, in other words, the dissemination of materials is most likely to be caused. and shows major module utilizing expansion, emancipation, equipping, and expediting. Speech data with knowledge analysis, human cognition, augmentation, and AI robot are analyzed in expansion set. Actuation and competitor design of emancipation is determined. Assistance and automation model uses the procedural knowledge and final declaration.

Methodology Employed

Robotic systems that utilize the making plans, observation, concurrence, and successive cognitive orientations review process acquire questionnaire questions from guardians and carry out the intellectual orienting examination control and experimental group. The robot then engages in a discussion with the user and gathers feedback. When the robot has finished evaluating the responses, it reports back to those same caregivers with the results .This section describes the cognitive assessment method and the communication mechanisms platform. Our Friend Robotic, a 3D-printed desk device, is fitted with a cognition assessment process. The capacitive touch screen is linked to an ARM-based microcomputer executing Android platform, and the interaction is shown on it. In addition to having a 3D camera, this robot is equipped with a vision circuit composed of an RGB-D camera for image recognition and four loudspeakers that help with sound localization. We have also included voice and physical movement detection in our robot arm.The cognitive orientation assessment method has seven critical features: a development tool, inquiry and response creation, agreement between two parties, excessive screen, Internet computer vision, answer appraisal, and intelligence score .An online dataset and native databases are required for the relational database. In the public cloud, Q&A worksheets containing users' accounts and summaries of memory score are stored, along with cognitive orientations evaluations. These may be revised and checked by a caretaker. The personal dataset provides the user's focus strategy, test timetables, and Q&A answers.

Modeling and Formulations of Comrade Robots

The study of bending moment enables one to approach performs of large masses. According to the current motion, one may see the position, orientations, and higher incidence as having evolved through time. Dynamics in robotics are used to build up basic equations of controls, with the dynamic transfer function for deceivers acting as the explanation governing motion. Torque is the mechanism that is responsible for producing the dynamic movement of both manipulating arms in a robot's arm .. Dynamic modeling is involved in the development of the differential equations of the manipulation as a function of something like the displacements acting on it. In dynamic modeling, the robotics manipulator's components are constrained to a set of forces and; as a result, the locations, velocities, and deceleration are determined:(i)People who have torque needed to achieve certain end-effector movements are all determined by this calculation (the direct dynamic problem) (ii)The elastic scattering issue is modeled mathematically, and there are a variety of control methods which use the model(iii)It enables the calculation of the real manipulation to be done usinga control scheme equations and manipulate Lagrange's movement. Joint characteristics and characteristics of the manipulation define the motion. A communication model with overall energy K and gravitational potential V is shown as follows. Lagrange refers to. It is a simple procedure using the Lagrangian differential equation derived. The general force that corresponds to the generalized coordinate qi is referred to as Qi. Connection I has kinetic and potential energy provided. A second-order linear evolution equation may be used to describe the Lagrangian equations of motion for the n-th links manipulators.where

Evaluation Process

Google has published a new open software speech recognition processing framework, known as SyntaxNet, to the public. Syntax Net's main purpose is to find out the words and phrases, and each word is clearly shown in phrase. A parser is capable of determining the morphological purpose of any single phrase, including conjunctions, in the phrase. In addition to providing an also before the model named Parse McParseface, Goggling also offers a grammar models, known as Parsey McParseface, that is developed. No matter how complicated the root of a phrase may be, SyntaxNet is able to recognize it is able to trace out the connection between the word meaning and each individual word in the phrase. This study aimed to use SyntaxNet, so that the customer's voice communication may be processed genuinely.

To illustrate, a phrase will be spoken, at which point the voice activation component will transform textual content, which is then processed by SyntaxNet for deeper comprehension. To put a POS on a word, SyntaxNet examines the whole phrase as well as the word's semantics. Similarly, since SyntaxNet can correctly predict the calculated value used when a machine evaluates the provided response with the right answer, assessing answers that utilize math is quite simple. The capabilities of SyntaxNet may also be utilized to detect whether there is negativity in the word but when the phrase has a pejorative perception.The programming language we use to describe paragraph characteristics is called SyntaxNet. Step one is answering the question, and step two is evaluating the response. Next, the input is examined and processed using SyntaxNet to identify both user responses and right answers. Long computational network and right answer structure are created from the interpreted results. Those trees stand for the concept of a "pos" and how words relate to one other . The second step in the algorithm is to connect two trees, and the saplings are compared using a mating Canadian land. A compatibility score is given for these tree trunks, depending on their resemblance.

The robot gives a score of 1 to a right answer tree and a score of 0 to an erroneous solution tree. A partial number may be given if the answer matches both trees; however, the progress and achievement are used to evaluate the two trees. To determine the user's cognitive score, the participant's characteristics and a caregiver-determined criterion are utilized.

Recognition state of robot has various questionnaires, which translates the audio data to text data. Depending on the availability of given response, the NLP is performed and messages are taken with NLP analysis model. The parsed text is extracted with the feature set of given database. These correlated results are analyzed and desired answers are taken for the task accomplishment. Feedbacks are saved; then the respective description database assessment result is produced.

In conlusion ,Artificial intelligence is a rapidly expanding area of research, which has implications in many sectors, such as medical services, and to provide pharmaceutical aid. It is well established that the area of healthcare is a dynamic market for AI. In this article, a robotics framework is created which uses human messages between a human and a robot to carry out cognitive orientation evaluation. SyntaxNet, which enables the robots to comprehend programming knowledge naturally, helped carry out natural language processing. The Comrade robot was created from the ground up to handle this entire ecosystem. We do not need outside assistance in order to conduct a cognitive orientation evaluation, since the system is capable of doing it. This research sought to elicit tasks where a certain robot aids with increasing the quality of life (QoL) and assisting with an autonomous, healthy ageing. This research presents occupations that are an important component of the lives of older people in all the secondary classrooms. This study demonstrates that it is possible to use technologies with an eye on improving the quality of life for older people. At a profound level, elderly people need robots to do more complex tasks. In the future, the research work may be adopted with big data analysis, image processing, and statistical analysis reviewed with comparative analysis of machine learning approach.

AI Robots- the future of technology

Artificial intelligence (AI) is the simulation of human intelligence in machines that programmed to think and act like humans. The machine associated with a human mind such as learning and problem-solving. The ideal characteristic of artificial intelligence is its ability to take action for the best chance of achieving a specific goal. The goals of artificial intelligence are based on learning, reasoning, and perception. Machines use a cross-disciplinary approach based on mathematics, computer science, linguistics, psychology, and more. Key points are as;-

- AI is the simulation of human intelligence in machines.
- The aim of artificial intelligence includes learning, reasoning, and perception.
- AI is used across different industries including finance and healthcare.
- Weak AI tends to be single-task oriented and strong AI is more complex and human-like.

AI Robots

Robotics is a domain in artificial intelligence with the study of creating intelligent and efficient robots. Robots are the artificial agents for the real-world environment. Robots manipulate the objects by perceiving, picking, moving, modifying the physical properties of objects, destroying it, or having an effect thereby freeing manpower from doing repetitive functions without getting bored, distracted, or exhausted. It is a branch of AI composed of Electrical Engineering, Mechanical Engineering, and Computer Science for designing, construction, and application of robots. The robots have mechanical construction designed to accomplish a particular task with power and control of the machinery. They contain some level of a computer program that determines what, when, and how a robot doing things.

Difference in Robot System and AI Program

Here is the difference between the two

- AI programs operate in computer-simulated worlds. The input of the AI program is in symbols and rules. They need general-purpose computers to operate the programs.
- Robots operate in the real physical world. The Inputs to robots is in analog signal in the form of speech waveform or images. They function with special hardware with sensors and effectors

Robot Locomotion

Locomotion is the mechanism where the robot is capable of moving in its environment. There are various types of locomotions

Legged

This type of locomotion consumes more power while doing walk, jump, trot, hop, climb up or down, etc. It requires several motors to accomplish a movement. It is suited for rough and smooth terrain wherein irregular or too smooth surface it consumes more power for wheeled locomotion. Sometimes it is a little difficult to implement because of stability issues. It comes with a variety of legs that is two, four, or six legs. Leg coordination is necessary for locomotion which has multiple legs. Gaits is a periodic sequence of lift and release events for each of the total legs. The total number of possible gaits where a robot travel depends upon the number of its legs. If a robot has k legs, then the number of possible events N (2k-1) . There are six possible different events

- Lifting the Left leg
- Releasing the Left leg
- Lifting the Right leg

- Releasing the Right leg
- Lifting both the legs together
- Releasing both the legs together

In the case of k 6 legs, there are 39916800 possible events. Hence, the complexity of robots is directly proportional to the number of legs.

Wheeled Locomotion

It requires fewer number of motors to complete a movement. It is easy to implement with less stability issues in case if there is more number of wheels. It is more efficient as compared to legged locomotion. The Standard wheel rotates around the wheel axle and the contact. The Castor wheel rotates around the wheel axle and the offset steering joint. Swedish 45o and Swedish 90o wheels rotate around the contact point, around the wheel axle, and the rollers. Ball or spherical wheel is the Omnidirectional wheel which is difficult to implement technically.

Slip Skid Locomotion

The robot is steered by moving the tracks with different speeds in the same or opposite direction. It has stability because of the large contact area of track and ground.

Components of a Robot

Robots are constructed with the following

- Power Supply The robots are powered by batteries, solar power, hydraulic
- Actuators – It converts energy into movement.
- Electric motors (AC/DC) – Motors are required for rotational movement.
- Pneumatic Air Muscles contract almost 40% when air is sucked in them.
- Muscle Wires contract by 5% when an electric current is passed through them.
- Piezo Motors and Ultrasonic Motors are the best for industrial robots.
- Sensors provide knowledge of the real-time information on the task environment

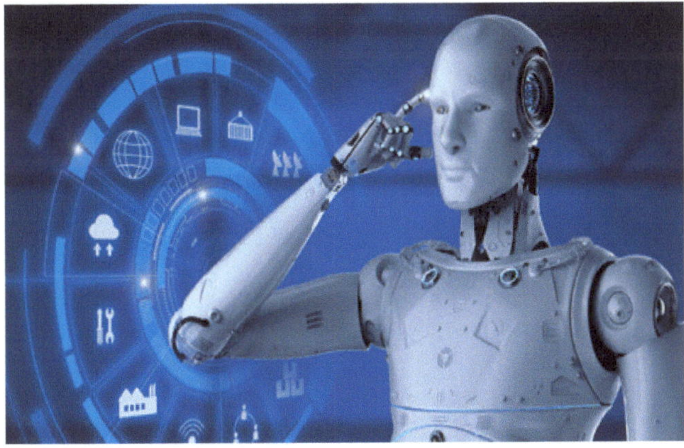

Fig.42.3 *Showing the features of a Robot in use*

Computer Vision

This is a technology of AI in which the robots can see. Vision plays a crucial role in the domains of safety, security, health, access, and entertainment. It automatically extracts, analyzes, and comprehends useful information from a single image or an array of images. This process accomplishes automatic visual comprehension.

Hardware of Computer Vision System

This involves Power supply, Image acquisition devices such as camera, processor, software, a Display device, accessories such as camera stands, cables, and connectors

Tasks of Computer Vision

- Optical Character Reader is a software to convert scanned documents into editable text, which accompanies a scanner.
- Face Detection comes with this feature, which enables to read the face and take the picture of perfect expression.
- Object Recognition is installed in supermarkets, cameras, high-end cars such as BMW, GM, and Volvo.
- Estimating the Position of an object to the camera as in the position of the tumor in the human body.

Application of Computer Vision

- Agriculture
- Autonomous vehicles
- Biometrics
- Character recognition
- Forensics, security, and surveillance
- Industrial quality inspection
- Face recognition
- Gesture analysis
- Geoscience
- Medical imagery
- Pollution monitoring
- Process control
- Remote sensing
- Robotics
- Transport

Applications of Robotic. The robotics has been instrumental in the various domains such as

- Industries Robots are used for handling material, cutting, welding, color coating, drilling, polishing, etc.
- Military – It reaches inaccessible and hazardous zones during the war. A robot named Daksh, developed by DRDO used to destroy life-threatening objects safely.
- Medicine – These robots carry hundreds of clinical tests simultaneously, rehabilitating permanently disabled people, and performing complex surgeries such as brain tumors.
- Exploration These robots used for space exploration, underwater drones used for ocean exploration.
- Entertainment Disney's have created hundreds of robots for animated movies.

Using AI to Help Care for Senior Citizens

- Providing Companionship
- Helping Seniors Live Securely and Independently in Their Homes
- Pose Detection for Preventive Care
- Trust Mindy Support for Your Medical Data Annotation Needs

As the world's population gradually becomes older, there is an increasing need to develop new technology to help provide better care for them. In fact, according to a report by the United Nations, there are 703 million people aged 65 and older, a number that is expected to more than double by 2050. Since the population of older adults is growing at such a rapid speed, there are various social, economic, and health challenges that must be addressed. This is an area where AI can be of great assistance since it can help the healthcare system deal with the increased demand for senior healthcare services. In this article, we will take a look at some of the ways AI is helping senior citizens take better care of themselves and maintain their independence.

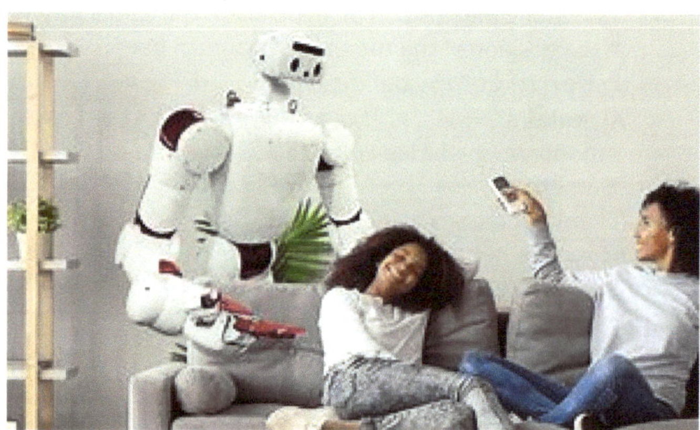

Fig.42.4 *Personal AI-based robots as lifetime human companions*

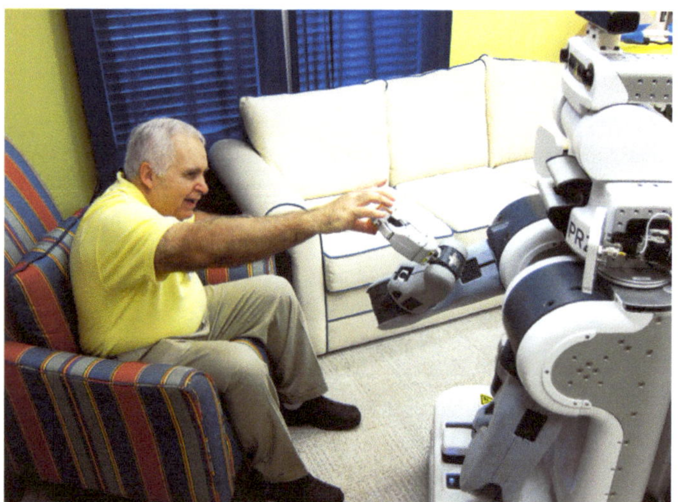

Fig, 42 5 *Scientists have created a robot that could help elderly people with dementia and other limitations live independently in their own homes*

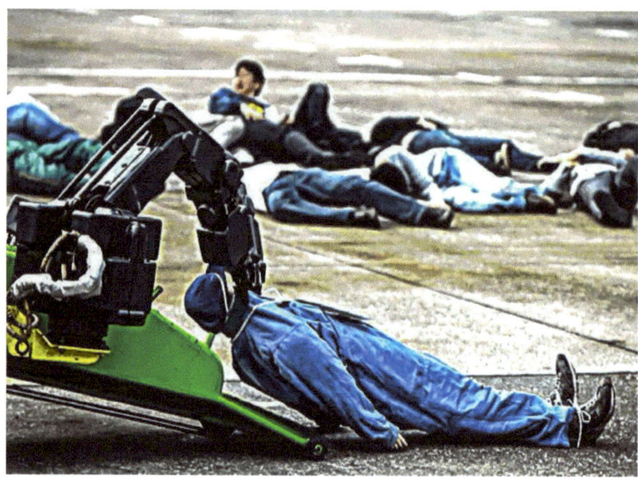

Fig. 42.6 *Robot is doing rescue-job*

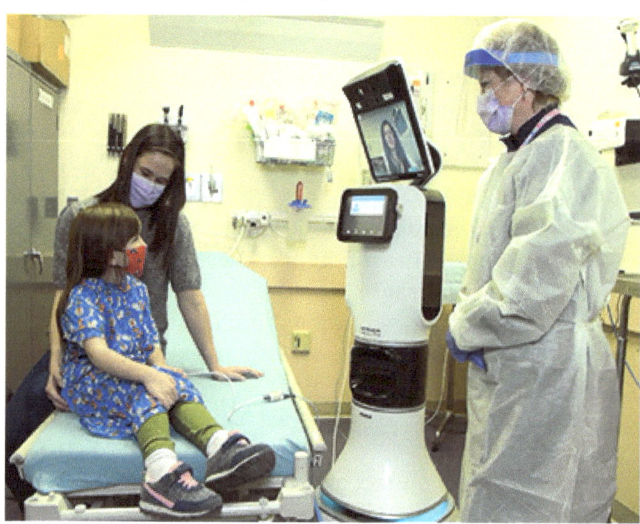

Fig.42 .7 *New robot helps care for kids in the emergency room*

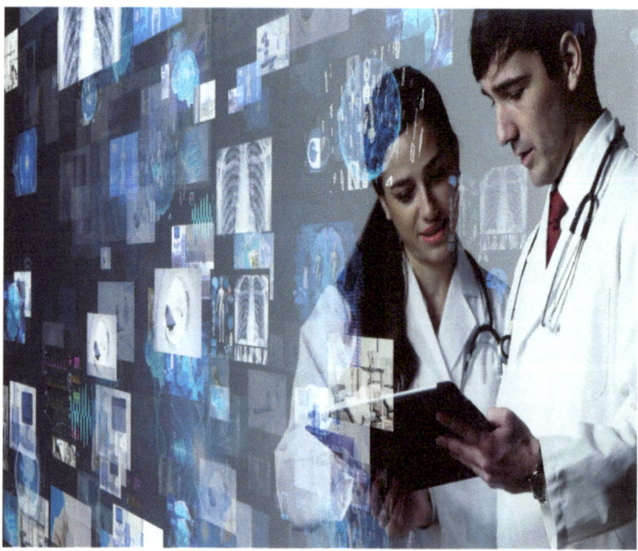

Fig. 42.8 *Using AI to Efficiently Diagnose and Reduce Medical Errors*

Pose Detection for Preventive Care

Falls are a leading cause of unintentional injuries and can result in devastating disabilities and fatalities when left undetected and not treated in time. In fact, worldwide, falls are a leading cause of unintentional injuries in adults older than 65 years old, with 37.3 million falls requiring medical attention and 646,000 resulting in deaths annually. Human pose detection can play a key role in elderly care for fast responses and preventing seniors from falling. A lot of studies have been done in Japan to create such pose detection software. For example, researchers at the Toyohashi University of Technology have done extensive research into estimating human poses using deep learning with depth data from twin camera systems in elderly care robots. The technology was able to generate data using computer graphics and motion capture technologies various poses that could signal a potential fall within acceptable reliability levels.

While fall prevention products are still being perfected, there are other products on the market, such as For example, in Canada there is a very useful tool called the AltumView's Cypress Smart Home Care Alert System that can call for help if a fall does occur. It can also provide a heat map of an area where falls have frequently occurred. This allows the caregiver to take measures, such as removing certain obstacles or blocking access to that location, to prevent similar accidents from happening again.

Trust Mindy Support for Your Medical Data Annotation Needs

Regardless of whether or not your dataset requires trained medical professionals to do the annotation or such work can be done without a medical background, Mindy Support can assemble a team for you to get the job done. Thanks to our skills and expertise, we can help you actually even the most daring and imaginative products. Contact us today to learn more about how we can help you.

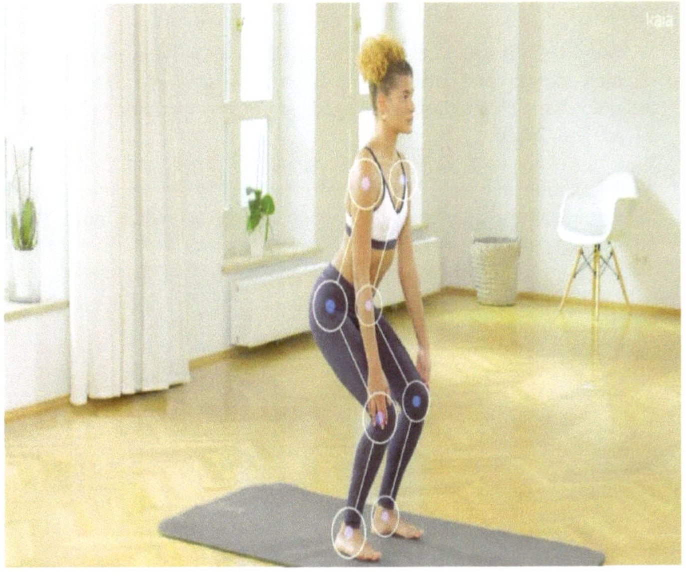

Fig. 42.9 *AI Pose Estimation Technology and How You Can Use It*

Helping Seniors Live Securely and Independently in Their Homes

According to a report from the AARP, 90% of seniors want to stay in their homes as they age. However, the homes of senior citizens often cannot accommodate their individual needs, posing many risks to their safety and wellness. This is why a lot of seniors in the US us various smart home devices to maintain their independence. This includes activity-based sensors that are connected to a smart security system and can trigger alarms and send help for potential break-ins, fires, and unsafe levels of carbon monoxide.

Another interesting feature is using machine learning to understand a senior's patterns and behaviors. If the system detects a change in their routine, such as the sensor on a medicine cabinet not being triggered when it's time to take a scheduled prescription, the AI spots this break in the pattern and notifies interested parties via email, text, and/or push notifications.

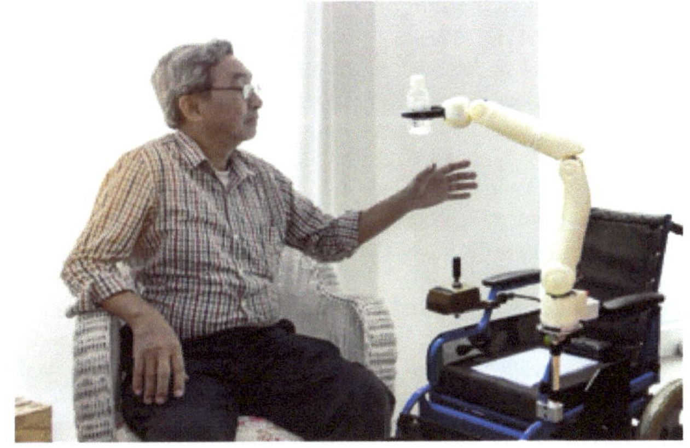

Fig.42.10 *AI helping seniors lve securely and independently in their homes*

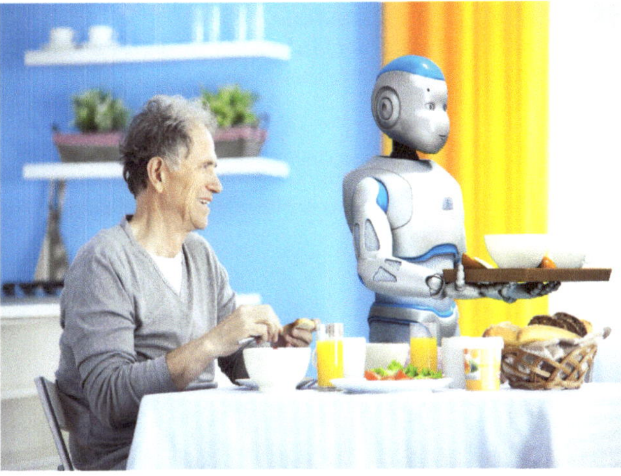

Fig. 42.11 *AI Romeo-An Intelligent French Robot To Help Elderly With Daily Tasks*

Bibliography and Acknowledgement

- Abubshait, E. Wiese, and Y. L. Human, "You look human, but act like a machine: agent appearance and behavior modulate different aspects of Human-Robot interaction," Frontiers in Psychology, vol. 8, 2017.
- B. Kartal, E. Nunes, J. Godoy, and M. Gini, "Monte Carlo tree search with branch and bound for multi-robot task allocation symposium conducted at the meeting of the the IJCAI-16 workshop on autonomous mobile service robots," vol. 30, no. 1, 2016.
- B. Zohuri and M. Moghaddam, "Neural network driven supper artificial intelligence based on internet of things and big data," Business Resilience System (BRS), vol. 1, 2018.
- D. SverreSyrdal, J. Saunders, and K. DautenhahnK. L. Koay and N. Burke, ""Teach me–show me""'—"end-user personalization of a smart home and comrade robot"," IEEE transactions on Human Machine Systems, vol. 46, no. 1, 2016.
  Davison, Introduction to Robotics, Department of Computing, Imperial College, London, UK, 2016.
- F. Al-Turjman and J. P. Lemayian, "Intelligence, security, and vehicular sensor networks in internet of things (IoT)-enabled smart-cities: an overview," Computers & Electrical Engineering, vol. 87, Article ID 106776, 2020.
- G. Viejo, D. D. Torrico, F. R. Dunshea, and S. Fuentes, "Development of artificial neural network models to assess beer acceptability based on sensory properties using a robotic pourer: a comparative model approach to achieve an artificial intelligence system," Beverages, vol. 5, 2019.
- G. Yang, Z. Pang, M. J. Deen et al., "Homecare robotic systems for healthcare 4.0: visions and enabling technologies," IEEE Journal of Biomedical and Health Informatics, vol. 24, pp. 2535–2549, 2020.
- H. Ashrafian, A. Darzi, and T. Athanasiou, "A novel modification of the Turing test for artificial intelligence and robotics in healthcare," International Journal of Medical Robotics and Computer Assisted Surgery, vol. 11, pp. 38–43, 2015.
- H. BozU. Kose, "Emotion extraction from facial expressions by using artificial intelligence techniques," Broad Research in Artificial Intelligence and Neuroscience, vol. 8, pp. 5–16, 2017.
- H. Manoharan, Y. Teekaraman, P. R. Kshirsagar, S. Sundaramurthy, and A. Manoharan, "Examining the effect of aquaculture using sensor-based technology with machine learning algorithm," Aquaculture Research, vol. 51, no. 11, pp. 4748–4758, 2020.
- J. Celis, S. Castro, and D. Guevara, "Voice processing with Internet of Things for a home automation system," in Proceedings of the International conference on Electronics, Electricalengineering and computing, pp. 8–10, IEEE, Lima, Peru, August 2018.
- J.Cowie, "Evaluation of a digital consultation and self-care advice tool in primary care: a multi-methods study," Inter. Jour.of Environ Res Public Health, vol. 15, 2018.Sensmeier, "Harnessing the power of artificial intelligence," Nursing Management, vol. 48, no. 11, pp. 14–19, 2017.
- Hameed, I. S. Bajwa, S. Ramzan, W. Anwar, and A. Khan, "An intelligent IoT based healthcare system using fuzzy neural networks," Scientific Programming, vol. 2020, Article ID 8836927, 15 pages, 2020.
- Pu, W. Moyle, C. Jones, and M. Todorovic, "The effectiveness of social robots for older adults: a systematic review and meta-analysis of randomized controlled studies," Gerontologist Jan, vol. 59, no. 1, pp. e37–51, 2019.
- M. M. A. D. Graaf, S. B. Allouch, and J. A. G. M. V. Dijk, "Why would I use this in my home? a model of domestic social robot acceptance," Human-Computer Interaction, vol. 34, pp. 115–173, 2019.
- M. Mortazavi, F. Aminiazad, H. Parsaei, and M. A. Mosleh-Shirazi, "An artificial neural network-based model for predicting annual dose in healthcare workers occupationally exposed to different levels of ionizing radiation," Radiation Protection Dosimetry, vol. 189, 2020.
- M. Sg, T. Ak, A. St, S. Sv, and O. Mj, "Role of artificial intelligence in health care," Biochemistry Ind Journal, vol. 11, no. 5, pp. 1–14, 2017.
  Mesko, "The role of artificial intelligence in precision medicine," Expert Rev Precis Med Drug Dev, vol. 2, pp. 239–241, 2017.
- P. R. Kshirsagar, H. Manoharan, F. Al-Turjman, and K. Kumar, "Design and testing of automated smoke monitoring sensors in vehicles," IEEE Sensors Journal, vol. 1, p. 1, 2020.
- P.-P. C. F. Rudzicz and S. Raimondo, "Ludwig: a conversational robot for people with alzheimer's," The Journal of the Alzheimer's Association, vol. 13, 2017.
- R. Bhatnagar and D. Batra, "Robotic process automation in healthcare-a review," International Robotics & Automation Journal, vol. 5, 2019.
  S. Montani, R. Bellazzi, A. Riva, C. Larizza, L. Portinale, and M. Stefanelli, "Artificial intelligence techniques for diabetes management: the T-IDDM project. ECAI," in Proceedings of the 14th European conerence on Artificial Intelligence, pp. 1–5, Berlin, Germany, August 2000.
- W. Moyle, C. Jones, L. Pu, and S. C. Chen, "Applying user-centred research design and evidence to develop and guide the use of technologies, including robots, in aged care," Contemporary Nurse, vol. 54, pp. 1–3, 2018.
- W. Yu, A. Kapusta, J. Tan, C. C. Kemp, G. Turk, and C. K. Liu, "Haptic simulation for robot-assisted dressing," in Proceedings of the IEEE International Conference on Robotics and Automation, pp. 6044–6051, Singapore, May 2017

Applications of ChatGPT In Medical Practice, Education and Research

ChatGPT, which can automatically generate written responses to queries using internet sources, soon went viral after its release at the end of 2022. The performance of ChatGPT on medical exams shows results near the passing threshold, making it comparable to third-year medical students. It can also write academic abstracts or reviews at an acceptable level. However, it is not clear how ChatGPT deals with harmful content, misinformation or plagiarism; therefore, authors using ChatGPT professionally for academic writing should be cautious. ChatGPT also has the potential to facilitate the interaction between healthcare providers and patients in various ways. However, sophisticated tasks such as understanding the human anatomy are still a limitation of ChatGPT. ChatGPT can simplify radiological reports, but the possibility of incorrect statements and missing medical information remain. Although ChatGPT has the potential to change medical practice, education and research, further improvements of this application are needed for regular use in medicine

ChatGPT (OpenAI, San Francisco, CA, USA) is an AI chatbot which was introduced in November 2022 and soon after went viral. ChatGPT has the ability to respond to various kinds of queries, automatically generating responses using internet sources. People across different fields, generations and continents started using ChatGPT, leading to a continuous increase in its popularity. Medicine is a field in which simplifying artificial intelligence (AI)-based technologies are highly important. It is obvious that applications such as ChatGPT have the potential to change medicine, with uses ranging from the automated extraction of electronic medical records to the development of sophisticated treatment plans. This article presents an overview of the early applications of ChatGPT in medicine.

ChatGPT in medical education

A recent study evaluated the performance of ChatGPT on the United States Medical Licensing Examination (USMLE). The study revealed that ChatGPT passed all three exams (Step 1, Step 2 CK, Step 3) near the passing threshold without any previous training. On the other hand, Gilson et al state that there is a significant decrease in performance with an increased difficulty of the questions.

However, the authors compare the performance of ChatGPT to a third-year medical student. Antaki et al tested ChatGPT for use in two multiple-choice question banks for the Ophthalmic Knowledge Assessment Program (OKAP) exam. The authors found similar results, with ChatGPT achieving 55.8% and 42.7% accuracy in the exams. Another study from Korea aimed at directly correlating the knowledge of Chat-GPT to that of medical students on the topic of parasitology. The authors revealed that the performance of ChatGPT was lower than medical students and concluded that ChatGPT's ability is not yet at an entirely acceptable level.

Academic writing

Gao et al tested ChatGPT's ability to write academic abstracts. They included 50 abstracts from five high-impact medical journals and asked ChatGPT to produce research abstracts using provided titles and journal requirements. The authors concluded that all ChatGPT-derived abstracts were acceptably written, but only 8% of them respected the formatting requirements of the journals. 68% of the generated abstracts by ChatGPT were correctly identified by the reviewers due to the 'vaguer' and more 'formulaic' type of writing. An AI output detector showed similar results in detecting the ChatGPT-derived abstracts.

In a recent article by Guo et al, the main attributes of ChatGPT's writing style are identified. The authors mention that ChatGPT writes in an organised manner and prefers a straightforward concept in the questions. Its answers are long and detailed, it shows less harmful information, and refuses to answer when it has no information about topics. However, it might 'fabricate facts' to give an answer, which should make users cautious regarding the professional use of ChatGPT. The authors observed that the main difference between ChatGPT's writing style and human writing is that the human writer is more subjective, colloquial and emotional, giving human abstracts a personal note.9 OpenAI warns that ChatGPT could sometimes 'responds to harmful instructions

A recent study evaluated ChatGPT's ability to generate a literature review on the concept of the 'digital twin' in

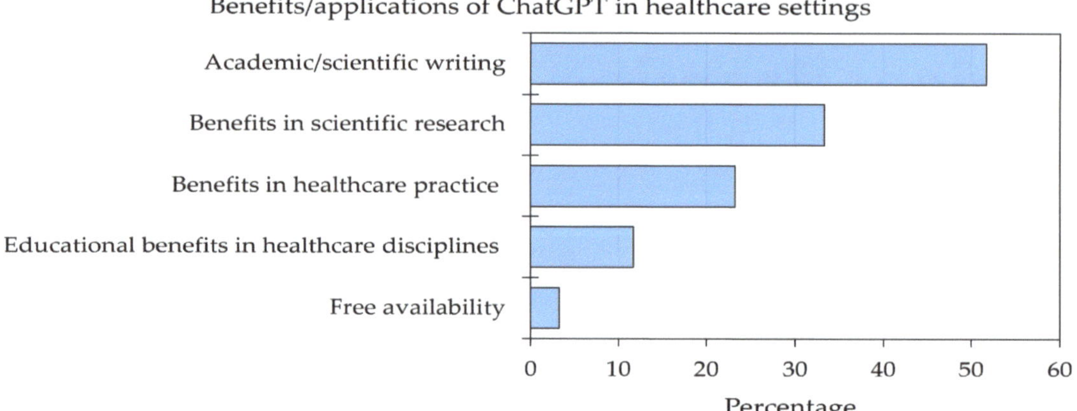

Fig. 43.1 *Summary of benefits/applications of ChatGPT in health care education, research, and practice based on the included records.*

healthcare, asking it to paraphrase selected literature from 2020 to 2022. Although the results were promising, the iThenticate plagiarism detection tool identified many plagiarism matches.

Interaction with Patients and Radiological Reporting

Thurzo et al reviewed AI-based applications, including ChatGPT, in the dental field. They concluded that ChatGPT could facilitate the interaction between healthcare providers and patients in various ways, from analysing patient messages to personalising the communication between healthcare professionals and patients. However, they found that ChatGPT has limitations in relation to sophisticated tasks such as understanding the human anatomy. Nov et al tested ChatGPT against healthcare providers' responses to patients. They found that ChatGPT had a similar rate of correct answers compared to the providers. In a case study conducted by Jeblick et al, radiologists had the task of evaluating the quality of simplified radiology reports generated with ChatGPT. The results showed that the reports were 'correct, complete, and not potentially harmful to patients'. However, incorrect statements and missing medical information that could potentially have led to harmful conclusions were also detected. Although this case study comprises small sample numbers, the authors emphasise the great potential of ChatGPT in radiology while also mentioning the need for further improvements.

The far-reaching consequences of ChatGPT among other LLMs can be described as a paradigm shift in academia and health care practice. The discussion of its potential benefits, future perspectives, and importantly, its limitations, appear timely and relevant . Therefore, the current review aimed to highlight these issues based on the current evidence.

The following common themes emerged from the available literature.

Benefits of ChatGPT in Scientific Research

ChatGPT, as an example of other LLMs, can be described as a

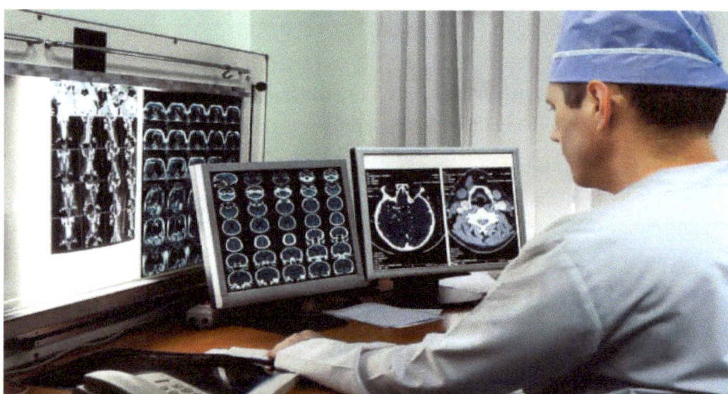

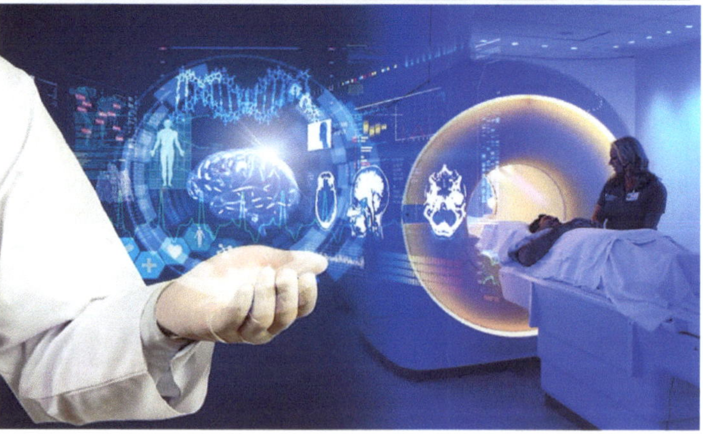

Fig.43.2 *A Radiology Information System (RIS) is a sophisticated EHR system designed specifically for use in a radiology practice. A radiology information system (RIS) is a networked software system for managing medical imagery and associated data. A RIS is especially useful for tracking radiology imaging orders and billing information, and is often used in conjunction with PACS to manage image archives, record-keeping and billing.*

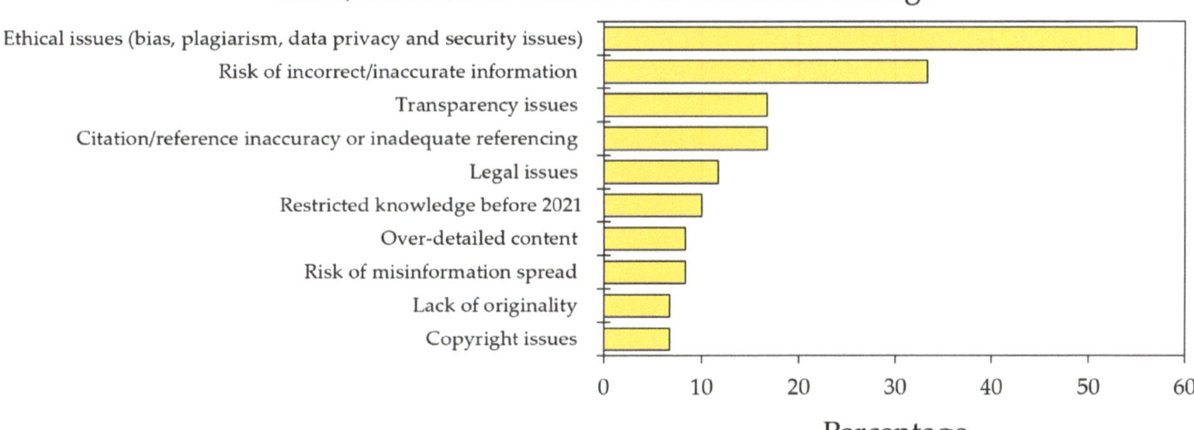

Fig.43.3 *Summary of risks/concerns of ChatGPT use in health care education, research, and practice based on the included records*

a promising or even a revolutionary tool for scientific research in both academic writing and in the research process itself. Specifically, ChatGPT was listed in several sources as an efficient and promising tool for conducting comprehensive literature reviews and generating computer codes, thereby saving time for the research steps that require more efforts from human intelligence (e.g., the focus on experimental design) . Additionally, ChatGPT can be helpful in generating queries for comprehensive systematic review with high precision, as shown by Wang et al., despite the authors highlighting the transparency issues and unsuitability for high-recall retrieval . Moreover, the utility of ChatGPT extends to involve an improvement in language and a better ability to express and communicate research ideas and results, ultimately speeding up the publication process with the faster availability of research results . This is particularly relevant for researchers who are non-native English speakers .Such a practice can be acceptable considering the already existent English editing services provided by several academic publishers. Subsequently, this can help to promote equity and diversity in research .

Limitations of ChatGPT Use in Scientific Research

On the other hand, the use of ChatGPT in academic writing and scientific research should be conducted in light of several limitations that could compromise the quality of research as follows.

First, superficial, inaccurate, or incorrect content was frequently cited as a shortcoming of ChatGPT use in scientific writing . The ethical issues including the risk of bias based on training datasets and plagiarism were also frequently mentioned, aside from the lack of transparency regarding content generation, which justifies the description of ChatGPT, on occasions, as a black box technology . Importantly, the concept of ChatGPT hallucination could be risky if the generated content is not thoroughly evaluated by researchers and health providers with proper expertise . This comes in light of the ability of ChatGPT to generate incorrect content that appears plausible from a scientific point of view .

Second, several records mentioned the current problems regarding citation inaccuracies, insufficient references, and ChatGPT referencing to non-existent sources .This was clearly shown in two recently published case studies with ChatGPT use in a journal contest . These case studies discouraged the use of ChatGPT, citing the lack of scientific accuracy, the limited updated knowledge, and the lack of ability to critically discuss the results . Therefore, the ChatGPT generated content, albeit efficient, should be meticulously examined prior to its inclusion in any research manuscripts or proposals for research grants.

Third, the generation of non-original, over-detailed, or excessive content can be an additional burden for researchers who should carefully supervise the ChatGPT-generated content This can be addressed by supplying ChatGPT with proper prompts (text input), since varying responses might be generated based on the exact approach of prompt construction .

Fourth, as it currently stands, the knowledge of ChatGPT is limited to the period prior to 2021 based on the datasets used in ChatGPT training . Thus, ChatGPT cannot be used currently as a reliable updated source of literature review . Nevertheless, ChatGPT can be used as a motivation to organize the literature in a decent format, if supplemented by reliable and up-to-date references .

Fifth, the risk of research fraud (e.g., ghostwriting, falsified or fake research) involving ChatGPT should be considered seriously ,as well as the risk of generating mis-

or disinformation with the subsequent possibility of infodemics,

Sixth, legal issues in relation to ChatGPT use were also raised by several records including copyright issues .

Finally, the practice of listing ChatGPT as an author does not appear to be acceptable based on the current ICMJE and COPE guidelines for determining authorship, as illustrated by Zielinski et al. and Liebrenz et al. This comes in light of the fact that authorship entails legal obligations that are not met by ChatGPT . However, other researchers have suggested the possibility of ChatGPT inclusion as an author in some specified instances .

A few instances were encountered in this review, where ChatGPT was listed as an author that can point to the initial perplexity of a few publishers regarding the role of LLM including ChatGPT in research . The disapproval of including ChatGPT or any other LLM in the list of authors was clearly explained in Science, Nature, and the Lancet editorials, which referred to such practice as scientific misconduct, and this view was echoed by many scientists . In the case of ChatGPT use in the research process, several records advocated the need for the proper and concise disclosure and documentation of ChatGPT or LLM use in the methodology or acknowledgement sections. A note worthy and comprehensive record by Borji can be used as a categorical guide for the issues and concerns of ChatGPT use, especially in the context of scientific writing .

Benefits of ChatGPT in Health Care Practice

From the health care practice perspective, the current review showed a careful excitement vibe regarding ChatGPT applications. The ability of ChatGPT to help in streamlining the clinical workflow appears promising, with possible cost savings and increased efficiency in health care delivery . This was illustrated recently by Patel and Lam, highlighting the ability of ChatGPT to produce efficient discharge summaries, which can be valuable to reduce the burden of documentation in health care .Additionally, ChatGPT, among other LLMs, can have a transforming potential in health care practice via enhancing diagnostics, prediction of disease risk and outcome, and drug discovery among other areas in translational research . Moreover, ChatGPT showed moderate accuracy in determining the imaging steps needed in breast cancer screening and in the evaluation of breast pain, which can be a promising application in decision making in radiology . ChatGPT in health care settings also has the prospects of refining personalized medicine and the ability to improve health literacy by providing easily accessible and understandable health information to the general public . This utility was demonstrated by ChatGPT responses, highlighting the need to consult health care providers among other reliable sources on specific situations .

Concerns Regarding ChatGPT Use in Health Care Practice

On the other hand, several concerns regarding ChatGPT use in health care settings were raised. Ethical issues including the risk of bias and transparency issues appeared as recurring major concerns Additionally, the generation of inaccurate content can have severe negative consequences in health care; therefore, this valid concern should be cautiously considered in health care practice . This concern also extends to involve the ability of ChatGPT to provide justification for incorrect decisions .

Other ChatGPT limitations including the issues of interpretability, reproducibility, and the handling of uncertainty were also raised, which can have harmful consequences in health care settings including health care research . In the area of personalized medicine, the lack of transparency and unclear information regarding the sources of data used for ChatGPT training are important issues in health care settings considering the variability observed among different populations in several health-related traits [69]. The issue of reproducibility between the ChatGPT prompt runs is of particular importance, which can be a major limitation in health care practice .

Medico-legal and accountability issues in the case of medical errors caused by ChatGPT application should be carefully considered . Importantly, the current LLMs including ChatGPT are unable to comprehend the complexity of biologic systems, which is an important concept needed in health care decisions and research [52,68]. The concerns regarding data governance, health care cybersecurity, and data privacy should draw specific attention in the discussion regarding the utility of LLMs in health care .

Other issues accompanying ChatGPT applications in health care include the lack of personal and emotional perspectives needed in health care delivery and research . However, ChatGPT emulation of empathetic responses was reported in a preprint in the context of hepatic disease . Additionally, the issue of devaluing the function of the human brain should not be overlooked; therefore, stressing the indispensable human role in health care practice and research is important to address any psychologic, economic, and social consequences that could accompany the application of LLM tools in health care settings .

Benefits and Concerns Regarding ChatGPT Use in Health Care Education

In the area of health care education, ChatGPT appears to have a massive transformative potential. The need to rethink and revise the current assessment tools in health care education comes in light of ChatGPT's ability to pass reputable exams (e.g., USMLE) and possibility of ChatGPT misuse, which would result in academic dishonesty .

Specifically, in ophthalmology examination, Antaki et al. showed that ChatGPT currently performed at the level of an average first-year resident . Such a result highlights the need to focus on questions involving the assessment of critical and problem-based thinking . Additionally, the utility of ChatGPT in health care education can involve tailoring education based on the needs of the student with immediate feedback .. Interestingly, a recent preprint by Benoit showed the promising potential of ChatGPT in rapidly crafting consistent realistic clinical vignettes of variable complexities that can be a valuable educational source with lower costs .Thus, ChatGPT can be useful in health care education including enhanced communication skills given proper academic mentoring . However, the copyright issues should be taken into account regarding the ChatGPT-generated clinical vignettes, aside from the issue of inaccurate references . Additionally, ChatGPT availability can be considered as a motivation in health care education based on the personalized interaction it provides, enabling powerful self-learning as well as its utility as an adjunct in group learning.

Other limitations of ChatGPT use in health care education include the concern regarding the quality of training datasets that could result in biased content and inaccurate information limited to the period prior to the year 2021. Additionally, other concerns include the current inability of ChatGPT to handle images as well as its low performance in some topics (e.g., failure to pass a parasitology exam for Korean medical students), and the issue of possible plagiarism .Despite ChatGPT versatility in the context of academic education , the content of ChatGPT in research assignments was discouraged, being currently insufficient, biased, or misleading .

Future Perspectives

As stated comprehensively in a commentary by van Dis et al., there is an urgent need to develop guidelines for ChatGPT use in scientific research, taking into account the issues of accountability, integrity, transparency, and honesty . Thus, the application of ChatGPT to advance academia and health care should be carried out ethically and responsibly, taking into account the potential risks and concerns it entails .

More studies are needed to evaluate the content of LLMs including its potential impact to advance academia and science with a particular focus on health care settings .In academic writing, a question arises as to whether authors would prefer an AI-editor and an AI-reviewer considering the previous flaws in the editorial and peer review processes . A similar question would also arise in health care settings involving the personal preference of emotional support from health care providers, rather than the potential efficiency of AI-based systems.

In health care education, more studies are needed to evaluate the potential impact of ChatGPT on the quality and efficiency of both educational content and assessment tools. ChatGPT utility to help in refining communication skills among health care students is another aspect that should be further explored as well as the applications of LLMs in the better achievement of the intended learning outcomes through personalized and instantaneous feedback for the students.

Conclusions

The imminent dominant use of LLM technology including the widespread use of ChatGPT in health care education, research, and practice is inevitable. Considering the valid concerns raised regarding its potential misuse, appropriate guidelines and regulations are urgently needed with the engagement of all stakeholders involved to ensure the safe and responsible use of ChatGPT powers. The proactive embrace of LLM technologies with careful consideration of the possible ethical and legal issues can limit the potential future complications. If properly implemented, ChatGPT, among other LLMs, have the potential to expedite innovation in health care and can aid in promoting equity and diversity in research by overcoming language barriers. Therefore, a science-driven debate regarding the pros and cons of ChatGPT is strongly recommended and its possible benefits should be weighed with the possible risks of misleading results and fraudulent research .

Based on the available evidence, health care professionals could be described as carefully enthusiastic regarding the huge potential of ChatGPT among other LLMs in clinical decision-making and optimizing the clinical workflow. "ChatGPT in the Loop: Humans in Charge" can be the proper motto to follow based on the intrinsic value of human knowledge and expertise in health care research and practice . An inspiring example of this motto could be drawn based on the relationship between the human character Cooper and the robotic character TARS from Christopher Nolan's movie Interstellar .

However, before its widespread adoption, the impact of ChatGPT from the health care perspective in a real-world setting should be conducted (e.g., using a risk-based approach) . Based on the title of an important perspective article "AI in the hands of imperfect users" by Kostick-Quenet and Gerke ,the real-world impact of ChatGPT among other LLMs should be properly evaluated to prevent any negative impact of its potential misuse. The same innovative and revolutionary tool can be severely deleterious if used improperly. An example to illustrate such severe negative consequences of ChatGPT misuse can be based on Formula 1 racing, as follows. In the 2004 Formula 1 season, the Ferrari F2004 (the highly successful Formula 1 racing car) broke several Formula 1 records in the hands of Michael Schumacher, one of the most successful Formula 1 drivers of all time. However, in my own hands —as a humble researcher without expertise in Formula 1 driving— the same highly successful car would only break walls and be damaged beyond repair.

Bibliography and Acknowledgement

- Aczel, B.; Wagenmakers, E. Transparency Guidance for ChatGPT Usage in Scientific Writing. PsyArXiv, 2023; Preprint. [Google Scholar] [CrossRef]
- Ahn, C. Exploring ChatGPT for information of cardiopulmonary resuscitation. Resuscitation 2023, 185, 109729. [Google Scholar] [CrossRef] [PubMed]
- Akhter, H.M.; Cooper, J.S. Acute Pulmonary Edema After Hyperbaric Oxygen Treatment: A Case Report Written With ChatGPT Assistance. Cureus 2023, 15, e34752. [Google Scholar] [CrossRef] [PubMed]
- Alberts, I.L.; Mercolli, L.; Pyka, T.; Prenosil, G.; Shi, K.; Rominger, A.; Afshar-Oromieh, A. Large language models (LLM) and ChatGPT: What will the impact on nuclear medicine be? Eur. J. Nucl. Med. Mol. Imaging, 2023; Online ahead of print. [Google Scholar] [CrossRef]
- Bašić, Ž.; Banovac, A.; Kružić, I.; Jerković, I. Better by You, better than Me? ChatGPT-3 as writing assistance in students' essays. arXiv, 2023; Preprint. [Google Scholar] [CrossRef]
- Benoit, J. ChatGPT for Clinical Vignette Generation, Revision, and Evaluation. medRxiv, 2023; Preprint. [Google Scholar] [CrossRef]
  Biswas, S. ChatGPT and the Future of Medical Writing. Radiology 2023, 223312. [Google Scholar] [CrossRef]
- Borji, A. A Categorical Archive of ChatGPT Failures. arXiv 2023, arXiv:2302.03494. [Google Scholar] [CrossRef]
  Brown, T.; Mann, B.; Ryder, N.; Subbiah, M.; Kaplan, J.D.; Dhariwal, P.; Neelakantan, A.; Shyam, P.; Sastry, G.; Askell, A. Language models are few-shot learners. Adv. Neural Inf. Process. Syst. 2020, 33, 1877–1901. [Google Scholar] [CrossRef]
- Cahan, P.; Treutlein, B. A conversation with ChatGPT on the role of computational systems biology in stem cell research. Stem. Cell. Rep. 2023, 18, 1–2. [Google Scholar] [CrossRef]
- Cascella, M.; Montomoli, J.; Bellini, V.; Bignami, E. Evaluating the Feasibility of ChatGPT in Healthcare: An Analysis of Multiple Clinical and Research Scenarios. J. Med. Syst. 2023, 47, 33. [Google Scholar] [CrossRef] [PubMed]
- Chatterjee, J.; Dethlefs, N. This new conversational AI model can be your friend, philosopher, and guide … and even your worst enemy. Patterns 2023, 4, 100676. [Google Scholar] [CrossRef] [PubMed]
- D'Amico, R.S.; White, T.G.; Shah, H.A.; Langer, D.J. I Asked a ChatGPT to Write an Editorial About How We Can Incorporate Chatbots Into Neurosurgical Research and Patient Care. Neurosurgery 2023, 92, 993–994. [Google Scholar] [CrossRef]
- De Angelis, L.; Baglivo, F.; Arzilli, G.; Privitera, G.P.; Ferragina, P.; Tozzi, A.E.; Rizzo, C. ChatGPT and the Rise of Large Language Models: The New AI-Driven Infodemic Threat in Public Health. SSRN, 2023; Preprint. [Google Scholar] [CrossRef]
- Deng, J.; Lin, Y. The Benefits and Challenges of ChatGPT: An Overview. Front. Comput. Intell. Syst. 2023, 2, 81–83. [Google Scholar]
- Domingos, P. The Master Algorithm: How the Quest for the Ultimate Learning Machine Will Remake Our World, 1st ed.; Basic Books, A Member of the Perseus Books Group: New York, NY, USA, 2018; p. 329. [Google Scholar]
- Fijačko, N.; Gosak, L.; Štiglic, G.; Picard, C.T.; John Douma, M. Can ChatGPT Pass the Life Support Exams without Entering the American Heart Association Course? Resuscitation 2023, 185, 109732.
  Gilson, A.; Safranek, C.W.; Huang, T.; Socrates, V.; Chi, L.; Taylor,
- R.A.; Chartash, D. How Does ChatGPT Perform on the United States Medical Licensing Examination? The Implications of Large Language Models for Medical Education and Knowledge Assessment. JMIR Med. Educ. 2023, 9, e45312. [Google Scholar] [CrossRef] [PubMed] Gordijn, B.; Have, H.t. ChatGPT: Evolution or revolution? Med. Health Care
- Philos. 2023, 26, 1–2. [Google Scholar] [CrossRef]
- Hallsworth, J.E.; Udaondo, Z.; Pedrós-Alió, C.; Höfer, J.; Benison, K.C.; Lloyd, K.G.; Cordero, R.J.B.; de Campos, C.B.L.; Yakimov, M.M.; Amils, R. Scientific novelty beyond the experiment. Microb. Biotechnol. 2023; Online ahead of print. [Google Scholar] [CrossRef]
- Harzing, A.-W. Publish or Perish. Available online: https://harzing.com/resources/publish-or-perish (accessed on 16 February 2023).
- Hisan, U.; Amri, M. ChatGPT and Medical Education: A Double-Edged Sword. Researchgate, 2023; Preprint. [Google Scholar] [CrossRef]
- Jeblick, K.; Schachtner, B.; Dexl, J.; Mittermeier, A.; Stüber, A.T.; Topalis, J.; Weber, T.; Wesp, P.; Sabel, B.; Ricke, J.; et al. ChatGPT Makes Medicine Easy to Swallow: An Exploratory Case Study on Simplified Radiology Reports. arXiv 2022, arXiv:2212.14882. [Google Scholar] [CrossRef]
- Johnson, K.B.; Wei, W.Q.; Weeraratne, D.; Frisse, M.E.; Misulis, K.; Rhee, K.; Zhao, J.; Snowdon, J.L. Precision Medicine, AI, and the Future of Personalized Health Care. Clin. Transl. Sci. 2021, 14, 86–93. [Google Scholar] [CrossRef] [PubMed]
- Jordan, M.I.; Mitchell, T.M. Machine learning: Trends, perspectives, and prospects. Science 2015, 349, 255–260. [Google Scholar] [CrossRef]
- Khan, A.; Jawaid, M.; Khan, A.; Sajjad, M. ChatGPT-Reshaping medical education and clinical management. Pak. J. Med. Sci. 2023, 39, 605–607. [Google Scholar] [CrossRef]
- Kim, S.G. Using ChatGPT for language editing in scientific articles. Maxillofac. Plast. Reconstr. Surg. 2023, 45, 13. [Google Scholar] [CrossRef] [PubMed]
- Kitamura, F.C. ChatGPT Is Shaping the Future of Medical Writing but Still Requires Human Judgment. Radiology 2023, 230171.
- Korteling, J.E.; van de Boer-Visschedijk, G.C.; Blankendaal, R.A.M.; Boonekamp, R.C.; Eikelboom, A.R. Human- versus Artificial Intelligence. Front. Artif. Intell. 2021, 4, 622364. [Google Scholar] [CrossRef] [PubMed]
- Kostick-Quenet, K.M.; Gerke, S. AI in the hands of imperfect users. Npj Digit. Med. 2022, 5, 197. [Google Scholar] [CrossRef] [PubMed]
  Kumar, A. Analysis of ChatGPT Tool to Assess the Potential of its Utility for Academic Writing in Biomedical Domain. Biol. Eng. Med. Sci. Rep. 2023, 9, 24–30. [Google Scholar] [CrossRef]
- Kung, T.H.; Cheatham, M.; Medenilla, A.; Sillos, C.; De Leon, L.; Elepaño, C.; Madriaga, M.; Aggabao, R.; Diaz-Candido, G.; Maningo, J.; et al. Performance of ChatGPT on USMLE: Potential for AI-assisted medical education using large language models. PLOS Digit. Health 2023, 2, e0000198. [Google Scholar] [CrossRef]
- Liebrenz, M.; Schleifer, R.; Buadze, A.; Bhugra, D.; Smith, A. Generating scholarly content with ChatGPT: Ethical challenges for medical publishing. Lancet Digit. Health 2023, 5, e105–e106.
- Lin, Z. Why and how to embrace AI such as ChatGPT in your academic life. PsyArXiv, 2023; Preprint. [Google Scholar]
- Lubowitz, J. ChatGPT, An Artificial Intelligence Chatbot, Is Impacting Medical Literature. Arthroscopy, 2023; in press. [Google Scholar]
- Lund, B.; Wang, S. Chatting about ChatGPT: How may AI and GPT impact academia and libraries? Library Hi. Tech. News, 2023; ahead-of-print. [Google Scholar] [CrossRef]
- Mann, D. Artificial Intelligence Discusses the Role of Artificial Intelligence in Translational Medicine: A JACC: Basic to Translational Science Interview With ChatGPT. J. Am. Coll. Cardiol. Basic Trans. Sci. 2023, 8, 221–223. [Google Scholar] [CrossRef]
- Manohar, N.; Prasad, S.S. Use of ChatGPT in Academic Publishing: A Rare Case of Seronegative Systemic Lupus Erythematosus in a Patient With HIV Infection. Cureus 2023, 15, e34616. [Google Scholar]

- Marchandot, B.; Matsushita, K.; Carmona, A.; Trimaille, A.; Morel, O. ChatGPT: The Next Frontier in Academic Writing for Cardiologists or a Pandora's Box of Ethical Dilemmas. Eur. Heart J. Open 2023, 3, oead007. [Google Scholar] [CrossRef]
- Margalida, A.; Colomer, M. Improving the peer-review process and editorial quality: Key errors escaping the review and editorial process in top scientific journals. PeerJ. 2016, 4, e1670. [Google Scholar] [CrossRef] [Green Version]
- Mavrogenis, A.F.; Quaile, A.; Scarlat, M.M. The good, the bad and the rude peer-review. Int. Orthop. 2020, 44, 413–415. [Google Scholar] [CrossRef] [Green Version]
- Mbakwe, A.B.; Lourentzou, I.; Celi, L.A.; Mechanic, O.J.; Dagan, A. ChatGPT passing USMLE shines a spotlight on the flaws of medical education. PLoS Digit. Health 2023, 2, e0000205. [Google Scholar] [CrossRef]
- McCarthy, J.; Minsky, M.L.; Rochester, N.; Shannon, C.E. A Proposal for the Dartmouth Summer Research Project on Artificial Intelligence, August 31, 1955. AI Mag. 2006, 27, 12. [Google Scholar] [CrossRef]
  Mijwil, M.; Aljanabi, M.; Ali, A. ChatGPT: Exploring the Role of Cybersecurity in the Protection of Medical Information. Mesop. J. CyberSecurity 2023, 18–21. [Google Scholar] [CrossRef]
- Moher, D.; Liberati, A.; Tetzlaff, J.; Altman, D.G. Preferred reporting items for systematic reviews and meta-analyses: The PRISMA statement. PLoS Med. 2009, 6, e1000097. [Google Scholar]
- Nachshon, A.; Batzofin, B.; Beil, M.; van Heerden, P.V. When Palliative Care May Be the Only Option in the Management of Severe Burns: A Case Report Written With the Help of ChatGPT. Cureus 2023, 15, e35649. [Google Scholar] [CrossRef] [PubMed]
- Nisar, S.; Aslam, M. Is ChatGPT a Good Tool for T&CM Students in Studying Pharmacology? SSRN, 2023; Preprint.
  Nolan, C. Interstellar; 169 minutes; Legendary Entertainment: Burbank, CA, USA, 2014. [Google Scholar]
- O'Connor, S. Open artificial intelligence platforms in nursing education: Tools for academic progress or abuse? Nurse Educ. Pract. 2023, 66, 103537. [Google Scholar] [CrossRef]
- Ollivier, M.; Pareek, A.; Dahmen, J.; Kayaalp, M.E.; Winkler, P.W.; Hirschmann, M.T.; Karlsson, J. A deeper dive into ChatGPT: History, use and future perspectives for orthopaedic research. Knee Surg. Sports Traumatol. Arthrosc. 2023;
- OpenAI. OpenAI: Models GPT-3. Available online: https://beta.openai.com/docs/models (accessed on 14 January 2023).
- Paranjape, K.; Schinkel, M.; Nannan Panday, R.; Car, J.; Nanayakkara, P. Introducing Artificial Intelligence Training in Medical Education. JMIR Med. Educ. 2019, 5, e16048. [Google Scholar] [CrossRef]
- Patel, S.B.; Lam, K. ChatGPT: The future of discharge summaries? Lancet Digit. Health 2023, 5, e107–e108. [Google Scholar] [CrossRef]
- Polonsky, M.; Rotman, J. Should Artificial Intelligent (AI) Agents be Your Co-author? Arguments in favour, informed by ChatGPT. SSRN, 2023; Preprint. [Google Scholar] [CrossRef]
- Quintans-Júnior, L.J.; Gurgel, R.Q.; Araújo, A.A.S.; Correia, D.; Martins-Filho, P.R. ChatGPT: The new panacea of the academic world. Rev. Soc. Bras. Med. Trop. 2023, 56, e0060.
- Rajpurkar, P.; Chen, E.; Banerjee, O.; Topol, E.J. AI in health and medicine. Nat. Med. 2022, 28, 31–38. [Google Scholar] [CrossRef]
- Rao, A.; Kim, J.; Kamineni, M.; Pang, M.; Lie, W.; Succi, M.D. Evaluating ChatGPT as an Adjunct for Radiologic Decision-Making. medRxiv 2023. [Google Scholar] [CrossRef]
- Sallam, M.; Salim, N.A.; Al-Tammemi, A.B.; Barakat, M.; Fayyad, D.; Hallit, S.; Harapan, H.; Hallit, R.; Mahafzah, A. ChatGPT Output Regarding Compulsory Vaccination and COVID-19 Vaccine Conspiracy: A Descriptive Study at the Outset of a Paradigm Shift in Online Search for Information. Cureus 2023, 15, e35029.
- Sallam, M.; Salim, N.A.; Barakat, M.; Al-Tammemi, A.B. ChatGPT applications in medical, dental, pharmacy, and public health education: A descriptive study. Narra J. 2023, 3, e103. [Google Scholar] [CrossRef]
- Sanmarchi, F.; Bucci, A.; Golinelli, D. A step-by-step Researcher's Guide to the use of an AI-based transformer in epidemiology: An exploratory analysis of ChatGPT using the STROBE checklist for observational studies. medRxiv, 2023; Preprint.
- Sarker, I.H. AI-Based Modeling: Techniques, Applications and Research Issues Towards Automation, Intelligent and Smart Systems. SN Comput. Sci. 2022, 3, 158. [Google Scholar] [CrossRef] [PubMed]
- Shahriar, S.; Hayawi, K. Let's have a chat! A Conversation with ChatGPT: Technology, Applications, and Limitations. arXiv 2023, arXiv:2302.13817. [Google Scholar] [CrossRef]
- Sharma, G.; Thakur, A. ChatGPT in Drug Discovery. ChemRxiv, 2023; Preprint. [Google Scholar] [CrossRef]
- Shen, Y.; Heacock, L.; Elias, J.; Hentel, K.D.; Reig, B.; Shih, G.; Moy, L. ChatGPT and Other Large Language Models Are Double-edged Swords. Radiology 2023, 230163. [Google Scholar] [CrossRef]
- Smith, R. Peer review: A flawed process at the heart of science and journals. J. R. Soc. Med. 2006, 99, 178–182.
  Stokel-Walker, C. AI bot ChatGPT writes smart essays—Should professors worry? Nature, 9 December 2022.
- Stokel-Walker, C. ChatGPT listed as author on research papers: Many scientists disapprove. Nature 2023, 613, 620–621. [Google Scholar]
- Stokel-Walker, C.; Van Noorden, R. What ChatGPT and generative AI mean for science. Nature 2023, 614, 214–216.
- Taecharungroj, V. "What Can ChatGPT Do?"; Analyzing Early Reactions to the Innovative AI Chatbot on Twitter. Big Data Cogn. Comput. 2023, 7, 35. [Google Scholar] [CrossRef]
- Tai, M.C. The impact of artificial intelligence on human society and bioethics. Tzu Chi. Med J. 2020, 32, 339–343. [
- Thorp, H.H. ChatGPT is fun, but not an author. Science 2023, 379, 313.
  Tobore, T.O. On Energy Efficiency and the Brain's Resistance to Change: The Neurological Evolution of Dogmatism and Close-Mindedness. Psychol. Rep. 2019, 122, 2406–2416.
- van Dis, E.A.M.; Bollen, J.; Zuidema, W.; van Rooij, R.; Bockting, C.L. ChatGPT: Five priorities for research. Nature 2023, 614, 224–226.
- Wang, S.; Scells, H.; Koopman, B.; Zuccon, G. Can ChatGPT Write a Good Boolean Query for Systematic Review Literature Search? arXiv 2023, arXiv:2302.03495. [Google Scholar] [CrossRef]
- Wogu, I.A.P.; Olu-Owolabi, F.E.; Assibong, P.A.; Agoha, B.C.; Sholarin, M.; Elegbeleye, A.; Igbokwe, D.; Apeh, H.A. Artificial intelligence, alienation and ontological problems of other minds: A critical investigation into the future of man and machines. In Proceedings of the 2017 International Conference on Computing Networking and Informatics (ICCNI), Lagos, Nigeria, 29–31 October 2017; pp. 1–10. [Google Scholar]
- Zielinski, C.; Winker, M.; Aggarwal, R.; Ferris, L.; Heinemann, M.; Lapeña, J.; Pai, S.; Ing, E.; Citrome, L. Chatbots, ChatGPT, and Scholarly Manuscripts WAME Recommendations on ChatGPT and Chatbots in Relation to Scholarly Publications. Maced J. Med. Sci. 2023, 11, 83–86. [Google Scholar] [CrossRef

INDEX

A

B

C

D

E

F

G

H

I

J

K

L

M

N

O

P

Q

R

S

T

U

V

W

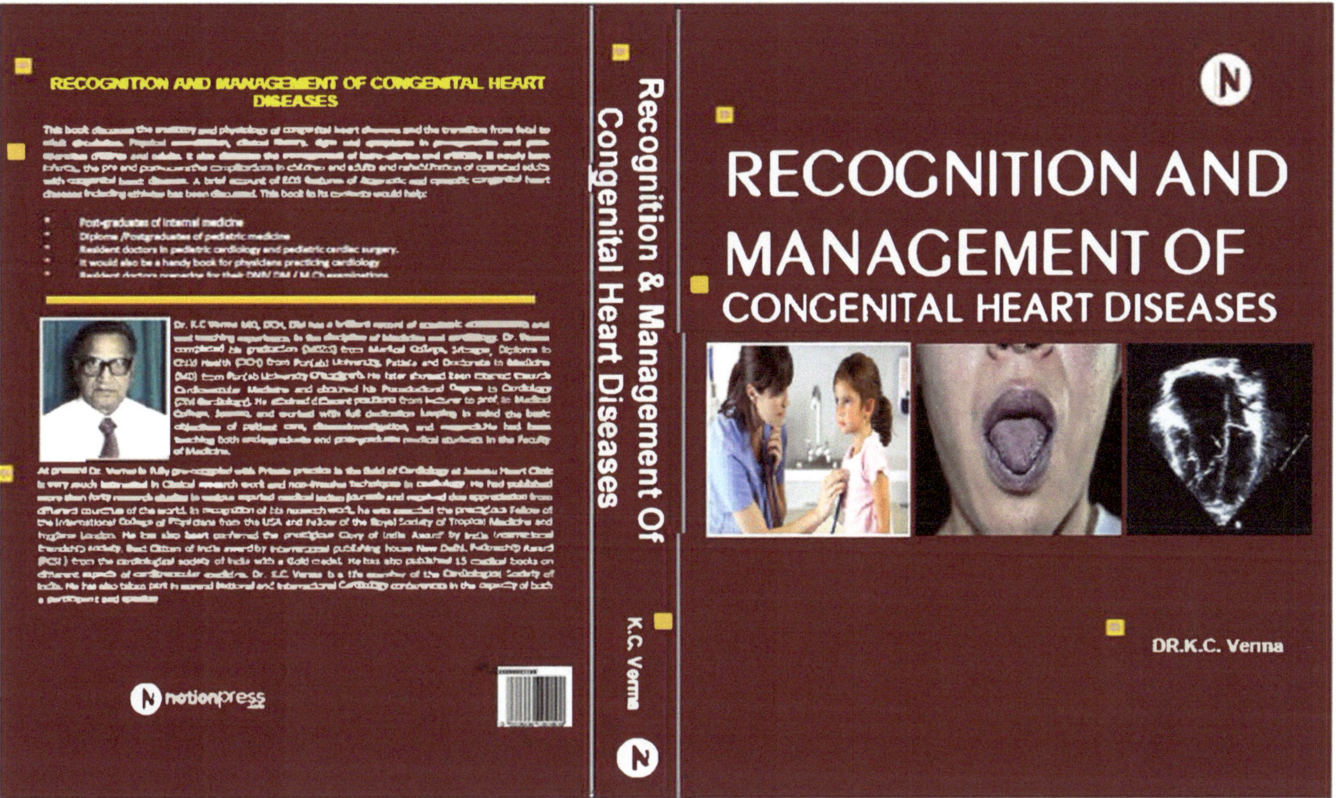
RECOGNITION AND MANAGEMENT OF CONGENITAL HEART DISEASES
Post-graduates of internal medicine
Diploma /Postgraduates of pediatric medicine
Resident doctors in pediatric cardiology and pediatric cardiac surgery.
It would also be a handy book for physicians practicing cardiology
notionpress
Recognition & Management Of Congenital Heart Diseases
K.C. Verma
RECOGNITION AND MANAGEMENT OF
CONGENITAL HEART DISEASES
DR.K.C. Verma

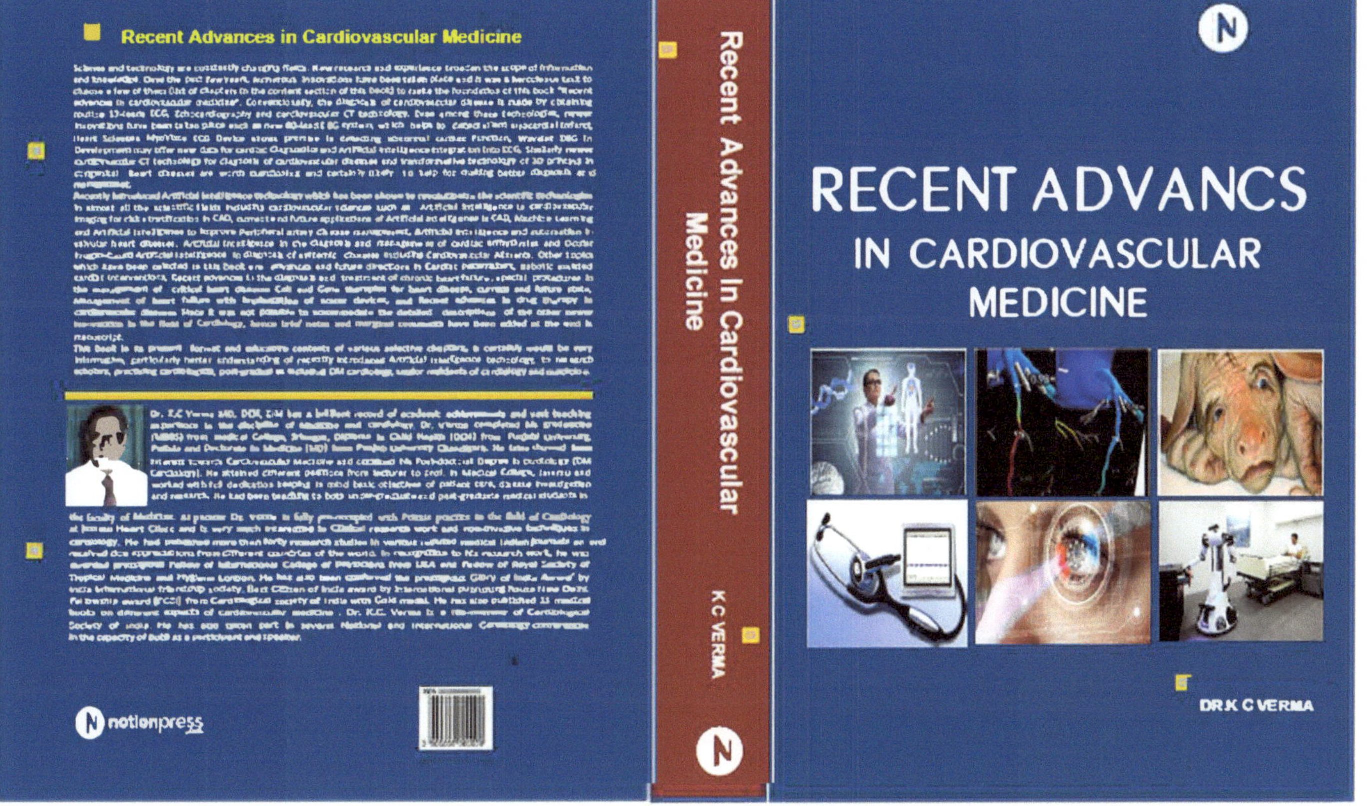
Recent Advances in Cardiovascular Medicine
notionpress
Recent Advances In Cardiovascular Medicine
K C VERMA
RECENT ADVANCS
IN CARDIOVASCULAR
MEDICINE
DR.K C VERMA

www.ingramcontent.com/pod-product-compliance
Ingram Content Group UK Ltd.
Pitfield, Milton Keynes, MK11 3LW, UK
UKHW060118300726
14090UKWH00002B/256

* 9 7 9 8 8 9 4 1 5 3 2 6 1 *